INFECTIOUS DISEASES OF THE HORSE

Edited by T.S. Mair and R.E. Hutchinson

A peer reviewed publication

ISBN 0-9545689-2-3

First published 2009

Equine Veterinary Journal Ltd.
Mulberry House, 31 Market Street, Fordham, Ely, Cambridgeshire CB7 5LQ, UK
Tel: 01638 720250 ■ Fax: 01638 720868 ■ Website: www.evj.co.uk

Front cover image:
A transmission electron micrograph of negatively stained Hendra virus.
Supplied by the Australian Biosecurity Microscopy Group (Australian Animal Health Laboratory, CSIRO, Geelong, Australia).

Typeset and published by:
Equine Veterinary Journal Ltd, Mulberry House, 31 Market Street, Fordham, Ely, Cambridgeshire CB7 5LQ, UK

Printed in Great Britain by:
Geerings Print Ltd, Ashford, Kent, UK.

CONTENTS

PREFACE

Abu Ali ibn Sina (Avicenna), the great 11th century Persian physician, is credited with the discovery of the contagious nature of infectious diseases. He introduced the concept of quarantine as a means of limiting the spread of contagious diseases in *The Canon of Medicine* (circa 1020). Since that time infectious diseases, caused by pathogenic viruses, bacteria, fungi, protozoa, multicellular parasites and prions, have continued to be major causes of disease in both man and domesticated animals.

In the late 1960s, the Surgeon General of the USA, William H. Stewart, stated that "...it is time to close the book on infectious diseases and pay more attention to chronic ailments such as cancer and heart disease" (Gibbs 2005). Unfortunately, the prediction that infectious diseases no longer pose the enormous threats to human and animal health that they did in the past proved to be mistaken. Many factors, including 'globalisation', increased international travel, intensification and monoculture in farming, ecosystem disruption, and possible climate change have resulted in an increasing rate of emergence of diseases and the ability of diseases to rapidly spread around the world, sometimes faster than the average time it takes for the disease to incubate and cause clinical signs. Furthermore, some of these diseases affecting animals are zoonotic or have the potential for becoming zoonotic. The emergence in recent years of new diseases such as SARS and Hendra virus, as well as the zoonotic potential of highly pathogenic influenza strains, highlight the importance of understanding the epidemiology of infectious diseases and the human-animal interactions required for the control and prevention of zoonotic diseases. Over the past 30 years, approximately 75% of new emerging infectious diseases have been zoonotic (Taylor *et al.* 2001). The threat of bioterrorism has also evolved from a possibility to a reality, thereby adding to the complexities of the epidemiology of some diseases.

Antibiotic and anthelmintic resistance are compounding the problems that some infectious diseases present us. Antibiotics changed the world. Since their discovery almost 8 decades ago, they have revolutionised the treatment of infections, transforming once deadly diseases into manageable health problems. The growing phenomenon of bacterial resistance to antibiotics, caused by the use and abuse of antibiotics and the simultaneous decline in research and development of new medicines, is now threatening to take us back to a pre-antibiotic era (Cars *et al.* 2008).

Equine practitioners remain at the frontline of the war against infectious diseases of the horse. The ability to recognise the clinical signs of infectious diseases is of vital importance in instituting timely and effective control. The objective of this Equine Veterinary Education peer reviewed publication is to provide the practitioner with an up-to-date review of the major equine infectious diseases, concentrating on diseases caused by viruses, bacteria, fungi and protozoa. We are indebted to all of the authors for their expert contributions. Special thanks go to Professor Peter Timoney and Professor James Wood for their invaluable advice and suggestions. Thanks also to the editorial staff at Equine Veterinary Journal Ltd. We hope that this publication will be a valuable resource for anyone faced with managing a case or an outbreak of infectious disease in horses.

Tim Mair
Bell Equine Veterinary Clinic, Mereworth, Maidstone, Kent ME18 5GS, UK

References

Cars, O., Högberg, L.D., Murray, M., Nordberg, O., Sivaraman, S., Lundborg, C.S., So, A.D. and Tomson, G. (2008) Meeting the challenge of antibiotic resistance. *Br. med. J.* **337**, a1438.

Gibbs, E.P.J. (2005) Emerging zoonotic epidemics in the interconnected global community. *Vet. Rec.* **157**, 673-679.

Taylor, L.H., Latham, S.M. and Woolhouse, M.E. (2001) Risk factors for human disease emergence. *Philos. Trans. R. Soc. Lond. B. Biol. Sci.* **356**, 983-989.

SPECIMEN SELECTION, SAMPLING AND SUBMISSION PROTOCOLS FOR THE LABORATORY DIAGNOSIS OF INFECTIOUS DISEASES

J. L. Hodgson*, K. J. Hughes† and D. R. Hodgson

Virginia-Maryland Regional College of Veterinary Medicine, Phase II Duckpond Drive, Virginia Tech, Blacksburg, Virginia 24061-0442, USA; and †Weipers Centre for Equine Welfare, Division of Companion Animal Sciences, Faculty of Veterinary Medicine, University of Glasgow, Bearsden Road, Glasgow G61 1QH, UK.

Keywords: horse; bacterial infection; diagnosis; sample collection; transportation

Summary

The ability to accurately diagnose an infectious disease is important for the equine clinician. Infections may be caused by a variety of agents (bacteria, fungi, viruses, parasites) and obtaining appropriate samples in a correct and timely manner is fundamental to determining the causative agent. Furthermore, transportation of samples to the laboratory must ensure that these agents survive and can be identified. This paper reviews a recommended diagnostic approach when infectious agents are suspected and the samples that may be obtained in order to confirm their presence.

Selection of cases for specimen collection

Before samples are collected for confirmation of an infectious disease, a number of issues should be addressed. First, samples should only be collected from cases where clinical evidence suggests an inflammatory process, and this inflammation should be specifically localised. Clinical signs suggestive of, but not pathognomonic for, bacterial, fungal and viral infections, may include fever, pain, heat, swelling and discharge. Clinicopathological findings consistent with bacterial or fungal infections include increased total white blood cell count with neutrophilia, possible left shift with toxic changes of neutrophils (bacteria), increased concentrations of fibrinogen and other acute phase proteins, and hyperglobulinaemia (Byrne 2007a). Viral infections may be associated with anaemia, lymphopenia, increased neutrophil: lymphocyte ratio and monocytosis (Oaks 2007). However, these clinicopathological changes do not occur in all cases of bacterial, fungal or viral infections, and their absence does not rule out the possibility of infectious disease. Alternatively, these clinical and clinicopathological changes may occur in other disease processes, and their presence should not be seen as confirmation of a microbial infection.

Another consideration when collecting samples is whether isolation and identification of the causative organism is required, or if empirical therapy may be implemented. Isolation and susceptibility testing of bacteria is not always indicated as some bacteria isolated from horses have a predictable sensitivity pattern. These bacteria include the β-haemolytic streptococci, *Pasteurella* spp. and most strict anaerobes (except *Bacteroides fragilis*) (Giguère 2006). Additionally, susceptibility testing might not be necessary for infections with a high level of efficacy for proven specific treatments (Morley *et al.* 2005). In such situations, selection of antimicrobial therapy should be based on results of earlier antimicrobial susceptibility testing, which may be derived from previous cases in a practice, or they may be obtained from information published in the veterinary literature. These sources provide rational, probability-based treatment options based on the

*Author to whom correspondence should be addressed.

organism likely to be isolated from a tissue site and its likely susceptibility patterns (Aucoin 2007).

Horses with serious or life-threatening infections, infections in sites that are difficult to treat or are nonresponsive to therapy, and infections where the suspected causative agent is known to have unpredictable susceptibility and probably antimicrobial resistance (e.g. *Escherichia coli, Pseudomonas aeruginosa, Staphylococcus aureus*) or requires nonroutine therapy (e.g. fungal infections) should have samples collected for culture and susceptibility testing. Samples should be collected as early in the course of the disease process as possible (Jones 2006), and wherever possible, specimens should be obtained before administration of antimicrobials. If it is not possible to collect the sample before antimicrobial agents have been administered, then the sample should be collected immediately before the next dose is given (when trough concentrations of antibiotic should exist). If antimicrobials are concentrated at the sampling site, such as in urine, it is best to wait at least 48 h after the last dose before specimen collection.

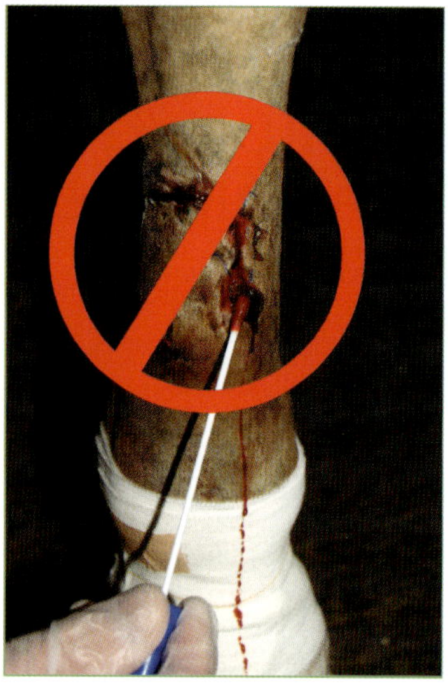

FIGURE 1: Samples should NOT be collected by swabbing the surface of wounds or inserting a swab into a draining tract. Samples obtained from deeper tissues (e.g. subcutaneous tissues) in cases of open wounds, or from the specific, localised site of infection (e.g. muscle, bone) in cases of draining tracts, should be obtained. These samples should be obtained by fine needle aspiration or biopsy.

Considerations for specimen collection

Specific localisation of the inflammatory process, and collection of samples from this site, is particularly important for bacterial infections due to the presence of normal flora. Many bacterial infections are caused by organisms that are present as part of the normal flora in sites that are close to, or contiguous with, the site of infection (Hirsh *et al.* 1999). It is therefore essential that samples are taken from the specific site where the disease process is occurring, rather than adjoining sites, so that the actual pathogen causing inflammation is isolated and not other bacteria that are part of the normal flora. Examples of this correct approach to sampling includes obtaining samples from the lower respiratory tract rather than a mucopurulent nasal discharge in cases of suspected bacterial pneumonia; obtaining uterine samples via guarded uterine swabs rather than a vaginal discharge in cases of suspected endometritis; and obtaining samples from subcutaneous tissues or bone rather than collecting samples from draining tracts or open wounds (**Fig 1**).

This principle of sample collection does not apply to viral infections, where obtaining samples from these sites may be appropriate. For example, equine influenza and equine herpesviruses are not part of the normal flora of the upper respiratory tract, therefore detection either through viral isolation or by detection of viral antigens and/or nucleic acids in nasal swabs, can be used to implicate the causative role of the virus in the disease process.

Once the site of infection has been specifically localised, it is necessary to establish if this site is normally considered sterile or has an indigenous bacterial flora. Sites with normal flora should be considered those that are adapted to having bacteria, fungi or parasites present and may even require their presence to have normal function. Alternatively, sites that should be considered sterile are not adapted to the presence of bacteria and have elaborate defence mechanisms to remove any bacteria that are introduced. Using this definition, sites such as the trachea, the urinary bladder and the uterus should be considered to be sterile even though bacteria may occasionally be isolated from these areas in normal horses. However, as these sites are not adapted for the presence of bacteria, any organisms gaining access to these areas are quickly and efficiently removed. As such, few if any bacteria are routinely isolated from these sites in normal horses, and collection of samples from these sites should use the same principles and techniques as for sterile sites.

Another consideration that should be assessed before samples are collected and submitted to the laboratory is whether anaerobes are likely to be present. If their presence is suspected, samples must be collected and transported in a manner that will ensure their survival. Clinical features that are consistent with anaerobic infections include gas and/or black discolouration of tissues, foul smell and infections near sites where anaerobes are part of the normal flora (e.g. gastrointestinal tract, respiratory tract, urogenital tract). In addition, anaerobes are more commonly isolated in severe, chronic infections such as tooth root or foot abscesses, and pleuropneumonia, where sufficient necrotic tissue exists to allow their invasion and multiplication. In these sites, anaerobes are frequently found as part of polymicrobial (mixed) infections.

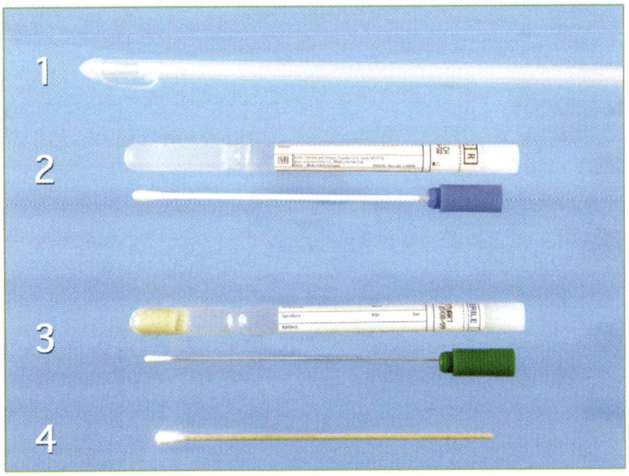

FIGURE 2: Swab collection devices used to collect samples for bacterial isolation and identification in horses: (1) guarded swab for collection of uterine samples; (2) swab collection device including media that will support growth of aerobic and anaerobic bacteria; (3) swab collection device with small (fine) swab suitable for collection of samples from the cornea or clitoral fossa (for isolation of Taylorella equigenitalis); (4) swabs without transport media are rarely suitable for use in equine practice.

Sampling different body sites

There are several sites that require specific samples to be collected in order to identify the causative agent.

Skin and subcutaneous tissues: In suspected cases of dermatophilosis, swab samples should be collected from underneath crusted lesions. The microscopic appearance of the bacteria (*Dermatophilus congolensis*) is pathognomonic. Hair samples may be collected in cases where dermatophytes (e.g. *Trichophyton equinum*) are suspected. All other cases of dermatitis should have a sample obtained by skin biopsy and/or aspiration of unruptured pustules/vesicles.

Samples from the centre of an abscess may be sterile, particularly if the process is chronic. Up to 3 ml should be collected from early lesions, if possible, together with a scraping from the wall of the abscess.

Uterus: Samples may be collected from the uterus via a guarded uterine swab (**Fig 2**) or an endometrial biopsy. However, swabs may be less diagnostic than biopsies for confirmation of endometritis (Lu and Morresey 2006).

Blood: Multiple blood samples are often required as bacteraemia can be intermittent and frequently only low numbers of bacteria are present (Byrne 2007a). If possible, at least one sample should be collected before administration of antibiotics or at the onset of fever. Ideally 2–3 more samples should be collected within 24 h from different collection sites, with the final sample(s) collected when trough antimicrobial concentrations occur (i.e. just prior to administration of the next dose). A 10 ml blood sample should be collected on each occasion to enhance the chance of isolation of causative agents. Special media is required for transportation and cultivation of these samples. These media also support growth of most fungal pathogens that cause fungaemia in horses, though these infections are very rare.

Blood samples may also be collected for isolation of viruses (e.g. equine herpesviruses - citrated or heparinised whole blood; equine arteritis virus - do not use heparinised blood, rather sodium citrate or ethylenediaminetetraacetic acid [EDTA] should be used as the anticoagulant) or for detection of nucleic acid (e.g. for *Anaplasma phagocytophilum*).

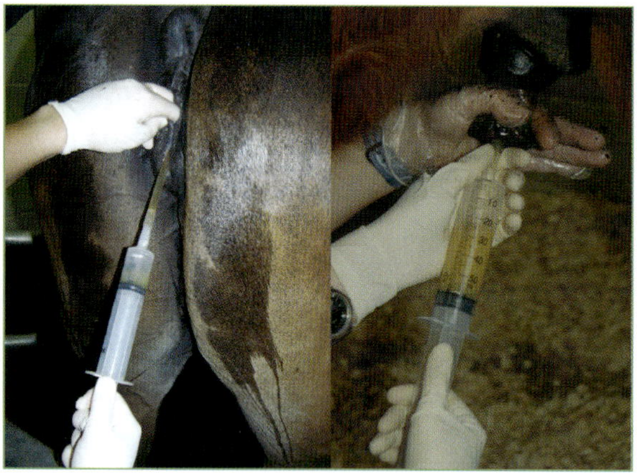

FIGURE 3: Urinary tract infections are rare. However, when suspected, samples for cultivation and sensitivity testing may be collected from the bladder by catheterisation.

Urine/kidney: Urinary tract infections in horses are rare (Frye 2006) and usually result from structural or functional inhibition of normal urine flow. Urine samples are usually best collected by catheterisation of the bladder (**Fig 3**), but mid-stream voided samples may also be used. Quantitation of urine cultures and concurrent cytological analysis are required for interpretation of isolated bacteria.

Lower respiratory tract and thorax: Tracheal wash samples should be collected using either the transtracheal technique or with a guarded catheter passed through an endoscope (Hodgson and Hodgson 2006) (**Fig 4**). It is important to ensure that the wash solution does not contain a bacteriostatic preservative (e.g. EDTA). Standardisation of collection technique, quantification of tracheal wash cultures, and cytological analysis are recommended for optimal interpretation (Hodgson and Hodgson 2006). To increase the sensitivity of diagnosis of Rhodococcus equi infections in foals, tracheal wash samples may also be submitted for PCR analysis (Hines 2007).

Bronchoalveolar lavage samples are rarely, if ever, indicated in cases of suspected bacterial pneumonia, but may be used in cases where fungal pathogens (e.g. *Pneumocystis carinii, Coccidioides immitis*) are suspected (Long 2007; Pappagianis and Higgins 2007).

Samples of pleural fluid should be obtained by thoracocentesis in addition to tracheal wash if concurrent pleuritis is suspected. Both sides of the thoracic cavity should be sampled as different bacteria may be isolated from each hemithorax.

Abdomen: Samples of peritoneal fluid should be collected using techniques to avoid enterocentesis. A portion of the sample should be immediately placed in fluid (blood) culture media to enhance isolation of the causative organism(s). If rupture of an abdominal viscus is suspected, and confirmed by cytology, culture and susceptibility testing is rarely warranted as normal flora of the GIT will be isolated.

Gastrointestinal tract: Multiple, fresh faecal samples (3–5 g) are preferred over rectal swabs as bacteria may be shed in low numbers and therefore missed on swabs. Rectal biopsy may increase the sensitivity of isolation of bacteria; however, this procedure is invasive and has an inherent risk to the horse (Feary and Hassel 2006). Specific tests may be required for diagnosis of enteric pathogens such as selective enrichment for *Salmonella* isolation, PCR for *Neorickettsia risticii*, *Lawsonia intracellularis* and *Salmonella*, toxin detection in cases of suspected clostridial enteritis, latex agglutination test for Rotavirus antigen and blood for serology in cases of *Lawsonia intracellularis.*

Eye: Gentle scraping of tissues at the edge of a corneal ulcer (using a Kimura spatula or blunt end of a scalpel blade) will provide the optimal sample for bacterial culture and susceptibility testing, while

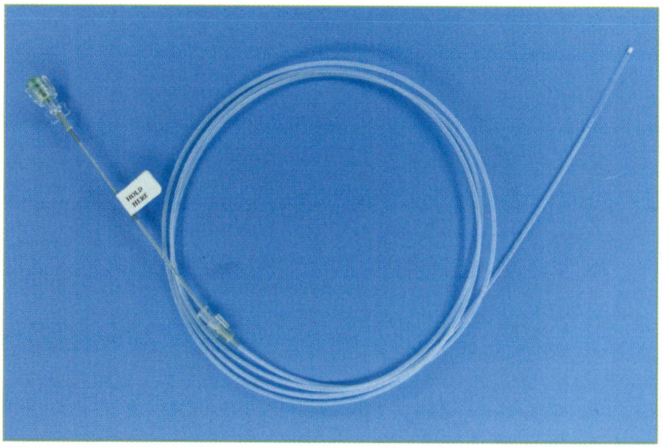

FIGURE 4: Collection of samples from the lower respiratory tract for bacterial cultivation must involve use of a guarded catheter if collection is through the biopsy port of an endoscope.

scrapings of the base of an ulcer are also useful for isolation of fungi. Alternatively, a fine cotton or Dacron-tipped swab (**Fig 2**), moistened with sterile saline, may be applied to regions of corneal ulceration; however, retrieval of microorganisms is expected to be less than when scrapings are obtained. Cytological evaluation of scrapings will aid in detection of inflammatory cells and diagnosis of fungal and/or bacterial keratitis. The collection of corneal scrapings is preferable for cytological examination; however, the use of a moistened swab is less traumatic and is recommended when extensive corneal compromise is present (e.g. keratomalacia).

Joints/bone: Isolation of bacteria from joints can be difficult as bacterial numbers can be low, especially in adults (Byrne 2007a). Samples should be inoculated into the same media used for blood cultures to enhance isolation. Biopsies of synovial membranes may improve bacterial isolation, but these samples are difficult to obtain and require more invasive procedures (i.e. arthroscopy/arthrotomy).

Meninges: Culture of cerebrospinal fluid (CSF) should be attempted in cases of suspected bacterial or fungal meningitis, but is frequently unrewarding (Seino 2007). Cytological evidence of inflammation (neutrophilic pleocytosis) and increased concentration of protein in the CSF, together with possible visualisation of the organism, is suggestive of infectious meningitis.

Some diseases causing neurological signs (e.g. botulism) rely on detection of toxin rather than isolation of bacteria.

Wounds: Culture of fresh wounds is rarely warranted, but culture of established wounds with signs of infection (heat, swelling, discharge) is clearly indicated. NEVER collect samples of the surface discharge or from draining tracts (**Fig 1**) as they will invariably be contaminated with local flora, which may include potential pathogens. Such samples are rarely possible to interpret correctly. Samples obtained from deeper tissues (e.g. subcutaneous, muscle, bone) in cases of open wounds, or from the specific, localised site of infection in cases of draining tracts, should be obtained. These latter samples should be obtained by fine needle aspiration or biopsy.

Methods for sample collection

There are a number of suitable ways to collect samples for bacterial, fungal and viral isolation and identification. The underlying principle of these techniques is to choose a method that will collect a sufficient volume of sample, using a system that will allow survival of the causative agent, whilst avoiding contamination from nearby sites with a normal flora.

In general, an adequate quantity of sample involves several millilitres of liquid or grams of tissue. All too frequently, an inadequate amount of material is obtained with a swab, making it nearly impossible for the laboratory to make appropriate smears and inoculate adequate culture material. A good rule is to assume that a swab should never be submitted *in lieu* of an aspirate, biopsy material, fluid or surgically removed tissue.

Multiple specimens should be submitted when lesions are large, present at several sites, or when more than one laboratory procedure is requested (e.g. bacterial and fungal cultures, PCR). Multiple samples may also be necessary for isolation of bacteria present in low numbers (e.g. in blood, joints, faeces).

Appropriate collection devices and specimen transport systems are needed to ensure survival of the microorganism, prevent overgrowth, and allow for optimal isolation and identification of the causative agent. Various containers are commercially available, ranging from simple swabs and plastic tube combinations to more complicated specimen collection devices.

Swabs: Swabs are rarely the best choice for sampling bacterial and fungal infections because they collect a small amount of material, the organisms can be adsorbed to swab fibres further decreasing the effective sample volume, and they can be made with substances that inhibit bacterial growth (Songer and Post 2005). In addition, samples submitted on swabs are prone to dessication and the relevant pathogen may not be viable on arrival at the laboratory. Thus, swabs are only acceptable for sample collection if samples are sent to a laboratory in a humidified transporting chamber or placed in a transport medium. Several swab-transport medium systems exist (**Fig 2**) and are best obtained from the diagnostic laboratory to which the sample will be sent. In addition, a number of newer transport

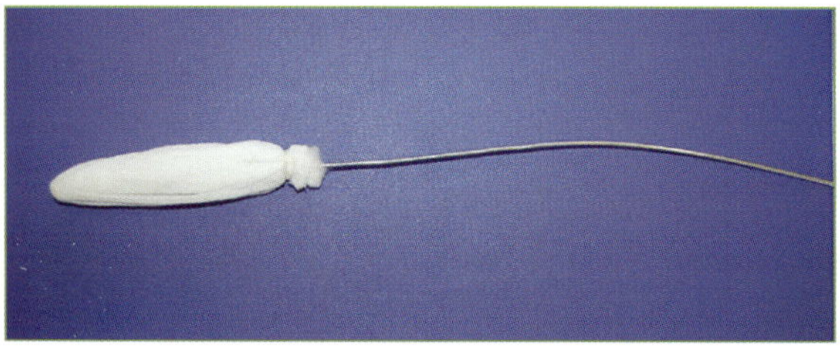

FIGURE 5: Nasopharyngeal swab suitable for isolation of respiratory viruses.

systems have been developed that aid survival of anaerobes and fastidious bacteria (Hindiyeh et al. 2001), though swabs are generally inferior for these bacteria. If submitting multiple samples, individual containers should be used to eliminate the possibility of cross contamination.

Swabs should never be used to collect samples from surface wounds (**Fig 1**) or from draining tracts. They are also usually of little value in collecting samples from sites with normal flora (e.g. upper respiratory tract) unless detection of a specific bacterium, fungus or virus is the goal of cultivation (e.g. in the case of strangles where isolation of *S. equi* ssp. *equi* is diagnostic, isolation of respiratory viruses, or isolation of *Cryptococcus neoformans*). In these cases, the surface of the mucous membrane can be gently wiped of any discharge and a swab used to collect the sample.

When swabs are used for isolation of viruses, care must be taken to use an appropriate type. For example, polyester swabs (**Fig 5**) should be used *in lieu* of cotton-tipped swabs when collecting nasal or nasopharyngeal samples for isolation of equine influenza virus as the virus can adhere to the latter type of swab.

Fine needle aspirates, washes and catheterisation: Samples collected by fine needle aspirate (**Fig 6**), washes or by catheterisation are good specimens for bacterial, fungal and occasionally viral isolation. These samples are relatively easy to collect and the larger sample size will increase the likelihood that a causative pathogen will be isolated. In addition, samples collected using these techniques are usually obtained in a more aseptic manner than for swabs. For all specimens obtained by fine needle aspiration skin decontamination should be performed as for surgery. Briefly, after clipping the site of collection, the area should be thoroughly disinfected by repeated application of 10% povidone-iodine or other suitable skin antiseptic solutions (e.g. 1% chlorhexidine gluconate) and allowed to dry. A final application of 70% isopropyl or ethyl alcohol should be applied to the skin and allowed to dry for at least 30 s.

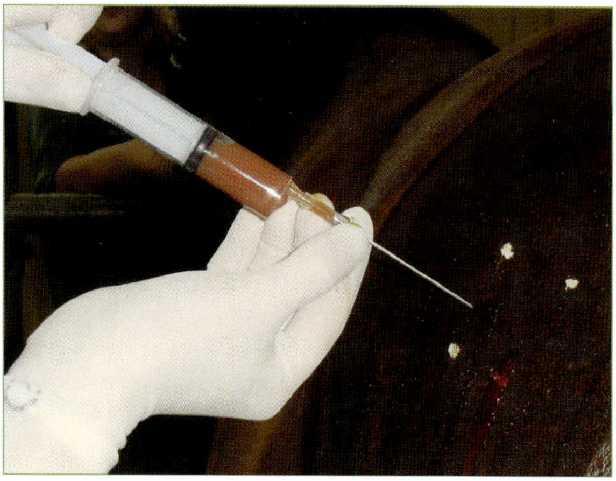

FIGURE 6: Fine needle aspirates, after a site has been surgically prepared, are a preferred method of sample collection for microbial cultivation and susceptibility testing.

Aspirates may also be used to collect samples from the lower respiratory tract through a catheter that is either passed transtracheally or through a guarded system using an endoscope (Hodgson and Hodgson 2006). Guarded catheters (**Fig 4**) must be used in these cases to prevent contamination of the sample with bacteria from the upper respiratory tract. These normal flora also cover the external surface of the endoscope during passage through the nasopharynx and care must be taken to avoid prior placement of the tip of the endoscope on the mucosa at the site of sampling.

Catheterisation of the bladder is preferred for collection of urine in cases where urinary tract infections are suspected (**Fig 3**). However, contamination of these samples with normal flora of the vagina or prepuce still occurs and quantification of the colony forming units in urine, in conjunction with urinary sediment cytology (i.e. >5 leucocytes/high power field), should be performed to assist interpretation (Hodgson *et al.* 2008).

Washes also may be used to obtain samples for detection of bacterial, fungal or viral antigens using a variety of immunoassays (e.g. ELISA, immunohistocytochemistry and immunofluorescence). Alternatively, nucleic acid may be detected in washes through polymerase chain reaction or DNA probes.

Biopsy or tissue samples: Surgical specimens or biopsies are often the preferred sample as they may represent the entire pathological process (Byrne 2007a). However, they are usually obtained at a considerable expense and some risk to the patient. If these procedures are performed, a portion of the tissue, rather than a swabbed specimen, should be submitted and they should be handled carefully to avoid contamination or dessication. Biopsies, tissue samples or aspirates are the preferred samples for the attempted isolation of anaerobes. These tissues should be placed in a commercially available system for anaerobes, such as Port-a-Cul[1] transport jars, which are inexpensive and easy to use.

In addition, biopsies and tissue samples may be used for *in situ* detection of viruses (e.g. immunohistochemistry, immunofluorescence and *in situ* DNA or RNA hybridisation) or histological examination of tissues for viral inclusion bodies.

Free catch: Samples collected by free catch (e.g. urine, milk) are more rarely collected in horses than other domestic species. However, if these samples are collected, procedures that minimise contamination should be used such as collection of mid stream samples and careful cleaning of the udder prior to sample collection. Faecal samples may be collected for cultivation of specific bacteria (e.g. *Salmonella* or *Clostridium difficile*) or detection of bacterial DNA in samples via PCR (e.g. *Neorickettsia risticii, Lawsonia intracellularis, Salmonella* spp.).

Cytological evaluation of samples for suitability for submission

Direct microscopic examination of collected samples is a simple and cost-effective procedure that should be performed on every sample collected, preferably before sample submission. Microscopic examination gives an indication of the likelihood of the presence of infection, the presence of a host inflammatory response, the possible pathogen, the predominant organism(s) in cases of mixed infection, and the suitability of the specimen for culture. This information also may be used for implementation of initial therapy and as a basis for interpretation of the significance of subsequent culture results. Finally, smears may provide the only information about the sample collected in cases where the causative agent cannot be cultured.

Smears should be made of the samples obtained using routine techniques (Tyler *et al.* 2002). Simple staining methods are suitable for most samples collected from equine infections and include Gram and Diff Quik[2] stains. Gram stained smears allow evaluation of the presence and type of bacteria (Gram reaction, number, size, shape) and fungi (yeasts) and Diff Quik stained smears allow evaluation of the type and intensity of inflammatory response, as well as the presence of toxic or degenerative changes in neutrophils consistent with a septic process. Diff Quik stain may also be used to detect filamentous fungi (e.g. *Aspergillus* spp.). Alternatively, periodic acid-Schiff (PAS)[3] stain may be used to detect both yeast and hyphae as this stain specifically stains the fungal cell wall pink (Byrne 2007b). Alternate forms of microscopy may be used for some organisms (e.g. dark field microscopy for detection of *Leptospira*).

At least 10^4–10^5 microorganisms per ml of fluid or g of tissue must be present in order to be detected microscopically, therefore failure to observe bacteria on a stained sample does not rule out an infection. The presence of intracellular bacteria is highly suggestive of a bacterial infection rather than mere contamination, especially in conjunction with cytological evidence of inflammation. Samples obtained from sites with normal flora will have many bacteria present, but these should not be accompanied by inflammatory cells if tissues are healthy. However, contamination of samples from sites of inflammation with normal flora will confuse interpretation, as inflammation will be present as will many bacteria. In these cases it is impossible to interpret cytological or culture results and emphasises the need for meticulous sample collection.

Some bacterial and fungal pathogens may have cytological features that allow definitive diagnosis. This includes the morphology of *Dermatophilus congolensis* (Gram-positive branching rods, with 'railroad track' appearance), and the presence of a capsule for *Cryptococcus neoformans*.

Principles of transportation

The major goals of sample transportation are to prevent further contamination, to maintain viability of pathogens and, if more than one type of microorganism is present, to maintain them in approximately the same ratio as occurred *in vivo*. Sample drying (all microorganisms), exposure to noxious atmosphere (oxygen for anaerobes) and excessive time delays are the major dangers in sample transportation.

Various types of transport devices that contain media (e.g. Stuart's medium[1]) may be used for transporting specimens to prevent dessication and maintain viability of bacteria and fungi. Essentially these contain buffered, non-nutritive salt solutions usually in a gelled matrix. As these media do not contain any nutrients, microorganisms multiply poorly if at all and thereby preserve the relative numbers and ratio of the original sample and minimise overgrowth by rapid-growing bacteria that may be present. However, bacteria do not remain viable in these media indefinitely, and more fastidious bacteria (e.g. β-haemolytic *Streptococcus* spp.) will not survive as long as *E. coli* or *Pseudomonas aeruginosa*.

Swab transport systems: Swabs should always be placed in transport medium, regardless of the expected time lapse between collection and processing. There are a number of different swab transport systems (**Fig 2**) that are best obtained from the diagnostic laboratory to which the sample will be sent. In addition, a number of newer systems have been developed (e.g. Copan Vi-Pak Amies agar gel collection and transport swabs)[1] (Hindiyeh et al. 2001) which maintain the viability of more fastidious organisms for longer (up to 24 h). These newer systems may also support anaerobes, though swabs are usually considered inferior for isolation of anaerobes. If submitting multiple samples, individual containers should be used to eliminate the possibility of cross contamination.

Broth transport systems: Nutrient broths are recommended for transportation of some samples (e.g. blood and synovial fluid) to help overcome bactericidal components of these fluids, to amplify bacteria that may be present in low numbers, and to help maintain viability of the bacteria present during transportation (Byrne 2007a). These systems may also be useful for transportation of fluids from the peritoneal or thoracic cavity in cases where low numbers of bacteria are anticipated (e.g. *Actinobacillus equuli* peritonitis). In general, the same systems are used for transportation as for cultivation in the laboratory (**Fig 7**). However, it is important to note that these fluids will support the growth of any organisms within the sample, and therefore can only be used when aspirates are collected from normally sterile body sites, and when great care has been taken to avoid contamination at the time of sampling. In addition, these fluids are rarely of use when polymicrobial infections are suspected, due to rapid overgrowth by less fastidious bacteria. Thus, their use should be restricted to cases where a single organism is probably involved, and when meticulous care has been used during sample collection.

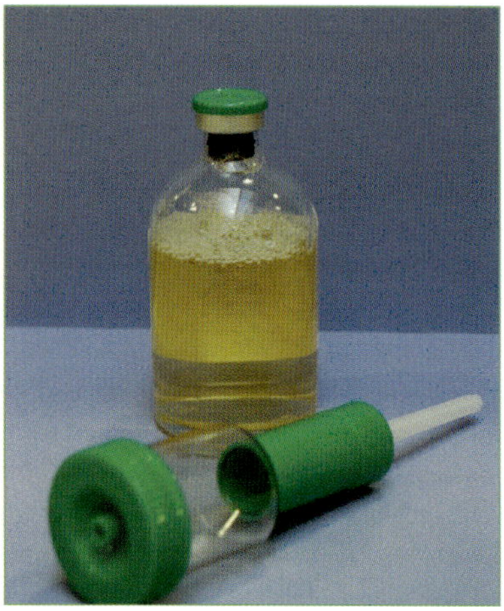

FIGURE 7: An example of a commercially available, conventional broth-based culture system that may be used for transportation and cultivation of fluid samples (e.g. blood, joint fluid).

Anaerobes: Samples that may include anaerobes must be inoculated into suitable transport media and sent to the laboratory as soon after collection as possible as many of these bacteria do not survive exposure to the oxygen in air for more than 20 min. If a swab is used for sampling sites with suspected anaerobes, it should be placed in semi-solid transport medium, such as the Port-a-Cul tube system for aerobic and anaerobic culture[1], to minimise air exposure. Alternatively, newer systems such as the Copan Vi-Pak Amies agar gel collection and transport swabs[1] (Hindiyeh *et al.* 2001) may be used, following modification by nitrogen gas flushing to keep an ideal (low) redox potential and to prevent oxidation of the transport medium. These media can support anaerobes and other fastidious bacteria for up to 24 h. If tissues or fluid samples are sampled, they should be placed in similar transport systems to those for swabs, and are also commercially available (e.g. Port-a-Cul jars and vials)[1].

Many of the blood culture systems can support the growth of anaerobes, but the conventional broth-based method will more reliably allow detection of anaerobic bacteria probably because the large volume of liquid preserves the anaerobic environment and allows proliferation of anaerobes that could be present in very low numbers (Byrne 2007a). Aerobic swabs are unacceptable for isolation of anaerobes and should not be submitted to the laboratory. However, because reduced oxygen is not lethal for aerobes and facultative anaerobes, anaerobic transport devices may be used for transportation of these bacteria in cases where mixed infections are suspected.

Media for transportation of specific bacterial pathogens: Swabs and discharges submitted for the isolation of *Taylorella equigenitalis* should be placed in Amies transport medium containing charcoal[1]. Cary Blair medium1 is routinely used for transportation of faecal samples where *Salmonella* are suspected. These samples should not be cooled during transportation.

Media for transportation of fungi: Almost all samples can be collected and transported as they would for bacterial cultures (Byrne 2007b).

Media for transportation of viruses: Swabs or tissues samples collected for viral isolation should be immediately placed in appropriate transport medium (cell culture medium or balanced salt solution containing 2–5% fetal bovine or calf serum). Samples should be refrigerated, or preferably frozen at -20°C or lower.

Packaging and temperature: Samples should always be submitted individually in separate leak-proof containers. A second container around the primary containers should be used in case leakage occurs - this should be packed with absorbent materials. Each container should be labelled with the identity of the animal, the type of specimen, and the date of collection. If transportation to the laboratory is delayed, most samples should be refrigerated at 4°C or stored on ice, but not frozen until the samples can be sent. Exceptions to this rule are samples obtained from cases where Salmonella spp. or anaerobes are suspected as these species do not tolerate cool temperatures. Fungal organisms do not withstand extreme heat or cold and should be protected appropriately during storage and transport to the laboratory.

Samples should be shipped to the laboratory as soon as possible after collection (e.g. same day or overnight). Frozen gel packs or ice can be used during transportation to maintain cool conditions without freezing. Obviously if the weather is warmer, more packs may be required. If possible samples should not be sent over the weekend, as there is an increased likelihood of delays during which temperature variations occur and bacterial viability is compromised.

If time of transportation is short, a fluid sample may be kept in the syringe used for collection, but the excess air should be expelled, the needle removed and the syringe capped with a sterile Luer bung (stopper) to avoid inadvertent injury and introduction of bacteria to personnel. However, because of occupational health and safety issues laboratories will often not accept samples presented in such a manner. Thus, it is wise to check prior to attempting sample submission in this way.

Information regarding signalment, case history and a tentative diagnosis should be submitted to the laboratory with the specimens to help laboratory staff to decide on the range of possible agents and thus select the appropriate media and procedures to identify the pathogen(s). It is recommended to always send an accompanying prepared smear for cytological evaluation as these represent a snapshot of the bacteria present at the time of sampling.

Manufacturers' addresses

[1]BD Diagnostic Systems, Oxford, UK.
[2]Baxter, Deerfield, Illinois, USA.
[3]Polysciences Inc., Warrington, Pennsylvania, USA.

References

Aucoin, D. (2007) *The Antimicrobial Reference Guide to Effective Treatment*, 3rd edn., North American Compendiums Inc., Port Huron. pp i-xiv.

Byrne, B.A. (2007a) Laboratory diagnosis of bacterial infections. In: *Equine Infectious Diseases*, Eds: D.C. Sellon and M.T. Long. W.B. Saunders, St Louis. pp 236-243.

Byrne, B.A. (2007b) Laboratory diagnosis of fungal diseases. In: *Equine Infectious Diseases*, Eds: D.C. Sellon and M.T. Long. W.B. Saunders, St Louis. pp 385-391.

Feary, D.J. and Hassel, D.M. (2006) Enteritis and colitis in horses. *Vet. Clin. N. Am.* **22**, 437-479.

Frye, M.A. (2006) Pathophysiology, diagnosis and management of urinary tract infection in horses. *Vet. Clin. N. Am.* **22**, 497-517.

Giguère, S. (2006) Antimicrobial drug use in horses. In: *Antimicrobial Therapy in Veterinary Medicine*, 4th edn., Eds: S. Giguere, J.F. Prescott, J.D. Baggot, R.D. Walker and P.M. Dowling, Blackwell Publishing, Ames. pp 449-462.

Hindiyeh, M. and Acevedo, V. and Carroll, K.C. (2001) Comparison of three transport systems (Starplex StarSwab II, the new Copan Vi-Pak Amies Agar Gel collection and transport swabs, and BBL Port-A-Cul) for maintenance of anaerobic and fastidious aerobic organisms. *J. Clin. Microbiol.* **39**, 377-380.

Hines, M.T. (2007) *Rhodococcus equi*. In: *Equine Infectious Diseases*, Eds: D.C. Sellon and M.T. Long, W.B. Saunders, St Louis. pp 281-295.

Hirsh, D.C., Zee, Y.C. and Castro, A.E. (1999) Laboratory diagnosis. In: *Veterinary Microbiology*, Blackwell Publishing, Oxford. pp 15-27.

Hodgson, J.L. and Hodgson, D.R. (2006) Collection and analysis of respiratory tract samples. In: *Equine Respiratory Medicine and Surgery*, Eds: B.C. McGorum, P.M. Dixon, N.E. Robinson and J. Schumacher, Elsevier, Edinburgh. pp 119-150.

Hodgson, J.L., Hughes, K.J. and Hodgson, D.R. (2008) Diagnosis of bacterial infections. Part 2: Bacterial cultivation, susceptibility testing and interpretation. *Equine vet. Educ.* **20**, 658-666.

Jones, R.L. (2006) Laboratory diagnosis of bacterial infections. In: *Infectious Disease of the Dog*, Ed: C. Greene, W.B. Saunders, St Louis. pp 267-273.

Long, M.T. (2007) Pneumocystis infections. In: *Equine Infectious Diseases*, Eds: D.C. Sellon and M.T. Long, W.B. Saunders, St Louis. pp 392-395.

Lu, K.G. and Morresey, P.R. (2006) Reproductive tract infections in horses. *Vet. Clin. N. Am.* **22**, 519-552.

Morley, P.S., Apley, M.D., Besser, T.E., Burney, D.P., Fedorka-Cray, P.J., Papich, M.G., Traub-Dargatz, J.D and Weese, J.S. (2005) Antimicrobial drug use in veterinary medicine. *J. vet. intern. Med.* **19**, 617-629.

Oaks, J.L. (2007) Laboratory diagnosis of viral infections. In: *Equine Infectious Diseases*, Eds: D.C. Sellon and M.T. Long, W.B. Saunders, St Louis. pp 116-124.

Pappagianis, D. and Higgins, J. (2007) Coccidiomycosis. In: *Equine Infectious Diseases*, Eds: D.C. Sellon and M.T. Long, W.B. Saunders, St Louis. pp 396-404.

Seino, K.K. (2007) Central nervous system infections. In: *Equine Infectious Diseases*, Eds: D.C. Sellon and M.T. Long, W.B. Saunders, St Louis. pp 46-57.

Songer, J.G. and Post, K.W. (2005) General principles of bacterial disease diagnosis. In: *Veterinary Microbiology: Bacterial and Fungal Agents of Animal Disease*, Eds: J.G. Songer and K.W. Post, W.B. Saunders, St Louis. pp 10-20.

Tyler, R.D., Cowell, R.L., MacAllister, C.G., Morton, R.J. and Caruso, K.J. (2002) Introduction. In: *Diagnostic Cytology and Haematology of the Horse*, 2nd edn., Eds: Cowell, R.L. and R.D. Tyler, Mosby, St Louis. pp 1-18.

GLOBALISATION OF TRADE AND THE SPREAD OF INFECTIOUS DISEASE

D. P. Leadon* and C. P. Herholz†

Irish Equine Centre, Johnstown, Naas, Co. Kildare, Ireland; and †Federal Veterinary Office, 3097 Bern-Liebefeld, Switzerland.

Keywords: horse; global statistics; trade, horse movements; international equestrian and racing events; spread of disease; syndromic surveillance

Summary

The importance of worldwide equine trade is reviewed and the examples in which equine movements or trade in equine-derived products have resulted in the introduction of pathogens in previously disease-free areas are presented. General awareness regarding unusual clinical signs needs to be promoted among horse owners and veterinarians as this is essential for early diagnosis and effective control and eradication.

Introduction

The traditional, and perhaps instinctive, view of the equine clinician is that the control and management of outbreaks of exotic and notifiable equine infectious diseases is the responsibility of international, national and local veterinary authorities. The principal organisations with responsibility for animal and international trade are the World Organization for Animal Health (OIE) (Anon 2008a), the Food and Agriculture Organization (FAO) (Anon 2008b) and the World Trade Organization (WTO) (Anon 1994). However, in reality, it is often the equine practitioner who is at the forefront of management of these conditions. The equine clinician's responsibility can thus far exceed the needs of the immediate clientele in this regard. Surveillance of equine diseases at a national level and prompt reporting to the relevant authorities and the OIE are critical to the effectiveness of national and international equine health control programmes and importation policies. This creates a need for clinicians to invest in self-education and awareness of horse populations, usage, transport and national and international equine infectious disease reporting.

Recognition of unusual presentations and clinical signs therefore needs to be promoted for both veterinarians and horse owners. Unexpected clinical syndromes are also of increasing importance for public health, as many of the emerging infectious diseases are zoonoses, such as West Nile encephalitis (Kahn 2006). The term 'syndromic surveillance' applies to the use of health-related data that precede diagnosis and signal a sufficient probability of a case or an outbreak to warrant further public health response. This type of surveillance has been shown to be a key element in detecting emerging diseases. As soon as recognition of exotic disease incursion has occurred and diagnosis has been achieved, counting of cases initiates the process of determining the disease pattern in regard to time and space. The pattern of disease occurrence may then be used as the basis for selecting approaches to disease investigation and disease control.

Horse populations

There are an estimated 58,372,106 horses in the world. The USA has a horse population of 9,500,000 (which includes Texas 978,822; California 698,345; Florida 500,124; Oklahoma 326,134; Kentucky 320,173; Ohio 306,898 and Missouri 281,255). The States with the fewest horses are Rhode Island (3509) and the District of Columbia, which reports a fluctuating total of around 33. Each of the primary use segments of the industry (recreational horse use being the largest segment with 3.9 million horses in this classification) creates an immense contribution

*Author to whom correspondence should be addressed.

to the overall economy, having a direct impact of $39 billion and an overall impact of $102 billion, when indirect and induced spending are included. The US horse industry supports 1.4 million equivalent full-time jobs.

Countries with horse population totals in excess of one million include: China (7,402,450); Mexico (6,260,000); Brazil (5,787,249); Argentina (3,655,000); Columbia (2,533,621); Mongolia (2,029,100); Ethiopia (1,655,383); Russian Federation (1,319,358); and Kazakhstan (1,163,500). Guam (20) and Grenada (30) had the lowest population totals. Two countries, Rwanda and Saint Helena, report a zero horse population.

The EU has an estimated horse population of 3.7 million (including: Romania 834,000; Germany 500,000; France 422,872; Poland 306,992; Italy 300,000; Spain 245,000; UK 185,000; Netherlands 128,500; Bulgaria 125,000; Sweden 95,700; Austria 85,000 and Ireland 79,900).

The horse industry is one of Australia's biggest industries and is worth more than Aus$8 billion a year with about 1.2 million horses used for racing, equestrian sports and recreation.

Although these are impressive totals, only a small fraction of the total horse populations are of sufficient economic value to justify investment in long distance transport, as it is estimated that 60% of the world's horses are working equids, based in developing countries.

The Thoroughbred sector contains the highest individual value segment of the horse industry. The highest producers of Thoroughbred foals are the USA (36,317); Australia (17,640) and Ireland (12,633). The Japan Thoroughbred foal crop was 7655 in 2006. Ireland produced more Thoroughbred foals in 2007 than the combined total of the UK (5843) and France (5269) and more than 40% of all EU Thoroughbred foals are Irish. Italy (2130) and Germany (1224) are the other principal EU producers. More than 40% of all Thoroughbred foals born in the USA are sired by Kentucky-based stallions - in 2006 - 14,801 live foals, which when placed in the above Kentucky total horse population context of 320,173 represents just 4.6% of the total. Other leading states ranked by number of state-sired live foals in 2007 include Florida (4063); California (3131); Louisiana (2016) and New York (1316).

Horse transport

There is extensive international and intercontinental trade in high value horses and also in horses destined for slaughter. General impressions of the extent of horse movements can be obtained from a variety of sources; e.g. the number of FEI sponsored equestrian competitions has more than doubled in recent years and a total of 4611 international and intercontinental movements of racehorses took place between 2001 and 2006 (Herholz *et al.* 2008). Weatherbys reported 1249 Thoroughbreds permanently exported and 1782 permanently imported into the UK in 2007. Although the numbers of horses transported for slaughter has been declining since 1995, 99,087 slaughter horses entered into and moved between the EU Member States in 2005 (**Fig 1**). However, much more comprehensive information on horse movements has become available since the implementation of the Trade Control and Expert System (TRACES) in the European Union. TRACES is an electronic system used to exchange information about intra-Community trade, importation or transit in the EU of live animals, semen and embryos as well as trade in mammalian animal waste and the importation of animal products. This system also documents transit of animals/animal products from a third country to another third country, imports from third countries and temporary imports. These data show that very large numbers of horses are being transported internationally and that these numbers have

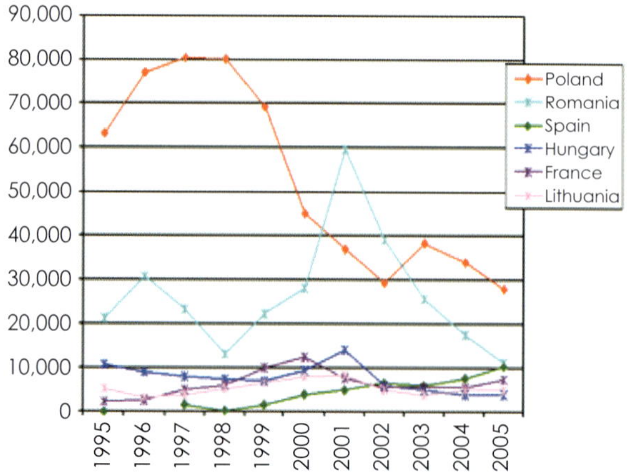

FIGURE 1: EU slaughter horse imports and countries of origin 1995–2005.

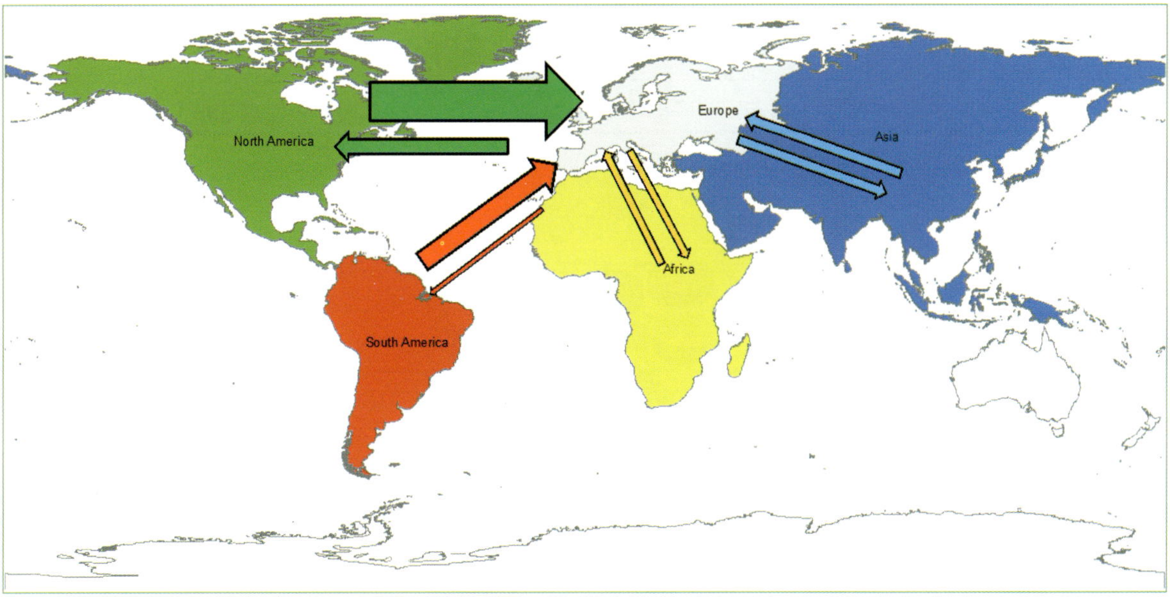

FIGURE 2: Worldwide movements of horses from and to Europe in 2008 (TRACES data 2008).

increased significantly during the last 4 years. In 2008, 14,386 horse movements took place from North- and South America, Africa and Asia to Europe (TRACES data 2008, **Fig 2**).

We have ranked the principal European horse importing countries under the continent of origin in **Table 1**. In all instances, equine imports, whether represented by live animals or animal products, are obliged to meet the pre- and post entry requirements stipulated by the importing country (Timoney 2007). These requirements vary depending on the disease situation in the country to which the horses are consigned. The total of horse imports from North- and South America, Africa and Asia into Europe from 2004 to 2008 are illustrated in **Figure 3**.

In shipping horses to non-EU countries (except Switzerland and Norway) it is important to note the requirements for re-entry into the original country. The health certificate for re-entry of registered horses for racing, competition and cultural events after temporary export is included in EU decision 93/195/EG.

TABLE 1: Principal European destination countries and number of horses* they imported from North and South America, Asia and Africa from 2004 to May 2008

North America		South America		Asia		Africa	
Ireland	**2255**	**Italy**	**6036**	**UK**	**1797**	**Spain**	**881**
Germany	2013	UK	3407	France	242	France	570
Italy	1450	Spain	715	Ireland	233	UK	294
Sweden	1365	France	614	Germany	167	Germany	118
Netherlands	1213	Belgium	250	Belgium	110	Portugal	105
France	1002	Netherlands	245	Netherlands	72	Belgium	102
Belgium	696	Germany	188	Italy	45	Netherland	80
UK	468	Portugal	67	Spain	42	Italy	12
Spain	401	Ireland	63	Portugal	23	Switzerland	9
Finland	397	Austria	57	Poland	18	Greece	6

*Equids certified as: registered equids; breeding/production; pets; other.

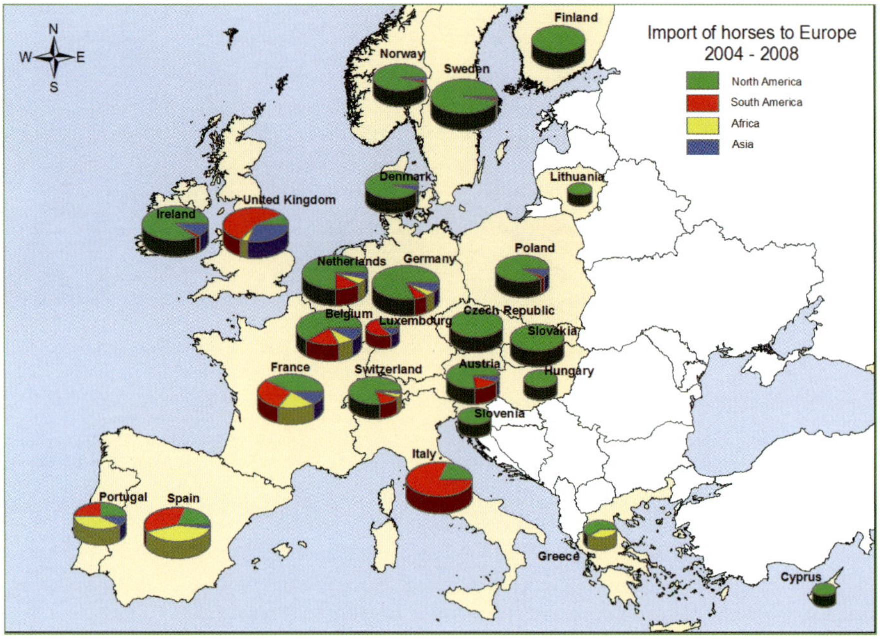

FIGURE 3: The total of horse imports from North and South America, Africa and Asia into Europe from 2004 to 2008 (source: Swiss Federal Veterinary Office).

The veterinary rules on importing horses (including other equids such as zebras and donkeys as well as their hybrids) from third countries into the EU, Switzerland and Norway can be found in different EU directives and at http://www.bvet.admin.ch/ein_ausfuhr/01210/01229/01232/index.html?lang=en.

The importance of strict pre- and post entry requirements stipulated by the importing country was highlighted by the recent outbreak of glanders in Brazil, in the urban area bordering the municipalities of Santo Andre and Sao Paulo in the Federal State of Sao Paulo. The Federal State of Sao Paulo is listed in Annex I to Decision 2004/2117EC as an area from where EU Member States allow all types of importation of categories of equids and their semen, ova and embryos. As soon as the outbreak of glanders was notified to the OIE on 5th September 2008, the animal health conditions for temporary admission of registered horses, permanent imports of equids and re-entry of EU registered horses of temporary export, were no longer extant and so imports of equids and equine products from all of Brazil were suspended for at least 6 months. Modification of requirements can be discussed and may be essential because several horses from Europe either were participating in competitions in Brazil or were scheduled to travel to Brazil to participate in other major equestrian events. Special quarantine and sanitation measures have been discussed to enable the return of these elite horses.

Spread of equine diseases

Despite enormous progress in scientific knowledge and improvements in sanitary standards, the world has recently seen several equine disease epidemics that have caused enormous economic losses.

TABLE 2: Main risks to biosecurity

Importation of live animals, meat and meat products	Legal Illegal Food companies Travellers
Livestock movement	
Animal to animal spread	
Extension of the range of disease vectors and/or change in vector competence	
Migrating birds or other wild animals	

Infectious diseases can be introduced into a country or region by various means. The main risk of introduction is considered to be the (illegal) importation of meat and meat products followed by livestock movement (**Table 2**, Vose 1997). Migratory birds can play an important role in the introduction of foreign animal diseases (Rappole *et al.* 2000). They have long been suspected as the principal means of introduction of West Nile virus into regions of the world in which it had not previously been present.

Global climate change may also result in alteration in the geographical distribution of equine diseases and in their transmission. Climate-driven changes in the size and activity of specific vector populations can enable transmission to become sustainable in previously nonendemic areas and *vice versa* (Khasnis and Nettleman 2005; Gould *et al.* 2006; Haines *et al.* 2006).

TABLE 3: Examples of equine disease outbreaks reported to the OIE from 2007 until September 2008 (source: WAHIS database)

	North America	South America	Africa	Asia	Europe
EIA	Clinical cases in limited zones	Clinical cases: Argentina, Brazil, Columbia, Ecuador, El Salvador, Guyana, Paraguay, Venezuela, Uruguay	Disease not reported	Clinical cases in limited zones Mongolia, China	Germany, Italy, France, Romania, Sicily, Sardinia
AHS	Disease never reported	Disease never reported	Senegal, South Africa, Lesotho, Ethiopia (19/09/08), Eritrea, Nigeria, Swaziland	Israel	Disease not reported
JE	Disease never reported	Disease never reported	Clinical disease never reported	Clinical cases Japan, China	Disease never reported
WEE	Suspicion not confirmed	Disease not reported	Disease not reported	Disease not reported	Disease not reported
VEE	Disease not reported	Clinical cases: Columbia, Guatemala	Disease never confirmed	Disease never confirmed	Disease never confirmed
WNV	Clinical cases	Guatemala, Columbia, Venezuela: Disease suspected, but not confirmed	Tunisia, Uganda	Israel	Russia, France Italy 22 Sep 2008
Equine influenza*	Disease not reported **	Disease not reported **	Egypt	Mongolia, China, Japan	Disease not reported **
EVA	Disease not reported	Disease not reported	Disease not reported	Disease not reported	Croatia
Glanders	Disease not reported	Brazil	Disease not reported	Iran (endemic)	Disease not reported
Equine piroplasmosis	Disease outbreak in a limited zone of Florida	Disease not reported**	Disease not reported**	Disease not reported**	Disease not reported**

EIA: equine infectious anaemia; AHS: African horse sickness; JE: Japanese encephalitis; WEE: Western equine encephalomyelitis; VEE: Venezuelan equine viral encephalomyelitis; WNV: West Nile virus; EVA: equine viral arteritis. *Reported from Australia, resolved 13.11.2007. ** Disease is in many countries not a compulsory notifiable disease.

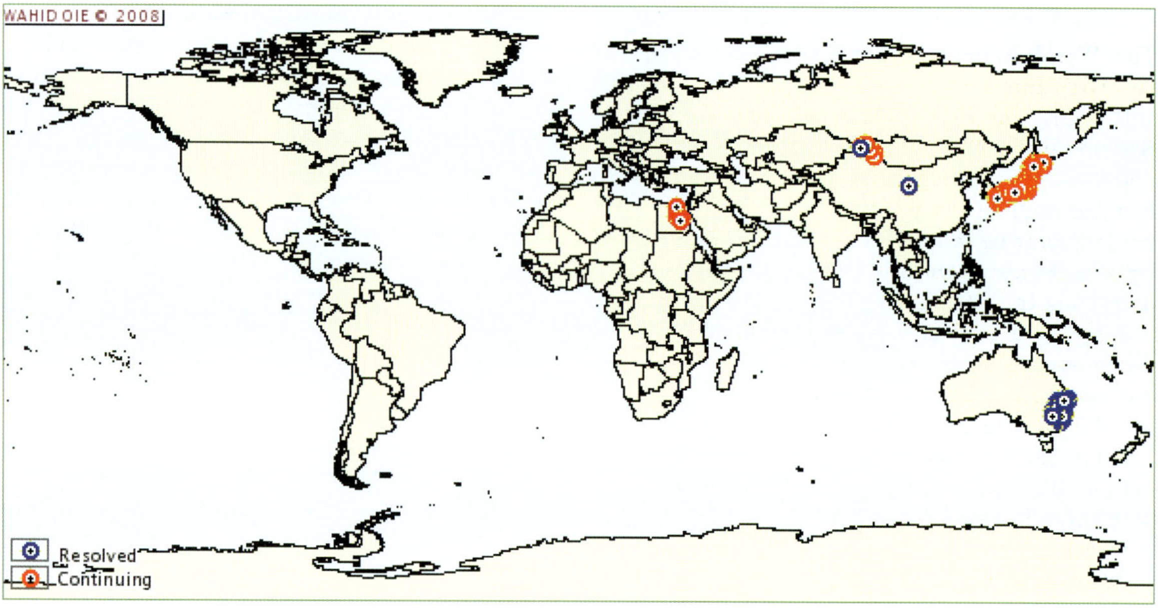

FIGURE 4: Outbreaks of equine influenza from January to June 2008 (source: OIE. WAHID).

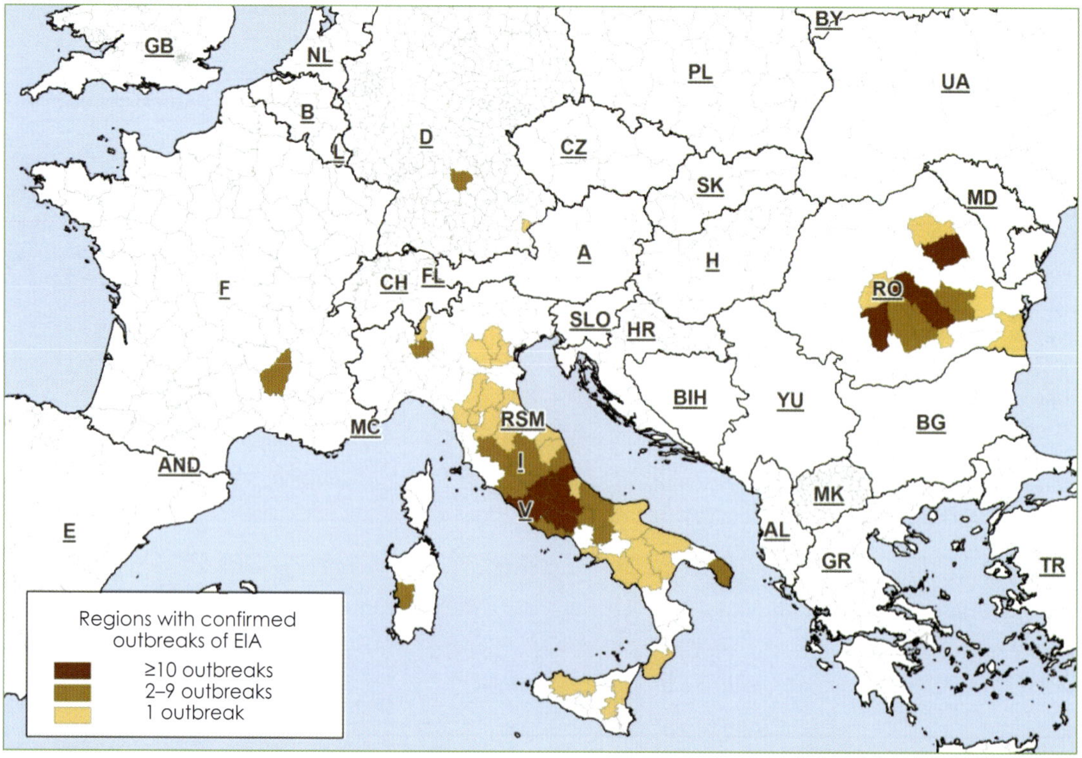

FIGURE 5: Outbreaks of equine infectious anaemia (EIA) in Europe from January to 15th September 2008 (source: Swiss Federal Veterinary Office).

Equine disease outbreaks

The World Animal Health Information Database (WAHID) Interface provides access to all data held within OIE's new World Animal Health Information System (Anon 2008b). This system provides immediate notifications and follow-up reports submitted by member countries in response to exceptional disease events occurring in these countries as well as follow-up reports about these events, 6 monthly reports describing the OIE-listed disease situations in each country and annual reports providing further background information on animal health, laboratory and vaccine production facilities. All member countries are obliged to notify disease outbreaks to the OIE as listed in the Terrestrial Animal Health Code. Disease data in this paper refer to the OIE WAHID database, with only a few exemptions. Important equine disease outbreaks reported to the OIE in 2007 and first half of 2008 are documented in **Table 3**.

The most recent example of a major equine disease outbreak that resulted from horse movement is the incursion of equine influenza into Australia in August 2007. The outbreak had a devastating economic impact on the racing and breeding industry. The disease was introduced into Australia by the importation of a sub-clinically infected stallion from Japan into the Sydney quarantine station, with subsequent spread within and then from, the quarantine facility. **Figure 4** shows the outbreaks of equine influenza notified to the OIE from January to June 2008.

Equine infectious anaemia (EIA) is endemic in many countries throughout the world; indeed, there are very few countries (*viz.* Greenland, Iceland and New Zealand) that have never reported EIA. In Europe, until September 2008 cases were reported in Italy, Romania, Germany, France, Sardinia and Sicilia (**Fig 5**). Ireland experienced an outbreak of EIA during 2006 where the probable source of primary infection was identified as hyperimmune plasma, imported from Italy without licence. More *et al.* (2008a,b) highlighted the modes of transition and spread of EIA in Ireland and the need for high standards of hygiene in the administration of medicines.

Equine disease control programmes

Vourc'h *et al.* (2006) recently described 'syndromic surveillance' systems with the goal of detecting emerging, atypical clinical diseases. Early detection of the unknown, unexpected and atypical clinical disease is essential in diagnosing emerging diseases (Anon 1998). Syndromic surveillance focuses on clinical features rather than clinical diagnosis. Therefore, clinical disease trends are monitored and grouped into syndromes. However, atypical disease case detection is limited by the experience of the field veterinarians (Cuenot *et al.* 2003). These surveillance systems must be sufficiently attractive for the practitioners to keep them engaged and to submit their case data (Vourc'h *et al.* 2006). Clinicians are then able to indicate unusual events that require additional measures. A number of emerging diseases are zoonotic and are potential future health problems (Kahn 2006). However, a lot of future work has to be done to evaluate the 'normal' disease event, to be able to differentiate between well known clinical diseases, rare disease events or emerging diseases (Grant and Olsen *et al.* 1999). The development of efficient and reliable surveillance systems is therefore challenging (Stärk *et al.* 2006).

It is uncommon to find a disease fitting the classic textbook description. The successful investigator thus requires a good knowledge and understanding of the ways in which a condition may behave to allow thoughtful comparison and consideration of options in differential diagnosis. The investigator must also recognise the potential complexity of a disease or production-limiting problem and consider those aspects of the environment, which are likely to influence its progression (Herholz *et al.* 2006).

Effective responses to emergency disease outbreaks require emergency disease planning at national, State/Territory and district level and the involvement of both animal health authorities and emergency management organisations. The basis for this planning is, for example, contained in the Australian Veterinary Emergency Plan (AUSVETPLAN) (Anon 2008c). AUSVETPLAN is a series of technical response plans that describe the proposed Australian approach to exotic disease incursion based on sound analysis, linking policy, strategies, implementation, coordination and emergency-management plans for African horse sickness (AHS), contagious equine metritis (CEM), equine influenza (EI) and Japanese encephalitis (JE) and other conditions. The Department of Environment Food and Rural Affairs (Defra) (Anon

2008d) in the UK provides also a wide range of information on disease outbreaks, disease surveillance and control. The management of the national programme to eradicate equine infectious anaemia from Ireland during 2006 was described by Brangan *et al.* (2008).

Conclusion

Globalisation of trade in horses and their biological products (e.g. semen, embryos, plasma) and increased international movement of horses, both legal and illegal, increases the risks of spread of a wide range of equine diseases. Countries can no longer consider themselves remote from the risk of introduction of infectious diseases of public health or veterinary significance (Brown 2006; Murray 2006; Timoney 2007; Herholz *et al.* 2008). Surveillance of equine diseases at a national level and prompt reporting to the relevant authorities and the OIE are critical to the effectiveness of national and international equine health control programmes and import policies.

References

Anon (1994) World Trade Organization (WTO) Agreement on the application of sanitary and phytosanitary measures. In: *The results of the Uruguay Round of Multilateral Trade Negotiations: The Legal Texts*, GATT, Geneva.

Anon (1998) Preventing emerging infectious diseases: A strategy for the 21st century. Overview of the updated CDC Plan. *CDC. MMWR Recomm. Rep.* **47**, (RR-15): 1-14.

Anon (2004) *Epidemiology: Some Basic Concepts and Definitions.* Food and Agriculture Organization (FAO). http://www.fao.org/Wairdocs/ILRI/x5436E/x5436e04.htm

Anon (2008a) *Terrestrial Animal Health Code.* Office International des Epizooties (OIE)7, http://www.oie.int/eng/normes/mcode/en_sommaire.htm Paris, World Organisation for Animal Health.

Anon (2008b) *World Animal Health Information Database (WAHID) Interface.* Office International des Epizooties (OIE), http://www.oie.int/wahid-prod/public.php?page=home, World Organisation for Animal Health, Paris.

Anon (2008c): *Australian Veterinary Emergency Plan (AUSVETPLAN)*: http://www.animalhealthaustralia.com.au/programs/eadp/ausvetplan_home.cfm

Anon (2008d) *International Disease Monitoring - Major Animal Diseases.* Defra, http://www.defra.gov.uk/animalh/diseases/monitoring/diseases.htm

Brangan, P., Bailey, D.C., Larkin, J.F., Myers, T. and More, S.J. (2008) Management of the national programme to eradicate equine infectious anaemia from Ireland during 2006: A review. *Equine vet. J.* **40**, 702-704.

Brown, C.C. (2006) Risks from emerging animal diseases. In: *Worldwide Risks of Animal Diseases, Vet. Ital.* **42**, 305-317.

Cuenot, M., Calavas, D., Abrial, D., Gasqui, P., Cazeau, G. and Ducrot, C. (2003) Temporal and spatial patterns of the clinical surveillance of BSE in France, analyzed from January 1991 to May 2002 through a vigilance index. *Vet. Res.* **34**, 261-272.

Gould, E.A., Higgs S., Buckley A. and Gritsun, T.S. (2006) Potential Arbovirus emergence and implications for the United Kingdom. www.cdc.gov/eid, *Emerg. Infect. Dis.* **12**, 549-555.

Grant, S. and Olsen, C.W. (1999) Preventing zoonotic diseases in immunocompromised persons: the role of physicians and veterinarians. *Emerg. Infect. Dis.* **12**, 159-163.

Haines, A., Kovats, R.S., Campbell-Lendrum, D. and Corvalan, C. (2006) Climate change and human health: Impacts, vulnerability and public health. *Public Health* **120**, 585-596.

Herholz, C., Jemmi, T., Stärk, K. and Griot, C. (2006) Patterns of animal diseases and their control. *Vet. Ital.* **42**, 295-303.

Herholz, C., Füssel, A., Timoney, P., Schwermer, H.P., Bruckner, L. and Leadon, D. (2008) Equine travellers to the Olympic Games in Hong Kong 2008: A review of worldwide challenges to equine health, with particular reference to vector-borne diseases. *Equine vet. J.* **40**, 87-95.

Kahn, LH. (2006) Confronting zoonoses, linking human and veterinary medicine. *Emerg. Infect. Dis.* [serial on the Internet]. 2006 Apr [date cited]. Available from http://www.cdc.gov/ncidod/EID/vol12no04/05-0956.htm

Khasnis, A. and Nettleman, M.D. (2005) Global warming and infectious disease. *Arch. Med. Res.* **36**, 689-696.

More, S.J., Aznar, I., Myers, T., Leadon, D.P. and Clegg, T.A. (2008) An outbreak of equine infectious anaemia in Ireland during 2006: The modes of transmission and spread in the Kildare cluster. *Equine vet. J.* **40**, 709-711.

More, S.J., Aznar, I., Bailey, D.C., Larkin, J.F., Leadon, D.P., Lenihan, P., Flahety, B., Forgarty, U. and Brangan, P. (2008) An outbreak of equine infectious anaemia in Ireland during 2006: Investigation methodology, initial source of infection, diagnosis and clinical presentation, modes of transmission and spread in the Meath Cluster. *Equine vet. J.* **40**, 706-708.

Murray, N. (2006) International trade and the spread of animal diseases: assessing the risks. In: *Worldwide Risks of Animal Diseases, Vet. Ital.* **42**, 319-336.

Rappole, J.H., Derrickson, S.R. and Hubálek, Z. (2000) Migratory birds and spread of West Nile virus in the western hemisphere. *CDC* **6**, No. 4. http://www.cdc.gov/ncidod/eid/vol6no4/rappole.htm

Stärk, K.D.C., Regula, G., Hernandez, J., Knopf, L., Fuchs, K., Morris, R.S. and Davies, P. (2006) Concepts for risk-based surveillance in the field of veterinary medicine and veterinary public health: Review of current approaches. *BMC Health Service Research,* **6**, 20; http://www.biomedcentral.com/1472-6963/6/20

Timoney, PJ. (2007) Infectious diseases and international movement of horses. In: *Equine Infectious Diseases,* Eds: D.C. Sellon and M.T. Long, W.B. Saunders, Philadelphia. pp 549-557.

Vose, D. (1997) Risk analysis in relation to the importation and exportation of animal products. *Rev. Sci. Tech.* **16**, 17-29.

Vourc'h, G., Bridges, V., Gibbens, J., De Groot, B.D., McIntyre, L., Poland, R. and Barnouin, J. (2006) Detecting emerging diseases in farm animals through clinical observations. *Emerg. Infect. Dis.* **12**, 204-210.

EQUINE INFLUENZA: A CONSTANTLY EVOLVING CHALLENGE

A. A. Cullinane

Virology Unit, Irish Equine Centre, Johnstown, Naas, Co. Kildare, Ireland.

Keywords: horse; influenza; epidemiology; diagnosis; vaccination; quarantine

Summary

H3N8 influenza viruses are a major cause of equine respiratory disease. The cost of the first Australian outbreak in 2007 was estimated to be several hundred million dollars. Equine influenza is endemic in Europe and North America where it is controlled by vaccination. In the UK and Ireland mandatory vaccination programmes for highly mobile horses serve as insurance for business continuity. Additional vaccination is required to provide optimal protection for individual yards. Vaccine efficacy is compromised by point mutations in the envelope proteins of the virus i.e. antigenic drift. The delay in updating vaccine strains as recommended by the Expert Surveillance Panel (ESP) is a cause of international concern. Protection against virus shedding correlates with the relatedness of the challenge virus to the strains in the vaccine. Many countries such as Australia have experienced epizootics of influenza associated with the importation of sub-clinically infected vaccinated horses. Such horses can be identified rapidly by RT-PCR for the detection of virus specific nucleic acid. Measurement of antibody to the virus haemagglutinin assists in the identification of susceptible horses that require vaccination. The strategic use of updated vaccines and sensitive diagnostic techniques minimises the risk of virus entry into populations that are free of equine influenza and the economic toll of the disease in countries where the virus is endemic.

Introduction

Equine influenza virus, an Orthomyxovirus, is categorised as an influenza A virus on the basis of antigenic properties of the nucleoprotein and matrix protein. Its single-stranded RNA genome consists of 8 segments, encoding structural and nonstructural proteins. Two structural proteins, haemagglutinin (HA) and neuraminidase (NA), project from the envelope and account for 25 and 10% of the viral protein mass, respectively. Virus neutralising antibodies are produced against the HA and viruses with variant HA molecules are selected to update vaccines.

Epidemiology

The primary natural reservoir of influenza A viruses are aquatic birds but these viruses occasionally transmit to poultry or jump the species barrier and infect man, swine, horses and seals (Horimoto and Kawaoka 2001). Interspecies transmission does not usually result in adaptation but sometimes the virus replicates efficiently in its new host, and over time establishes a host-specific stable lineage with distinct receptor-binding specificity.

There are currently 16 known HA subtypes and 9 known NA subtypes all of which infect aquatic birds (Fouchier *et al.* 2005). Many different combinations of HA and NA occur and influenza A viruses are divided into subtypes and named on the basis of these 2 proteins. Only 2 stable subtypes have been reported in horses: H7N7 and H3N8. They are considered to be of avian origin (Horimoto and Kawaoka 2001).

In aquatic birds, influenza viruses preferentially replicate in the cells of the intestinal tract and are transmitted by the faecal-oral route. In man, swine and horses influenza viruses replicate in the respiratory tract and are transmitted by the respiratory route. The first reported outbreak of equine respiratory disease to be confirmed as equine influenza occurred in 1956 in eastern Europe (Sovinova *et al.* 1958). The virus isolated was characterised as H7N7. Subsequently H7N7 viruses were identified as the cause of outbreaks in Europe,

Asia and the USA. Phylogenetic analysis of these viruses, indicate that they are the most ancient of all mammalian influenza virus lineages (Webster *et al.* 1992). Although H7N7 viruses co-circulated with H3N8 viruses in horses for many years, it is generally accepted that these viruses have not been active for a long period and may be extinct (Webster 1993). Phylogenetic analysis of nucleoprotein genes suggest that the H3N8 equine 2 virus genome originated in the late 19th century but the first isolation of a virus of this subtype took place in Florida in 1963 (Waddell *et al.* 1963). Since then, H3N8 influenza viruses have been recognised as the most important cause of equine respiratory disease in many of the major horse breeding and racing countries of the world.

Influenza viruses are highly mutable and undergo antigenic shift (major antigenic change) and antigenic drift (minor antigenic change). Antigenic shift may be caused by reassortment of the HA and NA genes when 2 different influenza viruses infect a cell at the same time or by direct transmission from another species. There is no evidence of genetic reassortment occurring in the viruses isolated from horses but there is evidence of interspecies transmission. Sequence analysis of a virus isolated in 1989 from horses during an influenza epidemic in North Eastern China established that the virus was more closely related to avian influenza viruses than to equine influenza viruses (Guo *et al.* 1992). However, it was a H3N8 virus, suggesting that this subtype of avian influenza viruses has a selective advantage over other subtypes for transmission to, and replication in, horses. Equine H3N8 viruses can also replicate and transmit in dogs (Crawford *et al.* 2005).

Antigenic drift refers to point mutations that occur in the HA and NA genes. Such changes occur less frequently in equine influenza viruses than in human viruses. However, a single nucleotide change can alter an antigenic site so that it is no longer recognised by the horse's immune system. In many countries, equine influenza is controlled by vaccination and antigenic drift impacts significantly on vaccine efficacy (Daly *et al.* 2003; Park *et al.* 2004). As a result of antigenic drift the H3N8 subtype has evolved into 2 distinct lineages designated the 'American-like' lineage and the 'European-like' lineage based on the initial geographical distribution of viruses (Daly *et al.* 1996). Three American sub-lineages have emerged the Argentina, Kentucky and Florida (Lai *et al.* 2001). The Florida sub-lineage has recently diverged into 2 clades. Clade 1 contains the Wisconsin/1/03, South Africa/4/03, Sydney/07 and Ibaraki/07 viruses and Clade 2 contains Newmarket/03 and other viruses that have been circulating in Europe since 2003 (http://www.oie.int/eng/publicat/BULLETIN%20PDF/Bull%202008-2-ENG.pdf).

To date, equine influenza outbreaks have been reported all over the world with the exception of a small number of island nations including New Zealand and Iceland.

Equine influenza has a low mortality rate but very high morbidity, which has a major economic effect, in that it leads to the disruption of equestrian activities. The disease is particularly contagious in immunologically naïve populations and occasionally causes large scale epidemics in partially immune populations. In Hong Kong in 1992, racing was suspended for one month and the estimated financial loss was close to $1 billion. In South Africa in 1986 racing was suspended for 2.5 months with a $70 million loss in betting revenue. In Australia in 2007 after the first incursion of equine influenza virus, a 72 h nationwide 'horse standstill' was imposed after which statewide bans were maintained in South Wales and Queensland prior to the introduction of zoning, vaccination and eventual eradication after several months (http://www.equineinfluenzainquiry.gov.au). The cost of the Australian outbreak was estimated to be several hundred million dollars. Equine influenza is a constant but fluctuating problem of economic significance in Europe and North America where it is controlled by widespread vaccination.

Three human pandemics of influenza occurred during the last century. All 3, the 1918 Spanish flu caused by H1N1, the 1957 Asian flu caused by H2N2 and the 1968 Hong Kong flu caused by H3N2 were associated with the introduction of a novel HA subtype into the population from nonhuman hosts (Cox and Subbarao 2000). Recent significant epidemics of equine influenza such as occurred in Australia and Japan in 2007 have been caused by Clade 1 viruses of the Florida sublineage i.e. viruses related to those in the vaccines and to which vaccinated horses and horses in endemic countries have partial pre-existing immunity (Bryant *et al.*

2008; Yamanaka *et al.* 2008a). The avian virus isolated in horses in China in 1989 (A/Equine/Jilin/1/89) failed to replicate in ducks, i.e. its receptor binding had become specific to horses. It was reported that over 13,000 horses were affected in this outbreak and that the mortality rate was up to 35% but it did not spread beyond China (Guo *et al.* 1995). If in the future a whole avian influenza virus became infective for horses without losing its ability to replicate in birds there would be a significant risk of global spread by aquatic birds during migratory flights. Such an event could lead to a pandemic of equine influenza.

Clinical features

The incubation period varies from 1–5 days and depends primarily on the size of the virus challenge and the immunological status of the horse. The most common clinical signs are pyrexia, a hacking cough and nasal discharge. Inappetance, depression,weight loss, myalgia, enlarged mandibular lymph nodes and limb oedema are also frequently observed (reviewed by Wilson 1993). The severity of the disease is related to the virulence of the virus strain and the immune status of the horses at the time of exposure (Newton *et al.* 2000a; Wattrang *et al.* 2003). Vaccinated horses may be only mildly or subclinically affected but can shed virus and serve as a source of virus to their cohorts (Daly *et al.* 2004).

Horses usually recover clinically from uncomplicated influenza within 10 days but coughing may persist for longer. The virus infects the ciliated respiratory epithelial cells and impairs the clearance mechanism. This increases the susceptibility of the respiratory tract to secondary bacterial invasion which, in turn, prolongs the recovery period. Pneumonia may occur. Sequelae of equine influenza can include chronic pharyngitis, chronic bronchiolitis, alveolar emphysema, which can contribute to COPD, sinusitis and guttural pouch infections. Pregnant mares may abort due to pyrexia. Sporadic cases exhibiting neurological signs have been reported but it has not been conclusively established that encephalopathy was caused by equine influenza virus infection (Daly *et al.* 2006). Equine influenza virus infection has been associated with peracute fatalities and respiratory disease in dogs (Crawford *et al.* 2005; Daly *et al.* 2008).

Diagnosis and identification of susceptible horses

Influenza in unvaccinated horses is easy to recognise clinically given its highly contagious nature and the characteristic persistent cough. However, vaccinated horses may show few, if any, clinical signs and laboratory analysis is required for diagnosis. In the past 2 decades many countries have experienced epizootics of equine influenza (for example, South Africa 1986 and 2003, India 1987, Hong Kong 1992, Dubai 1995 and Australia 2007), associated with the importation of sub-clinically infected vaccinated horses (Powell *et al.* 1995; Guthrie *et al.* 1999; Timoney 2000; King and Macdonald 2004; http://www.equineinfluenzainquiry.gov.au). Such horses are usually seropositive and shed only small quantities of virus. Fortunately, sensitive diagnostic techniques are available for the detection of equine influenza virus antigen and nucleic acid. The strategic use of these techniques is essential for the international control of the disease.

Traditionally, equine influenza was diagnosed by serology and virus isolation from nasal swabs. The virus can be isolated in embryonated hens' eggs or canine kidney cells. Some virus strains are difficult to isolate. It takes a minimum of 2 or 3 days and may take weeks depending on how many passages are required in the eggs. Virus isolation is important for characterising new strains but as a diagnostic technique for equine influenza it has been replaced by ELISAs to detect nucleoprotein and real time RT-PCR for the detection of virus specific nucleic acid.

A specific and highly sensitive antigen-capture ELISA developed by the Animal Health Trust (AHT) in Newmarket has been used in the UK since 1989 (Livesay *et al.* 1993). Because of the degree of conservation of the nucleoprotein among influenza viruses several kits for the diagnosis of human influenza including Directigen Flu-A and Espline have been used in the diagnosis of equine influenza (Chambers *et al.* 1994; Yamanaka *et al.* 2008b). These kits are easy to use and provide a rapid result. They have been used to test imported horses in quarantine in Dubai and Hong Kong. However, the sensitivity of such kits compares unfavourably with RT-PCR (Quinlivan *et al.* 2004, 2005a). RT-PCR is exquisitely sensitive and provides a diagnosis in hours. It was the technique used in the mass screening of horses during the 2007 outbreak in Australia (http://www.equineinfluenza inquiry.gov.au).

Antibody responses against the influenza HA can be measured by haemagglutination inhibition (HI) or single radial haemolysis (SRH). The SRH is more reproducible between laboratories (Mumford 2000) but the HI is more commonly used for diagnosis as it is less labour intensive. A definitive serological diagnosis of influenza requires the examination of paired serum samples for rising antibody levels and is thus usually retrospective. A clotted blood sample needs to be collected in the acute stage of the disease and tested with a second collected 10–14 days later. Veterinary advice is not always sought at the onset of clinical signs and where there is a delay, analysis of single samples may be useful. In unvaccinated horses an antibody titre against H3 indicates exposure to virus by natural infection at some time. In horses vaccinated with a vaccine containing both H7N7 and H3N8 strains, a much higher antibody level against H3 than against H7 may support a diagnosis of influenza. An ELISA to detect antibody to the nucleoprotein was used in the Australian outbreak in 2007 to differentiate infected horses from horses vaccinated (DIVA) with Proteq (http://www.equineinfluenzainquiry.gov.au). The nucleoprotein is produced during infection but not incorporated in vaccines such as Proteq Flu (Merial), which uses a canarypox vector to express only the HA genes (Edlund Toulemonde *et al.* 2005). The potential of this test to differentiate infected horses from horses vaccinated with other vaccines needs to be assessed.

Circulating antibodies against HA are the principle correlate of protection and horses can be blood tested to determine if they are at risk and require vaccination. In experimental challenge studies with whole inactivated and subunit vaccines SRH antibody levels of 120–154 mm^2 were shown to be required for virological protection against challenge with an antigenically similar virus (Mumford 1992). In influenza outbreaks protective antibody levels were estimated to be >160 mm^2 (Mumford 1992). Trainers should try to ensure that all horses in their yard have high antibody levels. Seronegative horses and horses with low antibody levels should be identified and vaccinated. Such horses are the most likely to become infected if exposed to virus and to introduce virus into a population (Newton *et al.* 2000b). Even if these horses are not the source of virus they play a major role in the onward spread of the virus. They are frequently the index cases as they are the most susceptible to influenza. When infected they rapidly amplify virus and serve as a source of significant virus challenge to their cohorts who may succumb despite being regularly vaccinated.

In specific circumstances, seronegative horses may be less susceptible to clinical disease than predicted. The immune response elicited by natural infection is different to that elicited by vaccination with conventional vaccines. Horses naturally infected with influenza virus may be protected against a repeat challenge despite having low antibody levels. Ponies experimentally infected were shown to be protected more than one year later and after their antibodies had waned (Hannant *et al.* 1988). Similarly, the modified-live virus intranasal vaccine (FluAvert IN) licensed in the USA does not induce antibodies that correlate with protection and there is currently no technique that can be readily employed in a diagnostic laboratory to evaluate the susceptibility of horses vaccinated with this product (Townsend *et al.* 2001).

Prevention and control

In countries where equine influenza virus is endemic the economic losses due to influenza can be minimised by vaccination of highly mobile horses. Congregation of horses at racetracks, horse shows, sales and other equestrian events is conducive to the spread of influenza and dispersal of horses after such events frequently leads to dissemination of virus over a large geographical area. In the UK and Ireland, the Jockey Club and Turf Club require that racehorses receive 2 primary vaccinations 21–92 days apart, followed by a third vaccination 150–215 days after the second, and thereafter annual vaccination. Since 2005 the Fédération Equestre Internationale (FEI) require that all horses competing in their competitions have been vaccinated in the previous 6 months. Many horse and pony societies require vaccination and it is a prerequisite for entry in many Thoroughbred sales. On the basis of the sales of vaccines it is roughly estimated that only around one third of the horse population in the UK and Ireland is vaccinated, yet no race meeting or major equestrian event has been cancelled in either country due to equine influenza since the introduction of mandatory vaccination for racehorses in 1981.

The Jockey Club and Turf Club Rules only require annual booster vaccination after the initial primary course and 6 month booster. Such a policy is effective in preventing a build-up of virus challenge of such magnitude that racing has to be suspended but it does not necessarily provide optimum protection for an individual training yard. Outbreaks of influenza occur most years in the UK and Ireland and there has been an increased incidence in vaccinated horses since 2003. Mandatory vaccination programmes act as insurance for business continuity, i.e. their primary aim is to induce sufficient herd immunity to protect equestrian events rather than individual horses or premises. Antibody against HA induced by exposure to virus by natural infection or by vaccination plays a primary role in the protection of horses against influenza (Mumford 1992; Daly *et al.* 2004). Therefore, serological studies have helped to determine when horses are most susceptible to influenza and when they benefit most from vaccination. Foals born to seropositive mares usually have equivalent levels of maternal antibodies within 48 h (Van Maanen *et al.* 1992; Cullinane *et al.* 2001). These antibodies persist for 3–6 months, although in some cases they may be more durable. It is advisable to vaccinate pregnant mares between the last 4–6 weeks of pregnancy to ensure their colostrum has protective levels of antibody (Cullinane *et al.* 2001). The vaccination of foals prior to the waning of maternal antibodies with inactivated or subunit vaccines fails to elicit an effective immune response (Van Maanen *et al.* 1992; Cullinane *et al.* 2001) and has been implicated in the inhibition of the humoural response of young horses to future vaccination (Newton *et al.* 2000b; Cullinane *et al.* 2001). However, vaccination of foals with maternal antibody using a canary pox recombinant vaccine (Proteq Flu) appears to stimulate an immunological memory and an improved response to subsequent vaccination when the maternal antibodies have waned (Minke *et al.* 2007).

The weakness and poor durability of the immune response of unprimed horses to 2 doses of vaccine has been repeatedly demonstrated and it is apparent that vaccination in accordance with the rules of the racing authorities in the UK and Ireland and vaccine manufacturers' recommendations, leaves horses at risk between their second and third vaccination (Van Oirschot *et al.* 1991; Van Maanen *et al.* 1992; Cullinane *et al.* 2001)

The inclusion of an additional booster 3–4 months after the second vaccination is indicated to afford greater protection (Cullinane *et al.* 2001). This is of particular benefit to horses being prepared for sales or entering training, i.e. those at increased risk from exposure to virus.

In young horses antibody levels tend to decline below a protective level within 4 months of booster vaccination (Newton *et al.* 2000b). Mathematical models suggest that 6 monthly rather than annual boosters reduce the risk of influenza infection in racehorses (Park *et al.* 2003) and this is consistent with unpublished observations in the field. In older horses serological monitoring assists in the timing of booster vaccination. Horses with high antibody levels often experience a decline in antibodies post booster vaccination. Vaccination of such horses should be delayed to optimise their response.

High levels of antibody are required to protect horses against infection with influenza virus. New arrivals in a yard should be serologically tested to determine if they require booster vaccination. Some trainers opt to administer a 'new' primary course to young racehorses. Newton *et al.* (2005) compared yearlings in one yard that were vaccinated 4–6 weeks apart with yearlings in another yard that extended the interval to 12 weeks. They concluded that increasing the interval between 2 doses of a 'new' primary course in previously primed horses led to a more durable antibody response.

In the last 2 decades new adjuvants and improved antigenic presentation systems have increased the effectiveness of conventional inactivated and subunit vaccines (reviewed by Paillot *et al.* 2006). Live attenuated such as the cold-adapted virus and recombinant vaccines such as the pox-based vaccines have been developed (Townsend *et al.* 2001; Edlund Toulemonde *et al.* 2005). These vaccines aim to stimulate an immune response more closely resembling that induced by natural infection. A live attenuated virus engineered by reverse genetics has the potential to be readily updated by the insertion of the HA and NA genes of a new strain (Quinlivan *et al.* 2005b). However, while significant progress has been made in vaccine development the speed with which the strains of virus in the vaccines have been updated is a cause of international concern. Strain specific antibody is more effective than cross-reactive antibody in providing protection. If there is a mismatch between the field virus and the strain in the vaccine the horse requires higher levels of antibody to confer protection (Newton *et al.* 1999). Since the introduction of mandatory vaccination in the UK in 1981, there have only been 2 large outbreaks of equine influenza: a countrywide epidemic in 1989 (Livesay *et al.* 1993) and a serious outbreak in the Newmarket area in 2003 (Newton *et al.* 2006). In both instances, the vaccine strains had been isolated 10 years earlier. Protection against virus shedding has been shown to correlate with the degree of antigenic relatedness of the vaccine strain to the challenge virus (Daly *et al.* 2003). The vaccinated horse(s) that introduced influenza into the Australian quarantine facility in 2007 had been vaccinated with outdated strains. In 2004 it was recommended by the Expert Surveillance Panel (ESP) including OIE and WHO experts that the vaccines be updated to include a South Africa 2003-like virus. At the time of writing this review only one vaccine in the EU and one in the USA have been updated in line with these recommendations. In 2008 an updated canary pox recombinant vaccine (Proteq Flu)[1] and an updated inactivated carbopol adjuvanted vaccine (Calvenza 03)[2] were licensed in the UK and USA respectively (http://www.aht.org.uk/equiflunet).

In 2008 the Australian Quarantine and Inspection Service (AQIS) revised their requirements for the importation of horses. Horses must now be vaccinated with a vaccine containing the strains recommended by the ESP prior to importation (www.aqis.gov.au) It is likely that there will be an increase in emphasis on the use of updated vaccines in horses being imported into countries that are free of equine influenza. Traditionally countries where influenza is not endemic have relied on vaccination to minimise the risk of virus entry and on post arrival quarantine to prevent virus escaping into the general horse population. These measures have repeatedly been shown to be inadequate (Guthrie *et al.* 1999; Timoney 2000; King and Macdonald 2004; http://www.equineinfluenzainquiry.gov.au). The risk of an infected horse leaving the quarantine facility can be significantly reduced by strategic RT-PCR testing as has been recently introduced in Australia (http://www.aqis.gov.au). However, in South Africa in 2003 (King and Macdonald 2004) and Australia in 2007 (http://www.equineinfluenzainquiry.gov.au) it was concluded that equine influenza virus escaped from the quarantine facility by indirect means such as personnel, vehicles or equipment. The identification of deficiencies in the biosecurity measures in place in both quarantine facilities has implications for people who have contact with infected horses in any circumstances. A better understanding of virus transmission, constant surveillance and timely updating of vaccines will be critical to minimising the economic toll of equine influenza in the future.

Manufacturers' addresses

[1]Merial, Duluth, Georgia, USA.

[2]Boehringer Ingelheim Animal Health Inc, Ingelheim, Germany.

References

Bryant, N., Rash, A., Lewis, N., Elton. D., Montesso, F., Ross, J., Newton, R., Paillot, R., Watson, J. and Jeggo, M. (2008) Australia equine influenza: vaccine protection in the UK. *Vet. Rec.* **162**, 491-492.

Chambers, T.M., Shortridge, K.F., Li, P.H., Powell, G. and Watkins, K.L. (1994) Rapid diagnosis of equine influenza by the Directigen Flu-A enzyme assay. *Vet. Rec.* **135**, 275-279.

Cox, N.J. and Subbarao, K. (2000) Global epidemiology of influenza, past and present. *Ann. Rev. Med.* **51**, 407-421.

Crawford., P.C., Dubovi, E.J., Castleman, W.L., Stephenson, I., Gibbs, E.P., Chen, L., Smith, C., Hill, R.C., Ferro, P., Pompey, J., Bright, R.A., Medina, M.J., Johnson, C.M., Olsen, C.W., Cox, N. J., Klimov, A.I., Katz, J.M. and Donis, R.O. (2005) Transmission of equine influenza virus to dogs. *Science* **310**, 482-485.

Cullinane, A., Weld, J., Osborne, M., Nelly, M., McBride, M. and Walsh, C. (2001) Field studies on equine influenza vaccination regimes in thoroughbred foals and yearlings. *Vet. J.* **161**, 186-193.

Daly, J.M., Newton, J.R. and Mumford, J.A. (2004) Current perspectives on control of equine influenza. *Vet. Res.* **35**, 411-423.

Daly, J.M., Lai, A.C.K., Binns, M.M., Chambers, T.M., Barrandeguy, M. and Mumford, J.A. (1996) Antigenic and genetic evolution of equine H3N8 influenza A viruses. *J. Gen. Virol.* **77**, 661-671.

Daly, J.M., Whitwell, K.E., Miller, J., Dowd, G., Cardwell, J.M. and Smith, K.C. (2006) Investigation of equine influenza cases exhibiting neurological disease: Coincidence or association. *J. comp. Pathol.* **134**, 231-235.

Daly, J.M., Yates, R.J., Browse, G., Swann, Z., Newton, J.R., Jessett, D., Davis-Poynter, N. and Mumford, J.A. (2003) Comparison of hamster and pony challenge models for evaluation of effect of antigenic drift on cross protection afforded by equine influenza vaccines. *Equine vet. J.* **35**, 458-462.

Daly, J.M., Blunden, A.S., Macrae, S., Miller, J., Bowman S.J., Kolodziejek, J., Nowotny, N. and Smith, K.C. (2008) Transmission of equine influenza virus to English foxhounds. *Emerg. Infect. Dis.* **14**, 461-464.

Edlund Toulemonde, C., Daly, J., Sindle, T., Guigal, P.M., Audonnet, J.C. and Minke, J.M. (2005) Efficacy of a recombinant equine influenza vaccine against challenge with an American lineage H3N8 influenza virus responsible for the 2003 outbreak in the United Kingdom. *Vet. Rec.* **156**, 367-371.

Fouchier, R.A., Munster, V., Wallesten, A., Bestebroer, T.M., Herfst, S., Smith, D., Rimmelzwaan, G.F., Olsen, B. and Osterhaus, A.D. (2005) Characterization of a novel influenza A virus hemagglutinin subtype (H16) obtained from black-headed gulls. *J. Virol.* **79**, 2814-2822.

Guo, Y., Wang, M., Zheng, G.S., Li, W.K., Kawaoka, Y. and Webster, R.G. (1995) Seroepidemiological and molecular evidence for the presence of two H3N8 equine influenza viruses in China in 1993-94. *J. Gen. Virol.* **76**, 2009-2014.

Guo.,Y., Wang., M., Kawaoka, Y., Gorman, O., Ito, T., Saito, T. and Webster, R.G. (1992) Characterisation of a new avian-like influenza A virus from horses in China. *Virology* **188**, 245-1255.

Guthrie, A.J., Stevens, K.B. and Bosman, P.P. (1999) The circumstances surrounding the outbreak and spread of equine influenza in South Africa. *Rev. Sci. Tech.* **18**, 179-185.

Hannant, D., Mumford, J.A. and Jesset, D.M. (1988) Duration of circulating antibody and immunity following infection with equine influenza virus. *Vet. Rec.* **122**, 125-128.

Horimito, T. and Kawaoka, Y. (2001) Pandemic threat posed by avian influenza A viruses. *Clin. Microbiol. Rev.* **14**, 129-149.

King, E.L. and Macdonald, D. (2004) Report of the Board of Inquiry appointed by the Board of the National Horseracing Authority to conduct enquiry into the causes of the equine influenza which started in the Western Cape in early December 2003 and spread to the Eastern Cape and Gauteng. *Aust. equine Vet.* **23**, 139-142.

Lai, A.C., Chambers, T.M., Holland, R.E. Jr, Morley, P.S., Haines, D.M., Townsend, H.G. and Barrandeguy, M. (2001) Diverged evolution of recent equine-2 influenza (H3N8) viruses in the Western Hemisphere. *Arch. Virol.* **146**, 1063-1074.

Livesay, G.J., O'Neil, T., Hannant, D., Yadav, M.P. and Mumford, J.A. (1993) The outbreak of equine influenza (H3N8) in Britain in 1989 and the use of antigen capture ELISA in the diagnosis of acute infection. *Vet. Rec.* **133**, 515-519.

Minke, J.M., Toulemonde, C.E., Dinic, S., Cozette, V., Cullinane, A. and Audonnet, J.C. (2007) Effective priming of foals born to immune dams against influenza by a canarypox-vectored recombinant influenza H3N8 vaccine. *J. comp. Pathol.* **137**, 76-80.

Mumford, J. (1992) Progress in the control of equine influenza. In: *Proceedings of the 6th International Conference on Equine Infectious Diseases, Cambridge,* Eds: W. Plowright, P.D. Rossdale and J.F. Wade, R&W Publications, Newmarket. pp 207-218.

Mumford, J. (2000) Collaborative study for the establishment of three European Pharmacopoeia Biological Reference Preparations for equine influenza horse antiserum. *Pharmeuropa* **Bio 2000-1**, 5-21.

Newton, J.R., Texier, M.J. and Shepherd, M.C. (2005) Modifying likely protection from equine influenza vaccination by varying dosage intervals within the Jockey Club Rules of Racing. *Equine vet. Educ.* **17**, 314-318.

Newton, J.R., Daly, J.M., Spencer, L. and Mumford, J.A. (2006) Description of the outbreak of equine influenza (H3N8) in the United Kingdom in 2003, during which recently vaccinated horses in Newmarket developed respiratory disease. *Vet. Rec.* **158**, 185-192.

Newton, J.R., Verheyen, K., Wood, J.L.N., Yates P.J. and Mumford, J.A. (1999) Equine influenza in the United Kingdom in 1998. *Vet. Rec.* **145**, 449-452.

Newton, J.R., Townsend, H.G., Wood, J.L., Sinclair, R., Hannant, D. and Mumford, J.A. (2000a) Immunity to equine influenza: relationship of vaccine-induced antibody in young thoroughbred racehorses to protection against field infection with influenza A/equine-2 viruses (H3N8). *Equine vet. J.* **32**, 65-74.

Newton, J.R., Lakhani, K.H., Wood, J.L. and Baker, D.J. (2000b) Risk factors for equine influenza serum antibody titres in young thoroughbred racehorses given an inactivated vaccine. *Prev. vet. Med.* **46**, 129-141.

Paillot, R., Hannant, D., Kydd, J.H. and Daly, J.M. (2006) Vaccination against equine influenza: Quid novi? *Vaccine* **24**, 4047-4061.

Park, A.W., Wood, J.L., Newton, J. R., Daly, J.M., Mumford, J.A. and Grenfell, B.T. (2003). Optimising vaccination strategies in equine influenza. *Vaccine* **21**, 2862-2870.

Park, A.W., Wood, J.L., Daly, J.M., Newton, J.R., Glass, K., Henley, W., Mumford, J.A. and Grenfell, B.T. (2004) The effects of strain heterology on the epidemiology of equine influenza in a vaccinated population. *Proc. Biol. Science* **271**, 1547-1555.

Powell, D.G., Watkins, K.L., Li, P.H. and Shortridge, K.F. (1995) Outbreak of equine influenza among horses in Hong Kong during 1992. *Vet. Rec.* **136**, 531-536.

Quinlivan, M., Dempsey, E., Ryan, F., Arkins, S. and Cullinane, A. (2005a) Real-time reverse transcription PCR for detection and quantitative analysis of equine influenza virus. *J. Clin. Microbiol.* **43**, 5055-5057.

Quinlivan, M., Zamarin, D., Garcia-Sastre, A., Cullinane, A., Chambers, T. and Palese, P. (2005b) Attenuation of equine influenza viruses through truncations of the NS1 protein. *J. Virol.* **79**, 8431-8439.

Quinlivan, M., Cullinane, A., Nelly, M., Van Maanen, K., Heldens, J. and Arkins, S. (2004) Comparison of sensitivities of virus isolation, antigen detection, and nucleic acid amplification for detection of equine influenza virus. *J. Clin. Microbiol.* **42**, 759-763.

Sovinova, O., Tumova, B., Pouska, F. and Nemec, J. (1958) Isolation of a virus causing respiratory disease in horses. *Acta Virol.* **2**, 52-61.

Timoney, P.J. (2000) Factors influencing the international spread of equine diseases. *Vet. Clin. N. Am.: Equine Pract.* **916**, 537-551.

Townsend, H.G., Penner, S.J., Watts, T.C., Cook, A., Bogdan, J., Haines, D.M., Griffin, S., Chambers, T., Holland, R.E., Whitaker-Dowling, P., Youngner, J.S. and Sebring, R.W. (2001) Efficacy of a cold-adapted, intranasal, equine influenza vaccine: challenge trials. *Equine vet. J.* **33**, 637-643.

Van Maanen, C., Bruin, G., de Boer-Luijtze, E., Smolders, G. and de Boer, G.F. (1992) Interference of maternal antibodies with the immune response of foals after vaccination against equine influenza. *Vet. Quart.* **14**, 13-17.

Van Oirschot, J.T., Bruin, G., Boer-Luytze, E. and Smolders, G. (1991) Maternal antibodies against equine influenza virus in foals and their interference with vaccination. *J. vet. Med. B* **38**, 391-396.

Waddell, G.H., Teigland, M.B. and Sigel, M.M. (1963) A new influenza virus associated with equine respiratory disease. *J. Am. vet. med. Ass.* **143**, 587-590.

Wattrang, E., Jessett, D.M., Yates, P., Fuxler, L. and Hannant, D. (2003) Experimental infection of ponies with equine influenza A2 (H3N8) virus strains of different pathogenicity elicits varying interferon and interleukin-6 responses. *Viral. Immunol.* **16**, 57-67.

Webster, R.G. (1993) Are equine 1 influenza viruses still present in horses? *Equine vet. J.* **25**, 537-538.

Webster, R.G, Bean, W.J., Gorman, O.T., Chambers, T.M. and Kawaoka, Y. (1992) Evolution and ecology of influenza A viruses. *Microbiol. Rev.* **56**, 152-179.

Wilson, W.D. (1993) Equine influenza. *Vet. Clin. N. Am.: Equine Pract.* **9**, 257-282.

Yamanaka, T., Hidekazu, N., Tsujimura, K., Kondo, T. and Matsumura, T. (2008a) Epidemic of equine influenza among vaccinated racehorses in Japan in 2007. *J. vet. med. Sci.* **70**, 623-625.

Yamanaka, T., Tsujimura, K., Kondo, T. and Matsumura, T. (2008b) Evaluation of antigen detection kits for diagnosis of equine influenza. *J. vet. med. Sci.* **70**, 189-192.

EQUINE VIRAL ARTERITIS

P. J. Timoney

Gluck Equine Research Center, University of Kentucky, Lexington, Kentucky 40546-0099, USA.

Keywords: horse; EVA; carrier stallion; manageable disease

Summary

Equine viral arteritis (EVA) is caused by equine arteritis virus (EAV), an enveloped, single-stranded, positive-sense RNA virus. The virus has a widespread global distribution and a significant level of infection in certain horse breeds. Typical clinical signs include fever, depression, leucopenia, dependent oedema and respiratory signs. EAV can also cause abortion in the pregnant mare and illness and death in young foals. A carrier state can occur in sexually mature intact males, i.e. colts and stallions, but not in mares, geldings or sexually immature colts. In the carrier stallion the virus is restricted to the reproductive tract where it localises primarily in certain of the accessory sex glands. Such stallions shed the virus constantly in the sperm-rich fraction of the ejaculate and are, therefore, a potential source of infection at time of breeding or release of seminal fluid. Transmission of EAV occurs readily by natural breeding or artificial insemination with fresh-cooled or cryopreserved semen.

Introduction

Equine viral arteritis, more popularly referred to as EVA, is a contagious disease of members of the equid family caused by equine arteritis virus (EAV) (Doll *et al.* 1957a), one of the 3 major viral respiratory pathogens of the horse (Timoney 2008a). Principally characterised by fever, depression, leucopenia, dependent oedema and respiratory signs, the disease is not typically life-threatening in otherwise healthy adult horses (Doll *et al.* 1957a; Jones 1969; Timoney and McCollum 1993a). However, EAV can cause abortion in the pregnant mare, and illness and death in young foals (Doll *et al.* 1957b; Golnik *et al.* 1981; Vaala *et al.* 1992; Del Piero *et al.* 1997). Equine viral arteritis derives its name from the widespread vasculitis involving the smaller blood vessels, especially the arterioles, that is characteristic of the disease (Jones *et al.* 1957; Jones 1969). Not unlike various other equine infectious diseases, many cases of primary EAV infection are asymptomatic (Timoney and McCollum 1986, 1993a).

Equine viral arteritis or a clinically very similar condition afflicted equine populations in Europe and possibly elsewhere for many years prior to 1953 (Pottie 1888; Clark 1892; Reeks 1902) when the aetiology and characteristic pathology of the disease were first determined by Doll *et al.* (1957a). For over 30 years, relatively little emphasis was placed on the veterinary medical and economic significance of EVA until it occurred on a widespread scale in central Kentucky in 1984, involving an estimated 41 Thoroughbred breeding farms (Timoney 1984; Timoney and McCollum 1991, 1993a). Immediate concerns were expressed at a national and international level by equine industries and regulatory authorities alike over the risk of spread of EVA to unprotected equid populations in the US and elsewhere (Timoney and McCollum 1993b). The threat of 'abortion storms' and of establishment of the carrier state in stallions led to the enactment of some of the most rigorous control measures on the international movement of horses by other major horse breeding countries, many of which remain in force today (Timoney and McCollum 1993a,b).

Notwithstanding the considerable amount of scientific information and knowledge currently available on EVA, there remains a great deal of misinformation, indeed total unawareness of the disease, among many in the equine industry (Anon 2000). Lack of familiarity with EVA is not restricted to the horse-owning community; however, it can also be encountered among some members of the veterinary profession.

In the past 40–50 years, EAV has become more geographically widespread due in major part to continued growth in the numbers of horses being transported both within and between countries worldwide (Timoney 2000a). Of special importance in this respect has been the shipment of stallions that are asymptomatic carriers of EAV (McCollum *et al.* 1999) and more recently, EAV infective semen (Balasuriya *et al.* 1998; Timoney *et al.* 1998; Timoney 2000b). The equine population in very few countries, such as Japan and Iceland, are known to be free of this infection (Matumoto *et al.* 1965; Konishi *et al.* 1975; Timoney and McCollum 1993a, 2004). The outcome of serological surveys has shown that the prevalence of infection can vary widely both between countries and between different breeds in the same country (McCollum and Bryans 1973; Moraillon and Moraillon 1978; Timoney and McCollum 1993a; Hullinger *et al.* 2001). Higher rates of infection are frequently found in Standardbreds and various Warmblood breeds (McCollum and Bryans 1973; van Maanen *et al.* 2005).

Notwithstanding the widespread global distribution of EAV and the significant level of infection in certain horse breeds, laboratory confirmed outbreaks of EVA have been relatively infrequent, being recorded only in North America and Europe (Timoney and McCollum 1993a). This situation would appear to be changing; however, with the frequency of reported outbreaks has been increasing in recent years. While a number of factors may have contributed to this including greater industry awareness of the disease and improved diagnostic capability, it is much more likely the result of increased international commerce in horses and semen (Timoney 2000a). Importation of carrier stallions and virus infective semen have been implicated in the introduction of EAV into various countries on numerous occasions (Balasuriya *et al.* 1998; McCollum *et al.* 1999; Timoney 2000b).

Aetiology

For many years, EAV was identified with a triad of viral pathogens historically linked to the 'equine influenza-abortion' syndrome, the others being equine herpesviruses 1 and 4 and equine influenza virus (Doll *et al.* 1957a). Subsequently, EAV was shown to be an enveloped, single-stranded, positive-sense RNA virus with quasi-species structure, and the prototype virus of the genus *Arterivirus*, family *Arteriviridae*, order *Nidovirales* (Cavanagh 1997; Snijder and Meulenberg 1998). Also included in this genus are porcine reproductive and respiratory syndrome virus, simian haemorrhagic fever virus, and lactic dehydrogenase elevating virus of mice, none of which are known to be of any public health significance (Plagemann and Moennig 1992).

Equine arteritis virus is a natural pathogen of equids, especially horses (Timoney and McCollum 1993a, 2004). Although there is a report of the detection of EAV nucleic acid in an aborted alpaca fetus, the significance of this finding has yet to be established (Weber *et al.* 2006).

All strains of EAV isolated so far are antigenically related (Fukunaga and McCollum 1977; Timoney and McCollum 1993a). While only one major serotype has been identified to date, there is ample evidence of differences in antigenicity and pathogenicity among temporally and geographically disparate isolates of the virus (Timoney and McCollum 1993a; Balasuriya *et al.* 1997; McCollum and Timoney 1999). Whereas some strains can cause frank disease, others only appear capable of inducing a mild febrile response (McCollum and Timoney 1999).

Equine arteritis virus is not very resistant outside the body; it is readily inactivated under conditions of heat, sunlight, low relative humidity or exposure to a range of commonly used disinfectants (Timoney and McCollum 1993a). However, infectivity of the virus can be maintained for very extended periods of time at or below freezing temperature (P.J. Timoney and W.H. McCollum, unpublished data). Equine arteritis virus can remain viable in cryopreserved semen for many years.

Clinical features

The clinical outcome of primary infection with EAV can vary with the virus strain, viral dose, route of exposure, age and physical condition of the horse or horses at risk and various other environmental factors (Timoney and McCollum 1993a, 2004). It should be emphasised that many cases of natural EAV infection are asymptomatic (Timoney and McCollum 1986). Since such individuals do not display the assemblage of clinical signs characteristic of EVA, strictly speaking they should not be considered cases of the disease (Doll *et al.* 1957a).

While EVA can affect horses of any age, clinical severity of the infection tends to be greater in very young or old animals or those in debilitated condition

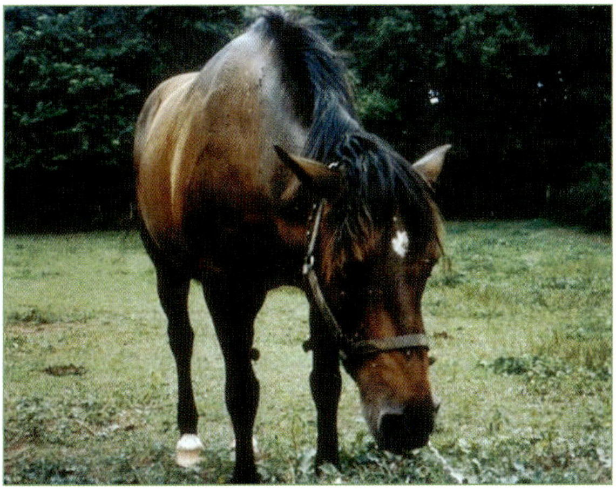

FIGURE 1: Depression in an experimental case of EVA. Reproduced with permission from IVIS.

(Timoney and McCollum 1993a). With 2 exceptions, death is a very uncommon sequel to infection in outbreaks of the disease (O'Connor 1993). Aside from abortion in the pregnant mare (Doll *et al.* 1957a,b; Golnik 1992; McCollum *et al.* 1999), fatal infection has been observed primarily in neonatal foals congenitally infected with the virus (Vaala *et al.* 1992) and in foals aged a few weeks to months that succumb from a fulminating, interstitial viral pneumonia or pneumoenteritis (Golnik *et al.* 1981; Del Piero *et al.* 1997; McCollum *et al.* 1999). Very rarely is EAV infection associated with mortality in otherwise healthy adult horses (O'Connor 1993). It should be noted that even without symptomatic treatment, the vast majority of naturally affected horses make complete and uneventful recoveries (Timoney and McCollum 1991, 1993a). Horses in training may experience a period of impaired performance during the acute and early convalescent phases of the infection (McCollum and Swerczek 1978; Timoney 2005).

The onset of clinical signs of EVA is preceded by an incubation period of 3–14 days, which varies with the route of exposure to the virus (Timoney and McCollum 1993a; Glaser *et al.* 1996). It is usually 6–8 days in horses infected by the venereal route (Timoney 1984). Typical cases of the disease can present with all or any combination of the following clinical signs: fever of up to 41°C of 2–10 days' duration, inappetance, depression (**Fig 1**), leucopenia (which becomes evident within 1–3 days of the onset of fever and can persist for 4–10 days), dependant oedema, especially of the lower limbs (**Fig 2**), scrotum, prepuce in the stallion (**Fig 3**) or the mammary glands in the mare (**Fig 4**), supra or periorbital oedema (**Fig 5**), nasal and/or lacrimal discharge (**Fig 6**), conjunctivitis, photophobia, an urticarial-type skin rash which is frequently localised to the sides of the head, neck or pectoral region (**Fig 7**) or may be generalised as a maculo-papular rash over the surface of the body. A range of other clinical signs have been infrequently observed in some outbreaks of EVA. These include: coughing, respiratory distress, submandibular lymphadenopathy, posterior paresis and ataxia, adventitious swelling in the intermandibular space, beneath the sternum, the shoulder region or other parts of the body, gingival and buccal erosions, icterus and diarrhoea (Doll *et al.*

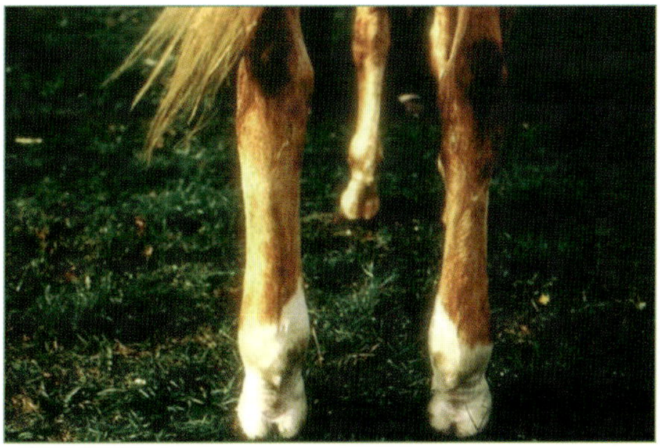

FIGURE 2: Severe lower limb oedema in an experimental case of EVA. Reproduced with permission from IVIS.

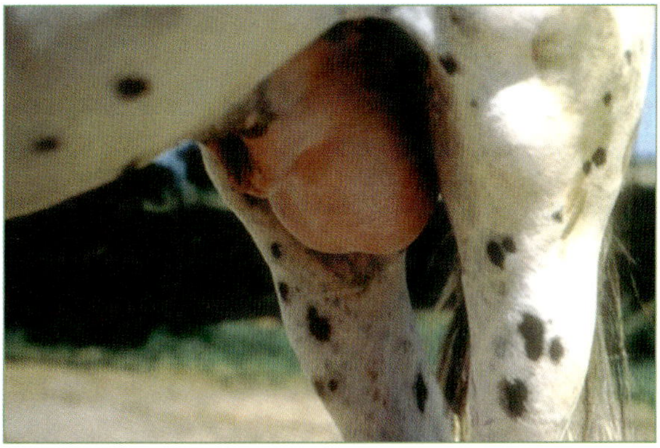

FIGURE 3: Scrotal and preputial oedema in an experimental case of EVA. Reproduced with permission from IVIS.

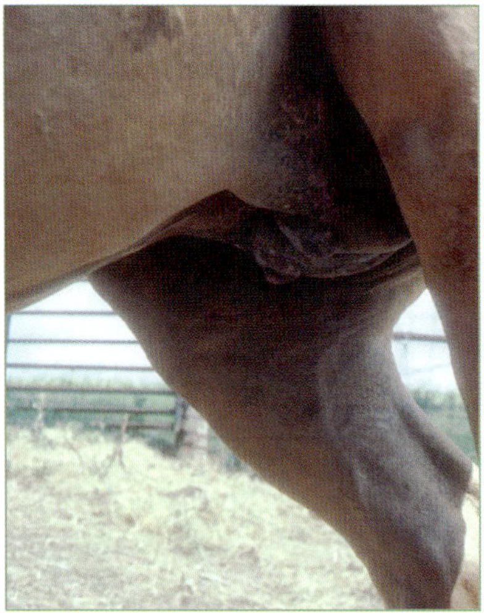

FIGURE 4: Oedema of the mammary glands in an experimental case of EVA. Reproduced with permission from IVIS.

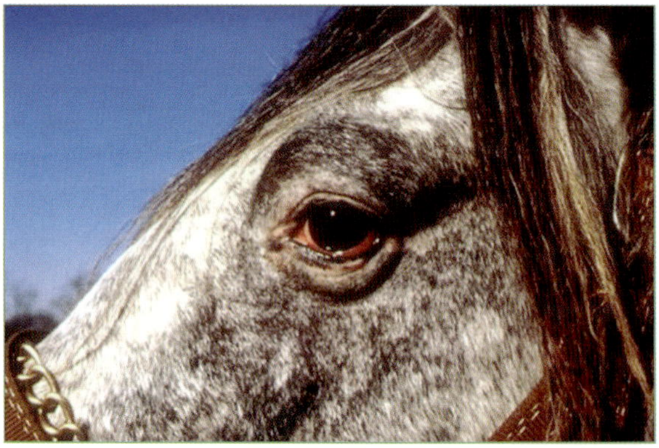

FIGURE 5: Periorbital oedema and conjunctivitis or 'pink-eye' in an experimental case of EVA. Reproduced with permission from IVIS.

1957a; Timoney 1984; Monreal *et al.* 1995). Compared to equine influenza and equine herpesvirus 1 and 4 infections, secondary bacterial infection of the respiratory tract is not a common feature in horses affected with EVA. Indeed, some outbreaks of the disease have been characterised by an absence of any clinical involvement of the respiratory system (Scollay and Foreman 1993). The duration of clinical illness can range from several days up to 2 weeks (Timoney and McCollum 1993a; Glaser *et al.* 1996). In many horses exposed to EAV for the first time, fever and leucopenia are often the only detectable signs of infection.

Of the various economic consequences of EAV infection, undoubtedly the one of greatest industry concern is abortion (Timoney and McCollum 1991). It is believed that many strains of the virus are abortigenic (Doll *et al.* 1957a; Golnik 1992; Timoney and McCollum 1993a; Balasuriya *et al.* 1998; McCollum *et al.* 1999). Abortion can be a sequel to clinical or asymptomatic infection, supervening late in the acute phase or early in the convalescent phase of the infection (Doll *et al.* 1957a,b; Golnik *et al.* 1981; McCollum and Timoney 1984). Under natural or experimental conditions, EAV-related abortion can occur in mares of 2 to >10 months' gestation (Timoney

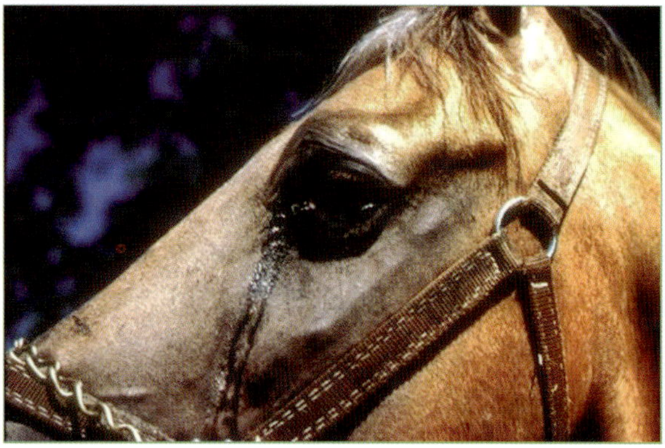

FIGURE 6: Epiphora in an experimental case of EVA. Reproduced with permission from IVIS.

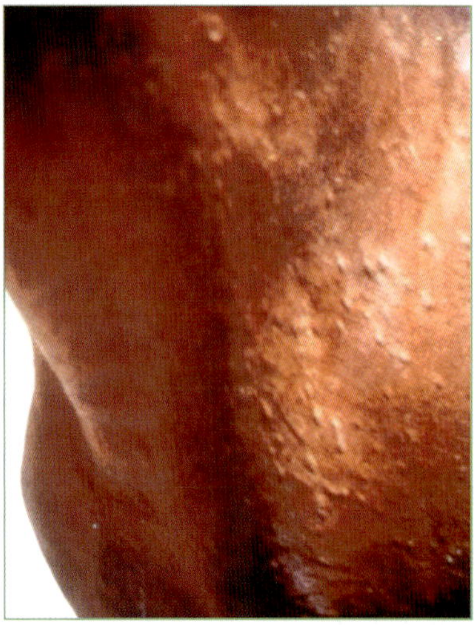

FIGURE 7: Urticarial rash over the neck and shoulder of an experimental case of EVA. Reproduced with permission from IVIS.

and McCollum 1993a, 2004). Abortion rates in unprotected mares can range from <10 to >70%. Where mares are exposed to EAV very late in pregnancy, they may not abort but carry to term and give birth to a congenitally infected foal (Vaala *et al.* 1992). When dealing with a case of EVA-related abortion or a congenitally infected foal, it should be emphasised that the placenta, placental fluids, aborted fetus or affected newborn foal are highly productive sources of virus and represent a significant risk to any unprotected mare or foal which may come into direct or indirect contact with them (Timoney and McCollum 2004).

A point of continued confusion among owners, breeders and even some veterinarians is whether an unprotected mare bred with EAV-infective semen can conceive while harbouring the virus in her reproductive tract and abort weeks and even months later from the infection (Timoney 2008a). There is no field or experimental evidence that this occurs. Abortion supervenes in mares that are already pregnant at time of exposure to the virus. This is believed to take place via the respiratory route through direct contact with an acutely infected horse, frequently but not invariably a mare recently bred with infective semen (Timoney and McCollum 2004; Timoney 2008a). Mares that abort from EAV infection do not appear to experience any impairment in fertility in subsequent breeding seasons.

Not always appreciated is the fact that the EVA-affected stallion that develops a significant febrile response and severe oedema of the scrotum and prepuce, may experience a period of temporary subfertility unless treated promptly to mitigate the fever and oedema (Neu *et al.* 1992; Timoney and McCollum 1993a). This subfertility is believed to result from prolonged elevation of the intrascrotal temperature and is not considered due to the direct effect of the virus. Stallion libido is usually diminished during the acute, clinical phase of the infection. There is a reduction in semen quality characterised by a decrease in sperm motility, sperm concentration, and percentage of morphologically normal sperm. These changes commence about a week after infection, reach their nadir about week 7, before returning to preinfection levels by week 16 in experimentally infected stallions (Neu *et al.* 1992). No long-term adverse effects on fertility have been noted in recovered stallions.

Epidemiology

The epidemiology of EVA involves a range of virus-, host- and environment-related factors (Timoney and McCollum 1993a; Glaser *et al.* 1997). Compared to the widespread global distribution of EAV, outbreaks of EVA are relatively infrequent and are most often associated with the movement of animals or the use of shipped semen (Timoney and McCollum 1993b). Furthermore, since many cases of primary infection are asymptomatic, transmission of the EAV can take place either on breeding farms, at racetracks, shows, performance events etc. without any clinical suggestion of presence of the virus much less of its possible widespread circulation. Among the factors known to be of importance in the epidemiology of this infection are: phenotypic variation among strains of EAV, modes of transmission during acute and chronic phases of the infection, occurrence of the carrier state in the stallion, nature and duration of acquired immunity to infection, and changing trends in the horse industry (Timoney and McCollum 2004).

Phenotypic variation

It has been known for many years that naturally occurring strains of EAV differ inherently from one another with respect to their ability to cause clinical disease (Timoney and McCollum 1993a). Limited experimental studies would indicate the existence of strains of varying pathogenicity, comprising those that are lentogenic, mesogenic and velogenic (McCollum and Timoney 1999). Of special importance in any consideration of virulence is whether all strains of EAV are indeed abortigenic and capable of establishing persistent infection in the stallion. As yet, this remains to be determined.

Modes of transmission

Transmission of EAV can occur by the respiratory, venereal, congenital or indirect routes (McCollum *et al.* 1971; Timoney 1984; Timoney *et al.* 1987a; Vaala *et al.* 1992; Timoney and McCollum 1993a; Glaser *et al.* 1997). Even though shed in various secretions and excretions by the acutely infected horse, EAV is present in very high concentration in respiratory tract secretions up to 1–3 weeks after the onset of infection (McCollum *et al.* 1971). It is not surprising, therefore, that respiratory transmission is of major importance in dissemination of EAV on breeding farms, at racetracks, sales and in veterinary hospitals or wherever horses are congregated together (Timoney and McCollum 1993a, 2004). EAV does not appear as readily contagious as equine influenza and equine herpesvirus 1 and 4 infections, however, unless under conditions of close physical contact as was amply demonstrated on many breeding premises during the 2006/07 multistate occurrence of EVA in the USA (Timoney *et al.* 2007a).

Aside from respiratory transmission, EAV can also be effectively spread by the venereal route by the acutely infected stallion or mare (Timoney 1984; McCollum and Timoney 1984).

The virus is no longer detectable in most body fluids and tissues beyond 28 days after infection, its disappearance coinciding with the development of a strong protective immune response in the infected individual (Timoney and McCollum 2004). The only exception being the sexually mature intact male, colt or stallion, that has become a carrier of EAV and that sheds the virus solely by the venereal route (Timoney *et al.* 1987a; Timoney and McCollum 1993a).

As previously mentioned, EAV can also be transmitted by the congenital route (Vaala *et al.* 1992). Unprotected mares in the final stage of pregnancy that are exposed to infection may not abort but give birth to a full-term foal that is congenitally infected with the virus, with little if any hope of survival (Timoney and McCollum 1993a).

Although seldom credited with the significance it deserves, EAV can also be spread on breeding farms, at racetracks etc. by indirect means through the use of shared tack or breeding shed equipment contaminated with the virus (Collins *et al.* 1987; Timoney and McCollum 1993a). Not to be overlooked in this regard is the risk of transmission of infection by individuals failing to observe appropriate sanitary measures after handling infected horses or virus-infective fluids such as semen (Timoney 2008a). The virus can be present on the hands of such individuals or on their clothing or on feed or water buckets, all potential sources of contamination.

Carrier state

Based on extensive field and experimental studies conducted since 1984, chronic infection with EAV or the carrier state has been found to occur only in sexually mature intact males, i.e. colts and stallions, but not in mares, geldings or sexually immature colts (Timoney and McCollum 1986, 1988; Timoney *et al.* 1987a; Holyoak *et al.* 1993; McCollum *et al.* 1994). Experimental studies have shown that predilection of the virus for the stallion is based on the testosterone-dependent nature of the carrier state (Little *et al.* 1992).

The carrier stallion is widely accepted as the natural reservoir of EAV and of major epidemiological importance in the dissemination and perpetuation of the virus (Timoney and McCollum 1988, 1993a, 2004). Frequency of the carrier state can vary from <10 to >70% (Timoney and McCollum 2000). Duration of viral persistence in the stallion can range from several weeks, to months, to many years, sometimes for the rest of a stallion's life (Timoney and McCollum 1993a, 2000, 2004). A variable percentage of stallions, even those that may have been persistently infected for years, can spontaneously clear themselves of the carrier state, with no evidence of reversion to a viral shedding state later (Timoney and McCollum 1993a, 2000). EAV in the carrier stallion is restricted to the reproductive tract where it localises primarily in certain of the accessory sex glands, especially the ampulla of the *vas deferens* (Neu *et al.* 1988; Little *et al.* 1992). Such stallions shed the virus constantly in the sperm-rich fraction of the ejaculate and are, therefore, a potential source of infection at the time of breeding or release of seminal fluid (Timoney *et al.* 1987a). It should be emphasised that they transmit the virus solely venereally and not by the respiratory or any other route. Transmission of EAV occurs readily by natural breeding or artificial insemination with fresh-cooled or cryopreserved semen (Timoney and McCollum 1993a, 2004; Timoney 2008a). Carrier stallions are invariably seropositive for antibodies to EAV, are clinically normal and appear to experience no impairment in their fertility (Timoney and McCollum 2000).

The role of the carrier stallion in the epidemiology of EVA is of considerable importance for 2 reasons. Firstly, it serves as the natural reservoir of EAV (Timoney and McCollum 2004) and secondly, it appears to provide the principal source of genotypic and phenotypic diversity among naturally occurring strains of the virus (Hedges *et al.* 1999).

Immunity

Compared to most other equine pathogens, EAV possesses the ability to stimulate a strongly protective, long-lasting immunity against EVA (Doll *et al.* 1968; McCollum 1970, 1986). Vaccination can also provide a level of immunity that protects against development of clinical disease and establishment of the carrier state in the stallion (Fukuaga *et al.* 1990, 1992, 1996; Whalen *et al.* 1999; Timoney and McCollum 2004; Timoney *et al.* 2007b). First-time vaccinates, however, may still undergo a limited reinfection cycle upon natural exposure to the virus (McCollum *et al.* 1988). Foals born of seropositive dams are passively protected against EVA for the first 3–5 months of life (McCollum 1976). Residual maternally acquired antibody titres can interfere with the response to vaccination in foals (P.J. Timoney and W.H. McCollum, unpublished data).

Industry trends

The global distribution of EAV has been impacted significantly over the past 30–50 years by 2 developments: firstly, the considerable growth that has occurred in the volume of international horse movements; and secondly, the ever expanding global trade in cryopreserved semen (Timoney 2007). There have been repeated instances where EAV has been introduced into countries through the importation of carrier stallions or virus-infective semen, on occasion, with very damaging economic consequences (Balasuriya *et al.* 1998; Timoney *et al.* 1998; McCollum *et al.* 1999; Timoney 2000b).

Diagnosis

Irrespective of how highly suggestive the clinical features of an outbreak of disease may be of EVA, they cannot serve *per se* as the basis for establishing a diagnosis (Timoney and McCollum 1993a). The simple reason for emphasising the importance of laboratory confirmation of a provisional diagnosis of the disease is that there are a range of other common, some less common and even several exotic infectious and noninfectious diseases of the horse that closely mimic the symptomatology of EVA. These include equine influenza, equine herpesvirus 1 and 4 infections, equine rhinitis A and B infections, purpura haemorrhagica, equine infectious anaemia, urticaria, and toxicosis caused by hoary alyssum (*Berteroa incana*). Of the exotic diseases that resemble EVA, Getah virus infection, dourine, surra and African horsesickness fever should not be overlooked in the context of a differential diagnosis of the disease (Timoney 2008b).

Laboratory confirmation of a provisional diagnosis of EVA should be pursued as early as possible in the clinical course of an outbreak. Verification of a diagnosis of the disease is based on EAV detection by virus isolation or polymerase chain reaction (PCR) assay, visualisation of viral antigen in the tissues of suspect cases of EVA-related abortion or death in young foals and finally, by demonstration of an antibody response by testing paired (acute and convalescent) sera collected 2–4 weeks apart (Timoney 2008b).

Appropriate specimens to collect from suspect cases of EAV infection include nasopharyngeal/nasal swabs or washings and unclotted (citrated or EDTA but not heparinised samples) as well as clotted blood samples. To optimise the chances of virus detection and confirmation, specimens should be obtained as early as possible after the onset of fever or other clinical signs. Upon collection, swabs should be transferred directly into viral transport medium and kept refrigerated or frozen at -20°C or lower in transit to a laboratory with proven competency and experience in testing for EAV infection. Unclotted blood samples should be transported refrigerated but not frozen.

When dealing with a suspect case(s) of EVA-related abortion, virus detection (by virus isolation or PCR) should be attempted from placental and fetal tissues and fluids, especially lung, thymus, spleen and liver (Timoney 2008b). Specimens should also be taken for histological and immunohistochemical examination for presence of the vascular lesions characteristically identified with EVA. A similar diagnostic approach should be taken when investigating a suspect case of EAV-related mortality in a foal or older horse.

Confirmation of the carrier state in a stallion that does not have a certified history of vaccination against EVA requires first of all, that the EAV serological status of the individual be determined. To date, the carrier state has only been found in virus neutralising antibody positive (titre ≥1:4) stallions (Timoney and McCollum 2000). In fact, the majority of carrier animals are strongly seropositive for antibodies to the virus. Confirmation of the carrier status of such stallions is based on detection of EAV in a collection of semen containing the sperm-rich fraction of the ejaculate either by virus isolation or PCR assay (Timoney *et al.* 1987a,b; Timoney 2008b). An alternative highly reliable, although more costly and time-consuming method, is to test breed a putative carrier stallion to 2 seronegative mares and to check these for seroconversion to EAV after 28 days (Timoney *et al.* 1987b).

Treatment

As yet, no specific antiviral treatment has been identified that is safe and effective for horses with EVA (Timoney and McCollum 1993a). Since the vast majority of cases of the disease make complete clinical recoveries, there is little indication for routine symptomatic treatment except to mitigate the severity of clinical signs in severely affected horses. This is especially important in the case of stallions that experience a high fever and extensive scrotal and preputial oedema. In order to minimise the risk of sperm damage and a period of subfertility, such individuals should be completely rested and given nonsteroidal anti-inflammatory drugs and a diuretic. Prophylactic antimicrobial treatment may also be indicated in severe cases of the disease. A gradual return to full activity is recommended for stallions as well as horses in training that have been affected with EVA, if adverse effects on performance are to be minimised or avoided.

Currently, there is no effective treatment for viral pneumonia or pneumoenteritis caused by EAV in newborn foals or those up to a few months (Timoney 2008a). Such cases invariably have a fatal outcome.

Nonsurgical treatments for promoting clearance of the carrier state in the stallion have met with mixed success. Current therapeutic approaches are based on inducing temporary downregulation of circulating testosterone levels either through the use of a GnRH antagonist (Fortier *et al.* 2002) or by GnRH immunisation of the stallion (Burger *et al.* 2006). While success has been claimed for each of these treatments, neither has yet been proven to be uniformly effective in eliminating the carrier state. It remains to be seen whether a period of down-regulation of GnRH production has any subsequent adverse effect on the fertility of treated stallions.

Recent studies have shown that it is possible to reduce but not completely eliminate EAV content in virus-infective semen through the use of density gradient centrifugation and a 'swim-up' protocol for treating such semen (Morrell and Geraghty 2006). A fully effective method for decontaminating semen without adversely affecting semen quality is not yet available.

Prevention and control

Equine viral arteritis can truly be considered a preventable and controllable disease in the context of what is known about the properties of the causal virus and the epidemiology of the infection (Timoney and McCollum 1993a; Glaser *et al.* 1997). Experience gained from past occurrences of EVA has served to emphasise the importance of sound management practices in conjunction with a targeted programme of vaccination, in achieving effective control of this disease (Timoney and McCollum 1993a, 2004). The success of such programmes is predicated in large measure on minimising or eliminating direct or indirect contact of susceptible horses with the secretions/ excretions of infected individuals.

Current EVA control programmes are aimed at preventing the dissemination of EAV in breeding horse populations and the concomitant risk of outbreaks of virus-related abortion, illness and death in young foals, or establishment of the carrier state in post pubertal colts and stallions (Timoney and McCollum 2004). While there have been a number of extensive occurrences of the disease at racetracks, sales, shows and other performance events, these are so sporadic and unpredictable, that no control programmes have yet been developed specifically to prevent the introduction and spread of EAV in such situations (Timoney 2005).

Of considerable benefit in advancing the control of EVA has been the availability of safe and effective vaccines against the disease. Two such vaccines have been developed: one, a modified live virus vaccine (Arvac)[1] and the other, an inactivated adjuvanted product (Artervac)[1] (McCollum 1969, 1970; Timoney and McCollum 1993a, 2004; Timoney 2008b).

Extensive field use of the modified live virus vaccine in North America since 1985 has confirmed its safety and immunogenicity in stallions and nonpregnant mares (McKinnon *et al.* 1986; Timoney *et al.* 1988; Timoney and McCollum 1993a). While it is contraindicated for use in pregnant mares and in foals aged <6 weeks, nonetheless, in the aftermath of the 2006/07 multistate occurrence of EVA in the USA, thousands of doses of the vaccine were used to immunise pregnant mares up to the final 2 months of gestation, without any reported adverse effects (Timoney *et al.* 2007b; P.J. Timoney, unpublished data). There is no evidence that the vaccine virus can establish the carrier state in the stallion (Timoney and McCollum 1993a, 2004). Vaccination confers a high degree of protective immunity that appears to last for one or more years (McCollum 1970, 1986). Following natural exposure to EAV, first time vaccinated horses may undergo a limited reinfection cycle with the possibility of short-term respiratory shedding of very small amounts of field virus (McCollum *et al.* 1988). Revaccination with this vaccine gives rise to a considerable anamnestic antibody response that would appear to persist for several years (Timoney and McCollum 1993a; Timoney *et al.* 2007b).

The inactivated, tissue-culture derived vaccine (Artervac)[1] is currently approved for use in several European countries (Timoney and McCollum 2004). The vaccine is safe for use in all categories of horses including pregnant mares. It is not as strongly immunogenic as the modified live virus vaccine, however, and 2 or more inoculations may be required to stimulate a detectable serum neutralising antibody response (Timoney 2008b). The duration of immunity produced by this vaccine is at least 6 weeks.

Equine viral arteritis can be successfully controlled on breeding farms through observance of sound management practices similar to those recommended for the prevention of equine herpesvirus and other respiratory infections, and by a targeted vaccination programme against the disease (Timoney and McCollum 1993a). Of critical importance in ensuring the effectiveness of such programmes is avoidance of direct or indirect contact between unprotected horses and infected individuals (Timoney and McCollum 2004). To minimise the risk of this happening, all horses arriving from other premises (farms, sales, training yards, veterinary clinics and shows) should be isolated from resident horses for 4 weeks. Neither teaser stallions nor nurse mares should be overlooked as a potential source of infection. Special consideration should be given to the management of pregnant mares which should be segregated and maintained in small groups until they foal. In the case of premises where it is not possible to isolate incoming horses from the resident population, it may be advisable to implement a policy of vaccination of all at-risk horses if the threat of an outbreak of EVA is to be avoided (Timoney 2008a).

Integral to the successful control of EAV infection in breeding populations is the need to identify any carrier stallions and to manage these appropriately (Timoney and McCollum 1993a, 2004). They should be physically isolated and special precautions taken when breeding or collecting them to prevent the inadvertent spread of the virus to other horses on the premises. Mares bred to such stallions by live cover or by AI should be seropositive to EAV either from previous natural infection or vaccination against EVA. The risk of introducing the disease onto a farm through the use of fresh-cooled (extended) or frozen semen can be significant (Balasuriya *et al.* 1998; Timoney 2000b). Under the circumstances, it is advisable to check the EAV status of semen to be used for AI, especially if imported. Mares inseminated with infective semen should be managed similarly to mares bred by live cover to a carrier stallion.

In view of the major importance of the carrier stallion in the epidemiology of EVA, a concerted effort should be made by the equine industry to curtail the natural reservoir of the virus. This requires a 2-fold approach if such a strategy is to maximally effective. Firstly, all noncarrier breeding stallions should be vaccinated annually against EVA between breeding seasons (Timoney and McCollum 1993a). Secondly, colt foals aged 6–12 months should be vaccinated, to minimise the risk of them becoming carriers at a later date. Over time, both of these measures would significantly reduce the reservoir of the virus, especially in breeds in which the infection is endemic.

When confronted with a suspect outbreak of EVA, regardless of circumstances surrounding its occurrence, the appropriate animal health regulatory authorities should be informed without delay. Affected and in-contact horses must be isolated and restrictions immediately placed on the movement of horses onto and off the affected premises (Timoney 2008a). It is essential to obtain laboratory confirmation of a provisional diagnosis of EVA as soon as possible. Where an outbreak has occurred on a breeding farm, all breeding activity whether involving live cover or AI should be suspended until further notice. Stalls and any tack or other equipment that may have come in contact with an infected horse should be thoroughly cleaned and sanitised with an appropriate disinfectant. Where there are a significant number of at-risk unprotected horses involved, consideration should be given to the immediate implementation of a vaccination program against EVA to curtail the further spread of the virus and hopefully, reduce the overall morbidity rate. This strategy has been adopted in a number of widespread occurrences of the disease in North America with no adverse consequences and reputedly, some success (Scollay and Foreman 1993). Restrictions on movement on and off an affected premises should remain in force until 3–4 weeks after the last clinical case or otherwise confirmed case of EAV infection.

Countries and equine industries differ greatly in how they perceive the significance of EVA. Some have adopted a 'zero tolerance' attitude towards the disease, frequently it would appear, in the absence of any knowledge of the status of their respective equine populations for this infection (Newton 2007). In contrast, others maintain a 'low key' stance over EVA, regarding it of relatively low veterinary medical or economic importance. Irrespective of how the disease is perceived by various countries, experience gained over the past 25 years has proven that EVA is a very preventable and controllable disease (Timoney and McCollum 1993a, 2004).

Manufacturer's address

[1]Fort Dodge Animal Health, Fort Dodge, Iowa, USA.

References

Anon (2000) *Equine Viral Arteritis (EVA) and the U.S. Horse Industry*. USDA:APHIS:VS, CEAH, National Animal Health Monitoring System (NAHMS), Fort Collins. #N315.0400.

Balasuriya, U.B.R., Evermann, J.F., Hedges, J.F., McKeirnan, A.J., Mitten, J.Q., Beyer, J.C., McCollum, W.H., Timoney, P.J. and MacLachlan, N.J. (1998) Serologic and molecular characterization of an abortigenic strain of equine arteritis virus isolated from infective frozen semen and an aborted equine fetus. *J. Am. vet. med. Ass.* **213**, 1586-1589.

Balasuriya, U.B.R., Patton, J.F., Rossitto, P.V., Timoney, P.J., McCollum, W.H. and MacLachlan, N.J. (1997) Neutralization determinants of laboratory strains and field isolates of equine arteritis virus: Identification of four neutralization sites in the amino-terminal ectodomain of the G_L envelope glycoprotein. *Virol.* **232**, 114-128.

Burger, D., Janett, F., Vidament, M., Stump, R., Fortier, G., Imboden, I. and Thun, R. (2006) Immunization against GnRH in adult stallions: Effects on semen characteristics, behavior and shedding of equine arteritis virus. *Animal reprod. Sci.* **94**, 107-111.

Cavanagh, D. (1997) *Nidovirales:* a new order comprising *Coronaviridae* and *Arteriviridae*. *Arch. Virol.* **142**, 629-633.

Clark, I. (1892) Transmission of pink-eye from apparently healthy stallions to mares. *J. comp. Pathol. Therapeut.* **5**, 261-264.

Collins, J.K, Kari, S., Ralston, S.L., Bennett, D.G., Traub-Dargatz, J.L., and McKinnon, A.O. (1987) Equine viral arteritis at a veterinary teaching hospital. *Prev. vet. Med.* **4**, 389-397.

Del Piero, F., Wilkins, P.A., Lopez, J.W., Glaser, A.L., Dubovi, E.J., Schlafer, D.H. and Lein, D.H. (1997) Equine viral arteritis in newborn foals: clinical, pathological, serological, microbiological and immunohistochemical observations. *Equine vet. J.* **29**, 178-185.

Doll, E.R., Bryans, J.T., McCollum, W.H. and Crowe, M.E.W. (1957a) Isolation of a filterable agent causing arteritis of horses and abortion by mares. Its differentiation from the equine abortion (influenza) virus. *Cornell Vet.* **47**, 3-40.

Doll, E.R., Knappenberger, R.E. and Bryans, J.T. (1957b) An outbreak of abortion caused by the equine arteritis virus. *Cornell Vet.* **47**, 69-75.

Doll, E.R., Bryans, J.T., Wilson, J.C. and McCollum, W.H. (1968) Immunization against equine viral arteritis using modified live virus propagated in cell cultures of rabbit kidney. *Cornell Vet.* **58**, 497-524.

Fortier, G., Vidament, M., deCraene, F., Ferry, B. and Daels, P.F. (2002) The effect of GnRH antagonist on testosterone secretion, spermatogenesis and viral excretion in EVA-virus excreting stallions. *Theriogenol.* **58**, 425-427.

Fukunaga, Y. and McCollum, W.H. (1977) Complement-fixation reactions in equine viral arteritis. *Am. J. vet. Res.* **38**, 2043-2046.

Fukunaga, Y., Wada, R., Matsumura, T., Sugiura, T. and Imagawa, H. (1990) Induction of immune response and protection from equine viral arteritis (EVA) by formalin inactivated-virus vaccine for EVA in horses. *J. vet. Med. B* **37**, 135-141.

Fukunaga, Y., Wada, R., Kanemaru, T., Imagawa, H., Kamada, M. and Samejima, T. (1996) Immune potency of lyophilized, killed vaccine for equine viral arteritis and its protection against abortion in pregnant mares. *J. equine vet. Sci.* **16**, 217-221.

Fukunaga, Y., Wada, R., Matsumura, T., Anzai, T., Imagawa, H., Sugiura, T., Kumanomido, T., Kanemaru, T. and Kamada, M. (1992) An attempt to protect against persistent infection of equine viral arteritis in the reproductive tract of stallions using formalin inactivated-virus vaccine. In: *Equine Infectious Diseases VI: Proceedings of the 6th International Conference*, Eds: W. Plowright, P.D. Rossdale and J.F. Wade, R&W Publications, Newmarket. pp 239-244.

Glaser, A.L., Chirnside, E.D., Horzinek, M.C. and de Vries, A.A.F. (1997) Equine arteritis virus. *Theriogenol.* **47**, 1275-1295.

Glaser, A.L., de Vries, A.A., Rottier, P.J., Horzinek, M.C. and Colenbrander, B. (1996) Equine arteritis virus: a review of clinical features and management aspects. *Vet. Quart.* **18**, 95-99.

Golnik, W. (1992) Viruses isolated from aborted foetuses and stillborn foals. In: *Equine Infectious Diseases VI: Proceedings of the 6th International Conference*, Eds: W. Plowright, P.D. Rossdale and J.F. Wade, R&W Publications, Newmarket. p 314.

Golnik, W., Michalska, Z. and Michalak, T. (1981) Natural equine viral arteritis in foals. *Schweizer Archiv Fur Tierheilkunde* **123**, 523-533.

Hedges, J.F., Balasuriya, U.B.R., Timoney, P.J., McCollum, W.H. and MacLachlan, N.J. (1999) Genetic divergence with emergence of novel phenotypic variants of equine arteritis virus during persistent infection of stallions. *J. Virol.* **73**, 3672-3681.

Holyoak, G.R., Little, T.V., McCollum, W.H. and Timoney, P.J. (1993) Relationship between onset of puberty and establishment of persistent infection with equine arteritis virus in the experimentally infected colt. *J. comp. Pathol.* **109**, 29-46.

Hullinger, P.J., Gardner, I.A., Hietala, S.K., Ferraro, G.L. and MacLachlan, N.J. (2001) Seroprevalence of antibodies against equine arteritis virus in horses residing in the United States and imported horses. *J. Am. vet. med. Ass.* **219**, 946-949.

Jones, T.C. (1969) Clinical and pathologic features of equine viral arteritis. *J. Am. vet. med. Ass.* **155**, 315-317.

Jones, T.C., Doll, E.R. and Bryans, J.T. (1957) The lesions of equine viral arteritis. *Cornell Vet.* **47**, 52-68.

Konishi, S., Akashi, H., Sentsui, H. and Ogata, M. (1975) Studies on equine viral arteritis. I. Characterization of the virus and trial survey on antibody with vero cell cultures. *Jap. J. Vet. Sci.* **37**, 259-267.

Little, T.V., Holyoak, G.R., McCollum, W.H. and Timoney, P.J. (1992) Output of equine arteritis virus from persistently infected stallions is testosterone-dependent. In: *Equine Infectious Diseases VI: Proceedings of the 6th International Conference*, Eds: W. Plowright, P.D. Rossdale and J.F. Wade, R&W Publications, Newmarket. pp 225-229.

Matumoto, M., Shimizu, T.T. and Ishizaki, R. (1965) Constation d'anticorps contre le virus de l'arterite equine dans le serum de juments indiennes. *Proceedings of the Societe Franco-Japonaise de Biologie*, Societe Franco-Japanaise de Biologie, France. pp 1262-1264.

McCollum, W.H. (1969) Development of a modified virus strain and vaccine for equine viral arteritis. *J. Am. vet. med. Ass.* **155**, 318-322.

McCollum, W.H. (1970) Vaccination for equine viral arteritis. In: *Equine Infectious Diseases II, Proceedings of the 2nd International Conference*, Karger, Basel. pp 143-151.

McCollum, W.H. (1976) Studies of passive immunity in foals to equine viral arteritis. *Vet. Microbiol.* **1**, 45-54.

McCollum, W.H. (1986) Responses of horses vaccinated with avirulent modified-live equine arteritis virus propagated in the E. Derm (NBL-6) cell line to nasal inoculation with virulent virus. *Am. J. vet. Res.* **47**, 1931-1934.

McCollum, W.H. and Bryans, J.T. (1973) Serological identification of infection by equine arteritis virus in horses of several countries. In: *Equine Infectious Diseases III, Proceedings of the Third International Conference on Equine Infectious Diseases*. S. Karger, Basel. pp 256-263.

McCollum, W.H. and Swerczek, T.W. (1978) Studies of an epizootic of equine viral arteritis in racehorses. *J. equine Med. Surg.* **2**, 293-299.

McCollum, W.H. and Timoney, P.J. (1984) The pathogenic qualities of the 1984 strain of equine arteritis virus. In: *Proceedings of the Grayson Foundation International Conference of Thoroughbred Breeders Organizations*. pp 34-47.

McCollum, W.H. and Timoney, P.J. (1999) Experimental observation on the virulence of isolates of equine arteritis virus. In: *Proceedings of the 8th International Conference on Equine Infectious Diseases*, Eds: U. Wernery, J.F. Wade, J.A. Mumford and O.-R. Kaaden, R&W Publications, Newmarket. pp 558-559.

McCollum, W.H., Prickett, M.E. and Bryans, J.T. (1971) Temporal distribution of equine arteritis virus in respiratory mucosa, tissues and body fluids of horses infected by inhalation. *Res. vet. Sci.* **2**, 459-464.

McCollum, W.H., Little, T.V., Timoney, P.J. and Swerczek, T.W. (1994) Resistance of castrated male horses to attempted establishment of the carrier state with equine arteritis virus. *J. comp. Pathol.* **111**, 383-388.

McCollum, W.H., Timoney, P.J., Roberts, A.W., Williard, J.E. and Carswell, G.D. (1988) Response of vaccinated and non-vaccinated mares to artificial insemination with semen from stallions persistently infected with equine arteritis virus. In: *Proceedings of the 5th International Conference on Equine Infectious Diseases*, Ed: D.G. Powell, The University Press of Kentucky, Lexington. pp 13-18.

McCollum, W.H., Timoney, P.J., Lee, J.W., Jr., Habacker, P.L., Balasuriya, U.B.R. and MacLachlan, N.J. (1999) Features of an outbreak of equine viral arteritis on a breeding farm associated with abortion and fatal interstitial pneumonia in neonatal foals. In: *Proceedings of the 8th International Conference on Equine Infectious Diseases*, Eds: U. Wernery, J.F. Wade, J.A. Mumford, and O.-R. Kaaden, R&W Publications, Newmarket. pp 559-560.

McKinnon, A.O., Colbern, G.T., Collins, J.K., Bowen, R.A., Voss, J.L. and Umphenour, N.W. (1986) Vaccination of stallions with a modified live equine viral arteritis virus. *J. equine vet. Sci.* **6**, 66-69.

Monreal, L., Villatoro, A.J., Hooghuis, H., Ros, I. and Timoney, P.J. (1995) Clinical features of the 1992 outbreak of equine viral arteritis in Spain. *Equine vet. J.* **27**, 301-304.

Moraillon, A. and Moraillon, R. (1978) Results of an epidemiological investigation on viral arteritis in France and some other European and Africa countries. *Annales de Recherches Veterinaires* **9**, 43-54.

Morrell, J.M. and Geraghty, R.M. (2006) Effective removal of equine arteritis virus from stallion semen. *Equine vet. J.* **38**, 224-229.

Neu, S.M., Timoney, P.J. and Lowry S.R. (1992) Changes in semen quality in the stallion following experimental infection with equine arteritis virus. *Theriogenol.* **37**, 407-431.

Neu, S.M., Timoney, P.J. and McCollum, W.H. (1988) Persistent infection of the reproductive tract in stallions experiementally infected with equine arteritis virus. In: *Equine Infectious Diseases V: Proceedings of the 5th International Conference*, Ed: D.G. Powell, The University Press of Kentucky, Lexington, pp 149-154.

Newton, J.R. (2007) Controlling EVA in the 21st century: 'zero tolerance' or 'live and let live'? *Equine vet. Educ.* **19**, 612-616.

O'Connor, B. (1993) Equine viral arteritis in a Thoroughbred filly. *Can. vet. J.* **34**, 506-507.

Plagemann, P.G.W. and Moennig, V. (1992) Lactate dehydrogenase-elevating virus, equine arteritis virus, and simian hemorrhagic fever virus: A new group of positive-strand RNA viruses. *Adv. Virus Res.* **4**, 99-192.

Pottie, A. (1888) The propagation of influenza from stallions to mares. *J. comp. Pathol. Therapeut.* **1**, 37-38

Reeks, H.C. (1902) The transmission of pink-eye from apparently healthy stallions to mares. *J. comp. Pathol. Therapeut.* **18**, 97-102.

Scollay, M.C. and Foreman, J.H. (1993) An overview of the 1993 equine viral arteritis outbreak at Arlington International Racecourse. *Proc. Am. Ass. equine Practnrs.* **39**, 255-256.

Snijder, E.J. and Meulenberg, J.J.M. (1998) The molecular biology of arteriviruses. *J. Gen. Virol.* **79**, 961-979.

Timoney, P.J. (1984) Clinical, virological and epidemiological features of the 1984 outbreak of equine viral arteritis in the Thoroughbred population in Kentucky, USA. In: *Proceedings of the Grayson Foundation International Conference of Thoroughbred Breeders Organizations on Equine Viral Arteritis*, Grayson Jockey Club Equine Research Foundation. pp 24-33.

Timoney, P.J. (2000a) Factors influencing the international spread of equine diseases. *Vet Clin. N. Am.: Equine Practice* **16**, 537-551.

Timoney, P.J. (2000b) Equine viral arteritis. AAEP Report March :7.

Timoney, P.J. (2005) Equine viral arteritis: how significant a threat to the horse? In: *Proceedings of the 15th International Conference of Racing Analysts and Veterinarians*, Eds: P.H. Albert, T. Morton and J.F. Wade, R & W Publications, Newmarket. pp 238-244.

Timoney, P.J. (2007) Infectious diseases and international movement of horses. In: *Infectious Diseases of Horses*, 1st edn., Eds: D. Sellon and M. Long, Saunders Elsevier, St. Louis. pp 549-556.

Timoney, P.J. (2008a) Equine viral arteritis. In: *Current Therapy in Equine Medicine*, 6th edn., Eds: N. Robinson and K. Sprayberry, Elsevier, St. Louis. pp 153-157.

Timoney, P.J. (2008b) Equine viral arteritis. In: *O.I.E. Manual of Standards for Diagnostic Tests and Vaccines for Terrestrial Animals*, 6th edn., Office International des Epizooties, Paris. pp 904-918.

Timoney, P.J. and McCollum, W.H. (1986) The epidemiology of equine viral arteritis. *Proc. Am. Ass. equine Practnrs.* **32,** 545-551.

Timoney, P.J. and McCollum, W.H. (1988) Equine viral arteritis - Epidemiology and control. *J. equine vet. Sci.* **8**, 54-59.

Timoney, P.J. and McCollum, W.H. (1991) Equine viral arteritis: Current clinical and economic significance. *Proc. Am. Ass. equine Practnrs.* **37**, 403-409.

Timoney, P.J. and McCollum, W.H. (1993a) Equine viral arteritis. *Vet. Clin. N. Am.: Equine Pract.* **9**, 295-309.

Timoney, P.J. and McCollum, W.H. (1993b) Equine viral arteritis in perspective in relation to international trade. *J. equine vet. Sci.* **13**, 50-52.

Timoney, P.J. and McCollum, W.H. (2000) Equine viral arteritis: further characterization of the carrier state in stallions. *J. Reprod. Fert., Suppl.* **56**, 3-11.

Timoney, P.J. and McCollum, W.H. (2004) Equine viral arteritis. In: *Infectious Diseases of Livestock with Special Reference to South Africa*, 2nd edn., Ed: K. Coetzer, Oxford University Press, Cape Town. pp 924-932.

Timoney, P.J., McCollum, W.H. and Vickers, M.L. (1998) The rationale for greater national control of EVA. *Equine Disease Quarterly*, October. pp 2-3.

Timoney, P.J., Umphenour, N.W. and McCollum, W.H. (1988) Safety evaluation of a commercial modified live equine arteritis virus vaccine for use in stallions. In: *Equine Infectious Diseases V: Proceedings of the 5th International Conference*, Ed: D.G. Powell, The University Press of Kentucky, Lexington. pp 19-27.

Timoney, P.J., Creekmore, L., Meade, B., Fly, D., Rogers, E. and King, B. (2007a) 2006 Multi-state occurrence of EVA. In: *Proceedings of the One Hundred and Tenth Annual Meeting of the United States Animal Health Association*. pp 354-362.

Timoney, P.J., Fallon, L., Shuck, K., McCollum, W., Zhang, J. and Williams, N. (2007b) The outcome of vaccinating five pregnant mares with a commercial equine viral arteritis vaccine. *Equine vet. Educ.* **19**, 606-611.

Timoney, P.J., McCollum, W.H., Murphy, T.W., Roberts, A.W., Willard, J.G. and Carswell, G.D. (1987a) The carrier state in equine arteritis virus infection in the stallion with specific emphasis on the venereal mode of virus transmission. *J. Reprod. Fert., Suppl.* **35**, 95-102.

Timoney, P.J., McCollum, W.H. and Roberts, A.W. (1987b) Detection of the carrier state in stallions persistently infected with equine arteritis virus. *Proc. Am. Ass. equine Practnrs.* **33,** 57-65.

Vaala, W.E., Hamir, A.N., Dubovi, E.J., Timoney, P.J. and Ruiz, B. (1992) Fatal, congenitally acquired infection with equine arteritis virus in a neonatal Thoroughbred. *Equine vet. J.* **24**, 155-158.

Van Mannen, C., Heldens, J., Cullinane, A.A., van den Hoven, R. and Westrate, M. (2005) The prevalence of antibodies against equine influenza virus, equine herpesvirus 1 and 4, equine arteritis virus and equine rhinovirus 1 and 2 in Dutch standardbred horses. *Vlaams Diergeneeskundig Tijdschrift* **74**, 140-145.

Weber, H., Beckmann, K. and Haas, L. (2006) Fallbericht: Equines Arteritisvirus (EAV) als Aborterreger bei Alpakas? *Deutsche Tierarztliche Wochenschrift* **113**, 162-163.

Whalen Jr., J.W., Hall, V.L., Srinivasappa, J., Ross, C., Eichmeyer, M. and Chu, S. (1999) An inactivated vaccine prevents persistent equine arteritis virus infection in stallions. In: *Proceedings of the Eighth International Conference on Equine Infectious Diseases*, Eds: U. Wernery, J.F. Wade, J.A. Mumford, and O.-R. Kaaden, R&W Publications, Newmarket. p 595.

EQUINE HERPESVIRUS-1: A REVIEW AND UPDATE

M. M. Brosnahan and N. Osterrieder*†

The Department of Microbiology and Immunology, Cornell University, College of Veterinary Medicine, Ithaca, New York 14853, USA; and †the Institut für Virologie, Freie Universität Berlin, 10115 Berlin, Germany.

Keywords: horse; EHV-1; herpesvirus; respiratory; neurological; abortion

Summary

Equine herpesvirus-1 (EHV-1) is ubiquitous in horse populations worldwide. The virus causes multiple clinical presentations, including respiratory disease, abortion, weak neonates and neurological disease. While currently available vaccinations may mitigate signs of respiratory and reproductive disease, they offer negligible protecction against the neurological form of the disease. In recent years, researchers have made strides in the development of improved diagnostic tests, but a vaccination producing long-term immunity against all forms of EHV-1 clinical disease remains elusive. Ongoing research continues to investigate the role of the host immune system in EHV-1 infection and disease, as well as the efficacy of novel metaphylaxis such as RNA interference. In the interim, clinicians are counselled to maintain ahigh index of suspicion in clinical cases where EHV-1 could be a factor, to make rapid, effective use of existing diagnostic tests, and to institute aggressive quarantine and treatment of potientially affected animals when indicated.

Introduction

Equine herpesvirus-1 (EHV-1) is a pervasive viral pathogen in horse populations worldwide. Active infection most commonly produces respiratory disease, with other clinical syndromes including abortion (Gilkerson *et al.* 1998), neonatal mortality (Murray *et al.* 1998) and neurological sequelae (Thorsen and Little 1975). Collectively these diseases cause significant impact to all aspects of the equine industry, particularly breeding and training facilities.

Despite being a longstanding target of the veterinary research community, many aspects of EHV-1 and its associated clinical entities remain incompletely understood. This unfortunately has resulted in less than perfect diagnostic tests but particularly prophylactic measures and treatment protocols being made available to equine practitioners. As incremental progress is made in fields relevant to this disease, the molecular knowledge prerequisite for subsequent improvements in the management of clinical EHV-1 infection is only slowly emerging.

The objectives of this article are to review for the equine practitioner salient information on the pathophysiology, epidemiology, clinical manifestations, diagnosis, treatment and prevention of clinical EHV-1 infection and to highlight areas in which current research shows promise for advances in the field and clinic settings.

Pathophysiology

Equine herpesvirus-1 is an alpha-herpesvirus with a double-stranded DNA genome. It is one of 9 herpesviruses known to infect horses. Other alpha-herpesviruses include the closely related but genetically distinct EHV-4 that primarily causes respiratory disease (Harless and Pusterla 2006), and EHV-3, the aetiological agent of the sexually transmitted disease equine coital exanthema (Kleiboeker and Chapman 2004). Equine herpesviruses 2 and 5 are gamma-herpesviruses that have been associated with keratoconjunctivitis (Kershaw *et al.* 2001) and severe respiratory disease (Diallo *et al.* 2008). These reports are, however, descriptive in nature and definitive proof as to the

*Author to whom correspondence should be addressed.

involvement of the viruses in disease still requires additional data.

Numerous strains of EHV-1 have been isolated and some of them have been thoroughly characterised. Importantly, recent research has focused on strain variations that are thought to be associated with the different forms of clinical disease (Allen *et al.* 1985; Ghanem *et al.* 2007; Goodman *et al.* 2007; Nugent *et al.* 2007). Generally speaking, necrotising vasculitis with ensuing hypoxia and malnutrition of tributary tissues, including fetal tissues, placenta and the central nervous system, is the common underlying pathophysiological mechanism responsible for the clinical manifestations associated with infection (Whitwell and Blunden 1992; Murray *et al.* 1998; Del Piero *et al.* 2000; Smith *et al.* 2004).

The typical life cycle of EHV-1 is outlined in **Figure 1**. Equine herpesvirus-1 is transmitted through nasal secretions and begins its initial round of replication upon entering respiratory epithelial cells. The receptor by which EHV-1 gains entry into cells has not yet been identified with certainty, but there is compelling evidence that the target receptor is not one of those known to be used by most other alpha-herpesviruses, although belonging to the nectin family of cell surface molecules (Frampton *et al.* 2005). Elucidation of this critical virus-host interaction may facilitate novel interventions at both prophylactic and therapeutic levels in the future.

Following initial replication the virus spreads to regional lymphatic tissues, primarily that of Waldeyer's ring and tributary lymph nodes, a process that frequently results in lymphadenopathy, particularly in young animals. The virus is then present in lymphocytes and a cell-associated viraemia ensues, enabling systemic transport of the virus via the blood stream. Cellular adhesion molecules are

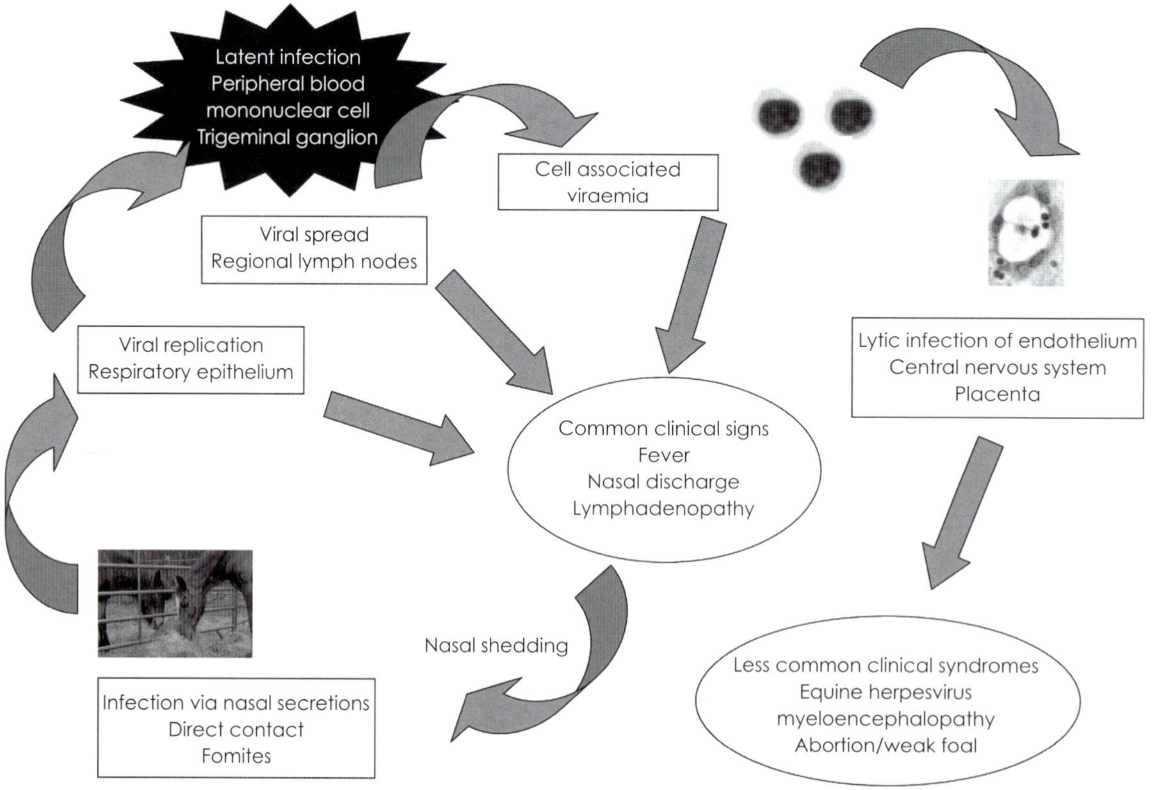

FIGURE 1: Typical life cycle of equine herpesvirus-1 resulting in associated clinical syndromes and persistence of the virus in equine populations worldwide (histopathology photographs courtesy of Drs Theresa Rizzi and Melanie Breshears).

then thought to mediate subsequent infection of endothelial cells (Smith *et al.* 2002) and lead to vasculitis in the pulmonary, CNS and placental vasculature and to the clinical syndromes observed. A genetic mutation has been identified in the DNA polymerase gene in one 'clade' of EHV-1 strains that appears to predispose for higher neurovirulence, possibly via increased efficiency of replication and subsequently higher levels of viraemia (Goodman *et al.* 2007; Nugent *et al.* 2007). Although the *post mortem* pathological findings associated with equine herpesvirus myeloencephalopathy (EHM) have typically been described as a necrotising myeloencephalopathy (Thorsen and Little 1975; Charlton *et al.* 1976; Little and Thorsen 1976), some authors have discussed the possibility of classical neurotropism found in other human and animal alpha-herpesviruses (Borchers *et al.* 2006).

Consistent with many herpesviruses, EHV-1 is able to establish a latent state in the host following initial infection, so that the virus may be found in both healthy and clinically affected animals. Presence of virus has been identified in lymphoid tissue and in the trigeminal ganglion of experimentally infected specific pathogen-free ponies by both culture and PCR (Slater *et al.* 1994). The virus may recrudesce in times of stress or immunosuppression, or may be iatrogenically activated following administration of immunosuppressive drugs such as corticosteroids. It is still unclear from which compartment latent EHV-1 is reactivated and subsequently spread within the population, but it seems logical that recrudescence could be initiated from both (trigeminal) neurons and peripheral blood mononuclear cells. Future studies will have to concentrate on the sites of latency and the frequency of reactivation observed in various tissues and how effectively virus can spread from animal-to-animal upon re-initiation of the lytic cycle.

A hallmark of infection of man and animals with all members of the herpesviruses is the evasion of the host's immune defences. EHV-1 has evolved numerous mechanisms to evade and to interfere with the host's immune response to viral threat. While a detailed discussion of these mechanisms is outside the scope of this review, broadly they include the production of proteins that inhibit leucocyte chemotaxis (van de Walle *et al.* 2007, 2008), as well as avoidance of antibody and cell-mediated lysis (van der Meulen *et al.* 2006). A number of proteins that the virus encodes in all stages of its replication have this capability, many of which are also serving other functions in virus replication. A thorough understanding of the immune evasion strategies of EHV-1 and other herpesviruses will be instrumental in the design of efficacious vaccines of the future.

Epidemiology

Equine herpesvirus-1 has been found in equids including horses, mules, donkey and zebras, and has been isolated from giraffe, onager and gazelle (Borchers and Frolich 1997; Hoenerhoff *et al.* 2006; Ibrahim *et al.* 2007; Ataseven *et al.* 2008). The epidemiology of EHV-1 varies across time and geographical region, and although the evolution of technologies employed in these analyses makes interpretive comparisons difficult, the reports collectively emphasise the ubiquity of the organism and the magnitude of the problem.

Epidemiological studies on the prevalence of EHV-1 variably rely on one or a combination of techniques including virus isolation, (quantitative) PCR and serology to define the presence, strain or movement of EHV-1 within a geographic area or a defined healthy or clinically affected population.

Serological studies of EHV-1 show variation in the prevalence of seropositive animals in different populations, but help to document the disease as one of international concern. It is important to note that various serological tests are used and that the results can vary in dependence of the test used. Very common are virus neutralisation (VN) assays, which represent a reasonably sensitive test system and are capable of detecting EHV-1 specific antibodies for extended periods. Both complement fixation assays (CFA) and a recently developed ELISA based on one of the viral surface glycoproteins, gG will reliably detect only recent infections that date back no more than 2–3 months. Further confounding serological analysis of EHV-1 is the fact that, with the exception of the gG ELISA, they are not capable of distinguishing between EHV-1- and EHV-4-specific antibodies. While the former induces a number of syndromes as outlined earlier, EHV-4 usually remains restricted to the upper respiratory tract and rarely causes systemic infection (Smith *et al.*

2003; Harless and Pusterla 2006). Using the gG ELISA in one Australian study, the prevalence of EHV-1 antibodies was 26.2% in mares while 11.4% of their foals were positive (Gilkerson *et al.* 1999a), whereas only 3 of 27 foals were seropositive in another study in California (Brown *et al.* 2007). Recent studies in Turkey showed that 12.5% of healthy horses tested were positive for EHV-1 specific antibodies by ELISA, as were 37.2% of mules and 24.2% of donkeys by virus neutralisation. In this same study, EHV-1 was isolated from 33.3% of horses with clinical respiratory disease (Ataseven *et al.* 2008).

The identification of EHV-1 DNA by different PCR assays also varies quite substantially across populations. Recent investigation of a Thoroughbred farm in California found only 4 of 1330 samples to be PCR positive for EHV-1 (Brown *et al.* 2007), and a report of 12 yearlings with clinical respiratory disease in Australia showed an absence of EHV-1 via quantitative, real-time PCR although EHV-4 and/or EHV-5 were present in all but one yearling (Diallo *et al.* 2008). By contrast, another study showed nearly all foals tested to be positive for EHV-1 by PCR (Foote *et al.* 2004).

In past years, the unavailability of a test that could distinguish between active and latent infections confounded epidemiological studies as well as diagnostic efforts, but recent advancements in technology have enabled this differentiation. A sophisticated nested PCR methodology applied to tissue from submandibular lymph nodes was used to evaluate EHV-1 status *post mortem* in broodmares in Kentucky. Latent infection was identified in 54% of the 132 mares examined thereby confirming data from earlier studies on the prevalence of the virus in equine populations (Allen *et al.* 2008). By contrast, in the only investigation of latency conducted during the course of an outbreak, 9 samples (5 blood, 4 swabs) with latency associated transcripts (LATs) were identified from 9 different horses at a Thoroughbred race track in California during the surveillance period, representing 12% of the 74 horses examined (Pusterla *et al.* 2007). As the technology to distinguish between lytic, nonreplicating and latent infections becomes more readily available for large scale studies, it is likely that geographic and other demographic variations in latent infection will be discovered.

Several theories exist to explain the transmission and perpetuation of EHV-1 in the equine population. There is a good body of evidence suggesting that initial infection often occurs within weeks after birth, and that unweaned foals are infected by asymptomatic but shedding dams in the herd, and subsequently by each other. It has been suggested that infection of dams by their offspring also occurs and there is compelling, statistically significant data that show an association of mares with foals on foot and the development of devastating neurological sequelae of infection. Taken together, these studies suggest that herds with newborns are an epidemiologically important component of EHV-1 persistence within the population (Gerber *et al.* 1977; Crowhurst *et al.* 1981; Gilkerson *et al.* 1999a,b; Foote *et al.* 2003; Studdert *et al.* 2003).

The underlying mechanisms have yet to be elucidated. Early experimental infection studies showed that the cell-mediated immune response to EHV-1 infection in pregnant mares is significantly diminished relative to nonpregnant controls (Gerber *et al.* 1977). More recent studies suggest that the nature of the cellular immune response in pregnant mares differs from other horses (Paillot *et al.* 2007). One possibility is that immune mediators present or absent in the pregnant mare relative to nonpregnant animals result in increased susceptibility to new or recrudescent infection. Continued research into the equine immune response to EHV-1 and the immunology of equine pregnancy is required to further characterise this important epidemiological observation.

Similarly, transmission of disease and persistence of the virus in the population at large is likely facilitated by shedding of recrudesced virus from latently infected horses. In experimental studies involving reactivation of latent EHV-1 infection, ponies showed no clinical signs, but continued to shed virus in nasal secretions for up to 10 days (Slater *et al.* 1994). Reservoirs of disease in other equids may also play a role in some communities, although there is a scarcity of systematic analyses concerning the prevalence and shedding of EHV-1 from e.g. donkeys and mules that have been suspected as a potential reservoir for EHV-1 (Ataseven *et al.* 2008). Recent evidence suggests that EHV-1 also may be transmissible during embryo transfer procedures (Hebia *et al.* 2007).

Clinical syndromes

Clinical presentations associated with EHV-1 infection encompass 3 major body systems and include respiratory disease, abortion and neonatal mortality, and neurological disease. Respiratory disease, usually restricted to the upper airways, is the most common manifestation of EHV-1 infection. In controlled experimental infection of naïve ponies or horses, consistent clinical signs have included pyrexia between 24–48 h after virus inoculation along with serous to mucopurulent nasal discharge and lymphadenopathy beginning around Day 4 and persisting through Days 7–10. Coughing has been observed only intermittently and rarely, it is not a common sign of infection (Chong and Duffus 1992; Sutton *et al.* 1998). Fever can be biphasic. A more severe, sporadic form of EVH-1 related respiratory disease has been reported within the past several years. Referred to as pulmonary vasculotropic EHV-1, these cases are characterised by multisystemic vasculitis with the pulmonary vasculature most severely affected (Hamir *et al.* 1994; Blunden *et al.* 1998; Del Piero *et al.* 2000; Del Piero and Wilkins 2001).

A second constellation of clinical signs that occurs with EHV-1 infection includes abortion and neonatal foal mortality. Abortion storms have long been known to result from EHV-1 infection and most commonly occur in late pregnancy (van Maanen *et al.* 2008). Abortion in these cases may involve infection of the fetus; however, pathology may be limited to the placenta and endometrium with the correlate of endothelial cell infection and vasculatis, and the fetus consequently is negative for virus. While these cases are rare, diagnostic procedures in the case of abortions have to ensure inclusion of the secundinae (Smith *et al.* 2004; Irwin *et al.* 2007). Abortions due to EHV-1 infection frequently occur as 'red-bag' or premature placental separation deliveries (Irwin *et al.* 2007).

Neonatal mortality resulting from EHV-1 infection has been reported to occur in the absence of readily visible signs. Upon pathological examination, necrotising bronchopneumonia and fibrinous degeneration are the primary *post mortem* finding (Murray *et al.* 1998).

The neurological sequel to EHV-1 infection has received increasing attention in recent years, and has been given consideration as an emerging infectious disease by the United States Department of Agriculture's Animal and Plant Health Inspection Service. The number of outbreaks reported in the USA and the UK increased from one in the 5-year period from 1970–1975 to 32 in the years from 2001–2005 (Anon 2007). A recent epidemiological study in Kentucky showed that 18% of latently infected broodmares were infected with strains belonging to the 'neurological clade' of EHV-1 (see below). In the Netherlands and likely in Europe as a whole, EHM is now considered the most common cause of equine infectious neurological disease (Goehring *et al.* 2006).

The clinical syndrome EHM encompasses a constellation of neurological signs including ataxia that may progress to paresis and recumbency, head pressing, depression, hyperaesthesia, decreased tail and anal tone and urinary incontinence. Other signs reported in horses with EHM include fever, lymphadenopathy, inappetence and limb oedema. The disease may but does not reliably occur following other indications of EHV-1 infection such as respiratory disease or abortion, and often occurs in outbreaks at training and breeding facilities. The index case in these situations is often one horse with a recent history of presence at a sale or competition. Onset of neurological signs has been reported variably at 24–72 h and 4–8 days after the onset of fever. Seasonal clustering has been reported between mid-November and mid-May in one report, which probably is a consequence of abortion storms that occur during that time and with which the most neurological outbreaks have been shown to be associated (Friday *et al.* 2000; Goehring *et al.* 2006). The morbidity for EHM within reported EHV-1 outbreaks varies. Neurological signs were reported in 8 of 9 pregnant, lactating mares and 2 of 8 other horses in one study while in 2 recent large outbreaks 34% and 41% of horses became neurological (Crowhurst *et al.* 1981; Friday *et al.* 2000; Henninger *et al.* 2007).

The development of neurological disease in a subset of horses within an outbreak is probably the result of a complex interplay between the viral strain and the genetic makeup and the immune system of individual animals. So far, however, no correlation of disease incidence or severity with haplotype or other elements of host genetics has been shown. On the side of the agent, however, there is growing evidence that a genetic mutation affecting the DNA polymerase gene (D752) is related to a greater likelihood of neurological disease in infected horses (Goodman *et al.* 2007), but not all horses infected with representatives of the neurological genotype or clade develop neurological disease. Conversely, neurological disease can also be caused, albeit at greatly reduced odds ratios, by N752 variant strains that appear to represent the majority of EHV-1 strains circulating at least in the USA. Individual and environmental risk factors associated with the development of neurological disease are inconsistent in existing literature. Mares were more likely to develop severe neurological disease in one report (Goehring *et al.* 2006), but gender was not a factor in another large scale report (Henninger *et al.* 2007). In both of these reports being in an older age group was associated with the development of neurological disease. The number of vaccines received prior to the outbreak, and the use of immune stimulants have also been considered to be associated with increased predisposition for the development of EHM, but statistical significance with either of the factors could not be established (Henninger *et al.* 2007).

Diagnosis

Historically, virus isolation, which is considered the diagnostic gold standard for many virus diseases including EHV-1, and either paired acute and convalescent sera demonstrating a 4-fold rise in titre or a single titre of >1:256 were the tests available for diagnosis of EHV-1. However, these tests require much time, and are not ideal in situations of abortion storms or EHM where accurate diagnosis and rapid containment are imperative. Cross-reactivity of antibodies between EHV-1 and EHV-4 further limits the usefulness of serology, and a major advancement came with the development of a type specific ELISA test that distinguishes between EHV-1 and EHV-4 (Crabb *et al.* 1995). It is unclear how reliable this test is in identifying seropositive or latently infected animals and how early after infection horses can be unequivocally identified as harbouring EHV-1 or EHV-4.

Numerous protocols of employing polymerase chain reaction (PCR) have been developed to improve the speed and accuracy with which EHV-1 and EHV-4 may be diagnosed. The described assays that are offered by many diagnostic laboratories worldwide include differentiation of EHV-1 and EHV-4 (Diallo *et al.* 2007), rapid detection of neuropathogenic EHV-1 (Allen 2007), quantification of viraemia and nasal shedding (Hussey *et al.* 2006; Perkins *et al.* 2008), and differentiation between active and latent infections (Allen *et al.* 2008). Other advancements providing for more rapid or efficient diagnostics include validation of automated vs. manual procedures (Mapes *et al.* 2008) and nasal swabbing techniques (Pusterla *et al.* 2008). Coordinated use of select diagnostic tests can result in rapid diagnosis, effective management and response to treatment in outbreak situations, as well as significant contribution to the overall understanding of the pathogenesis of EHV-1 (Pusterla *et al.* 2007; Studdert *et al.* 2003).

As a general recommendation, the veterinarian should stay with one diagnostic laboratory to ensure consistency and comparability of results, especially with respect to the serological procedures. Serological titres can vary substantially between laboratories and wrong conclusions may be drawn from results if laboratories are switched, especially with regard to serum pairs that still are a reliable method for the identification of acute infections.

Treatment and prognosis

Historically, treatment of EHV-1 infection has been limited to supportive care including anti-inflammatory medication with nonsteroidal anti-inflammatory drugs such as flunixin meglumine or treatment with dimethylsulphoxide (DMSO), treatment of secondary bacterial infection with antibiotics as required, urinary catheterisation if indicated and padding or slinging to prevent pressure necrosis and ulceration in recumbent animals.

More recently attention has been given to the use of antiviral medications in the treatment of clinical EHV-1 infection, particularly in cases of EHM. Acyclovir, a potent drug widely used in human herpesvirus infections, successfully reduces viral plaque size and number *in vitro* (Garre *et al.* 2007a), but has shown poor bioavailability on oral administration (Bentz *et al.* 2006). Nonetheless, clinical use of acyclovir was reported in 2 large outbreaks of EHM. In one the use of acyclovir in a given animal was associated with survival (Henninger *et al.* 2007), and in the other the efficacy of this drug was considered inconclusive due to inadequate data (Friday *et al.* 2000). Newer research investigating the use of valacyclovir, a prodrug of acyclovir, suggests promise for clinical efficacy due to better bioavailability (Garre *et al.* 2007b; Maxwell *et al.* 2008). A rapid decline in viral load was attributed to the use of oral valacyclovir in one case of EHM (Pusterla *et al.* 2007). However, a recent treatment study of experimental infection seems to prove poor performance of the drug in ponies and horses with respect to clinical signs, virus shedding and viraemia (Garre *et al.* 2009). The only significant difference observed was a lower peak fever in treated vs. untreated ponies. It is difficult to assess the effect of this drug on EHM in this study, as the groups were small and no ponies in either the treated or untreated groups developed signs of neurological disease.

The prognosis for horses with EHM varies across published reports. In general, horses that become recumbent for greater than 24 h have a very poor prognosis (McCartan *et al.* 1995). Some horses with severe neurological signs are reported to recover completely, while others continue to suffer from residual deficits including ataxia and incontinence. In one large outbreak, overall mortality was 12%, while mortality among horses developing neurological signs was 30% (Henninger *et al.* 2007). In another case, overall mortality was 2% and mortality among neurological animals was 5%. A report of a smaller outbreak indicated 2 of 10 (20%) horses developing neurological signs died or were subject to euthanasia (Crowhurst *et al.* 1981).

Novel approaches to metaphylactic or post exposure management of viral infections are currently being researched. One of these is so-called RNA interference, a mechanism for silencing viral gene expression. Such potential drugs, given locally (intranasally) or systemically could prevent virus replication at the site of entry, virus dissemination via the bloodstream, and interanimal spread (Stevenson 2004). Conceptionally more conventional although technically novel would be a reported treatment with recombinant neutralising antibodies, a method having shown promise in initial trials (Molinkova *et al.* 2008).

Prevention and management

The development and application of an EHV-1 vaccine resulting in both sustained immunity and protection against neurological sequelae would provide a cornerstone for the universal control of EHV-1 related infection, yet this goal remains elusive. With a response to natural infection that confers only 3–6 months of immunity for affected animals (Kydd *et al.* 2006), the equine immune system has so far resisted attempts at artificially inducing long-term protection. The best that has been achieved to date by existing vaccines is a mitigation of clinical signs and viral shedding upon infection and some improvement in EHV-1 associated abortions with no apparent protection against EHM.

Evidence suggests that long-lasting immunity to EHV-1 related diseases will require stimulation of both humoural and cell-mediated components at local (mucosal) and systemic levels. It is clear from observations of both natural exposure as well as experimental infection that humoural immunity alone is not adequate to prevent infection. Following infection, complement fixation (CF) antibodies continue to provide protection for up to 3 months, while virus neutralising (VN) antibodies may be present for up to a year (Kydd *et al.* 2006). Despite this, the rapid cell-associated viraemia that occurs upon infection or re-infection probably protects virus from the effects of these serum antibodies.

One example that clearly demonstrates the failure of humoural immunity to provide protection at an individual or population level is the documentation of infection in neonatal foals despite the presence of adequate maternal antibodies. In one report, virus was identified by PCR and ELISA in vaccinated mares and their unvaccinated neonatal foals on a Thoroughbred farm in Australia (Foote *et al.* 2004). Other studies have demonstrated that high levels of maternal antibodies do not protect from infection, but mitigate clinical disease on initial infection (Kydd *et al.* 2006). Foals may subsequently be reinfected, or recrudesce and infect others, thereby enabling the virus to persist in the population.

There is increasing evidence accumulating that supports the theory that a strong cellular immune response is critical in controlling EHV-1 infection. Repeated exposures to EHV-1 under natural or experimental conditions result in increasing numbers of cytotoxic T-lymphocytes (Kydd *et al.* 2003) and immunity that becomes stronger over time. Studies have shown in pregnant mares that the presence of higher levels of cellular immunity in the form of virus-specific cytotoxic T-lymphocytes is significantly correlated with resistance to abortion on challenge with EHV-1; and similar resistance to disease has also been demonstrated in non-pregnant adults (Kydd *et al.* 2003). It is likely that a strong cellular immune response decreases the magnitude of the cell-associated viraemia necessary for the development of abortions or neurological disease, thus lowering the chance for these clinical signs to occur (Patel and Helden 2005). It has also been determined that mucosal antibody production in the form of IgA occurs upon infection, and although this protection is short-lived, the ability to stimulate mucosal immunity is desired in an effective vaccine protocol (Kydd *et al.* 2006).

Currently available traditional vaccines, including inactivated and modified live virus varieties, fail to achieve all of these goals (Patel and Helden 2005). While the severity of respiratory disease and viral shedding may be decreased in vaccinated animals, and there is some evidence that appropriate vaccination of pregnant mares can decrease the incidence of abortion, incidence of EHM seems mockingly unmitigated by vaccination. Numerous reports document outbreaks in horses with current vaccination status (Friday *et al.* 2000; Henninger *et al.* 2007). Furthermore, epidemiological studies suggest that the presence of EHV-1 in a population of horses appears to be independent of the herd's vaccination status, a property that may illustrate the daunting task at hand (Foote *et al.* 2003). Of note is the association of both frequent vaccination and the use of immunostimulants with neurological disease in one report, although a causal relationship is difficult to formally be established (Henninger *et al.* 2007).

Nonetheless, until such time that the ideal EHV-1 vaccine becomes a reality, and in spite of the sometimes conflicting evidence on the impact of vaccination protocols, it seems prudent for the veterinarian to devise strategic vaccination protocols for horses in high risk populations such as in the management of large numbers of horses in breeding and training facilities. Although one recent study showed that a modified live vaccine provided better protection compared to an inactivated combination product, (Goodman *et al.* 2006), the variability in available vaccines worldwide precludes definitive conclusions based upon this single criterion.

Novel approaches to vaccination are currently being investigated as alternatives, including virus deletion mutants that are devoid of e.g. immunomodulatory functions, live vectored vaccines delivering other (viral) antigens together with the EHV-1 vaccine, and so-called DNA vaccines that are based on application of nucleic acid that will result in production of the immunogen *in vivo* in the vaccinated horse (Minke *et al.* 2004, 2006). Because of some of its unique characteristics such as the ability to carry large amounts of DNA and to enter many different types of cells, EHV-1 is currently being investigated as a vector of immunisation for a variety of human and animal diseases (Trapp *et al.* 2005; Rosas *et al.* 2008). It is likely that in the process of refining the use of EHV-1 as a vector, new information will be learned about EHV-1 host-virus interactions that will result in improved vaccine strategies against EHV-1 itself.

In the interim, practitioners must rely onthe use of rapid diagnosis, isolation and hygiene regimens with the goal of containment as the next best approach for controlling disease caused by EHV-1. Intensive clinical management of EHV-1 may be facilitated by developments such as the recent investigation into the feasibility of air testing for aerosolised EHV-1 and may give hints as to where interventions have to be initiated to be effective (Pusterla and Mapes 2008).

Conclusion

It is fair to say that EHV-1, a ubiquitous pathogen of the horse, still presents many challenges for practitioners and researchers alike. While researchers are attempting to unravel the mysteries behind EHV-1 immune evasion with the goal of developing prophylaxis able to provide both long-term immunity and immunity against the neurological form of disease, practitioners are faced with an exponential increase in the number of neurovirulent EHV-1 outbreaks they are required to manage. A successful battle against EHV-1 morbidity and mortality and associated economic losses will require the coordinated best efforts of both parties.

It is an unfortunate reality that currently available EHV-1 vaccines and vaccination regimes do not prevent infection, although they may mitigate clinical signs and viral shedding. Considering these facts, the next best defence against devastating outbreaks is a high index of suspicion in appropriate circumstances that will allow rapid, accurate diagnosis and containment of disease. The presence of an index case with a history of outside exposure is common but not invariable in EHM outbreaks and cases of abortion. Hence, acute onset of neurological disease or abortions should be viewed with a high degree of suspicion, particularly in large training or breeding facilities (Henninger *et al.* 2007). Immediate quarantine of suspected EHM animals as well as in-contact animals is ideal until EHV-1 infection is ruled in or out, as a high degree of viral shedding has been documented in clinical cases of acute EHM (Pusterla *et al.* 2007).

Similarly, because some cases of EHV-1 abortion present with lesions in the placenta only, examination of fetal membranes, and not just fetal tissues, should be routine in all cases of abortion so that an atypical index case does not go undiagnosed. Premature placental separation is a common feature of neonatal EHV-1 infection. Consequently, all 'red bag' deliveries should be treated as suspicious, particularly in circumstances where other known risk factors such as ingestion of fescue are not present (Smith *et al.* 2004; Irwin *et al.* 2007). Neonatal mortality has been reported in the absence of a history of respiratory disease or abortion on the premises, so testing for EHV-1 should be considered in cases of neonatal mortality.

On the part of researchers, every effort must be made to comprehensively test novel diagnostic tools, therapies and preventive preparations, and make breakthroughs in diagnostic and therapeutic technology commercially available as soon as is sensible and feasible. For example, rapid diagnostic tests and the ability to distinguish between active and latent infections will enable practitioners to use caution while minimising the risk of unnecessary quarantines. If met with the necessary knowledge and care by researchers and veterinarians alike, EHV-1 infections will hopefully present a historic disease in the not too distant future.

Acknowledgements

We wish to acknowledge our colleagues, Drs Armando Damiani, Gillian Perkins and Gerlinde van de Walle for our common efforts in drug research and vaccine development. Research on equine herpesvirus-1 disease in the authors' laboratory is kindly supported by the Grayson Jockey Club Research Foundation, the Morris Animal Foundation, the Harry M. Zweig Memorial Fund for Equine Research at Cornell University, and the Deutsche Forschungsgemeinschaft (DFG Os 143/4-1). Dr Brosnahan's work at Cornell University is supported by an institutional training grant from the National Institutes of Health.

References

Allen, G.P. (2007) Development of a real-time polymerase chain reaction assay for rapid diagnosis of neuropathogenic strains of equine herpesvirus-1. *J. vet. diag. Invest.* **19**, 69-72.

Allen, G.P., Yeargan, M.R., Turtinen, L.W. and Bryans, J.T. (1985) A new field strain of equine abortion virus (equine herpesvirus-1) among Kentucky horses. *Am. J. vet. Res.* **46**, 138-140.

Allen, G.P., Bolin, D.C., Bryant, U., Carter, C.N., Giles, R.C., Harrison, L.R., Hong, C.B., Jackson, C.B., Poonacha, K., Wharton, R. and Williams, N.M. (2008) Prevalence of latent neuropathogenic equine herpesvirus-1 in the Thoroughbred broodmare population of central Kentucky. *Equine vet. J.* **40**, 102-103.

Anon (2007) *Equine herpesvirus myeloencephalopathy: a potentially emerging disease,* USDA APHIS Information Sheet.

Ataseven, V.S., Daglap, S.B., Guzel, M., Basaran, Z., Tan, M.T. and Geraghty, B. (2008) Prevalence of equine herpesvirus-1 and equine herpesvirus-4 infections in *Equidae* species in Turkey as determined by ELISA and multiplex nested PCR. *Res. vet. Sci.* **86**, 339-344.

Bentz, B.G., Maxwell, L.K., Erkert, R.S., Royer, C.M., Davis, M.S., MacAllister, C.G. and Clarke, C.R. (2006) Pharmacokinetics of acyclovir after single intravenous and oral administration to adult horses. *J. vet. intern. Med.* **20**, 589-594.

Blunden, A.S., Smith, K.C., Whitwell, K.E. and Dunn, K.A. (1998) Systemic infection by equid herpesvirus-1 in a Grevy's zebra stallion (*Equus grevyi*) with particular reference to genital pathology. *J. comp. Pathol.* **119**, 485-493.

Borchers, K. and Frolich, K. (1997) Antibodies against equine herpesviruses in free-ranging mountain zebras from Namibia. *J. Wildlife Dis.* **33**, 812-817.

Borchers, K., Thein, P. and Sterner-Kock, A. (2006) Pathogenesis of equine herpesvirus-associated neurological disease: a revised explanation. *Equine vet. J.* **38**, 283-287.

Brown, J.A., Mapes, S., Ball, B.A., Hodder, A.D., Liu, I.K. and Pusterla, N. (2007) Prevalence of equine herpesvirus-1 infection among Thoroughbreds residing on a farm on which the virus was endemic. *J. Am. vet. med. Ass.* **231**, 577-580.

Charlton, K.M., Mitchell, D., Girard, A. and Corner, A.H. (1976) Meningoencephalomyelitis in horses associated with equine herpesvirus 1 infection. *Vet. Pathol.* **13**, 59-68.

Chong, Y.C. and Duffus, W.P.H. (1992), Immune responses of specific pathogen free foals to EHV-1 infection. *Vet. Microbiol.* **32**, 215-228.

Crabb, B.S., MacPherson, C.M., Reubel, G.H., Browning, G.F., Studdert, M.J. and Drummer, H.E. (1995) Epitopes of glycoprotein G of equine herpesvirus 4 and 1 located near the C terminal elicit type-specific antibody response in the natural host. *J. Virol.* **67**, 6332-6338.

Crowhurst, F.A., Dickinson, G. and Burrows, R. (1981) An outbreak of paresis in mares and geldings associated with equid herpesvirus-1. *Vet. Rec.* **109**, 527-528.

Del Piero, F. and Wilkins, P.A. (2001) Pulmonary vasculotropic EHV-1 infection in equids. *Vet. Pathol.* **38**, 474-475.

Del Piero, F., Wilkins, P.A., Timoney, P.J., Kadushin, J., Vogelbacker, J., Lee, J.W., Berkowitz, S.J. and La Perle, K.M.D. (2000) Fatal nonneurological EHV-1 infection in a yearling filly. *Vet. Pathol.* **37**, 672-676.

Diallo, I.S., Hewitson, G., Wright, L.L., Kelly, M.A., Rodwell, B.J. and Corney, B.G. (2007) Multiplex real-time PCR for the detection and differentiation of equid herpesvirus 1 (EHV-1) and equid herpesvirus 4 (EHV-4). *Vet. Microbiol.* **123**, 93-103.

Diallo, I.S., Hewitson, G.R., de Jong, A., Kelly, M.A., Wright, D.J., Corney, B.G. and Rodwell, B.J. (2008) Equine herpesvirus infections in yearlings in South-East Queensland. *Arch. Virol.* **153**, 1643-1649.

Foote, C.E., Gilkerson, J.R., Whalley, J.M. and Love, D.N. (2003) Seroprevalence of equine herpesvirus 1 in mares and foals on a large Hunter Valley stud farm in years pre and post vaccination. *Aust. vet. J.* **81**, 283-288.

Foote, C.E., Love, D.N., Gilkerson, J.R. and Whalley, J.M. (2004) Detection of EHV-1 and EHV-4 DNA in unweaned Thoroughbred foals from vaccinated mares on a large stud farm. *Equine vet. J.* **36**, 341-345.

Frampton, A.R., Goins, W.F., Cohen, J.B., von Einem, J., Osterrieder, N., O'Callaghan, D.J. and Glorioso, J.C. (2005) Equine herpesvirus 1 utilizes a novel herpesvirus entry receptor. *J. Virol.* **79**, 3169-3173

Friday, P., Scarratt, W.K., Elvinger, F., Timoney, P.J. and Bonda, A. (2000) Ataxia and paresis with equine herpesvirus type 1 infection in a herd of riding school horses. *J. vet. intern. Med.* **14**, 197-201.

Garre, B., Gryspeerdt, A., Croubels, S., De Backer, P. and Nauwynck, H. (2009) Evaluation of orally administered valacyclovir in experimentally EHV1-infected ponies. *Vet. Microbiol.* **135**, 214-221.

Garre, B., van der Meulen, K., Nugent, J., Neyts, J., Croubels, S., De Backer, P. and Nauwynck, H. (2007a) *In vitro* susceptibility of six isolates of equine herpesvirus 1 to acyclovir, ganciclovir, cidofovir, adefovir, PMEDAP and foscarnet. *Vet. Microbiol.* **122**, 43-51.

Garre, B., Shebany, K., Gryspeerdt, A., Baert, K., van der Meulen, K., Nauwynck, H., Deprez, P., De Backer, P. and Croubels, S. (2007b) Pharmacokinetics of acyclovir after intravenous infusion of acyclovir and after oral administration of acyclovir and its prodrug valacyclovir in healthy adult horses. *Antimicrob. Agents Chemother.* **51**, 4308-4314.

Gerber, J.D., Marron, A.E., Bass, E.P. and Beckenhauer, W.H. (1977) Effect of age and pregnancy on the antibody and cell-mediated immune responses of horses to equine herpesvirus 1. *Can. J. Comp. Med.* **41**, 471-478.

Ghanem, Y.M., Ibrahim, E.M., Yamada, S., Matsumura, T., Osterrieder, N., Yamaguchi, T. and Fukushi, H. (2007) Molecular characterization of the equine herpesvirus 1 strains Rac11 and Kentucky D. *J. vet. med. Sci.* **69**, 573-576.

Gilkerson, J.R., Love, D.N. and Whalley, J.M. (1998) Epidemiology of equine herpesvirus abortion: searching for clues to the future. *Aust. vet. J.* **76**, 675-676.

Gilkerson, J.R., Whalley, J.M., Drummer, H.E., Studdert, M.J. and Love, D.N. (1999a) Epidemiology of EHV-1 and EHV-4 in the mare and foal populations on a Hunter Valley stud farm: are mares the source of EHV-1 for unweaned foals. *Vet. Microbiol.* **68**, 27-34

Gilkerson, J.R., Whalley, J.M., Drummer, H.E., Studdert, M.J. and Love, D.N. (1999b) Epidemiological studies of equine herpesvirus 1 (EHV-1) in Thoroughbred foals: a review of studies conducted in the Hunter Valley of New South Wales between 1995 and 1997. *Vet. Microbiol.* **68**, 15-25.

Goehring, L.S., van Winden, S.C., van Maanan, C. and Sloet van Oldruitenborgh-Oosterbaan, M.M. (2006) Equine herpesvirus type 1-associated myeloencephalopathy in the Netherlands: a four year retrospective study (1999-2003). *J. vet. intern. Med.* **20**, 601-607.

Goodman, L.B., Wagner, B., Flaminio, M.J.B.F., Sussman, K.H., Metzger, S.M., Holland, R. and Osterrieder, N. (2006) Comparison of the efficacy of inactivated combination and modified-live virus vaccines against challenge infection with neuropathogenic equine herpesvirus type 1 (EHV-1). *Vaccine* **24**, 3636-3645.

Goodman, L.B., Loregian, A., Perkins, G.A., Nugent, J., Buckles, E.L., Mercorelli, B., Kydd, J.H., Palu, G., Smith, K.C., Osterrieder, N. and Davis-Poynter, N. (2007) A point mutation in a herpesvirus polymerase determines neuropathogenicity. *PLoS Pathogens* **3**, 1583-1592.

Hamir, A.N., Vaala, W., Heyer, G. and Moser, G. (1994) Disseminated equine herpesvirus-1 infection in a two-year-old filly. *J. vet. diag. Invest.* **6**, 493-496.

Harless, W. and Pusterla, N. (2006) Equine herpesvirus 1 and 4 respiratory disease in the horse. *Clin. Tech. Equine Pract.* **5**, 197-202.

Hebia, I., Fieni, F., Duchamp, G., Destrumelle, S., Pellerin, J.L., Zientara, S., Vautherot, J.F. and Bruysas, J.F. (2007) Potential risk of equine herpes virus 1 (EHV-1) transmission by equine embryo transfer. *Theriogenol.* **67**, 1485-1491.

Henninger, R.W., Reed, S.M., Saville, W.J., Allen, G.P., Hass, G.F., Kohn, C.W. and Sofaly, C. (2007) Outbreak of neurologic disease caused by equine herpesvirus-1 at a university equestrian center. *J. vet. intern. Med.* **21**, 157-165.

Hoenerhoff, M.J., Janovitz, E.B., Richman, L.K., Murphy, D.A., Butler, T.C. and Kiupel, M. (2006) Fatal herpesvirus encephalitis in a reticulated giraffe (*Giraffa camelopardalis reticulata*). *Vet. Pathol.* **45**, 769-772.

Hussey, S.B., Clark, R., Breathnach, C., Soboll, G., Whalley, J.M. and Lunn, D.P. (2006) Detection and quantification of equine herpesvirus-1 viremia and nasal shedding by real-time polymerase chain reaction. *J. vet. diag. Invest.* **18**, 335-342.

Ibrahim, E.S.M., Kinoh, M., Matsumura, T., Kennedy, M., Allen, G.P., Yamaguchi, T. and Fukushi, H. (2007) Genetic relatedness and pathogenicity of equine herpesvirus 1 isolated from onager, zebra and gazelle. *Arch. Virol.* **152**, 245-255.

Irwin, V.L., Traub-Dargatz, J.L., Newton, J.R., Scase, T.J., Davis-Poynter, N.J., Nugent, J., Creis, L., Leaman, T.R. and Smith, K.C. (2007) Investigation and management of an outbreak of abortion related to equine herpesvirus type 1 in unvaccinated ponies. *Vet. Rec.* **160**, 378-380.

Kershaw, O., von Oppen, T., Glitz, F., Deegan, E., Lugwig, H. and Borchers, K. (2001) Detection of equine herpesvirus type 2 (EHV-2) in horses with keratoconjunctivitis. *Virus Res.* **80**, 93-99.

Kleiboeker, S.B. and Chapman, R.K. (2004) Detection of equine herpesvirus 3 in equine skin lesions by polymerase chain reaction. *J. vet. diag. Invest.* **16**, 74-79.

Kydd, J., Townsend, H.G.G. and Hannant, D. (2006) The equine immune response to equine herpesvirus-1: the virus and its vaccines. *Vet. Immunol. Immunopathol.* **111**, 15-30.

Kydd, J.H., Wattrang, E. and Hannant, D. (2003) Pre-infection frequencies of equine herpesvirus-1 specific cytotoxic T lymphocytes correlate with protection against abortion following experimental infection of pregnant mares. *Vet. Immunol. Immunopathol.* **96**, 207-217.

Little, P.B. and Thorsen, J. (1976) Disseminated necrotizing myeloencephalitis: a herpes associated neurological disease of horses. *Vet. Pathol.* **13**, 161-171.

Mapes, S., Leutenegger, C.M. and Pusterla, N. (2008) Nucleic acid extraction methods for detection of EHV-1 from blood and nasopharyngeal secretions. *Vet. Rec.* **162**, 857-859.

Maxwell, L.K., Bentz, B.G., Bourne, D.W.A. and Erkert, R.S. (2008) Pharmacokinetics of valacyclovir in the adult horse. *J. vet. Pharmacol. Therap.* **31**, 312-320.

McCartan, C.G., Russell, M.M., Wood, J.L. and Mumford, J.A. (1995) Clinical, serological and virological characteristics of an outbreak of paresis and neonatal foal disease due to equine herpesvirus-1 on a stud farm. *Vet. Rec.* **136**, 7-12.

Minke, J.M., Audonnet, J.C. and Fischer, L. (2004) Equine viral vaccines: the past, present and future. *Vet. Res.* **35**, 425-443.

Minke, J.M., Fischer, L., Baudu, P., Guigal, P.M., Sindle, T., Mumford, J.A. and Audonnet, J.C. (2006) Use of DNA and recombinant canarypox viral (ALVAC) vectors for equine herpes virus vaccination. *Vet. Immunol. Immunopathol.* **111**, 47-57.

Molinkova, D., Skladal, P. and Celer, V. (2008) *In vitro* neutralization of equid herpesvirus 1 mediated by recombinant antibodies. *J. Immunol. Methods* **333**, 186-191.

Murray, M.J., Del Piero, F., Jeffrey, S.C., Davis, M.S., Furr, M.O., Dubovi, E.J. and Mayo, J.A. (1998) Neonatal equine herpesvirus type 1 infection on a Thoroughbred breeding farm. *J. vet. intern. Med.* **12**, 36-41.

Nugent, J., Birch-Machin, I., Smith, K.C., Mumford, J.A., Swann, Z., Newton, J.R., Bowden, R.J., Allen, G.P. and Davis-Poynter, N. (2007) Analysis of equid herpesvirus 1 strain variation reveals a point mutation of the DNA polymerase strongly associated with neuropathogenic versus nonneuropathogenic disease outbreaks. *J. Virol.* **80**, 4047-4060.

Paillot, R., Daly, J.M., Luce, R., Montesso, F., Davis-Poynter, N., Hannant, D. and Kydd, J.H. (2007) Frequency and phenotype of EHV-1 specific, IFN-gamma synthesising lymphocytes in ponies: The effects of age, pregnancy and infection. *Dev. Comp. Immunol.* **31**, 202-214.

Patel, J.R. and Helden, J. (2005) Equine herpesviruses 1 (EHV-1) and 4 (EHV-4) - epidemiology, disease and immunoprophylaxis: A brief review. *Vet. J.* **170**, 14-23.

Perkins, G.A., Goodman, L.B., Dubovi, E.J., Kim, S.G. and Osterrieder, N. (2008) Detection of equine herpesvirus-1 in nasal swabs of horses by quantitative real time PCR. *J. Am. vet. med. Ass.* **22**, 1234-1238.

Pusterla, N. and Mapes, S. (2008) Evaluation of an air tester for the sampling of aerosolized equine herpesvirus type 1. *Vet. Rec.* **163**, 306-308.

Pusterla, N., Mapes, S. and Wilson, W.D. (2008) Diagnostic sensitivity of nasopharyngeal and nasal swabs for the molecular detection of EHV-1. *Vet. Rec.* **162**, 520-521.

Pusterla, N., Wilson, W.D., Mapes, S., Finno, C., Isbell, D., Arthur, R. and Ferraro, G.L. (2007) Characterization of viral loads, strain and state of equine herpesvirus-1 using real-time PCR in horses following natual exposure at a racetrack in California. *Vet. J.* **179**, 230-239.

Rosas, C., Van de Walle, G.R., Metzger, S.M., Hoelzer, K., Dubovi, E.J., Kim, S.G., Patel, J.R. and Osterrieder, N. (2008) Evaluation of a vectored equine herpesvirus type 1 (EHV-1) vaccine expressing H3 haemagglutinin in the protection of dogs against canine influenza. *Vaccine* **26**, 2335-2343.

Slater, J.D., Borchers, K., Thackray, A.M. and Field, H.J. (1994) The trigeminal ganglion is a location for equine herpesvirus 1 latency and reactivation in the horse. *J. gen. Virol.* **75**, 2007-2016.

Smith, D., Hamblin, A. and Edington, N. (2002) Equid herpesvirus 1 infection of endothelial cells requires activation of putative adhesion molecules: an *in vitro* model. *Clin. Experimental Immunol.* **129**, 281-287.

Smith, K.C., Blunden, A.S., Whitwell, K.E., Dunn, K.A. and Wales, A.D. (2003) A survey of equine abortion, stillbirth and neonatal death in the UK from 1988 to 1997. *Equine vet. J.* **35**, 496-501.

Smith, K.C., Whitwell, K.E., Blunden, A.S., Bestbier, M.E., Scase, T.J., Geraghty, R.J., Nugent, J., Davis-Poynter, N. and Cardwell, J.M. (2004) Equine herpesvirus-1 abortion: atypical cases with lesions largely or wholly restricted to the placenta. *Equine vet. J.* **36**, 79-82.

Stevenson, M. (2004) Therapeutic potential of RNA interference. *New Engl. Med.* **351**, 1772-1777.

Studdert, M.J., Hartley, C.A., Dynon, K., Sandy, J.R., Slocombe, R.F., Charles, J.A., Milne, M.E., Clarke, A.F. and El-Hage, C. (2003) Outbreak of equine herpesvirus type 1 myeloencephalitis: new insights from virus identification by PCR and the application of an EHV-1-specific antibody detection ELISA. *Vet. Rec.* **153**, 417-423.

Sutton, G.A., Viel, L., Carman, P.S. and Boag, B.L. (1998) Pathogenesis and clinical signs of equine herpesvirus-1 in experimentally infected ponies *in vivo*. *Can. J. vet. Res.* **62**, 49-55.

Thorsen, J. and Little, P.B. (1975) Isolation of equine herpesvirus type 1 from a horse with an acute paralytic disease. *Can. J. Comp. Med.* **39**, 358-359

Trapp, S., von Einem, J., Hofmann, H., Kostler, J., Wild, J., Wagner, R., Beer, M. and Osterrieder, N. (2005) Potential of equine herpesvirus 1 as a vector for immunization. *J. Virol.* **79**, 5445-5454.

Van de Walle, G.R., May, M.L., Sukhumavasi, W., von Einem, J. and Osterrieder, N. (2007) Herpesvirus chemokine-binding glycoprotein G (gG) efficiently inhibits neutrophil chemotaxis *in vitro* and *in vivo*. *J. Immunol.* **179**, 4161-4169.

Van de Walle, G.R., Sakamoto, K. and Osterrieder, N. (2008) CCL3 and viral chemokine binding protein gG modulate pulmonary inflammation and virus replication during equine herpesvirus-1 infection. *J. Virol.* **82**, 1714-1722.

van der Meulen, K.M., Favoreel, H.W., Pensaert, M.B, and Nauwynck, H.J. (2006) Immune escape of equine herpesvirus 1 and other herpesviruses of veterinary importance. *Vet. Immunol. Immunopathol.* **111**, 31-40.

van Maanen, C., Willink, D.L., Smeenk, L.A., Brinkhof, J., Terpstra, C. (2008) An equine herpesvirus 1 (EHV-1) abortion storm at a riding school. *Vet. Quart.* **22**, 83-87.

Whitwell, K.E. and Blunden, A.S. (1992) Pathological findings in horses dying during an outbreak of the paralytic form of equid herpesvirus type 1 (EHV-1) infection. *Equine vet. J.* **24**, 13-19.

RHINITIS AND ADENOVIRUS INFECTIONS OF HORSES

J. L. N. Wood*, J. R. Newton† and K. Smith‡

Department of Veterinary Medicine, University of Cambridge, Madingley Road, Cambridge CB3 0ES; †Animal Health Trust, Lanwades Park, Kentford, Newmarket CB8 7NN, Suffolk; and ‡Department of Veterinary Clinical Sciences, The Royal Veterinary College, Hawkshead Lane, North Mymms, Hatfield, Hertfordshire AL9 7TA, UK.

Keywords: horse; rhinitis; adenovirus; respiratory disease; rhinovirus

Summary

Equine rhinitis and adenoviruses typically cause mild, self limiting respiratory infections in all equids. More disease is seen in younger rather than older animals, in which natural immunity is thought to develop. The various viruses, their specific disease associations and their diagnosis, epidemiology and management are described in this review.

Equine rhinitis viruses

Equine rhinitis virus A and B were previously classified as equine rhinovirus-1, -2 and -3. They are common in horse populations but knowledge of their epidemiology, pathogenesis and association with disease is poor. Here they are referred to as rhinitis viruses.

The viruses

Several different picornaviruses have been isolated from horses (Plummer 1962; Studdert and Gleeson 1977; Mumford and Thomson 1978; Fukunaga *et al.* 1983); most are rhinitis viruses, which have been isolated from the respiratory tract, mouth, blood and faeces and most of which were previously referred to as rhinoviruses.

The rhinitis viruses were originally grouped into 3 categories, equine rhinovirus-1 (ERV-1), ERV-2 and ERV-3. ERV-1 has now been reclassified as equine rhinitis virus A (ERAV) (Varrasso *et al.* 2001). ERAV is one of 2 apthoviruses, the other being foot and mouth disease virus (Stanway *et al.* 2005). ERV-2 has been renamed equine rhinitis-B virus (ERBV) and has been reclassified as an *Erbovirus*, a new genus in the Picornaviridae (Hinton and Crabb 2001); detailed phenotypic and genetic analyses demonstrate division of ERBV into 3 distinct phylogenetic groups (Black and Studdert 2006), although it is likely that there is no direct clinical significance of this serologically cross reacting virus. ERV-3 has also recently been classified as an *Erbovirus* and named ERBV2 in view of its close sequence homology with ERBV (Huang *et al.* 2001). Another group of viruses, 'acid stable picornavirus' (ASPV) have also been isolated from the respiratory tract of horses in UK (Mumford and Thomson 1978) and Japan (Fukunaga *et al.* 1983). ASPV has now been reclassified as ERBV3 on the basis of sequence homology with other ERBVs (Black and Studdert 2006).

Infection with ERAV stimulates a long lasting neutralising antibody response, which is thought to prevent further disease, although repeated infections in racehorses in training can occur (Mumford 1994). Infection with ERAV does not stimulate cross reactive neutralising antibody to either ERBV (Mumford 1994; Mumford and Thomson 1978; Steck *et al.* 1978). There is little information on cell mediated immune responses to equine picornaviruses.

Clinical signs and pathogenesis

Both natural and experimental infection of seronegative horses with ERAV has been associated with pyrexia (<40.4°C) for up to 5 days, nasal discharge and swelling of pharyngeal lymph nodes and a moist cough (Plummer 1962; Plummer and Kerry 1962). Natural infections may frequently be

*Author to whom correspondence should be addressed.

sub-clinical, particularly in seropositive animals (Studdert and Gleeson 1978). ERAV has recently also been reported to be the cause of an abortion storm in dromedaries (Wernery *et al.* 2008).

Although ERBV infections may sometimes cause slight pyrexia and mild respiratory signs (Steck *et al.* 1978), infections are usually sub-clinical and infection of gnotobiotic foals failed to induce clinical signs of respiratory disease (Mumford and Thomson 1978). There is little or no information on the ability of ERBV2 to cause disease.

Equine rhinitis virus B3 was initially isolated from a Thoroughbred racehorse in training, although it was not showing signs of respiratory disease at the time (Mumford and Thomson 1978). Experimental infection of a gnotobiotic foal failed to produce signs of respiratory disease, but seroconversion did occur and virus was recovered from the animal. Serological investigations of naturally occurring outbreaks of respiratory disease have produced confusing results and there is little evidence that this virus is a cause of equine respiratory disease, although the very limited amount of work reported precludes firm conclusions from being drawn.

Diagnosis

Equine rhinitis virus infections may be diagnosed by isolation of virus in tissue culture, detection of viral RNA by PCR (Li *et al.* 1997; Black *et al.* 2007) or through demonstration of viral seroconversion using either CF or VN tests (Mumford and Thomson 1978).

Epidemiology

Equine rhinitis virus A has a world-wide distribution. Infection can spread by respiratory contact and outbreaks of disease associated with ERAV have been reported (Mumford 1994; Li *et al.* 1997). Prolonged excretion of ERAV in urine in racehorses is common, particularly in 2- and 3-year-olds (McCollum and Timoney 1992) and is probably an important source of infection.

Many foals in the UK remain seronegative to ERAV and racehorses usually experience their first ERAV infection in their second or third year, whilst in training (Powell *et al.* 1974). A similar situation has also been reported elsewhere, including North America (Holmes *et al.* 1978). During outbreaks, ERAV is highly contagious and transmission rates in naive populations may approach 100% (Holmes *et al.* 1978; Studdert and Gleeson 1978). Initial infections are usually associated with clinical signs (Burrows 1979; Li *et al.* 1997; Klaey *et al.* 1998), but repeated infections with ERAV, detectable in racehorses using the CF test (Mumford and Thomson 1978), are frequently not associated with signs of disease. Most foals become infected with ERBV during the first few months of life (Holmes *et al.* 1978; Burrows 1979) and repeated infections are frequently observed. It is clear that infections with ERBV and ERBV2 are common in Australia, where they have been most often studied (Huang *et al.* 2001). Most infections are not associated with obvious clinical signs.

Prevention

No commercially available equine rhinitis vaccines currently exist. However, ERAV infection stimulates such strong clinical immunity and immunisation with inactivated virus stimulates VN antibody and protection against experimental infection (Burrows 1979).

Due to the lack of commercially available vaccines, controlled infection programmes with ERAV in racehorses have been suggested as a means of ensuring that disease does not occur shortly before important race meetings, but so far have not been reported (Klaey *et al.* 1998).

No information is available on stimulation of immunity to ERBV or ERBV2, but natural infection may be associated with prolonged excretion (Fukunaga *et al.* 1983) and virus neutralising antibody levels are not maintained at high levels, suggesting that natural immunity may be poor.

Equine adenovirus

There are several reports of the isolation of equine adenovirus from foals (Wilks and Studdert 1972; Studdert *et al.* 1974; Dutta 1975; Whitlock *et al.* 1975; Konishi *et al.* 1977) and, less frequently, from adult horses, with pneumonia or signs of upper respiratory disease (unpublished observations). In some situations, the infection has been associated with diarrhoea (Studdert and Blackney 1982) or a loosening of faecal material (Powell *et al.* 1974; unpublished observations). While isolates are antigenically similar (Studdert 1978), there are 2 equine adenoviruses. (EqAdV1 and EqAdV2).

EqAdV1 has been isolated from the respiratory tracts of foals and horses in a wide variety of geographic locations. EqAdv2 has been isolated from lymph nodes and faeces of cases of diarrhoea (Studdert and Blackney 1982) and respiratory disease (Horner and Hunter 1982).

The infection can be diagnosed by isolation of virus, detection of viral DNA (Bell *et al.* 2006), or by demonstration of seroconversion using serum neutralisation tests or haemagglutination inhibition assays (Newton *et al.* 2003).

Equine adenovirus is a very important cause of morbidity and mortality in Arabian foals suffering from severe combined immunodeficiency (SCID) (Whitlock *et al.* 1975; Thompson *et al.* 1976; Perryman *et al.* 1978). In addition, the virus has been isolated from the spinal cord of a few horses with *cauda equina* neuritis (Edington *et al.* 1984), but its role, if any, in this rare disease, remains unclear.

Experimental infection studies have demonstrated that the virus can cause signs of respiratory disease, including mild nasal discharge, rhinitis, tracheitis, bronchopneumonia and an interstitial pneumonia (McChesney *et al.* 1974; Pascoe *et al.* 1974; Gleeson *et al.* 1978). Signs of disease were worsened in colostrum deprived foals and also diminished in foals aged >2 months compared to those aged 48 h. Clinical signs had largely resolved, even in colostrum deprived animals, within 10 days (McChesney *et al.* 1974).

Different serological surveys have demonstrated that antibodies to EqAdV1 are common in many horse populations, often being close to 100% (Studdert 1996). Antibodies to EqAdV2 also appear to be common (Studdert 1996). However, despite this, structured studies in both foals (Hoffman *et al.* 1993; Dunowska *et al.* 2002) and young Thoroughbred racehorses (Burrell *et al.* 1996; Christley *et al.* 2001; Dunowska *et al.* 2002; Newton *et al.* 2003; Wood *et al.* 2005) have failed to demonstrate any association between clinical respiratory disease and the presence of virus or seroconversion. Occasional outbreaks of respiratory disease or pyrexia in adult animals associated with adenovirus infection do undoubtedly occur, but, in the authors' experience, are not common.

Infection with equine adenovirus may be common, but the virus does not generally appear to be an important cause of equine disease, particularly in the adult. The advent of genetic tests that have markedly reduced the numbers of Arab foals born with SCID reduces the apparent significance of equine adenovirus further.

References

Bell, S.A., Leclere, M., Gardner, I.A. and Maclachlan, N.J. (2006) Equine adenovirus 1 infection of hospitalised and healthy foals and horses. *Equine vet. J.* **38**, 379-381.

Black, W.D., Hartley, C.A., Ficorilli, N.P. and Studdert, M.J. (2007) Reverse transcriptase-polymerase chain reaction for the detection equine rhinitis B viruses and cell culture isolation of the virus. *Arch. Virol.* **152**, 137-149.

Black, W.D. and Studdert, M.J. (2006) Formerly unclassified, acid-stable equine picornaviruses are a third equine rhinitis B virus serotype in the genus *Erbovirus*. *J. Gen. Virol.* **87**, 3023-3027.

Burrell, M.H., Wood, J.L., Whitwell, K.E., Chanter, N., Mackintosh, M.E. and Mumford, J.A. (1996) Respiratory disease in thoroughbred horses in training: the relationships between disease and viruses, bacteria and environment. *Vet. Rec.* **139**, 308-313.

Burrows, R. (1979) Equine rhinovirus and adenovirus infections. *Proc. Am. Ass. equine Practnrs.* **24**, 299-306.

Christley, R.M., Hodgson, D.R., Rose, R.J., Wood, J.L., Reids, S.W., Whitear, K.G. and Hodgson, J.L. (2001) A case-control study of respiratory disease in Thoroughbred racehorses in Sydney, Australia. *Equine vet. J.* **33**, 256-264.

Dunowska, M., Wilks, C.R., Studdert, M.J. and Meers, J. (2002) Equine respiratory viruses in foals in New Zealand. *N.Z. vet. J.* **50**, 140-147.

Dutta, S.K. (1975) Isolation and characterization of an adenovirus and isolation of its adenovirus-associated virus in cell culture from foals with respiratory tract disease. *Am. J. vet. Res.* **36**, 247-250.

Edington, N., Wright, J.A., Patel, J.R., Edwards, G.B. and Griffiths, L. (1984) Equine adenovirus 1 isolated from *cauda equina* neuritis. *Res. vet. Sci.* **37**, 252-254.

Fukunaga, Y., Kumanimodo, T., Kamada, M. and Wada, R. (1983) Equine picornavirus: isolation of virus from the oral cavity of healthy horses. *Bulletin of the Equine Research Institute* **20**, 103-109.

Gleeson, L.J., Studdert, M.J. and Sullivan, N.D. (1978) Pathogenicity and immunologic studies of equine adenovirus in specific-pathogen-free foals. *Am. J. vet. Res.* **39**, 1636-1642.

Hinton, T.M. and Crabb, B.S. (2001) The novel picornavirus equine rhinitis B virus contains a strong type II internal ribosomal entry site which functions similarly to that of encephalomyocarditis virus. *J. Gen. Virol.* **82**, 2257-2269.

Hoffman, A.M., Viel, L., Prescott, J.F., Rosendal, S. and Thorsen, J. (1993) Association of microbiologic flora with clinical, endoscopic, and pulmonary cytologic findings in foals with distal respiratory tract infection. *Am. J. vet. Res.* **54**, 1615-1622.

Holmes, D.F., Kemen, M.J. and Coggins, L. (1978) Equine rhinovirus infection - serological evidence of infection in selected United States horse populations. In: *Proceedings of the Fourth International Conference on Equine Infectious Diseases*, Eds: J.T. Bryans and H. Gerber, Veterinary Publications, Lyon. pp 315-319.

Horner, G.W. and Hunter, R. (1982) Isolation of two serotypes of equine adenovirus from horses in New Zealand. *N. Z. vet. J.* **30**, 62-64.

Huang, J.A., Ficorilli, N., Hartley, C.A., Wilcox, R.S., Weiss, M. and Studdert, M.J. (2001) Equine rhinitis B virus: a new serotype. *J. Gen. Virol.* **82**, 2641-2645.

Klaey, M., Sanchez-Higgins, M., Leadon, D.P., Cullinane, A., Straub, R. and Gerber, H. (1998) Field case study of equine rhinovirus 1 infection: clinical signs and clinicopathology. *Equine vet. J.* **30**, 267-269.

Konishi, S.I., Harasawa, R., Mochizuki, M., Akashi, H. and Ogata, M. (1977) Studies on equine adenovirus. I. Characteristics of an adenovirus isolated from a Thoroughbred colt with pneumonia. *Nippon Juigaku Zasshi* **39**, 117-125.

Li, F., Drummer, H.E., Ficorilli, N., Studdert, M.J. and Crabb, B.S. (1997) Identification of noncytopathic equine rhinovirus 1 as a cause of acute febrile respiratory disease in horses. *J. clin. Microbiol.* **35**, 937-943.

McChesney, A.E., England, J.J., Whiteman, C.E., Adcock, J.L., Rich, L.J. and Chow, T.L. (1974) Experimental transmission of equine adenovirus in Arabian and non-Arabian foals. *Am. J. vet. Res.* **35**, 1015-1023.

McCollum, W.H. and Timoney, P.J. (1992) Studies on the seroprevalence and frequency of equine rhinovirus-I and -II infection in normal horse urine. In: *Proceedings of the Sixth International Conference on Equine Infectious Diseases*, Eds: W. Plowright, P.D. Rossdale and J.F. Wade, R&W Publications, Newmarket. pp 83-87.

Mumford, J.A. (1994) Equine rhinovirus infections. In: *Infectious Diseases of Livestock with Special Reference to South Africa*, Eds: J.A.W. Coetzer, G.R. Thomson, R.C. Tustin and N.P.J. Kriek, Oxford University Press, Oxford. pp 820-822.

Mumford, J.A. and Thomson, G.R. (1978) Studies on picornaviruses isolated from the respiratory tract of horses. In: *Proceedings of the Fourth International Conference on Equine Infectious Diseases*, Eds: J.T. Bryans and H. Gerber, Veterinary Publications, Lyon. pp 419-429.

Newton, J.R., Wood, J.L. and Chanter, N. (2003) A case control study of factors and infections associated with clinically apparent respiratory disease in UK Thoroughbred racehorses. *Prev. vet. Med.* **60**, 107-132.

Pascoe, R.R., Harden, T.J. and Spradbrow, P.B. (1974) Letter: Experimental infection of a horse with an equine adenovirus. *Aust. vet. J.* **50**, 278-279.

Perryman, L.E., McGuire, T.C. and Crawford, T.B. (1978) Maintenance of foals with combined immunodeficiency: causes and control of secondary infections. *Am. J. vet. Res.* **39**, 1043-1047.

Plummer, G. (1962) An equine respiratory virus with enterovirus properties. *Nature* **195**, 519-520.

Plummer, G. and Kerry, J.B. (1962) Studies on an equine respiratory virus. *Vet. Rec.* **74**, 967-970.

Powell, D.G., Burrows, R. and Goodridge, D. (1974) Respiratory viral infections among thoroughbred horses in training during 1972. *Equine vet. J.* **6**, 19-24.

Stanway, G., Brown, F., Christian, P., Hovi, T., Hyypiä, T., King, A.M.Q., Knowles, N.J., Lemon, S.M., Minor, P.D. *et al.* (2005) Family Picornaviridae. In: *Virus Taxonomy. Eighth Report of the International Committee on Taxonomy of Viruses*, Eds: C.M. Fauquet, M.A. Mayo, J. Maniloff, U. Desselberger and L.A. Ball, Elsevier/Academic Press, Amsterdam. pp 757-778.

Steck, F., Hofer, B., Schaeren, B., Nicolet, J. and Gerber, H. (1978) Equine rhinoviruses: new serotypes. In: *Proceedings of the Fourth International Conference on Equine Infectious Diseases,* Eds: J.T. Bryans and H. Gerber, Veterinary Publications, Lyon. pp 321-328.

Studdert, M.J. (1978) Antigenic homogeneity of equine adenoviruses. *Aust. vet. J.* **54**, 263-264.

Studdert, M.J. (1996) Equine adenovirus infections. In: *Virus Infections of Equines*, Ed: M.J. Studdert, Elsevier Science, Amsterdam. pp 67-80.

Studdert, M.J. and Blackney, M.H. (1982) Isolation of an adenovirus antigenically distinct from equine adenovirus type 1 from diarrheic foal feces. *Am. J. vet. Res.* **43**, 543-544.

Studdert, M.J. and Gleeson, L.J. (1977) Isolation of equine rhinovirus type 1. *Aust. vet. J.* **53**, 452.

Studdert, M.J. and Gleeson, L.J. (1978) Isolation and characterisation of an equine rhinovirus. *Zentralbl Veterinarmed B.* **25**, 225-237.

Studdert, M.J., Wilks, C.R. and Coggins, L. (1974) Antigenic comparisons and serologic survey of equine adenoviruses. *Am. J. vet. Res.* **35**, 693-699.

Thompson, D.B., Spradbrow, P.B. and Studdert, M. (1976) Isolation of an adenovirus from an Arab foal with a combined immunodeficiency disease. *Aust. vet. J.* **52**, 435-437.

Varrasso, A., Drummer, H.E., Huang, J.A., Stevenson, R.A., Ficorilli, N., Studdert, M.J. and Hartley, C.A. (2001) Sequence conservation and antigenic variation of the structural proteins of equine rhinitis A virus. *J. Virol.* **75**, 10550-10556.

Wernery, U., Knowles, N.J., Hamblin, C., Wernery, R., Joseph, S., Kinne, J. and Nagy, P. (2008) Abortions in dromedaries (*Camelus dromedarius*) caused by equine rhinitis A virus. *J. Gen. Virol.* **89**, 660-666.

Whitlock, R.H., Dellers, R.W. and Shively, J.N. (1975) Adenoviral pneumonia in a foal. *Cornell Vet.* **65**, 393-401.

Wilks, C.R. and Studdert, M.J. (1972) Isolation of an equine adenovirus. *Aust. vet. J.* **48**, 580-581.

Wood, J.L., Newton, J.R., Chanter, N. and Mumford, J.A. (2005) Association between respiratory disease and bacterial and viral infections in British racehorses. *J. clin. Microbiol.* **43**, 120-126.

EQUINE INFECTIOUS ANAEMIA

R. F. Cook*, S. J. Cook and C. J. Issel

Department of Veterinary Science, Gluck Equine Research Center, University of Kentucky, Lexington, Kentucky 40546, USA.

Keywords: horse; lentivirus; pathogenesis; epidemiology; transmission; diagnosis and control; Coggins test

Summary

Equine infectious anaemia (EIA) is a disease caused by an equid-specific lentivirus related to HIV-1. Although EIA virus (EIAV) can induce considerable morbidity and sometimes mortality, persistent infection does not result in chronic immunodeficiency. In fact, the immune system of most exposed equids will eventually acquire the power to limit the extent of viral replication and thus prevent the recurrence of disease, resulting in the so-called 'inapparent carrier' stage of EIA. However, while these animals may appear healthy, they remain infected and therefore reservoirs of the virus. Transmission of EIA is mainly via contaminated blood. Although under natural conditions this is accomplished primarily by large blood-feeding insects such as horseflies, man is by far the most efficient vector of this virus. In the absence of effective vaccines, control of EIA is reliant on identification and segregation of infected individuals. A summary of the most important EIA facts is shown in **Table 1**.

TABLE 1: Snapshot facts about equine infectious anaemia (EIA)

Causative agent	Equine lentivirus EIA virus
Duration of infection	Persists for life
Clinical signs	Recurring fever, petechia, anaemia, cachexia (most infections are found in equids without overt clinical signs)
Transmission	Blood-borne by man and insects (mechanical)
Diagnosis	Detection of specific antibody in ELISA and AGID (Coggins) tests
Control	Testing and segregation by 200 yards (183 m)
Treatment/vaccine	None available

Virus properties

Equine infectious anaemia virus (EIAV) is classified within the lentivirus genus of the *Retroviridae* family, with a host range restricted to members of the *Equidae*. In terms of genetic organisation, EIAV is the simplest known lentivirus resulting in it being dubbed the 'country cousin' of HIV (Leroux *et al.* 2004). Despite this seemingly inferior designation, EIAV utilises a sophisticated array of strategies to avoid elimination by the immune responses of its host and establish persistent infections.

Equine infectious anaemia (EIA) was one of the first diseases proven to have a viral aetiology (Vallée and Carré 1904). Electron microscopy of the virus reveals oval or circular particles having mean diameter of 115 nm with a conical internal core structure that is typical of lentiviruses, surrounded by a proteinaceous matrix and bounded by a lipid membrane (**Fig 1**) containing numerous 6–8 nm projections (Matheka *et al.* 1976; Weiland *et al.* 1977). Within the core are 2 copies of the single stranded RNA genome that at approximately 8.1 kb is 17% smaller than the genome of HIV-1. In common with all members of the *Retroviridae* this genome contains (**Fig 2**) 3 major structural genes (*gag*, *pol* and *env*) flanked by repeated elements containing regulatory sequences. In addition to these major genes, all lentiviruses encode ancillary proteins that vary from 3 in EIAV (Tat, S2 and Rev) to 6 in complex lentiviruses such as HIV-1. The EIAV Tat and Rev are involved in viral replication and while S2 is essential for virulence its function is unknown (Li *et al.* 2000). **Table 2** shows a summary of the properties of all EIAV encoded proteins.

Replication of wild-type EIAV isolates occurs primarily in cells of the monocyte/macrophage lineage (McGuire *et al.* 1971; McConnel *et al.* 1977; Evans *et*

*Author to whom correspondence should be addressed.

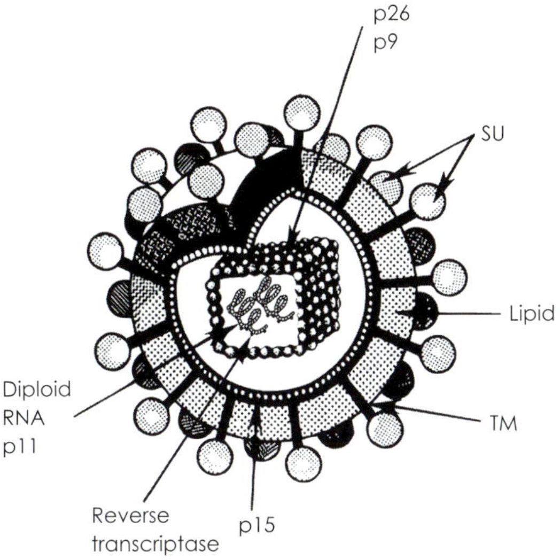

FIGURE 1: Structural model of the EIAV particle showing probable locations of the major structural antigens. Organisation of the envelope glycoproteins (depicted as monomers) is unknown although they form a trimeric structure in HIV-1.

al. 1984; Sellon *et al.* 1992) although some strains can replicate in endothelial cells (Maury *et al.* 1998; Oaks *et al.* 1999). EIAV will not replicate in fibroblastic cell-types without adaptation, a process that is associated with extensive genetic and phenotypic changes including loss of virulence (Malmquist *et al.* 1973; Gutekunst and Becvar 1979; Orrego *et al.* 1982; Carpenter and Chesebro 1989). When EIAV infects monocytes, viral proteins are not produced and the viral replication cycle is not completed until differentiation into a mature tissue macrophage occurs (Sellon *et al.* 1992; Maury 1994). Consequently, once internalised by monocytes EIAV is not exposed to immunological surveillance. As a result these cells may act as efficient 'stealth carriers' for disseminating the virus around the body. EIAV enters its host cell following attachment of the viral surface unit (SU) envelope glycoprotein to a molecule on the cell surface (equine lentivirus receptor 1, ELR1) recently identified as a member of the tumour necrosis factor family of receptor proteins (Zhang *et al.* 2005). This

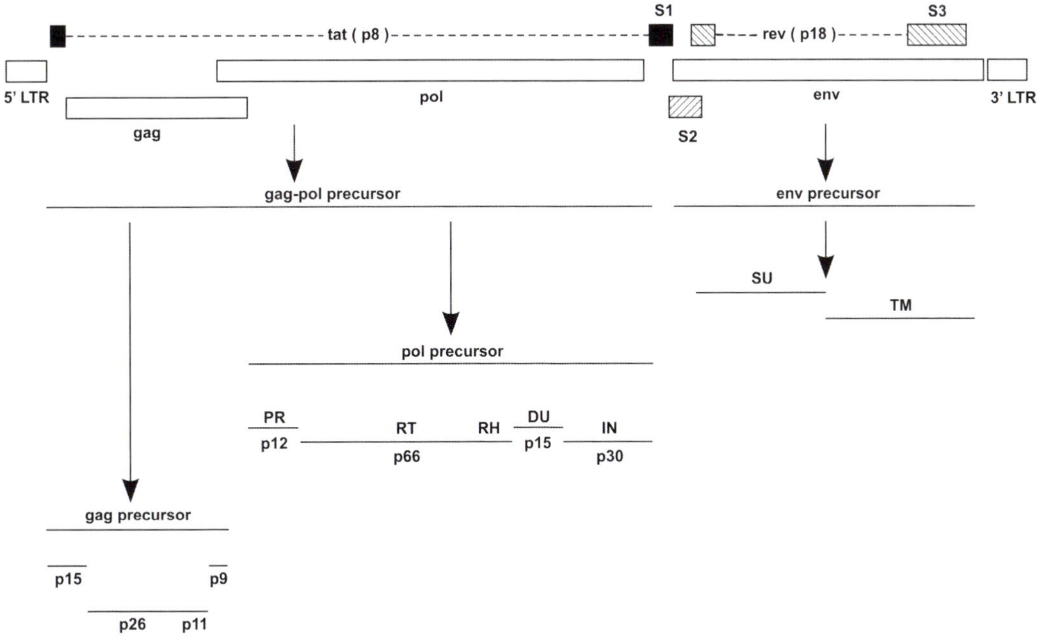

FIGURE 2: EIAV proviral genome organisation. The structural proteins of EIAV are produced from polyprotein precursor molecules. Individual Gag and Pol proteins are cleaved by a virally encoded Protease whereas the SU and TM envelope glycoproteins are produced by the action of host-cell specified proteases. LTR, long terminal repeat; PR, protease; RT-RH, reverse transcriptase-RNase H; DU, dUTPase; IN, integrase; tat, transcriptional trans-activator; rev, regulator of viral mRNA splicing and transport; SU, surface unit glycoprotein; TM, transmembrane glycoprotein.

TABLE 2: Structural and regulatory proteins specified by the EIAV genome. The apparent molecular weights (kDa) and functional properties of these proteins are reviewed previously by Leroux *et al.* (2004) or described in text

Gene	Product	kDa	Functional properties
Gag	Matrix	15	Structural protein. Critical for virus assembly.
	Capsid (p26)	26	Structural protein. Predominant component of the viral core.
	Nucleocapsid	11	Structural protein. Binds to the viral RNA genome. Also has topoisomerase 1 activity.
	p9	9	Structural protein. Contains YPDL late domain required for virus particle budding. N-terminal 32 amino acid important in viral DNA production.
Pol	Protease	12	Cleavage and processing of the *gag* and *pol* polyprotein precursors.
	Reverse transcriptase (RT)	66 51	Converts the single stranded viral RNA genome into a double-stranded DNA copy following infection of the host cell. Also degrades viral RNA during the process of dsDNA synthesis (RNase H activity). RT exists as homo- and heterodimers of p66 and p51 subunits. Although both subunits have polymerase activity, only p66 has RNase H activity.
	dUTPase	15	Hydrolyses dUTP to dUMP and inorganic phosphate. Essential for efficient replication *in vivo*.
	Integrase	30	Promotes integration of viral cDNA into host cell chromatin.
Env	Surface unit (SU) Transmembrane (TM)	90 45	The SU and TM glycoproteins are produced from an envelope polyprotein. following cleavage with host-specified proteases. SU binds to equine lentivirus receptor-1 (ELR1) while TM promotes fusion between viral and endocytotic vesicle membranes.
S1	Second exon of the transactivator (tat) protein	8	Regulates viral transcription.
S2	S2	7	Not known but S2 viral deletion mutants have attenuated pathogenicity.
S3	Second exon of *rev*	18	Regulates viral RNA splicing.

interaction triggers clathrin-mediated endocytosis and once inside the endocytotic vesicle the resultant low pH stimulates fusion between the viral and vesicle lipid membranes (Brindley and Maury 2005, 2008) thereby releasing the viral core into the cytoplasm where the single-stranded viral RNA genome is transformed into a double stranded DNA copy by the viral reverse transcriptase. Eventually, this 'proviral DNA' will be transported to the nucleus where it may subsequently be integrated into host cell chromosomal DNA by the virally specified integrase enzyme. Host cell transcription factors, RNA polymerase II and the cellular protein synthesis machinery are responsible for producing all the viral components required to complete the replication cycle.

Clinical features

Classical cases of EIA progress through 3 distinct clinical phases. The initial or acute episode is generally transitory, lasting 1–3 days in which the main clinical signs are fever and thrombocytopenia. Although reductions in platelets can promote petechial haemorrhaging on mucous membranes, they are not usually sufficient to produce overt defects in the coagulation cascade. Therefore, acute episodes of EIA may be overlooked or misdiagnosed. The initial febrile episode may then be followed by a prolonged period (generally 12 months but can be longer) of recurring disease cycles termed the chronic phase in which fever and thrombocytopenia are accompanied by anaemia, oedema, depressed neurological reactions and cachexia. If the animal survives, the frequency of disease episodes will gradually diminish until it enters a very prolonged period (that can last for the remainder of the animal's life) where obvious signs of disease are completely absent. This phase is the inapparent carrier stage because the animal appears clinically normal but as it is infected with EIAV, it remains a reservoir for transmission. Although this description of EIA is the one commonly found in textbooks the actual clinical signs associated with EIAV exposure are highly variable and may range from a completely asymptomatic infection to severe peracute disease where the animal is unable to control primary viral replication, resulting in constant fever, plummeting platelet levels and eventually death. A consequence of the extensive variation in clinical signs is that they are not a reliable indicator of EIA. Factors

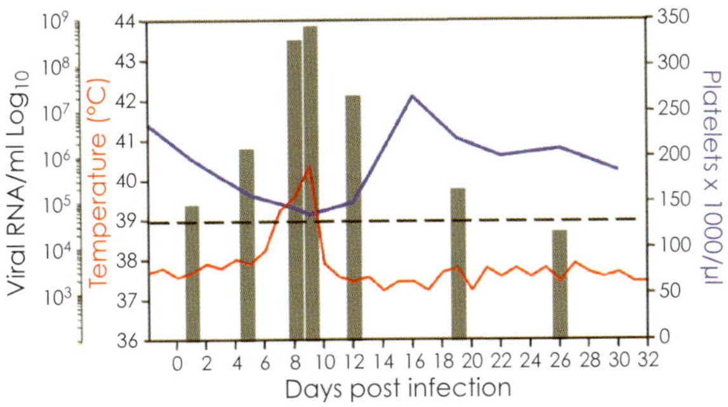

FIGURE 3: Correlation between plasma-associated viral RNA burden and clinical signs of acute EIA. The rectal temperature (red) and platelet level (blue) expressed as platelets/µl of blood are shown in comparison with plasma-associated EIAV RNA burden (log_{10}/ml, solid bars).

responsible for significant variation in clinical signs are discussed below.

Pathogenesis of disease

In animals infected with EIAV, there is a very close relationship between overt signs of disease and amounts of virus present (**Fig 3**). Tissue associated viral burdens are at their highest levels during febrile episodes and decline several orders of magnitude concomitant with the resolution of clinical signs. It has been demonstrated that amounts of tissue-associated EIAV must reach a critical or threshold value in order to trigger disease (Cook *et al.* 2003). The observed variation in clinical signs may therefore be interpreted in the context of threshold viral burdens. Following acute infection, disease in normal, fully immunocompetent horses will only be produced if the inoculum strain of EIAV reaches or exceeds the threshold viral burden level before primary immune responses effectively limit viral replication. Therefore, to induce disease the infecting virus must possess sufficient replicative potential within its host. Although the spectrum of virulence among naturally occurring EIAV strains has not been rigorously determined it is known that any mutation in the viral genome that reduces viral replication rates *in vivo* will attenuate pathogenicity (Threadgill *et al.* 1993; Lichtenstein *et al.* 1995; Cook *et al.* 1998, 2003). In addition to viral replicative ability, differences between individual animals and between species of equid also play a significant role in the appearance of clinical signs following infection with EIAV. For example, in an experiment involving infection of horses/ponies with identical amounts of a pathogenic strain of EIAV derived from an infectious molecular clone it was observed that some animals could control acute viral replication more efficiently and as a result had no obvious disease signs (Cook *et al.* 2003). Furthermore, a comparison between different species of equid infected with horse virulent EIAV strains showed that donkeys remained clinically unaffected and that their peak viral titres were at least 1000-fold lower than in horses or ponies (Cook *et al.* 2001). A supplemental conclusion from research in different species is that once EIAV has been adapted to one equid host it may not replicate optimally in another equid species.

Many of the clinical signs associated with acute EIA are caused by pro-inflammatory mediators released in response to tissue associated viral burdens reaching the threshold level and are not dependent on the development of viral-specific adaptive immune responses. This is demonstrated by the fact acute EIA signs occur in foals that lack mature T or B cells because of inherited severe combined immunodeficiency (SCID) disease (Crawford *et al.* 1996; Tornquist *et al.* 1997). The pathology of lentiviral-mediated disease is augmented by the fact that infection of macrophages by this group of viruses disrupts the regulation of host-cell gene expression to produce increases in the production of pro-inflammatory molecules such as tumour necrosis factor alpha (TNFα), interleukin 1 (IL-1α and IL-1β) and interleukin 6 (IL-6) (Yoo *et al.* 1996; Esser *et al.* 1996; Lechner *et al.* 1997; Swardson *et al.* 1997; Lim *et al.* 2005). This has been demonstrated in equine monocyte-derived macrophage cultures where infection with pathogenic strains of EIAV produces significant increases in the production of these cytokines (Lim *et al.* 2005) and during acute disease where significantly elevated blood levels of TNFα, IL-6 and transforming growth factor β (TGFβ) have been observed (Costa *et al.* 1997; Tornquist *et al.* 1997; Sellon *et al.* 1999). IL-1, IL-6 and TNFα can induce febrile responses by activating the arachidonic pathway to increase production of prostaglandin E2 (PGE2). In addition to inducing febrile reactions, the cytokines released in response to EIAV infection may also cause thrombocytopenia. For example, TNFα and TGFβ have both been shown to suppress equine megakaryocyte colony growth (Tornquist and Crawford 1997) and in the mouse model injection with

TNFα alone induces a profound thrombocytopenia by stimulating cells expressing the widely distributed 55 kDa tumour necrosis factor receptor 1 (TNFR1) to release platelet agonists such as thrombin, plasmin and serotonin (Tacchini-Cottier *et al.* 1998). Excessive TNFα production may also contribute to anaemia in EIAV infected animals because it has the ability to suppress erythropoiesis (Moldawer *et al.* 1989; Zamai *et al.* 2000; Dufour *et al.* 2003; Felli *et al.* 2005). However, it is not the only mechanism because extensive phagocytosis of complement C3 coated erythrocytes also occurs in these animals, resulting in the presence of haemosiderin granules in the macrophages found in organs such as the liver, spleen and lymph nodes (Perryman *et al.* 1971; Sentsui and Kono 1987).

While clinical signs of acute EIA can be attributable to the storm of pro-inflammatory cytokines released in response to the burden of tissue-associated EIAV attaining the critical threshold level, adaptive immune responses, when present, also play a role in the pathogenesis of EIA. For example, platelets from EIAV infected horses have significant levels of bound IgG or IgM and so become destined for immune mediated destruction contributing to splenomegaly and hepatomegaly (Banks *et al.* 1972; Clabough *et al.* 1991). Furthermore, the glomeruli in the kidneys of chronically infected animals often show thickening of the glomerular tufts with both mesangial and epithelial cell proliferation. These diseased glomeruli have both immunoglobulin and complement C3 deposited at the basement membranes and mesangial areas (Henson and McGuire 1971).

EIAV and genetic variation

The ability to undergo rapid, extensive genetic variation is one of the main factors contributing to pathogenesis and persistence in lentiviral infections. This ability enables lentiviruses to respond quickly to environmental pressures such as those exerted by the immune system. Each febrile episode in an EIAV infected animal is caused by a different antigenic variant as defined by antibody neutralisation studies (Kono 1969; Kono *et al.* 1973; Montelaro *et al.* 1984; O'Rourke *et al.* 1989; Leroux *et al.* 2001). In addition, this phenomenon of 'antigenic drift' also extends to the viral epitopes recognised by cytotoxic T cells (CTL), particularly if these cells have the high-avidity binding phenotype associated with the efficient clearance of infected cells (Mealey *et al.* 2003). Therefore, EIAV infections are characterised by constantly changing viral populations whose evolution is driven by selective forces consisting of immunological pressure and the requirement for efficient replication, a phenomenon known as biological fitness. Mutational studies with EIAV have demonstrated that these forces are sometimes diametrically opposed in that genetic changes associated with antigenic variation will significantly decrease replication rates unless they are accompanied by complimentary nucleotide substitutions elsewhere in the viral genome (R.F. Cook, unpublished observations). As a result, the viral populations associated with each febrile episode represent a unique solution to balance avoidance of host immune responses with replicative efficiency. The twin engines driving this dynamic evolutionary process are genetic recombination, facilitated by the presence of 2 copies of the viral genome per virus particle and properties associated with the viral reverse transcriptase. This enzyme has no proofreading ability and has been shown to have an error rate of one nucleotide substitution for every 10,000 incorporated (Preston *et al.* 1988; Roberts *et al.* 1988; Bakhanashvili and Hizi 1993). Effectively, this means that during every replication cycle there is a high probability that at least one nucleotide substitution will introduced during proviral DNA synthesis. Therefore, the process of EIAV replication rapidly transforms a single infectious particle into a swarm of related but genetically distinct viruses called a 'quasispecies'. This type of progressively divergent population increases the probability that viral variants will be generated that can respond to new environmental selection pressures. The quasispecies is therefore an excellent substrate for the evolutionary process.

Host immune responses

Antibodies against EIAV may be detected in sensitive immunoblot or ELISA tests as early as 14–28 days post infection (PI) although most reports indicate they are non-neutralising. Strain specific neutralising antibodies are not generally observed until 38–87 days PI and may not reach maximal levels until

90–148 days PI (Kono *et al.* 1973; O'Rourke *et al.* 1988; Rwambo *et al.* 1990; Ball *et al.* 1992; Hammond *et al.* 1997), generally long after the acute disease episode has been resolved. As cytotoxic lymphocytes (CTL) can be detected in experimental infections at 14 days pi (Mealey *et al.* 2005) it is currently believed that cell-mediated and not humoural immune responses are responsible for initial control of EIAV infections. Once acute viral replication has been controlled the animal will remain free of overt clinical signs until a variant virus emerges that can evade immunological surveillance.

If EIAV has seemingly limitless mutational capacity, what terminates the recurring disease cycles and how do animals attain inapparent carrier status?

At one time it was thought there might be selective pressure to limit pathogenicity in the host and to ensure the progressive attenuation of EIAV (Belshan *et al.* 1998). However, viruses transferred from inapparent carrier equids often produce disease in naïve recipients. Furthermore, recrudescence of clinical signs can be induced in carriers by immunosuppression with corticosteroids (Kono *et al.* 1976; Tumas *et al.* 1994; Craigo *et al.* 2002; Howe *et al.* 2005). These observations suggest the immune system and not viral attenuation is primarily responsible for the eventual cessation of clinical signs in EIAV infected animals. To envisage how this might occur, it is necessary to consider evolution the mammalian immune system in response to lentiviral infections. Cell-mediated and humoural immune responses to new infections are restricted by the phenomenon of immunodominance to just a handful of the many potential epitopes within microbial pathogens (Borysiewicz *et al.* 1988; Pamer *et al.* 1991; Busch and Pamer 1998; Rodriguez *et al.* 2002; Yu *et al.* 2002; Kedl *et al.* 2003). Furthermore, immunodominance does not always translate into an effective immune response. EIAV epitopes recognised by high-avidity immunodominant CTL are subject to rapid mutational changes with the original sequences disappearing from the viral population (Mealey *et al.* 2003).

In contrast, low or even moderate avidity immunodominant CTL do not appear to have substantially detrimental effects on the survival of EIAV and epitopes bound by these less efficient T cells can persist in the viral population (Mealey *et al.* 2003, 2005). Therefore, the initial adaptive immune response to EIAV is likely to consist of the eventual appearance of strain specific neutralising antibodies coupled with a very limited number of effective CTLs. While this is apparently sufficient to resolve acute disease, it is easy to envisage how a highly mutable virus such as EIAV could evade these initial immune responses by producing escape mutants with the replicative capacity to induce additional clinical episodes. As such, it appears the immune system is locked into a constant cycle of 'catch-up'. However, this cycle may be broken by a gradual broadening of the immune responses leading to the recognition of a greater number of epitopes including some that may be conserved because of functional constraints.

The result of these enhanced responses is that complete escape from immunological surveillance becomes extremely difficult unless there is suppression of the immune system. For example, the number of CTL epitopes recognised in some HIV positive patients increases from 2 during symptomatic acute infection to 27 after 18 months (Yu *et al.* 2002). The fact that relatively large numbers of T-helper and CTL epitopes can be identified within just the viral envelope glycoproteins 7 months after infection with an attenuated EIAV strain (Tagmyer *et al.* 2007) suggests a similar broadening of the immune response occur in the horse. An important additional consideration is that unlike HIV, EIAV does not infect T-helper cells and does not produce immunodeficiency. Therefore, in the case of EIAV infected equids broader cell-mediated immune responses are likely to remain protective for very long periods consistent with inapparent carrier status. In addition, antibody responses in EIAV infected animals gradually evolve from low-avidity interactions with linear epitopes to high-avidity binding with predominantly conformational epitopes (Hammond *et al.* 1997). Neutralising antibodies also evolve from being highly strain specific to more generally reactive. However, while more broadly reactive cell-mediated and humoural immune responses may eventually restrict EIAV replication and prevent disease they are not sufficient to completely eradicate the virus.

Epidemiology

EIAV has a worldwide distribution. In regions where the virus has been endemic for many years, it is likely that the majority of cases will be inapparent carriers. Furthermore, when new infections occur in such regions they may go unnoticed because of mild or variable clinical signs and so local owners may be completely unaware of the extent of the infection.

Although EIA is best thought of as a blood-borne infection all tissues and body fluids should be considered as potentially infectious especially during clinical episodes when viral burdens are high. Viral nucleic acids have been detected in nasal swabs and swabs taken from the buccal cavity and genitalia (Quinlivan *et al.* 2007). Infectious virus has also been detected in milk by inoculation in susceptible horses (Stein and Mott 1942, 1946) although foals allowed to nurse from this material remained noninfected suggesting virus is not absorbed through the gut. EIAV may also be transmitted *in utero* although this only seems to occur if the mare experiences a clinical episode during gestation (Kemen and Coggins 1972) suggesting that high viral burdens are essential before EIAV can cross the placenta. The fact that foals of inapparent carriers have proven to be at low risk of acquiring the infection either during pregnancy or through weaning, even in areas of high vector populations, provides support for this hypothesis (McConnico *et al.* 2000; Issel and McConnico 2001). An observation that stallions had a higher incidence of the infection within a feral horse population suggests yet another potential mechanism for the dissemination of EIAV is via behavioural characteristics such as fighting/biting (Issel *et al.* 1998).

Although different modes of EIAV transmission are recognised, the most important is by the transfer

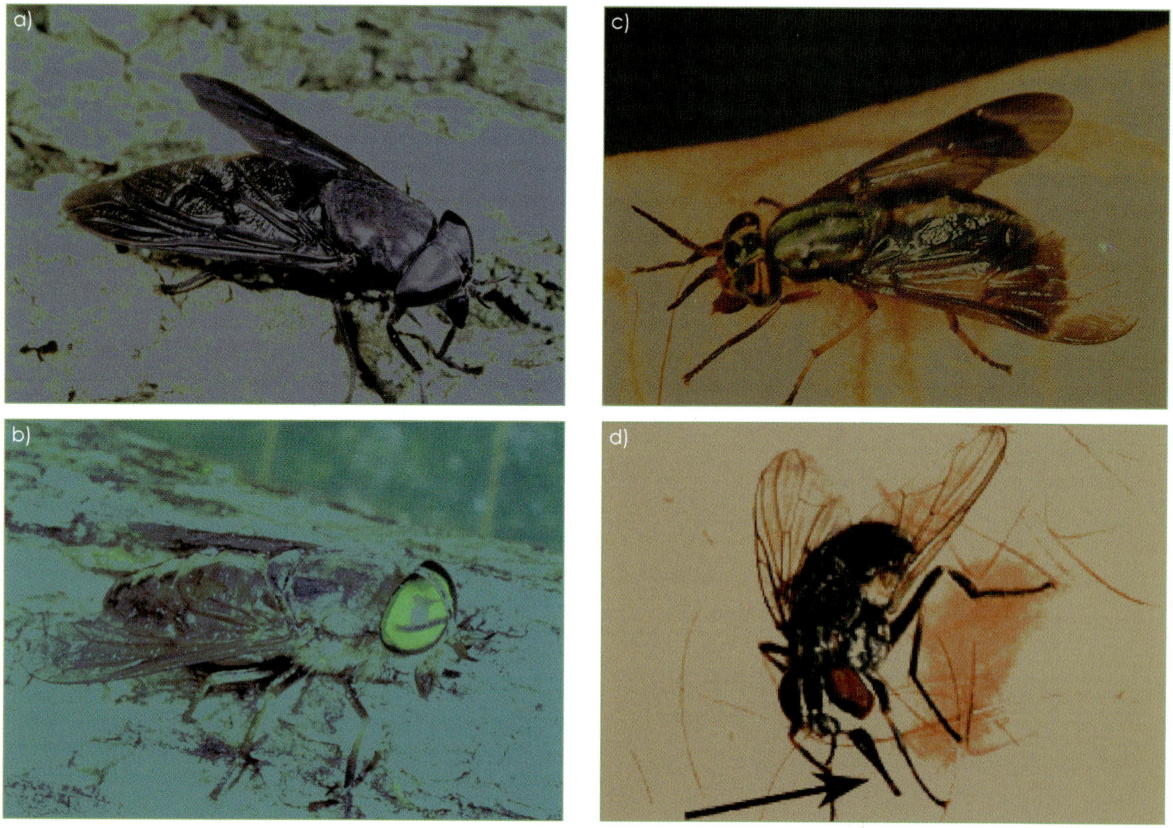

FIGURE 4: Haematophagous insects implicated in EIAV transmission. Tabanids shown are 2 horse fly species (a and b) and a deer fly species (c), photos provided by Dr R. Bessin, Department of Entomology, University of Kentucky. A stable fly (Stomoxys calcitrans), photograph by Dr L. Higley Department of Entomology, University of Nebraska-Lincoln, is shown in d) with arrow pointing at the stout proboscis.

of contaminated blood, conducted under natural conditions primarily by blood-feeding insects (**Fig 4**). EIAV does not replicate in insects or in insect cell lines (Shen *et al.* 1978; Williams *et al.* 1981; Issel and Foil 1984) demonstrating that transmission by arthropods is purely mechanical. This means that the probability of transmission is directly proportional to the volume of blood retained on the mouthparts after feeding and so it is not surprising that only larger biting flies of the order *Diptera* (stable flies, *Stomoxys calcitrans*; deer flies, *Chrysops* spp.; and horse flies *Tabanus* spp., *Hybomitra* spp. *et al.*) are implicated as vectors (Stein *et al.* 1942; Hawkins *et al.* 1973, 1976; Kemen *et al.* 1978; Foil *et al.* 1983; Issel and Foil 1984). Despite one published account (Stein *et al.* 1943) mosquitoes are not thought to be important for transmission and secretions from their mouthparts may actually rapidly inactivate EIAV (Williams *et al.* 1981). For mechanical transmission to occur the fly must initiate feeding on an EIAV-infected subject and then be interrupted (for example by defensive movements) so that it transfers to a new susceptible host. If an insect feeds to repletion it will not generally seek a second host and thus ceases being a potential vector. Although many insects in the order *Diptera* are strong fliers, once their feeding is interrupted, the decision to return to the original or seek a new host is based on proximity. From experimental measurements it has been extrapolated that 99% of horse flies will return to the original host if an alternative is 50 or more metres away (Issel and Foil 1984). This provides strong support for the 200 yard segregation distance imposed by many state regulatory agencies in the USA for the quarantine of EIAV infected equids.

Successful insect mediated transmission of EIAV is dependent on levels of virus present in blood at the time of feeding and on the amounts carried on the mouthparts. For example, the blood volume retained on the mouthparts of *Tabanus fuscicostatus* is 10 ± 5 nl (Foil *et al.* 1987). Therefore, if this insect feeds on a horse during a clinical episode when the blood-associated titre of EIAV may equal or exceed 10^6 horse infectious doses (HID_{50})/ml there could be as many as 5–15 infectious viruses retained on the mouthparts suggesting the possibility of transmission by a single fly-bite. Experimental studies in which *T. fuscicostatus* was permitted to feed on donor animals with clinical EIA before being transferred to naïve recipient ponies have demonstrated the probability that EIAV can be transmitted by a single fly-bite under optimal conditions is 1 in 7 (Hawkins *et al.* 1976). This experiment demonstrates there is a very high risk of transmission when animals experiencing clinical episodes of EIA are present in the population. Furthermore, this risk increases dramatically in regions where insect vector densities are high and where thousands of vector feeding attempts may occur on one horse during a 24 h period (Foil *et al.* 1985). In contrast to animals with clinical signs of EIA, inapparent carriers frequently have blood associated EIAV titres of about 1 HID_{50}/ml (Issel *et al.* 1982). At a titre of 1 HID_{50}/ml the probability of an EIAV particle being present on the mouthparts of a single *T. fuscicostatus* after interrupted feeding is only 1 in 67,000–200,000.

Although insect-mediated transfer from EIAV infected animals with high viraemia burdens is relatively efficient by far the most effective vector of this virus is man. Occasionally, human transmission may involve fomites such as riding bits or tooth-rasps but the greatest threat is via iatrogenic transfer. Infectious EIAV can be recovered from hypodermic needles for periods up to 96 h in contrast to the <4 h from insect mouthparts (Hawkins *et al.* 1976; Williams *et al.* 1981). Furthermore, the residual volumes of blood left in hypodermic syringes and needles is likely to be 1000- or even 10,000-fold greater than that transferred by insects. A particularly graphic illustration of iatrogenic transfer recently occurred in Europe where the 2006 EIA outbreaks in Ireland and Italy are believed to have been caused by inoculation of EIAV-contaminated plasma produced for the treatment of *Rhodococcus equi* infections in foals (Cullinane *et al.* 2007). This highlights the inherent dangers in using blood or tissue products from untested equine populations.

A previously undocumented form of EIAV transmission may have also occurred during the 2006 EIA outbreak in Ireland when all 14 adult horses and 2 of 7 foals present in a veterinary hospital over a 12 h period became infected. There were no reports of significant infestations of haematophagous insects in this establishment at the time and conventional iatrogenic transmission appears unlikely as some mares were present only because of their sick foals and did not receive treatment. The one factor linking these cases was a mare admitted to the hospital with

```
                                          V1
US Day 0      MVSIAFYGGIPGGISTPITQQSE--KSKCEENTMFQPYCYNNDSKNSMAE
US Day 106    MVSIAFYGGIPGGISTPITQQSE--KSRCEENTMFQPYCYNNDSKNSMAE
Liaoning SU   MVSIAFYGGIPGGISTPITQQTKSTDTQKGDHMVYQPYCYNDSHKAEMAE

US Day 0      SKEARDQEMNLKEESKEE-KRRNDWWKIGMFLLCLAGTTGGILWWYEGLP
US Day 106    SKEARDQEMNLKEESKEE-KRRNDWWKIGMFLLCLAGTTGGILWWYEGLP
Liaoning SU   ARDTRYQEEMNRKEEKEDNKRRNNWWKIGMFLLCLLGTTGGFLWWYEGQK
                                                               V2
US Day 0      QQHYIGLVAIGGRLNGSGQSNAIECWGSFPGCRPFQNYFSYETNRSMHMD
US Day 106    QQHYIGLVAIGGRLNGSGQSNAIECWGSFPGCRPFQNYFSYETNRSMHID
Liaoning SU   HSHYIGLVTIGGRLNGSGMTSAIECWGSFPGCRPFTNYFSYETNRTISRD
                                                              V3
US Day 0      NNTATLLEAYHREITFIYKSSCTDSDHCQEYQCKKVNLNSSDSSNSVRVE
US Day 106    NNTATLLEAYHREITFIYKSSCTDSDHCQEYQCKKVNL------------
Liaoning SU   NNTATLLDAYQREVTNIYRTSCVDSDHCQEYKCKQVQLRENSSNIIMNNC
                                                         V4
US Day 0      DVMNTTEYWGFKWLECNQTENFKTILVPENEMVNINDTDTWIPKGCNETW
US Day 106    --MNTTEYWGFKWLECNQTENFKTILVPENEMVNINDNDTWIPKGCNETW
Liaoning SU   SNNSCEEFWGFSWLECNQTENAITILVPEVEMQ-----------------
                                                V5
US Day 0      ARVKRCPIDILYGIHPIRLCVQPPFFLVQE-KGIANTSRIGNCGPTIFLG
US Day 106    ARVKRCPIDILYGIHPIRLCVQPPFFLAQE-KGIANTSRIGNCGPTIFLG
Liaoning SU   -------MDLLYGINRIRMCVQPPFFLFKQNDTSNNTSILSNCGPLVFLG
                         V6
US Day 0      VLEDNKGVVRGNYTACNVSRLKINRKDYTGIYQVPIFYTCNFTNITSCNN
US Day 106    VLEDNKGVVRGNYTACNVSHLKINRKDYTGIYQVPIFYTCNFTNITSCNN
Liaoning SU   ILEDNKAAIQN--GSCTLHRTNIKRPDYSGFYQVPIFYICNLTGLQSCNN
                                        V7
US Day 0      EPIISVIMYETNQVQYLLCNNNNSN-----NYNCVVQSFGVIGQAHLELP
US Day 106    ESIISVIMYETNQVQYLLCNNNNSN-----NYNCVVQSFGVIGQAHLELP
Liaoning SU   GSIISIIMSESNVQYLLCNTSNTNSTNNATVSCVVQSFGVIGQAHVALP
                        V8
US Day 0      RPNKRIRNQNFNQYNCSINNKTELETWKLVKTSGITPLPISSEANTGLIR
US Day 106    RPNKRIRNQSFNQYNCSINNKTELETWKLVKTSGITPLPISSEANTGLIR
Liaoning SU   RKNKRLQSPKFAHYNCTINNKTELRQWQLVKTSGITPLPISSTANTGLVR

US Day 0      HKR
US Day 106    HKR
Liaoning SU   HKR
```

FIGURE 5: Conserved and variable domains in the SU glycoprotein. Comparison of the predicted SU amino acid sequence (single letter code) of a North American EIAV strain (US Day 0, GenBank accession number AF005113) used in a pony infection experiment with SU sequences of a virus isolated from the same pony during a febrile episode at 106 days post infection (US Day 106, GenBank accession number AF005116) and the Liaoning (China) strain (GenBank accession number AF327877). Hypervariable regions V1 to V8 were identified by Leroux et al. (1997).

suspected liver disease that began bleeding profusely from the nostrils and was eventually subjected to euthanasia because of the extensive uncontrollable blood loss estimated to be approximately 20 litres. Cleaning and removal of this very large amount of blood was accomplished at least in part using a pressure washer. Unfortunately, later tests demonstrated the cause of excessive bleeding was thrombocytopenia resulting from a particularly severe clinical episode of EIA and it has been suggested pressure washing may have aerosolised the EIAV contaminated blood. If pressure washing had produced EIAV containing particles in the 0.5–1 µm size range, these would be capable of reaching the alveoli where they would be in close proximity to suitable host cells in the form of alveolar macrophages. Although this is, at present, just a hypothesis respiratory transmission does occur with the Maedi-Visna lentivirus.

Molecular epidemiology

Tracing the source of an outbreak, designing diagnostic tests and formulating effective vaccines are all dependent on understanding the extent of variation that occurs between different isolates of an infectious agent. Early studies on sequential samples taken from individual EIAV infected horses, demonstrated that Gag and Pol were extensively conserved (Salinovich *et al.* 1986), while Rev and the envelope glycoproteins, especially SU, varied significantly (Salinovich *et al.* 1986; Payne *et al.* 1989; Leroux *et al.* 1997; Zheng *et al.* 1997a,b; Belshan *et al.* 1998; Leroux *et al.* 2001). Therefore, the general belief was that the overall structure of the envelope glycoproteins (particularly SU) facilitated antigenic variation whereas greater functional constraints imposed significant restrictions on amino acid substitutions within Gag and Pol. However, nucleotide sequence information for EIAV isolates from several different countries has recently become available. In the case of Env it appears that significant variation occurs in SU between geographically distinct EIAV isolates but the amino acid substitutions are limited primarily to the same 8 hypervariable domains (Leroux *et al.* 1997, 2001) seen in sequential viral isolates from a single animal (**Fig 5**). Extensively conserved blocks of amino acid sequence separate these variable domains, which explains the somewhat counterintuitive observation (Issel *et al.* 1999; Cullinane *et al.* 2007) that serological diagnosis of EIAV infections from many different parts of the world can be accomplished using immunoblot assays with viral antigens, including SU, prepared from a North American fibroblast-adapted strain.

The overall homology between *gag* sequences from North American, European and Asian EIAV isolates is approximately 80% at the predicted amino acid level and as such is much lower than suggested by earlier studies (Salinovich *et al.* 1986). However, variation is not evenly distributed between the *gag* encoded proteins with p26 and p11 being the most conserved at 91.9 and 90.4%, respectively (**Fig 6**) while p15 varies by 26% and p9 (**Fig 7**) is only 48.3%

```
Can 1   PIIIDGAGNRNFRPLTPRGYTTWVNTIQTNNLLNEASVNLFGILSVDCTS
Jap     PIMIDGAGNRNFRPLTPRGYTTWVNTIQTNGLLNEASQNLFGILSVDCTS
Wyo     PIMIDGAGNRNFRPLTPRGYTTWVNTIQTNGLLNEASQNLFGILSVDCTS
Can 3   PIMIDGAGNRNFRPLTPRGYTTWVNTIQANNLLNEASVNLFGILSVDCTS
Lia     PIMIDGAGNRNFRPLTPRGYTTWVNTIQQNNLLNEASVNLFGILSVDCTS
Ita     PIMIDGAGNRNFRPLTPRGYTTWVNTIQQNNLLNEASVNLFGILSVDCTS
Ire     PIMIDGAGNRNFRPLTPRGYTTWVNTIQQNNLLNEASVNLFGILSVDCTS
Can 10  PIIIDGAGNRNFRSLTPRGYTTWVNTIQTNGLLNEASQNLFGILSVDCTS
Can 7   PIIVDGAGNRNFRPLTPRGYTTWVNTIQTNNLLNEASVNLFGILSVDCTS

Can 1   EEMNAFLDVVPGQAGQKQVLLDLLDKIAEDWDNRHPLPNAPLVAPPQGPI
Jap     EEMNAFLDVVPGQAGQKQILLDAIDKIAEDWDNRHPLPNAPLVAPPQGPL
Wyo     EEMNAFLDVVPGQAGQKQILLDAIDKIADDWDNRHPLPNAPLVAPPQGPI
Can 3   EEMNAFLDVVPGQAGQKQVLLDILEKIAEAWDNKHPLPNAPLVAPPQGPI
Lia     EEMNAFLDVVPGQAGQKQVLLDNLDKIAEEWDRRHPMPNPPLVAPPQGPI
Ita     EEMNAFLDVVPGQAGQKQVLLDLLEKIAQDWDNAHPLPNAPMVAPPQGPI
Ire     EEMNAFLDVVPGQAGQKQVLLDLLDKIAQDWDNAHPLPNAPMVAPPQGPI
Can 10  EEMNAFLDVVPGQAGQKQVLLDAIEKIAEDWDNRHPLPNAPLVAPPQGPI
Can 7   EEMNAFLDVVPGQAGQKQVLLDLLDKIAEDWDNRHPLPNAPLVAPPQGPI

Can 1   PMTARFIRGLGVPRERQMEPAFDQFRQTYRQWIIEAMTEGIKIMIGKPKA
Jap     PMTARFIRGLGVPRERQMEHAFDQFRQTYRQWIIEAMSEGIKVMIGKPKA
Wyo     PMTARFIRGLGVPRERQMEPAFDQFRQTYRQWIIEAMSEGIKVMIGKPKA
Can 3   PMTARFIRGLGVPRERQMEPAFDQFRQTYRQWIIEAMTEGIKIMIGKPKA
Lia     PMTARFIRGLGVPRERQMEPAFDQFRQTYRQWIIEAMTEGIKIMIGKPKA
Ita     PMTARFIRGLGVPRERQMEPAFDQFRQTYRQWIIEAMTEGIKIMIGKPKA
Ire     PMTARFIRGLGVPRERQMEPAFDQFRQTYRQWIIEAMTEGIKIMIGKPKA
Can 10  PMTARFIRRLGVPRERQMEPAFDQFRQTYRQWIIDAMSEGIKIMIGKPKA
Can 7   PMTARFIRGLGVPRERQMEPAFDQFRQTYRQWIIDAMTEGIKIMIGKPKA

Can 1   QNIRQGPKEPYSEFIDRLLSQIKSEGHPSEITKFLTDTLTIQNANEECRN
Jap     QNIRQGVKEPYPEFIDRLLSQIKSEGHPQEISKFLTDTLTIQNANEECRN
Wyo     QNIRQGAKEPYPEFVDRLLSQIKSEGHPQEISKFLTDTLTIQNANEECRN
Can 3   QNIRQGPKEPYPDFVDRILSQIKSEGHPAEITKFLIDTLTIQNANEECRS
Lia     QNIRQGPKEPYPEFVDRLLSQIKSEGHPADITKFLTDTLTIQNANDECKS
Ita     QNIRQGPKEPYPDFVDRLLSQVKSEGHPSEITKFLTDTLTIQNANEECKA
Ire     QNIRQGPKEPYPDFVDRLLSQVKSEGHPSEITKFLTDTLTIQNANEECKA
Can 10  QNIRQGPKEPYPDFIDRLLSQIKSEGHPAEIAKFLTDTLTIQNANEECKA
Can 7   QNIRQGPKEPYPDFIDRLLSQIKSEGHPTEITKFLTDTLTIQNANEECKN

Can 1   AMRHLRPEDTLEEKMYACRDIGSTKQKMLLLARAL
Jap     AMRHLRPEDTLEEKMYACRDIGTTKQKMMLLAKAL
Wyo     AMRHLRPEDTLEEKMYACRDIGTTKQKMMLLAKAL
Can 3   AMRHLRPEDTLEEKMYACRDIGTVKQKMMLLARAL
Lia     AMRHLRPEDTLEEKMYACRDIGTMKQKMALLAKAL
Ita     AMRHLRPEDTLEEKLYACRDIGTTKQKMMLLARAL
Ire     AMRHLRPEDTLEEKLYACRDIGTTKQKMMLLARAL
Can 10  AMRHLRPEDTLEEKLYACRDIGTTKQKMMLLARAL
Can 7   AMRHLRPEDTLEEKLYACRDIGTVKQKMMLLARAL
```

FIGURE 6: Homology in Gag p26 between EIAV isolates from different countries. A comparison of predicted amino acid sequences (single letter code) between Canadian (Can 1, GenBank accession number EF418582; Can 3, GenBank accession number EF418583; Can 7 GenBank accession number EF418584; Can 10, GenBank accession number EF418585), Chinese (Lia, GenBank accession number AF327877), Japanese (Jap, GenBank accession number AB008197), Italian (Ita, GenBank accession number EU240733), Irish (Ire, Quinlivan et al. 2007) and the United States (Wyo, GenBank accession number AF033820).

homologous. The fact that p26 is relatively conserved is reassuring because this is the primary antigen in diagnostic assays for the serological detection of EIAV infections including the agar gel immunodiffusion (AGID or Coggins) test (Issel and Cook 1993; Issel *et*

```
Can 1   PVQQKGQHQGNATQETPQVQNLYPDLSKLKKEYKVKEETQIDQEELNLSSLWE
Ita     PIQQKGQQMTQQGG-PKESQGLYPDLTQMKQEYKLEKKSQEEVEDLNLNSLWE
Ire     PIQQKGQQMTQQGG-PKESQGLYPDLTQMKQEYKLEKKSQEEVEDLNLNSLWE
Lia     PVQKESMNKTQKE--EKQQGTLYPDLSQMKQEYKIKE--EENQEDLNLDSLWE
Jap     PIQQKSQHNKSVVQETPQTQNLYPDLSEIKKEYNVKEKDQVDQEDLNLDSLWE
Wyo     PIQQKSQHNKSVVQETPQTQNLYPDLSEIKKEYNVKEKDQV--EDLNLDSLWE
Can 10  PVQQKSQRKESVKQERSQVQNLYPDLSKLKEEYNVKEEIQADQEDLNLSSLWE
Can 3   PVQQKSQSKESTTQKTPQSQNLYPDLSKLKVEYNVKEEVQADQEDLNLSSLWE
Can 7   PVQQRSQNKESITQETSQAQSLYPDLSKLKQEYNVRKEAQQEQEDLNLSSLWE
```

FIGURE 7: Amino acid variation in Gag p9. The isolates compared are as described in Figure 6.

al. 1999). On the other hand, the extent of variation in p9 was unexpected with the only significant homology (**Fig 7**) being at the carboxyl terminus and the tyrosine (Y)-proline (P)-aspartic acid (D)-leucine (L) motif that is critical for progeny virus budding from the host cell plasma membrane (Puffer *et al.* 1997, 1998; Chen *et al.* 2005). This extensive variation occurs despite the fact that p9 is important for the efficient progression of cytoplasmic linear proviral DNA into the circular form found within the cell-nucleus, a property that is dependent on the N-terminal 32 amino acids (Jin *et al.* 2005).

Comparison of complete *gag* gene sequences from the viruses responsible for the 2006 outbreaks of EIAV in Ireland and Italy (Quinlivan *et al.* 2007; Felicetti *et al.* 2008) demonstrate extensive homology in p15 (98.4%), p26 (99.6%), p11 (98.7%) and p9 (100%) providing convincing support for the widely held belief that these viruses were derived from the same source. In addition, the similarities between these isolates in the potentially highly variable p9 suggest that the molecular characterisation of this antigen may be an extremely useful epidemiological tool for studying the source and progression of future EIA outbreaks.

EIA treatment and prevention

Effective vaccines against even the relatively simple lentiviruses such as EIAV are not available. In many cases of infectious disease, fully protective immune responses are induced that eliminate the pathogen from the body and prevent re-infection. The goal of a successful vaccine therefore, is to duplicate the naturally occurring protective immune responses. Unfortunately, lentiviruses have evolved to persist in the presence of strong immune responses and do not normally induce sterilising immunity. In many cases of EIAV infection partial protection in terms of disease prevention is only accomplished, as discussed above, after the immune system has been exposed to actively replicating virus for months or even years. Under these circumstances, it is perhaps not surprising that attempts to use conventional vaccine technologies against lentiviruses have not been very successful, although live attenuated viruses have at times shown some promise and were reportedly used successfully in China (Shen *et al.* 1979). However, additional studies have highlighted problems with the efficacy of the Chinese vaccine (Zhang *et al.* 2007) and studies with a genetically engineered attenuated EIAV strain in the USA demonstrated that post incubation periods of 7 months were not sufficient to protect against challenge by virulent viruses with antigenic differences in only a single viral protein (Craigo *et al.* 2007). Consequently, if vaccines are to be successful against lentiviruses they will probably have to stimulate responses that go beyond those normally produced by the mammalian immune system, an achievement that is unlikely in the near future.

Anti-retroviral drugs can delay progression to AIDS in human patients infected with HIV and similar compounds could be developed for use in EIAV infected horses that may lower the probabilities of transmission by reducing tissue-associated viral burdens. However, current drugs only suppress rather than eliminate lentiviral infections and although controlling the spread of EIA by reducing the probability of transmission may be theoretically possible, the cost of developing and administrating such a programme would be prohibitively high. Therefore, the only currently available, practical option for controlling the spread of EIAV is to use proven management techniques based on the identification of infected individuals. Unfortunately, this cannot be accomplished with conventional virus isolation techniques as the virus does not replicate in continuous cell cultures found in most diagnostic virology laboratories and primary horse leucocyte cultures are not sufficiently sensitive for routine use. In many cases a viable alternative to virus isolation is the detection of viral genetic material using highly sensitive polymerase chain reaction (PCR) based techniques and this has been used successfully to detect EIAV infected individuals. However, these techniques require prior nucleotide sequence information and are very vulnerable to nucleotide substitutions. Therefore, it would be unwise to use PCR-based assays in situations where the EIAV strain was uncharacterised. For example, a real-time reverse transcriptase PCR (Cook *et al.* 2002) designed to quantitate viral RNA from several North American EIAV isolates was not able to detect viral RNA from the viruses responsible for the 2006 Irish outbreak (Quinlivan *et al.* 2007). Additionally, many inapparent carriers of EIAV carry such low burdens of EIAV that they may be reported falsely as negative in many PCR-based assays.

As our knowledge about the extent of genetic variation in EIAV increases, it may one day be possible to design 'universal' PCR assays capable of detecting all strains of this virus with exquisite sensitivity. However, until then serological methods of detection remain the method of choice for identification of EIAV infected equids.

Diagnosis and control

The agar gel immunodiffusion (AGID or Coggins) test and EIA-ELISA tests are widely used for the detection of antibody against EIAV. Although, these assays are based on different technologies there is a very high degree of agreement between EIA-ELISA and AGID test results. The AGID requires at least one day to complete and is probably the least sensitive technique; however, it is the only method that has been shown to correlate with the presence of virus in horse inoculation tests (Pearson *et al.* 1971; Coggins *et al.* 1972). For this reason all positive EIA-ELISA results must be confirmed by immunodiffusion before regulatory actions are taken. Furthermore, the fact that AGID test results have been correlated with the presence of virus has led many countries to recognise it as the official diagnostic test for EIA. In comparison to AGID, EIA-ELISA tests are generally more sensitive and can be completed in a few hours. Within the USA, 4 ELISA test kits (Vira-CHEK[1], SA-ELISA II[2], VMRD ELISA[3] and CELISA[4]) are currently approved by the USDA and these were found to be effective during the 2006 Irish outbreak (Cullinane *et al.* 2007). The immunoblot test for EIA is an important research tool that is gaining wider use to help explain the few cases where AGID and EIA-ELISA test results do not agree. The immunoblot is one of the most sensitive assays and unlike other serological tests, detects antibody reactivity to multiple (usually SU, TM and p26) viral proteins (Issel *et al.* 1999). The disadvantage of this test is that it is not yet commercially available.

The diagnosis of EIA can be improved by combining the strengths of the current serological tests. For example, the rapidity and sensitivity of ELISA tests make them ideal for screening suspected cases of EIA for subsequent confirmation by AGID. Furthermore, utilisation of multiple serological test formats can resolve the extremely small number of cases when a single test may produce 'false positive' or 'false negative' results. 'False positive' reactions can occur for a variety of reasons including exposure to retroviruses other than EIAV. This is because the capsid protein is the most conserved antigen among the *Retroviridae* and contains interspecies determinants that may produce cross-reactive antibodies with EIAV p26. Usually these cross-reactive antibodies are present in low levels and so the frequency of detection is higher in the relatively sensitive EIA-ELISA tests compared with AGID. This highlights the fact the AGID test correlates with higher specificity in terms of an extremely low rate of false positive reactions. In addition, serum from these animals will react exclusively with p26 in immunoblots and can be interpreted as negative for EIA, if after retesting at 30–60 days reactivity with additional viral antigens is not detected (Issel and Cook 2004; Issel *et al.* 2007). At the other end of the spectrum a small number of EIAV-infected individuals have been identified with very low antibody titres and have been reported as 'falsely negative' in AGID. However, serum samples from these animals produce positive reactions in more sensitive EIA-ELISA and immunoblot (reactivity with 2 or more EIAV antigens) tests (Issel and Cook 2004; Issel *et al.* 2007). As a result, of the increased sensitivity of EIA-ELISA formats these authors recommend wider acceptance/use of negative results in these assays when testing equids prior to interstate/international travel.

Although serological testing has been used with considerable success for over 35 years to control EIA outbreaks in many countries, a recognised limitation of this approach is the potentially lengthy delay between the time of exposure to EIAV and the first positive serological result. This determines the duration of restrictions that regulatory authorities may impose to control EIA outbreaks such as limiting the movements of equids for commerce or the quarantine of suspected cases. The incubation period for EIA is generally defined as the time from exposure to the virus until the first serological evidence of infection. Under carefully controlled experimental conditions with known virus strains, this occurs within 45 days (Issel and Cook 1993). To allow for differences in expected field exposures retesting after 60 days of quarantine is recommended and widely accepted (http://www.aphis.usda.gov/vs/nahss/equine/eia/eia_umr_jan_10_ 2007.pdf). In field outbreaks, it may be impossible to determine the initial date of exposure to EIAV. Furthermore, the spread of EIAV may continue among groups of animals placed under quarantine unless the possibility of transmission by insects or man is eliminated by the imposition of strict handling and segregation protocols. As a result, EIA incubation periods longer than 45 days may be recorded. However, the incubation period of EIA could also be more variable under field conditions because of differences in the route of exposure, the immune responses of individual hosts and the plethora of viral variants present in nature. During the 2006 EIA outbreak in Ireland, for example, incubation periods as long as 157 days were reported (Cullinane *et al.* 2007).

Following identification, the next step is the removal of EIAV infected animals from susceptible contacts. As equids are the only known hosts for this virus it should be possible to eradicate the infection/disease and, therefore in some states in the USA, euthanasia of EIA seropositive individuals is recommended. However, for economic, social and political reasons, comprehensive testing and eradication programmes are not always possible. This will almost certainly be the case in regions of the world where equids provide much of the motive power for the agricultural and transportation industries. However, it is possible to break transmission of EIAV by segregation. Separation of seropositive from nonseropositive horse herds has been used effectively by maintaining a strict 200 yard separation distance from susceptible equids. An obvious disadvantage of the segregation technique is that it requires relatively large amounts of space. However, even in situations where control programmes are difficult to instigate, the probability of natural transmission from most inapparent carrier animals is relatively small because of low viral burdens, the miniscule amounts of blood retained on insect mouthparts and insect behaviour. Under these circumstances, man remains the greatest threat as an agent for transmission and education is therefore one of the most important tools for controlling the spread of EIAV. Owners and veterinarians need to adhere to strict aseptic practices including treating all body fluids and particularly blood from equids as potentially infectious. The realisation that a healthy horse does not always mean an EIA-free horse begs for the adoption of standard/universal precautions to prevent the spread of blood-borne agents in equids.

The recent outbreaks of EIA in Western Europe produced many valuable lessons ranging from the dangers of using blood products from untested or nonapproved sources to the need for vigilance and active surveillance. Although adequate testing programmes are difficult and expensive to instigate they are essential for identifying those populations where EIA is endemic and for preventing spread to regions that may be free of the infection. Unfortunately, the chances of spreading EIA, especially during the inapparent carrier phase, can only increase as traditional borders become more porous and the international movement of equids more prevalent.

Acknowledgements

The authors thank Diane Furry for help with the preparation of this manuscript.

Manufacturers' addresses

[1]Synbiotics, Kansas City, Missouri, USA.
[2]Centaur, Overland Park, Kansas, USA.
[3]VMRD, Pullman, Washington, USA.
[4]IDEXX, Westbrook, Maine, USA.

References

Bakhanashvili, M. and Hizi, A. (1993) Fidelity of DNA synthesis exhibited *in vitro* by the reverse transcriptase of the lentivirus equine infectious anemia virus. *Biochem.* **32**, 7559-7567.

Ball, J.M., Rushlow, K.E., Issel, C.J. and Montelaro, R.C. (1992) Detailed mapping of the antigenicity of the surface unit glycoprotein of equine infectious anemia virus by using synthetic peptide strategies. *J. Virol.* **66**, 732-742.

Banks, K.L., Henson, J.B. and McGuire, T.C. (1972) Immunologically mediated glomerulitis of horses. I. Pathogenesis in persistent infection by equine infectious anemia virus. *Lab. Invest.* **26**, 701-707.

Belshan, M., Harris, M.E., Shoemaker, A.E., Hope, T.J. and Carpenter, S. (1998) Biological characterization of Rev variation in equine infectious anemia virus. *J. Virol.* **72**, 4421-4426.

Borysiewicz, L.K., Hickling, J.K., Graham, S., Sinclair, J., Cranage, M.P., Smith, G.L. and Sissons, J.G. (1988) Human cytomegalovirus-specific cytotoxic T cells. Relative frequency of stage-specific CTL recognizing the 72-kD immediate early protein and glycoprotein B expressed by recombinant vaccinia viruses. *J. expt. Med.* **168**, 919-931.

Brindley, M.A. and Maury, W. (2005) Endocytosis and a low-pH step are required for productive entry of equine infectious anemia virus. *J. Virol.* **79**, 14482-14488.

Brindley, M.A. and Maury, W. (2008) Equine infectious anemia virus entry occurs through clathrin-mediated endocytosis. *J. Virol.* **82**, 1628-1637.

Busch, D.H. and Pamer, E.G. (1998) MHC class I/peptide stability: implications for immunodominance, *in vitro* proliferation, and diversity of responding CTL. *J. Immunol.* **160**, 4441-4448.

Carpenter, S. and Chesebro, B. (1989) Change in host cell tropism associated with *in vitro* replication of equine infectious anemia virus. *J. Virol.* **63**, 2492-2496.

Chen, C., Vincent, O., Jin, J., Weisz, O.A. and Montelaro, R.C. (2005) Functions of early (AP-2) and late (AIP1/ALIX) endocytic proteins in equine infectious anemia virus budding. *J. Biol. Chem.* **280**, 40474-40480.

Clabough, D.L., Gebhard, D., Flaherty, M.T., Whetter, L.E., Perry, S.T., Coggins, L. and Fuller, F.J. (1991) Immune-mediated thrombocytopenia in horses infected with equine infectious anemia virus. *J. Virol.* **65**, 6242-6251.

Coggins, L., Norcross, N.L. and Nusbaum, S.R. (1972) Diagnosis of equine infectious anemia by immunodiffusion test. *Am. J. vet. Res.* **33**, 11-18.

Cook, R.F., Cook, S.J., Li, F.L., Montelaro, R.C. and Issel, C.J. (2002) Development of a multiplex real-time reverse transcriptase-polymerase chain reaction for equine infectious anemia virus (EIAV). *J. Virol. Methods* **105**, 171-179.

Cook, R.F., Leroux, C., Cook, S.J., Berger, S.L., Lichtenstein, D.L., Ghabrial, N.N., Montelaro, R.C. and Issel, C.J. (1998) Development and characterization of an *in vivo* pathogenic molecular clone of equine infectious anemia virus. *J. Virol.* **72**, 1383-1393.

Cook, R.F., Cook, S.J., Berger, S.L., Leroux, C., Ghabrial, N.N., Gantz, M., Bolin, P.S., Mousel, M.R., Montelaro, R.C. and Issel, C.J. (2003) Enhancement of equine infectious anemia virus virulence by identification and removal of suboptimal nucleotides. *Virol.* **313**, 588-603.

Cook, S.J., Cook, R.F., Montelaro, R.C. and Issel, C.J. (2001) Differential responses of *Equus caballus* and *Equus asinus* to infection with two pathogenic strains of equine infectious anemia virus. *Vet. Microbiol.* **79**, 93-109.

Costa, L.R., Santos, I.K., Issel, C.J. and Montelaro, R.C. (1997) Tumor necrosis factor-alpha production and disease severity after immunization with enriched major core protein (p26) and/or infection with equine infectious anemia virus. *Vet. Immunol. Immunopathol.* **57**, 33-47.

Craigo, J.K., Leroux, C., Howe, L., Steckbeck, J.D., Cook, S.J., Issel, C.J. and Montelaro, R.C. (2002) Transient immune suppression of inapparent carriers infected with a principal neutralizing domain-deficient equine infectious anaemia virus induces neutralizing antibodies and lowers steady-state virus replication. *J. Gen. Virol.* **83**, 1353-1359.

Craigo, J.K., Zhang, B., Barnes, S., Tagmyer, T.L., Cook, S.J., Issel, C.J. and Montelaro, R.C. (2007) Envelope variation as a primary determinant of lentiviral vaccine efficacy. *Proc. Natl. Acad. Sci. USA* **104**, 15105-15110.

Crawford, T.B., Wardrop, K.J., Tornquist, S.J., Reilich, E., Meyers, K.M. and McGuire, T.C. (1996) A primary production deficit in the thrombocytopenia of equine infectious anemia. *J. Virol.* **70**, 7842-7850.

Cullinane, A., Quinlivan, M., Nelly, M., Patterson, H., Kenna, R., Garvey, M., Gildea, S., Lyons, P., Flynn, M., Galvin, P., Neylon, M. and Jankowska, K. (2007) Diagnosis of equine infectious anaemia during the 2006 outbreak in Ireland. *Vet. Rec.* **161**, 647-652.

Dufour, C., Corcione, A., Svahn, J., Haupt, R., Poggi, V., Beka'ssy, A.N., Scime, R., Pistorio, A. and Pistoia, V. (2003) TNF-alpha and IFN-gamma are overexpressed in the bone marrow of Fanconi anemia patients and TNF-alpha suppresses erythropoiesis *in vitro*. *Blood* **102**, 2053-2059.

Esser, R., Glienke, W., von Briesen, H., Rubsamen-Waigmann, H. and Andreesen, R. (1996) Differential regulation of proinflammatory and hematopoietic cytokines in human macrophages after infection with human immunodeficiency virus. *Blood* **88**, 3474-3481.

Evans, K.S., Carpenter, S.L. and Sevoian, M. (1984) Detection of equine infectious anemia virus in horse leukocyte cultures derived from horses in various stages of equine infectious anemia viral infection. *Am. J. vet. Res.* **45**, 20-25.

Felicetti, M., Capomaccio, S., Cappelli, K., Marenzoni, M.L., Verini Supplizi, A., Coletti, M., and Passamonti, F. (2008) Gag genetic diversity of equine infectious anemia in infected horses in Italy. GenBank [Accession number EU24073]. .

Felli, N., Pedini, F., Zeuner, A., Petrucci, E., Testa, U., Conticello, C., Biffoni, M., Di Cataldo, A., Winkles, J.A., Peschle, C. and De Maria, R. (2005) Multiple members of the TNF superfamily contribute to IFN-gamma-mediated inhibition of erythropoiesis. *J. Immunol.* **175**, 1464-1472.

Foil, L., Stage, D., Adams, W.V. Jr. and Issel, C.J. (1985) Observations of tabanid feeding on mares and foals. *Am. J. vet. Res.* **46**, 1111-1113.

Foil, L.D., Adams, W.V., McManus, J.M. and Issel, C.J. (1987) Bloodmeal residues on mouthparts of *Tabanus fuscicostatus* (*Diptera: Tabanidae*) and the potential for mechanical transmission of pathogens. *J. med. Entomol.* **24**, 613-616.

Foil, L.D., Meek, C.L., Adams, W.V. and Issel, C.J. (1983) Mechanical transmission of equine infectious anemia virus by deer flies (*Chrysops flavidus*) and stable flies (*Stomoxys calcitrans*). *Am. J. vet. Res.* **44**, 155-156.

Gutekunst, D.E. and Becvar, C.S. (1979) Responses in horses infected with equine infectious anemia virus adapted to tissue culture. *Am. J. vet. Res.* **40**, 974-977.

Hammond, S.A., Cook, S.J., Lichtenstein, D.L., Issel, C.J. and Montelaro, R.C. (1997) Maturation of the cellular and humoural immune responses to persistent infection in horses by equine infectious anemia virus is a complex and lengthy process. *J. Virol.* **71**, 3840-3852.

Hawkins, J.A., Adams, W.V., Cook, L., Wilson, B.H. and Roth, E.E. (1973) Role of horse fly (*Tabanus fuscicostatus Hine*) and stable fly (*Stomoxys calcitrans L.*) in transmission of equine infectious anemia to ponies in Louisiana. *Am. J. vet. Res.* **34**, 1583-1586.

Hawkins, J.A., Adams, W.V. Jr., Wilson, B.H., Issel, C.J. and Roth, E.E. (1976) Transmission of equine infectious anemia virus by *Tabanus fuscicostatus*. *J. Am. vet. med. Ass.* **168**, 63-64.

Henson, J.B. and McGuire, T.C. (1971) Immunopathology of equine infectious anemia. *Am. J. clin. Pathol.* **56**, 306-313.

Howe, L., Craigo, J.K., Issel, C.J. and Montelaro, R.C. (2005) Specificity of serum neutralizing antibodies induced by transient immune suppression of inapparent carrier ponies infected with a neutralization-resistant equine infectious anemia virus envelope strain. *J. Gen. Virol.* **86**, 139-149.

Issel, C.J. and Cook, R.F. (1993) A review of techniques for the serologic diagnosis of equine infectious anemia. *J. vet. diag. Invest.* **5**, 137-141.

Issel, C.J. and Cook S.J. (2004) Equine infectious anemia testing and control of EIA: how much is enough? *US An. Health Assn. Proc.* **108**, 316-327.

Issel, C.J. and Foil, L.D. (1984) Studies on equine infectious anemia virus transmission by insects. *J. Am. vet. med. Ass.* **184**, 293-297.

Issel, C.J. and McConnico, R.S. (2001) The risk of EIA in foals. *Equine Disease Quarterly Newsletter* **9**, 3-4.

Issel, C.J., Cordes, T. and Halstead, S. (2007) Control of equine infectious anemia should take new directions. *US An, Health Assn. Proc.* **111**, 90-99.

Issel, C.J., Adams, W.V. Jr., Meek, L. and Ochoa, R. (1982) Transmission of equine infectious anemia virus from horses without clinical signs of disease. *J. Am. vet. med. Ass.* **180**, 272-275.

Issel, C.J., Cook, S.J., Cook, R.F. and Cordes, T.R. (1999) Optimal paradigms to detect reservoirs of equine infectious anemia virus (EIAV). *J. equine vet. Sci.* **19**, 728-732.

Issel, C.J., Cook, S.J., Howell, D., Nitschke Sinclear, J., Gardner, D., Mathis, J.G., Marshall, M.R. and Rogers, L.E. (1998) Equine infectious anemia in wild free-roaming horses in Utah. *US An. Health Assn. Proc.* **102**, 376-384.

Jin, S., Chen, C. and Montelaro, R.C. (2005) Equine infectious anemia virus Gag p9 function in early steps of virus infection and provirus production. *J. Virol.* **79**, 8793-8801.

Kedl, R.M., Kappler, J.W. and Marrack, P. (2003) Epitope dominance, competition and T cell affinity maturation. *Curr. Opin. Immunol.* **15**, 120-127.

Kemen, M.J. Jr. and Coggins, L (1972) Equine infectious anemia: transmission from infected mares to foals. *J. Am. vet. med. Ass.* **161**, 496-499.

Kemen, M.J., McClain, D.S. and Matthysse, J.G. (1978) Role of horse flies in transmission of wquine infectious anemia from carrier ponies. *J. Am. vet. med. Ass.* **172**, 360-362.

Kono, Y. (1969) Viremia and immunological responses in horses infected with equine infectious anemia virus. *Natl. Inst. anim. Health Quart.* **9**, 1-9.

Kono, Y., Kobayashi, K. and Fukunaga, Y. (1973) Antigenic drift of equine infectious anemia virus in chronically infected horses. *Arch Gesamte Virusforsch* **41**, 1-10.

Kono, Y., Hirasawa, K., Fukunaga, Y. and Taniguchi, T. (1976) Recrudescence of equine infectious anemia by treatment with immunosuppressive drugs. *Natl. Inst. anim. Health Quart.* **16**, 8-15.

Lechner, F., Machado, J., Bertoni, G., Seow, H.F., Dobbelaere, D.A. and Peterhans, E. (1997) Caprine arthritis encephalitis virus dysregulates the expression of cytokines in macrophages. *J. Virol.* **71**, 7488-7497.

Leroux, C., Cadore, J.L. and Montelaro, R.C. (2004) Equine infectious anemia virus (EIAV): what has HIV's country cousin got to tell us? *Vet. Res.* **35**, 485-512.

Leroux, C., Issel, C.J. and Montelaro, R.C. (1997) Novel and dynamic evolution of equine infectious anemia virus genomic quasispecies associated with sequential disease cycles in an experimentally infected pony. *J. Virol.* **71**, 9627-9639.

Leroux, C., Craigo, J.K., Issel, C.J. and Montelaro, R.C. (2001) Equine infectious anemia virus genomic evolution in progressor and nonprogressor ponies. *J. Virol.* **75**, 4570-4583.

Li, F., Leroux, C., Craigo, J.K., Cook, S.J., Issel, C.J. and Montelaro, R.C. (2000) The S2 gene of equine infectious anemia virus is a highly conserved determinant of viral replication and virulence properties in experimentally infected ponies. *J. Virol.* **74**, 573-579.

Lichtenstein, D.L., Rushlow, K.E., Cook, R.F., Raabe, M.L., Swardson, C.J., Kociba, G.J., Issel, C.J. and Montelaro, R.C. (1995) Replication *in vitro* and *in vivo* of an equine infectious anemia virus mutant deficient in dUTPase activity. *J. Virol.* **69**, 2881-2888.

Lim, W.S., Payne, S.L., Edwards, J.F., Kim, I. and Ball, J.M. (2005) Differential effects of virulent and avirulent equine infectious anemia virus on macrophage cytokine expression. *Virol.* **332**, 295-306.

Malmquist, W.A., Barnett, D. and Becvar, C.S. (1973) Production of equine infectious anemia antigen in a persistently infected cell line. *Arch Gesamte Virusforsch* **42**, 361-370.

Matheka, H.D., Coggins, L., Shively, J.N. and Norcross, N.L. (1976) Purification and characterization of equine infectious anemia virus. *Arch. Virol.* **51**, 107-114.

Maury, W. (1994) Monocyte maturation controls expression of equine infectious anemia virus. *J. Virol.* **68**, 6270-6279.

Maury, W., Oaks, J.L. and Bradley, S. (1998) Equine endothelial cells support productive infection of equine infectious anemia virus. *J. Virol.* **72**, 9291-9297.

McConnel, M.B., Katada, M., McConnell, S. and Moore, R. (1977) Demonstration of equine infectious anemia virus in primary leukocyte cultures by electron microscopy. *Am. J. vet. Res.* **38**, 2067-2069.

McConnico, R.S., Issel, C.J., Cook, S.J., Cook, R.F., Floyd, C. and Bisson, H. (2000) Predictive methods to define infection with equine infectious anemia virus in foals out of reactor mares. *J. equine vet. Sci.* **20**, 387-392.

McGuire, T.C., Crawford, T.B. and Henson, J.B. (1971) Immunofluorescent localization of equine infectious anemia virus in tissue. *Am. J. Pathol.* **62**, 283-294.

Mealey, R.H., Zhang, B., Leib, S.R., Littke, M.H. and McGuire, T.C. (2003) Epitope specificity is critical for high and moderate avidity cytotoxic T lymphocytes associated with control of viral load and clinical disease in horses with equine infectious anemia virus. *Virol.* **313**, 537-552.

Mealey, R.H., Sharif, A., Ellis, S.A., Littke, M.H., Leib, S.R. and McGuire, T.C. (2005) Early detection of dominant Env-specific and subdominant Gag-specific CD8+ lymphocytes in equine infectious anemia virus-infected horses using major histocompatibility complex class I/peptide tetrameric complexes. *Virol.* **339**, 110-126.

Moldawer, L.L., Marano, M.A., Wei, H., Fong, Y., Silen, M.L., Kuo, G., Manogue, K.R., Vlassara, H., Cohen, H., Cerami, A. *et al.* (1989) Cachectin/tumor necrosis factor-alpha alters red blood cell kinetics and induces anemia *in vivo. FASEB Journal* **3**, 1637-1643.

Montelaro, R.C., Parekh, B., Orrego, A. and Issel, C.J. (1984) Antigenic variation during persistent infection by equine infectious anemia virus, a retrovirus. *J. biol. Chem.* **259**, 10539-10544.

O'Rourke, K., Perryman, L.E. and McGuire, T.C. (1988) Antiviral, anti-glycoprotein and neutralizing antibodies in foals with equine infectious anaemia virus. *J. Gen. Virol.* **69**, 667-674.

O'Rourke, K.I., Perryman, L.E. and McGuire, T.C. (1989) Cross-neutralizing and subclass characteristics of antibody from horses with equine infectious anemia virus. *Vet. Immunol. Immunopathol.* **23**, 41-49.

Oaks, J.L., Ulibarri, C. and Crawford, T.B. (1999) Endothelial cell infection *in vivo* by equine infectious anaemia virus. *J. Gen. Virol.* **80**, 2393-2397.

Orrego, A., Issel, C.J., Montelaro, R.C. and Adams, W.V. Jr. (1982) Virulence and in vitro growth of a cell-adapted strain of equine infectious anemia virus after serial passage in ponies. *Am. J. vet. Res.* **43**, 1556-1560.

Pamer, E.G., Harty, J.T. and Bevan, M.J. (1991) Precise prediction of a dominant class I MHC-restricted epitope of *Listeria monocytogenes. Nature* **353**, 852-855.

Payne, S.L., Rushlow, K., Dhruva, B.R., Issel, C.J. and Montelaro, R.C. (1989) Localization of conserved and variable antigenic domains of equine infectious anemia virus envelope glycoproteins using recombinant env-encoded protein fragments produced in *Escherichia coli. Virol.* **172**, 609-615.

Pearson, J.E., Becvar, C.S. and Mott, L.O. (1971) Evaluation of the immunodiffusions test for the diagnosis of equine infectious anemia. *Proc. US anim. Health Ass.* **74**, 259-267.

Perryman, L.E., McGuire, T.C., Banks, K.L. and Henson, J.B. (1971) Decreased C3 levels in a chronic virus infection: equine infectious anemia. *J. Immunol.* **106**, 1074-1078.

Preston, B.D., Poiesz, B.J. and Loeb, L.A. (1988) Fidelity of HIV-1 reverse transcriptase. *Science* **242**, 1168-1171.

Puffer, B.A., Watkins, S.C. and Montelaro, R.C. (1998) Equine infectious anemia virus Gag polyprotein late domain specifically recruits cellular AP-2 adapter protein complexes during virion assembly. *J. Virol.* **72**, 10218-10221.

Puffer, B.A., Parent, L.J., Wills, J.W. and Montelaro, R.C. (1997) Equine infectious anemia virus utilizes a YXXL motif within the late assembly domain of the Gag p9 protein. *J. Virol.* **71**, 6541-6546.

Quinlivan, M., Cook, R.F. and Cullinane, A. (2007) Real-time quantitative RT-PCR and PCR assays for a novel European field isolate of equine infectious anaemia virus based on sequence determination of the gag gene. *Vet. Rec.* **160**, 611-618.

Roberts, J.D., Bebenek, K. and Kunkel, T.A. (1988) The accuracy of reverse transcriptase from HIV-1. *Science* **242**, 1171-1173.

Rodriguez, F., Harkins, S., Slifka, M.K. and Whitton, J.L. (2002) Immunodominance in virus-induced CD8(+) T-cell responses is dramatically modified by DNA immunization and is regulated by gamma interferon. *J. Virol.* **76**, 4251-4259.

Rwambo, P.M., Issel, C.J., Adams, W.V. Jr., Hussain, K.A., Miller, M. and Montelaro, R.C. (1990) Equine infectious anemia virus (EIAV) humoural responses of recipient ponies and antigenic variation during persistent infection. *Arch. Virol.* **111**, 199-212.

Salinovich, O., Payne, S.L., Montelaro, R.C., Hussain, K.A., Issel, C.J. and Schnorr, K.L. (1986) Rapid emergence of novel antigenic and genetic variants of equine infectious anemia virus during persistent infection. *J. Virol.* **57**, 71-80.

Sellon, D.C., Perry, S.T., Coggins, L. and Fuller, F.J. (1992) Wild-type equine infectious anemia virus replicates *in vivo* predominantly in tissue macrophages, not in peripheral blood monocytes. *J. Virol.* **66**, 5906-5913.

Sellon, D.C., Russell, K.E., Monroe, V.L. and Walker, K.M. (1999) Increased interleukin-6 activity in the serum of ponies acutely infected with equine infectious anaemia virus. *Res. vet. Sci.* **66**, 77-80.

Sentsui, H. and Kono, Y. (1987) Phagocytosis of horse erythrocytes treated with equine infectious anemia virus by cultivated horse leukocytes. *Arch. Virol.* **95**, 67-77.

Shen, D.T., Gorham, J.R., Jones, R.H. and Crawford, T.B. (1978) Failure to propagate equine infectious anemia virus in mosquitoes and *Culicoides variipennis*. *Am. J. vet. Res.* **39**, 875-876.

Shen, R.X., Xu, Z.D., He, X.S. and Zhang, S.X. (1979) Study on immunological methods of equine infectious anemia. *China Agricult. Sci.* **4**, 41-115.

Stein, C.D. and Mott, L.O. (1942) Studies on congenital transmission of equine infectious anemia. *Vet. Med.* **37**, 370-377.

Stein, C.D. and Mott, L.O. (1946) Equine infectious anemia in brood mares and their offspring. *Vet. Med.* **41**, 274-278.

Stein, C.D., Lotze, J.C. and Mott, L.O. (1942) Transmission of equine infectious anemia by the stablefly, *Stomoxys calcitrans*, the horse fly, *Tabanus sulcifrons* (Macquart), and by injection of minute amounts of virus. *Am. J. vet. Res.* **3**, 183-193.

Stein, C.D., Lotze, J.C. and Mott, L.O. (1943) Evidence of transmission of inapparent (subclinical) form of equine infectious anemia by mosquitos (*Psorophora columbiae*), and by injection of the virus in extremely high dilution. *J. Am. vet. med. Ass.* **102**, 163-169.

Swardson, C.J., Lichtenstein, D.L., Wang, S., Montelaro, R.C. and Kociba, G.J. (1997) Infection of bone marrow macrophages by equine infectious anemia virus. *Am. J. vet. Res.* **58**, 1402-1407.

Tacchini-Cottier, F., Vesin, C., Redard, M., Buurman, W. and Piguet, P.F. (1998) Role of TNFR1 and TNFR2 in TNF-induced platelet consumption in mice. *J. Immunol.* **160**, 6182-6186.

Tagmyer, T.L., Craigo, J.K., Cook, S.J., Issel, C.J. and Montelaro, R.C. (2007) Envelope-specific T-helper and cytotoxic T-lymphocyte responses associated with protective immunity to equine infectious anemia virus. *J. Gen. Virol.* **88**, 1324-1336.

Threadgill, D.S., Steagall, W.K., Flaherty, M.T., Fuller, F.J., Perry, S.T., Rushlow, K.E., Le Grice, S.F. and Payne, S.L. (1993) Characterization of equine infectious anemia virus dUTPase: growth properties of a dUTPase-deficient mutant. *J. Virol.* **67**, 2592-2600.

Tornquist, S.J. and Crawford, T.B. (1997) Suppression of megakaryocyte colony growth by plasma from foals infected with equine infectious anemia virus. *Blood* **90**, 2357-2363.

Tornquist, S.J., Oaks, J.L. and Crawford, T.B. (1997) Elevation of cytokines associated with the thrombocytopenia of equine infectious anaemia. *J. Gen. Virol.* **78**, 2541-2548.

Tumas, D.B., Hines, M.T., Perryman, L.E., Davis, W.C. and McGuire, T.C. (1994) Corticosteroid immunosuppression and monoclonal antibody-mediated CD5+ T lymphocyte depletion in normal and equine infectious anaemia virus-carrier horses. *J. Gen. Virol.* **75**, 959-968.

Vallée, H. and Carré, H. (1904) Sur la nature infectieuse de l'anémie du cheval. *C. R. Acad. Sci.* **139**, 331-333.

Weiland, F., Matheka, H.D., Coggins, L. and Hatner, D. (1977) Electron microscopic studies on equine infectious anemia virus (EIAV). Brief report. *Arch. Virol.* **55**, 335-340.

Williams, D.L., Issel, C.J., Steelman, C.D., Adams, W.V. Jr. and Benton, C.V. (1981) Studies with equine infectious anemia virus: transmission attempts by mosquitoes and survival of virus on vector mouthparts and hypodermic needles, and in mosquito tissue culture. *Am. J. vet. Res.* **42**, 1469-1473.

Yoo, J., Chen, H., Kraus, T., Hirsch, D., Polyak, S., George, I. and Sperber, K. (1996) Altered cytokine production and accessory cell function after HIV-1 infection. *J. Immunol.* **157**, 1313-1320.

Yu, X.G., Addo, M.M., Rosenberg, E.S., Rodriguez, W.R., Lee, P.K., Fitzpatrick, C.A., Johnston, M.N., Strick, D., Goulder, P.J., Walker, B.D. and Altfeld, M. (2002) Consistent patterns in the development and immunodominance of human immunodeficiency virus type 1 (HIV-1)-specific CD8+ T-cell responses following acute HIV-1 infection. *J. Virol.* **76**, 8690-8701.

Zamai, L., Secchiero, P., Pierpaoli, S., Bassini, A., Papa, S., Alnemri, E.S., Guidotti, L., Vitale, M. and Zauli, G. (2000) TNF-related apoptosis-inducing ligand (TRAIL) as a negative regulator of normal human erythropoiesis. *Blood* **95**, 3716-3724.

Zhang, B., Jin, S., Jin, J., Li, F. and Montelaro, R.C. (2005) A tumor necrosis factor receptor family protein serves as a cellular receptor for the macrophage-tropic equine lentivirus. *Proc. Natl. Acad. Sci. USA*, **102**, 9918-9923.

Zhang, X., Wang, Y., Liang, H., Wei, L., Xiang, W., Shen, R. and Shao, Y. (2007) Correlation between the induction of Th1 cytokines by an attenuated equine infectious anemia virus vaccine and protection against disease progression. *J. Gen. Virol.* **88**, 998-1004.

Zheng, Y.H., Nakaya, T., Sentsui, H., Kameoka, M., Kishi, M., Hagiwara, K., Takahashi, H., Kono, Y. and Ikuta, K. (1997a) Insertions, duplications and substitutions in restricted gp90 regions of equine infectious anaemia virus during febrile episodes in an experimentally infected horse. *J. Gen. Virol.* **78**, 807-820.

Zheng, Y.H., Sentsui, H., Nakaya, T., Kono, Y. and Ikuta, K. (1997b) *In vivo* dynamics of equine infectious anemia viruses emerging during febrile episodes: insertions/duplications at the principal neutralizing domain. *J. Virol.* **71**, 5031-5039.

AFRICAN HORSE SICKNESS

A. J. Guthrie* and M. Quan

Equine Research Centre, Faculty of Veterinary Science, University of Pretoria, Onderstepoort 0110, Republic of South Africa.

Keywords: horse; African horse sickness; virus; AHSV

Summary

African horse sickness (AHS) is a noncontagious, infectious, insect-borne disease of equids caused by African horse sickness virus (AHSV), which can result in 90% mortality in naïve horses. The area in which orbivirus infections occur has expanded recently probably due to changes in vector biology associated with climate change. Currently, modified live virus AHS vaccines are commercially available for use in endemic areas but the suitability of these vaccines for use in epizootics has been questioned. The increased risk of AHS outbreaks in areas usually free of the disease along with the current lack of inactivated or recombinant vaccines is of concern particularly in areas that are considered to be at highest risk, including Europe and the Middle East. This paper reviews the aetiology, epidemiology, clinical signs, pathology, diagnosis, treatment and control of AHS.

Introduction

African horse sickness (AHS) is a noncontagious, infectious, insect-borne disease of equids caused by African horse sickness virus (AHSV). In horses the disease is usually peracute to acute and in naive animals more than 90% of those affected die. Clinically, the disease is characterised by pyrexia, oedema of the lungs, pleura and subcutaneous tissues and haemorrhages on the serosal surfaces of organs. Mules are less susceptible than horses, and donkeys and zebras rarely show clinical signs of disease.

The first known historical reference to a disease resembling AHS was reported in Yemen in 1327 (Henning 1956). Documents reporting on the travels of Portuguese explorers in East Africa in 1569 reported AHS affecting horses imported from India (Henning 1956). Neither horses nor donkeys were indigenous to southern Africa but were introduced shortly after the arrival of the first settlers of the Dutch East India Company in the Cape of Good Hope in 1652 (Henning 1956). Dutch East India Company records make frequent reference to 'perreziekte' or 'pardeziekte' in the Cape of Good Hope (Theiler 1921). In 1719 about 1700 horses died due to AHS in the Cape of Good Hope. Major epizootics of AHS occurred in southern Africa prior to the 1950s at intervals of roughly 20–30 years. Severe losses were reported in 1780, 1801, 1839, 1855, 1862, 1891, 1914, 1918, 1923, 1940, 1946 and 1953 (Henning 1956). The 1854/55 epizootic was the most severe with almost 70,000 horses (40% of the population) dying in the Cape of Good Hope (Bayley 1856).

In the early 1900s, M'Fadyean (M'Fadyean 1900), Theiler, Nocard and Sieber (Henning 1956) all succeeded in transmitting AHS with a bacteria free filtrate of blood from infected horses confirming that the disease was caused by a virus. Sir Arnold Theiler described the plurality of 'immunologically distinct strains' of AHSV since immunity acquired against one 'strain' did not always afford protection against infection by 'heterologous strains' (Theiler 1921). Alexander and coworkers (Alexander 1933) showed that viscerotropic isolates of AHSV became neurotropic but did not lose their immunogenicity after serial intracerebral passage in mice. This led to the development of the first polyvalent vaccine against AHS in the 1930s (Alexander 1936). The proposal by Pitchford and Theiler that AHS may be transmitted by biting insects (Pitchford and Theiler 1903) was finally confirmed in 1944 when Du Toit showed that *Culicoides* species were probably vectors of both AHS and bluetongue viruses (Du Toit 1944).

*Author to whom correspondence should be addressed.

In endemic areas, severe losses due to AHS have ceased since the development of the polyvalent vaccine. However, epizootics in countries outside the endemic regions in Africa (Lubroth 1988; Anderson *et al.* 1989) serve as a warning that AHS may spread to areas traditionally free of the disease. AHS is one of the important diseases to consider when moving equids internationally but movement can be accomplished safely following appropriate quarantine and testing procedures (Anon 2008a,b). The recent outbreaks of bluetongue in Europe, associated with changes in vector range and capacity due to climate change, suggest that the epidemiology of AHSV may be very different if an epizootic of AHS were to recur in Europe (Dufour *et al.* 2008).

Aetiology

African horse sickness virus is a member of the genus *Orbivirus* in the family Reoviridae and as such is morphologically similar to other orbiviruses such as bluetongue virus (BTV) of ruminants and equine encephalosis virus (EEV) (Verwoerd *et al.* 1979). The virion is about 70 nm in diameter. The genome comprises 10 double stranded RNA segments, each of which encodes at least one polypeptide (Grubman and Lewis 1992). The core particle comprises 2 major proteins, VP 3 and 7 which are highly conserved among the 9 AHSV serotypes, and 3 minor proteins, VP 1, 4 and 6 (Bremer *et al.* 1990). Together these proteins make up the group specific epitopes (Roy *et al.* 1994). The core particle is surrounded by the outer capsid, which is composed of VP 2 and 5. VP 2 is responsible for antigenic variation (Burrage *et al.* 1993; Martinez-Torrecuadrada and Casal 1995). At least 3 nonstructural proteins have been identified (NS 1, 2 and 3/3a) (Devaney *et al.* 1988).

Nine antigenically distinct serotypes have been described (McIntosh 1958; Howell 1962). While there may be some cross relatedness between the serotypes there is no field evidence of any intratypic variation (McIntosh 1958; Howell 1962). All 9 serotypes have been documented in eastern (Davies *et al.* 1993) and southern Africa (McIntosh 1958; Howell 1962; Blackburn and Swanepoel 1988a) while serotype 9 is more widespread and appears to predominate in the northern parts of sub-Saharan Africa (Adeyefa and Hamblin 1995; Sailleau *et al.* 2000a). Serotypes 2, 6 and 7 have been isolated in Senegal, Nigeria and Ethiopia in 2007 and 2008 indicating that the plurality of serotypes in this region may be increasing.

Epidemiology

The ASHV is biologically transmitted by *Culicoides* spp., of which *C. imicola* and *C. bolitinos* have been shown to play an important role in Africa (Meiswinkel *et al.* 2000). The disease has a seasonal occurrence and its prevalence is influenced by climatic and other conditions that favour the breeding of *Culicoides* spp. Although other insects have been suggested as possible vectors of AHSV, none have been shown to play a role under natural conditions. AHSV can be transmitted between horses by parenteral inoculation of infective blood or organ suspensions and it is more readily transmitted by the intravenous than by the subcutaneous route (Henning 1956).

A continuous transmission cycle of AHSV between *Culicoides* midges and zebras exists in the Kruger National Park in South Africa (Barnard 1993). Under such circumstances a sufficiently large zebra (*Equus burchelli*) population can act as a reservoir for virus (Barnard 1998). Donkeys may play a similar role in parts of Africa where there are large donkey populations (Hamblin *et al.* 1998). In view of the high mortality in horses, this species is regarded as an accidental or indicator host. Animals that have been infected with AHSV do not remain carriers of the virus, which explains the failure of the disease to become established outside tropical Africa, despite the occurrence of many epizootics (Henning 1956).

African horse sickness is endemic in eastern and central Africa (Theiler 1921) and spreads regularly to southern Africa. In endemic areas, different serotypes of AHS may be active simultaneously but one serotype usually dominates during a particular season. AHS has been recorded in Egypt in 1928, 1943, 1953, 1958 and 1971 (Salama *et al.* 1981), Yemen in 1930 and Palestine, Syria, Lebanon and Jordan in 1944 (Alexander 1948). In 1959, AHS serotype 9 occurred in the south eastern regions of Iran. This was followed by outbreaks during 1960 in Cyprus, Iraq, Syria, Lebanon and Jordan as well as Afghanistan, Pakistan, India and Turkey. Between 1959 and 1961 this region lost more than 300,000 equids (Howell 1960, 1963; Reid 1961). In 1965 AHS occurred in Libya, Tunisia, Algeria and Morocco and subsequently spread to Spain in 1966 (Hazrati 1967). Between 1987 and 1990, AHS serotype 4 occurred in Spain with the virus being introduced by zebra imported from Namibia (Lubroth 1988; Rodriguez *et al.* 1992). AHS was also confirmed in southern Portugal in 1989 and Morocco between 1989 and 1991 with these outbreaks being extensions of the outbreak in Spain (Zientara *et al.* 1998). In 1989 an outbreak of AHS serotype 9 occurred in Saudi Arabia (Anderson *et al.* 1989). AHS was also reported in Saudi Arabia and Yemen in 1997 and on the Cape Verde Islands in 1999. Serotypes 6 and 9 of AHSV were isolated from samples collected from equids in Ethiopia in 2003 (Zeleke *et al.* 2005) and serotype 2 resulted in the death of approximately 2000 horses in Ethiopia in 2008. Serotypes 2 and 7 of AHSV were isolated in Senegal in 2007 and serotype 2 was isolated in Nigeria in 2007. AHS was also reported in The Gambia in 2007. AHS can be distributed over great distances if equids incubating the disease are translocated by land, sea or air (Lubroth 1988; Rodriguez *et al.* 1992). Spread of AHS has been reported to occur as a result of windborne spread of infected vectors (Sellers *et al.* 1977).

African horse sickness is not endemic in parts of South Africa but each year the disease appears in the north eastern part of the country, occasionally during December but usually in January, from where it spreads southwards. The extent of the southerly spread is influenced by the extent of favourable climatic conditions for the breeding of *Culicoides* midges (Bosman *et al.* 1995). Early and heavy rains followed by warm, dry spells favour the occurrence of epizootics. The first cases of AHS usually occur at the beginning of February, but the most serious outbreaks commonly occur in March and April. Following the first frosts, which usually occur at the end of April or in May, the disease disappears abruptly. However, in the north-eastern parts of South Africa, where the occurrence of frost is less common, deaths may continue to occur into May and June (Henning 1956). In recent years the southerly spread of AHS has been less extensive, probably as a result of the widespread use of a more effective vaccine, which became available in 1974 (Bosman *et al.* 1995). Approximately 300,000 doses of polyvalent AHS vaccine are sold annually by Onderstepoort Biological Products, Onderstepoort. It is speculated that immunisation of horses in these regions establishes a fairly effective 'immune barrier' that seems to impede the southerly spread of the disease (Bosman *et al.* 1995). Outbreaks of AHS associated with the introduction of infected animals have been reported in the Cape Peninsula in 1967 (Bosman *et al.* 1995), 1990 (Du Plessis *et al.* 1991), 1999 (Bell 1999) and 2004.

Horses are most susceptible to the disease (mortality of 70–95%), but mules are less so (mortality of 50–70%). Most infections of donkeys and zebras are subclinical (Theiler 1921). Generally, horses of all breeds are equally susceptible to AHS but variation in susceptibility to the same virus in individual breeds has been reported (Theiler 1921). Some indigenous horses in North and West Africa, which descend from animals that have been present there since at least 2000 BC, have apparently acquired natural resistance to AHS (Bourdin 1973). Foals born to immune mares acquire passive immunity by the ingestion of colostrum (Alexander and Mason 1941). This passive immunity progressively declines and is completely lost after about 4–6 months. Donkeys in the Middle East appear to be more susceptible to AHS (mortality of 3–10%) than southern African donkeys (Alexander 1948). Zebras are highly resistant to AHS and only show a mild fever following experimental infection (Erasmus *et al.* 1978).

Dogs are the only other species that contract a highly fatal form of AHS (Theiler 1906; Haig *et al.* 1956). All reported clinical cases in dogs have resulted from the ingestion of infected carcass material from horses that have died from AHS (Bevan 1911; Piercy 1951). However, it is doubtful that dogs play any role in the spread or maintenance of AHSV, as *Culicoides* spp. do not readily feed on them (McIntosh 1955). Besides zebras (Davies and Oteino 1977; Erasmus *et al.* 1978; Binepal *et al.* 1992; Barnard 1997), no other wildlife or domestic ruminants have been shown to play a significant role in the epidemiology of AHS.

Clinical signs

The clinical findings of natural and experimental cases of AHS have been described by various workers (Theiler 1921; Lubroth 1988). In experimental cases, the incubation period is usually 5–7 days, but it may be as short as 2 days and rarely as long as 10 days. The duration of the incubation period depends on the virulence of the virus and the dose of virus received.

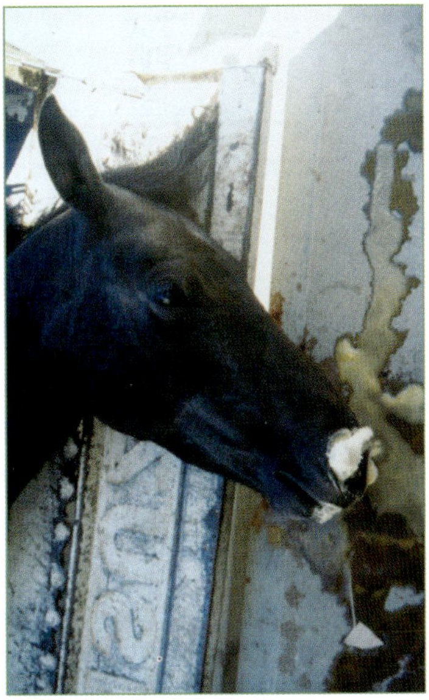

FIGURE 1: 'Pulmonary' or 'dunkop' form of African horse sickness with froth and serous fluid at nostrils due to severe alveolar oedema.

'Dunkop' or 'pulmonary' form

This is the peracute form of AHS and occurs when AHSV infects fully susceptible horses, with recovery being exceptional. In endemic areas it is also common in foals that have lost their maternally derived passive immunity. It is also the usual form in dogs that become infected following the ingestion of AHSV infected carcass material.

The incubation period is short (3–4 days) and is followed by a rapid rise in temperature over a day or 2, with the body temperature reaching 40–41°C. This form is characterised by very marked and rapidly progressive respiratory failure and the respiratory rate may exceed 50 breaths/min. The animal tends to stand with its forelegs spread apart, its head extended, and the nostrils dilated. Expiration is frequently forced with the presence of abdominal heave lines. Profuse sweating is common, and paroxysmal coughing may be observed terminally often with frothy, serofibrinous fluid exuding from the nostrils (**Fig 1**). The onset of dyspnoea is usually very sudden and death occurs within 30 min to a few hours of its appearance. Sometimes an apparently healthy horse, at work, becomes listless, suddenly severely dyspnoeic and dies shortly thereafter. Initially, the appetite of affected animals remains good, despite the high fever and respiratory distress. The prognosis for horses suffering from the 'dunkop' form is extremely grave (<5% recover). If animals recover, the fever subsides gradually but the breathing remains laboured for a number of days.

'Dikkop' or 'cardiac' form

The incubation period in this form of AHS is longer (5–7 days) followed by a fever of 39–41°C that persists for 3–4 days. The more typical clinical symptoms do not appear until the fever has begun to decline. At first the supraorbital fossae fill as the underlying adipose tissue becomes oedematous and raises the skin well above the level of the zygomatic arch (**Figs 2** and **3**). The oedema can later extend to the conjunctiva (**Fig 4**), lips, cheeks, tongue, intermandibular space and laryngeal region, and may extend a variable distance down the neck towards the chest, often obliterating the jugular groove. As the swellings increase, dyspnoea and cyanosis may supervene. However, ventral oedema and oedema of the lower limbs are not observed. Unfavourable prognostic signs include petechial haemorrhages on the conjunctivae and on the ventral surface of the tongue. These, if they occur, become evident shortly before death. Some animals may show signs of severe colic, repeatedly lie down, are restless when standing

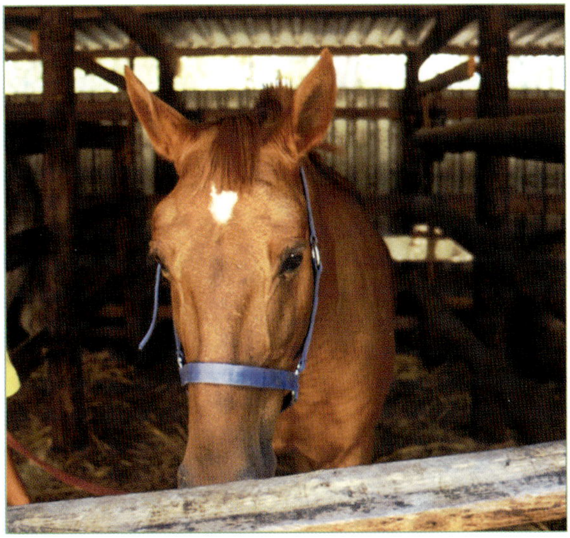

FIGURE 2: 'Cardiac' or 'dikkop' form of African horse sickness with filling of supraorbital fossae.

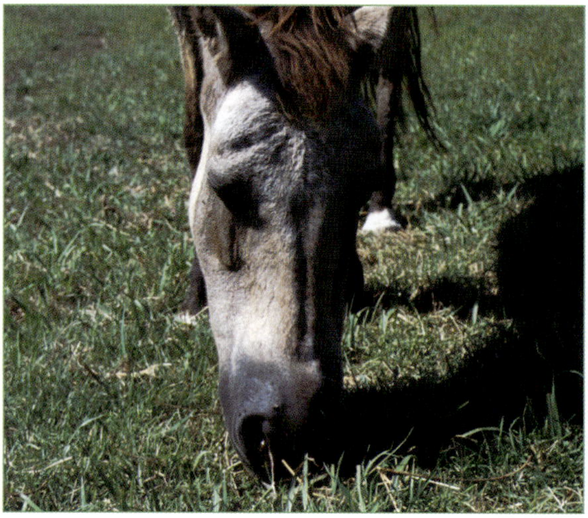

FIGURE 3: Severe oedema of the head associated with the 'cardiac' form of African horse sickness.

and frequently paw the ground. The course of the 'dikkop' form of AHS is always more protracted and milder than in the 'dunkop' form, with a mortality rate of >50%. Death usually occurs within 4–8 days after the onset of the febrile reaction. In cases that recover, swellings gradually subside over a period of 3–8 days. Paralysis of the oesophagus may be a complication, particularly in those cases with severe oedematous swellings of the head, resulting in dysphagia (Theiler 1920). In severely affected animals the oesophagus becomes distended and animals may die from inhalation pneumonia. Equine piroplasmosis is a common complication of AHS during recovery (Henning 1956). In such cases icterus, anaemia and constipation are evident.

'Mixed' form

Although this is the most common form of AHS, it is rarely diagnosed clinically. It is seen at necropsy in the majority of fatal cases of AHS in horses and mules. Initial pulmonary signs of a mild nature that do not progress are followed by oedematous swellings and effusions, and death results from cardiac failure. More commonly, the subclinical cardiac form is suddenly followed by marked dyspnoea and other signs typical of the pulmonary form. Death usually occurs 3–6 days after the onset of the febrile reaction.

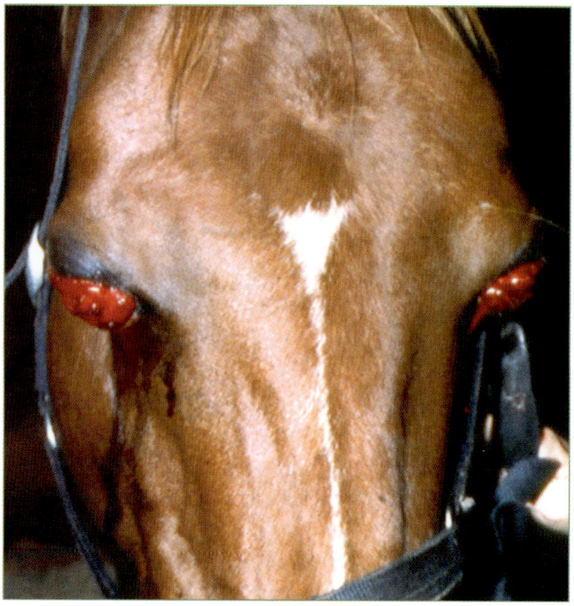

FIGURE 4: Severe conjunctival oedema and hyperaemia with some haemorrhage in a horse suffering from African horse sickness.

Horse sickness fever

This is the mildest form of AHS and is frequently not diagnosed clinically. The incubation period is 5–9 days after which the temperature gradually rises over a period of 4–5 days to 40°C followed by a drop in temperature to normal, and recovery. Apart from the febrile reaction, other clinical signs are rare and inconspicuous. Some animals may be depressed with partial loss of appetite, congestion of the conjunctivae, slightly laboured breathing and increased heart rate, but these signs are transient. This form of the disease is usually observed in donkeys and zebra or in immune horses infected with a heterologous serotype of AHSV.

Pathology

'Dunkop' or 'pulmonary' form macroscopic pathology

The most striking finding is diffuse, severe, subpleural and interlobular oedema of the lungs (**Fig 5**). Severe hydrothorax is common with the pleural cavity containing several litres of transparent, pale yellow, gelatinous fluid. Subcutaneous and intermuscular oedema is usually

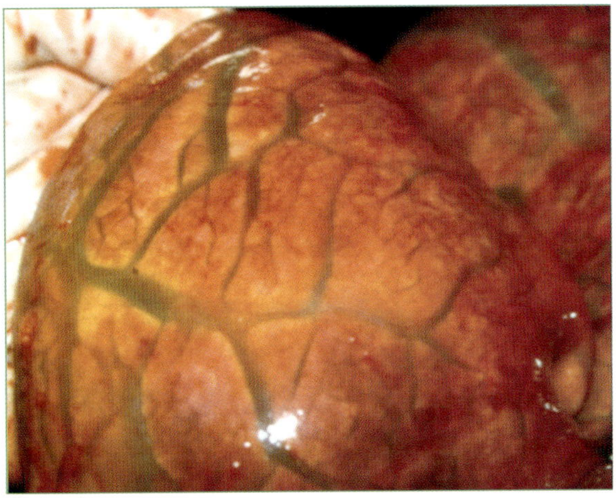

FIGURE 5: Severe septal oedema of lungs.

'Dikkop' or 'cardiac' form macroscopic pathology

The most characteristic finding in this form is the presence of distinctly yellow oedema of the subcutaneous and intermuscular connective tissues. The oedema is particularly severe around the *ligamentum nuchae*. In mild cases only the head and neck are involved, but in severe cases the oedema involves the lower parts of the neck, the thorax and shoulders. The eyelids, supraorbital fossae and lips are commonly involved. The tongue may have petechiae or ecchymoses on its ventral surface and is occasionally swollen and cyanotic. Severe hydropericardium is almost invariably present. Sub-

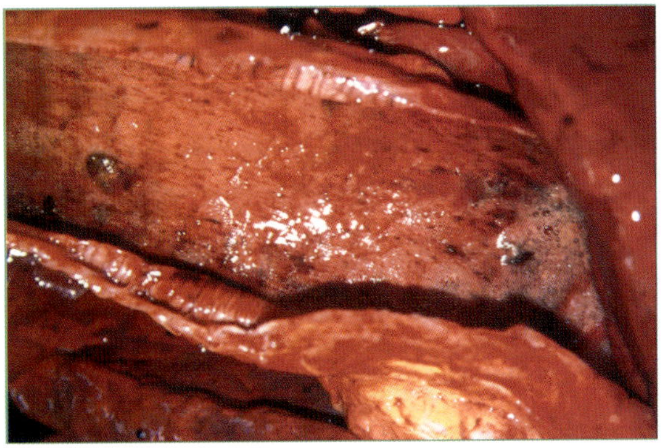

FIGURE 6: Froth and serosal haemorrhages in trachea.

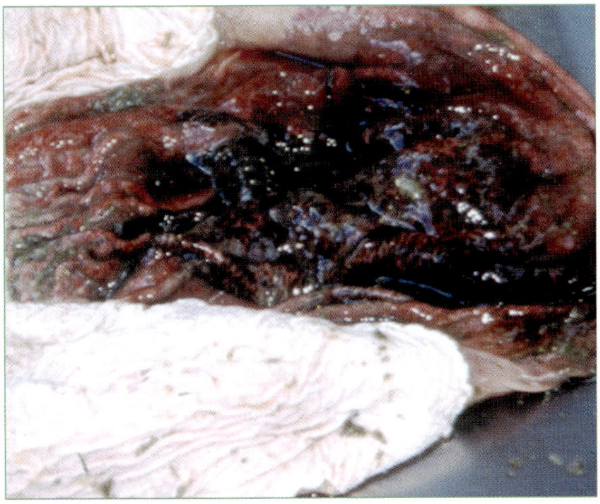

FIGURE 7: Congestion of glandular part of the stomach.

absent. Oedema may also involve the mediastinum, base of the heart and the parietal pleura. Serous fluid oozes from the cut surface of the lung. The trachea and bronchi usually contain large amounts of froth and yellow serous fluid. Petechiae and ecchymoses are sometimes present on the mucosa of the trachea (**Fig 6**). The bronchial and mediastinal lymph nodes are severely swollen and oedematous. The spleen is normal in size with the white pulp being more prominent than usual. Moderate, diffuse congestion of the mucosa of the glandular part of the stomach is a consistent finding (**Fig 7**). Patchy congestion of the serosal surface of the small intestine and scattered petechiation on the intestinal serosa are common (**Fig 8**). There is usually some degree of ascites.

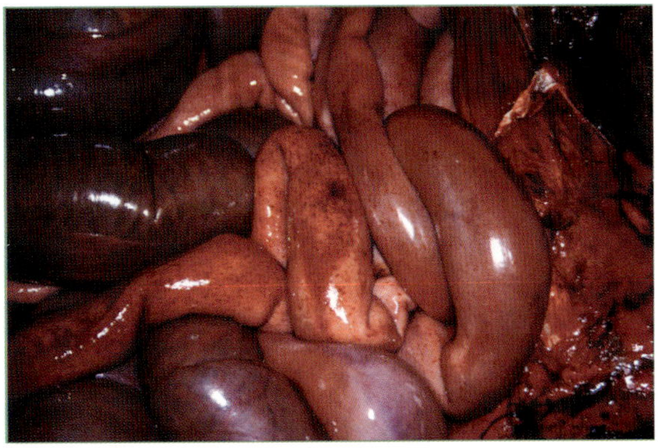

FIGURE 8: Petechiation on surfaces of small and large intestines.

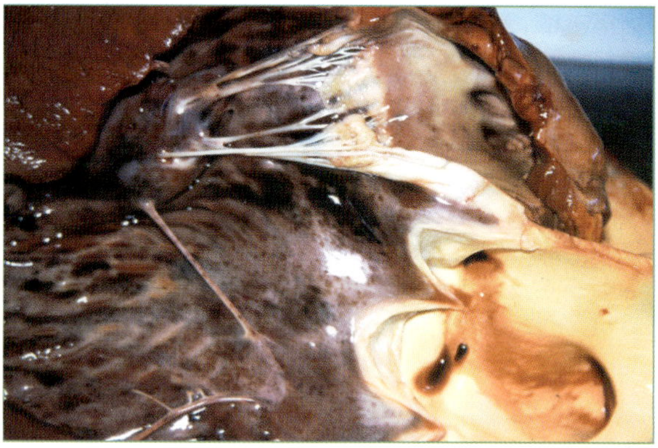

FIGURE 9: Sub-endocardial haemorrhages in left ventricle of the heart.

epicardial petechiation and sub-endocardial ecchymoses, particularly over the papillary muscles, are usually present (**Fig 9**). Pale grey areas of varying size may occur in the myocardium of horses with severe myocardial damage. The lungs are usually normal or slightly congested and hydrothorax is rare. The lymph nodes are swollen and oedematous. Mild nephrosis may be present. Moderate to severe oedema, congestion and petechiation of the mucosa of the caecum, colon and rectum are common (**Fig 8**). In cases with oesophageal paralysis, the oesophagus is distended with a variable amount of compressed food.

'Mixed' form

Lesions described for the pulmonary and cardiac forms of AHS and oedematous infiltration are found together in animals that die of this form of the disease.

Diagnosis

A definitive diagnosis of AHS is virtually impossible from clinical signs during the early febrile phase of the disease. Haematological abnormalities include leucopenia, thrombocytopenia, elevated packed cell volume, erythrocyte count and haemoglobin concentration. Haemostatic abnormalities include increased concentration of fibrin degradation products, prolonged prothrombin, activated partial thromboplastin and thrombin clotting times (Skowronek *et al.* 1995). A presumptive diagnosis should be possible once the characteristic clinical signs have developed. The typical macroscopic lesions of AHS on necropsy are often sufficiently specific to allow a provisional diagnosis of the disease to be made. The clinical signs of AHS may be confused with those of equine encephalosis. Many of the epidemiological features of the 2 infections are similar. Horses with swelling of the supraorbital fossae, eyelids or lips as a result of equine encephalosis cannot be differentiated clinically from the 'cardiac' form of AHS. However, the mortality rate of AHS is much higher than that of equine encephalosis. Virus isolation and identification are essential to confirm either diagnosis.

The disseminated petechiation associated with the 'cardiac' form of AHS may be very similar to that found in cases of purpura haemorrhagica and equine viral arteritis. However, the subcutaneous oedema observed in these conditions tends to be more ventral than that observed in cases of AHS. In purpura haemorrhagica, haemorrhages tend to be more severe, numerous and widespread than in AHS. The early stages of piroplasmosis may occasionally be confused with AHS. AHS may also be complicated by piroplasmosis and, in such cases, ventral oedema may be severe.

African horse sickness is foreign to almost all countries outside of sub-Saharan Africa and is an OIE listed disease. Suspected cases of AHS must, therefore, be reported to the State Veterinary Authority and must always be subject to laboratory confirmation. Blood samples collected in heparin and/or EDTA during the febrile stage of the disease or specimens of the lungs, spleen and lymph nodes collected at necropsy and kept at 4°C can be used for virus isolation and agent identification by antigen capture enzyme-linked immunosorbent assay (ELISA) or polymerase chain reaction (PCR) (Anon 2004).

A number of PCR assays (Stone-Marschat *et al.* 1994; Wilson 1994; Zientara *et al.* 1994; Sailleau *et al.* 1997; Aradaib *et al.* 2006; Aguero *et al.* 2008; Rodriguez-Sanchez *et al.* 2008; Fernandez-Pinero *et al.* 2008) have been described for the detection of AHSV and to differentiate between serotypes (Sailleau *et al.* 2000b; Koekemoer and van Dijk 2004; Koekemoer 2008). Molecular techniques have also been described to provide for further genetic characterisation of specific viruses (Koekemoer *et al.* 2003; Quan *et al.* 2008). These assays are rapid, sensitive and versatile, and they may supplement or replace some of the conventional methods.

Treatment and control

There is no specific treatment for AHS. Affected animals should be provided with supportive therapy, nursed and rested as the slightest exertion may result in death. Animals that survive should be rested for at least 4 weeks following recovery before being returned to light work. They should also be carefully monitored for complications such as piroplasmosis.

Since the demonstration in the early 1930s that AHSV could be attenuated by serial intracerebral passage in mice, the immunisation of horses against the disease has been greatly simplified and improved (Alexander and van der Vyfer 1935; Alexander 1936). The first highly effective attenuated vaccine was produced in 1936 (Alexander *et al.* 1936). Virus attenuation occurs faster during passage in cell culture than in mouse brain (Mirchamsy and Taslimi 1964). The size of plaques in cell culture has been found to be a marker of the virulence of AHS viruses and therefore, large plaque variants are now selected as candidate vaccine strains (Erasmus 1973; Anon 2004). In endemic areas, annual vaccination of horses in late winter or early summer is a very practical means of control. Unfortunately, prophylactic immunisation against AHS cannot be relied upon to fully protect all horses against infection or disease. However, horses that have received 3 or more courses of immunisation are usually well protected against AHS. Onderstepoort Biological Products currently produces a polyvalent vaccine containing attenuated strains prepared in 2 components, one trivalent (serotypes 1, 3 and 4) and the other quadrivalent (serotypes 2, 6, 7 and 8) (Du Plessis *et al.* 1998). Immunisation consists of the administration of these component vaccines at least 3 weeks apart. Serotype 5 and 9 are not included in the vaccines as serotype 8 and 6, respectively, are reported to afford adequate cross protection. Generally, immunisation has little or no side effects. A slight temperature response may occur 5–13 days after vaccination as a result of virus replication. Occasionally, individual animals vaccinated for the first time may show a severe vaccine reaction and may develop clinical signs of AHS. The simultaneous administration of several serotypes of attenuated AHS in horses usually results in the production of antibody against each serotype, although the response of individual horses may vary, and in some animals, antibody against one or more of the serotypes may not be detectable by neutralisation test (Alexander and Mason 1941; Blackburn and Swanepoel 1988b). This is possibly because of interference between viruses in the polyvalent vaccine or over attenuation of vaccine strains (McIntosh 1958; Erasmus 1978). During the outbreak of AHS in Spain, about 10% of animals immunised for the first time with a monovalent attenuated AHS virus serotype 4 vaccine failed to seroconvert. However, at least some of these animals appeared to be resistant to challenge (Hamblin *et al.* 1991).

The antibody acquired from colostrum correlates well with the antibody level of the dams and determines the duration of passive immunity (Alexander and Mason 1941; Blackburn and Swanepoel 1988b). Because of possible interference of passive immunity with response to vaccination in foals born to immune mares, it is recommended that foals should not be immunised before they are aged 6 months. However, some foals acquire low levels of antibody to one or more AHS virus serotypes via the colostrum and neutralising antibody to individual serotypes may decline to undetectable levels shortly after birth with the result that these foals can become susceptible to infection well before age 6 months (Blackburn and Swanepoel 1988b).

Various approaches have been used unsuccessfully in an attempt to develop new generation vaccines for AHS including baculovirus-expressed subunits of VP2 (Du Plessis *et al.* 1998), a DNA vaccine for VP2 (Romito *et al.* 1999) and an Alphavax vectored vaccine containing genes expressing VP2 and VP5 (MacLachlan *et al.* 2007). Recently, a canarypox virus vectored vaccine expressing the genes for VP2 and VP5 of Bluetongue has been shown to provide high level protection in sheep (Boone *et al.* 2007). The results of this study suggest that this approach to the development of recombinant vaccines may be applicable for orbivirus infections and warrants further investigation for AHSV.

The risk of infection of susceptible horses can be reduced significantly by stabling them from before dusk until after sunrise as *Culicoides* spp. are nocturnal and are not inclined to enter buildings (Blackburn and Swanepoel 1988b). The application of insect repellants and the use of insecticides on animals also reduces the risk of infection.

Following a suspected outbreak of AHS in a country that has previously been free of the disease, attempts should be made to limit further transmission of the virus and to achieve eradication as soon as possible. It is important that control measures be instituted immediately. The control measures in epizootic situations include: 1) delineation of the area of infection; 2) strict movement controls within, into and out of the infected area; 3) stabling of all equids from at least dusk to dawn; 4) insect control measures; 5) temperatures of all equids should be measured for early detection of infected animals; 6) vaccination of all susceptible animals with a relevant monovalent or polyvalent vaccine should be seriously considered; 7) all vaccinated animals should be identified; and 8) the World Oorganisation for Animal Health (OIE) should be notified of the outbreak of disease.

The Terrestrial Animal Health Code (Anon 2008a) provides guidelines for the importation of domestic horses from AHS infected countries or zones. These include the housing of animals in vector-protected quarantine facilities for a period of at least 40 days and testing for the absence of AHSV or demonstration of a stable or declining AHS antibody titre.

References

Adeyefa, C.A. and Hamblin, C. (1995) Continuing prevalence of African horse sickness in Nigeria. *Rev. Elev. Med. Vet. Pays Trop.* **48**, 31-33.

Aguero, M., Gomez-Tejedor, C., Angeles, C.M., Rubio, C., Romero, E. and Jimenez-Clavero, A. (2008) Real-time fluorogenic reverse transcription polymerase chain reaction assay for detection of African horse sickness virus. *J. vet. diag. Invest.* **20**, 325-328.

Alexander, R.A. (1933) Preliminary note on the infection of white mice and guinea pigs with the virus of horsesickness. *J. S. Afr. vet. med. Ass.* **4**, 1-9.

Alexander, R.A. (1936) Studies on the neurotropic virus of horsesickness. V. The antigenic response of horses to simultaneous trivalent immunization. *Onderstepoort J. vet. Sci. Anim. Ind.* **7**, 11-16.

Alexander, R.A. (1948) The 1944 epizootic of horsesickness in the Middle East. *Onderstepoort J. vet. Sci. Anim. Ind.* **23**, 77-92.

Alexander, R.A. and Mason, J.H. (1941) Studies on the neurotropic virus of horsesickness. VII. Transmitted immunity. *Onderstepoort J. vet. Sci. Anim. Ind.* **16**, 19-32.

Alexander, R.A. and van der Vyfer, B. (1935) Horsesickness field experiments with neurotropic vaccine during the season 1933-34. *J. S. Afr. vet. med. Ass.* **6**, 33-38.

Alexander, R.A., Neitz, W.O. and Du Toit, P.J. (1936) Horsesickness: Immunization of horses and mules in the field during the season 1934-1935 with a description of the technique of preparation of polyvalent mouse neurotropic vaccine. *Onderstepoort J. vet. Sci. Anim. Ind.* **7**, 17-30.

Anderson, E.C., Mellor, P. and Hamblin, C. (1989) African horse sickness in Saudi Arabia. *Vet. Rec.* **125**, 489.

Anon (2004) *Manual of Diagnostic Tests and Vaccines for Terrestrial Animal (Mammals, Birds and Bees)*, Office Internationale des Epizooties, Paris.

Anon (2008a) African horse sickness. In: *Terestrial Animal Health Code*, Office International des Epizooties, Paris.

Anon (2008b) Commission Decision of 8 August 2008 on the temporary admission and imports into the Community of registered horses from South Africa (2008/698/EC). *Off. J. Eur. Un.* L235, 16-25.

Aradaib, I.E., Mohemmed, M.E., Sarr, J.A., Idris, S.H., Ali, N.O., Majid, A.A. and Karrar, A.E. (2006) Short communication: a simple and rapid method for detection of african horse sickness virus serogroup in cell cultures using RT-PCR. *Vet. Res. Comm.* **30**, 319-324.

Barnard, B.J.H. (1993) Circulation of African horsesickness virus in zebra (*Equus burchelli*) in the Kruger National Park, South Africa, as measured by the prevalence of type specific antibodies. *Onderstepoort J. vet. Res.* **60**, 111-117.

Barnard, B.J.H. (1997) Antibodies against some viruses of domestic animals in southern African wild animals. *Onderstepoort J. vet. Res.* **64**, 95-110.

Barnard, B.J.H. (1998) Epidemiology of African horse sickness and the role of the zebra in South Africa. *Arch. Virol., Suppl.* **14**, 13-19.

Bayley, T.B. (1856) *Notes on the Horse-Sickness at the Cape of Good Hope, in 1854-55*, Saul Solomon & Co., Cape Town. pp 1-124.

Bell, R.A. (1999) Outbreak of African horse sickness in the Cape Province of South Africa. *Vet. Rec.* **144**, 483.

Bevan, L.E.W. (1911) The transmission of African horsesickness to the dog by feeding. *Vet. J.* **67**, 402-408.

Binepal, V.S., Wariru, B.N., Davies, F.G., Soi, R. and Olubayo, R. (1992) An attempt to define the host range for African horse sickness virus (Orbivirus, Reoviridae) in East Africa, by a serological survey in some Equidae, Camelidae, Loxodontidae and Carnivore. *Vet. Microbiol.* **31**, 19-23.

Blackburn, N.K. and Swanepoel, R. (1988a) African horse sickness in Zimbabwe: 1972 to 1981. *Trop. Anim. Health Prod.* **20**, 169-176.

Blackburn, N.K. and Swanepoel, R. (1988b) Observations on antibody levels associated with active and passive immunity to African horse sickness. *Trop. Anim. Hlth. Prod.* **20**, 203-210.

Boone, J.D., Balasuriya, U.B., Karaca, K., Audonnet, J.C., Yao, J., He, L., Nordgren, R., Monaco, F., Savini, G., Gardner, I.A. and MacLachlan, N.J. (2007) Recombinant canarypox virus vaccine co-expressing genes encoding the VP2 and VP5 outer capsid proteins of bluetongue virus induces high level protection in sheep. *Vaccine* **25**, 672-678.

Bosman, P., Bruckner, G.K. and Faul, A. (1995) African horse sickness surveillance systems and regionalization/zoning: the case of South Africa. *Rev. sci. tech. Off. int. Epiz.* **14**, 645-653.

Bourdin, P. (1973) Ecology of African horsesickness. In: *Equine Infectious Diseases III*, Ed: H. Gerber, Karger SA, Basel. pp 12-30.

Bremer, C.W., Huismans, H. and Van Dijk, A.A. (1990) Characterization and cloning of the African horsesickness virus genome. *J. Gen. Virol.* **71**, 793-799.

Burrage, T.G., Tevejo, R., Stone-Marschat, M. and Laegreid, W.W. (1993) Neutralizing epitopes of African horsesickness virus serotype 4 are located on VP2. *Virol.* **196**, 799-803.

Davies, F.G. and Oteino, S. (1977) Elephants and zebras as possible reservoir hosts for African horse sickness virus. *Vet. Rec.* **100**, 291-292.

Davies, F.G., Soi, R.K. and Binepal, V.S. (1993) African horse sickness viruses isolated in Kenya. *Vet. Rec.* **132**, 440.

Devaney, M.A., Kendall, J. and Grubman, M.J. (1988) Characterization of a nonstructural phosphoprotein of two orbiviruses. *Virus Res.* **11**, 151-164.

Du Plessis, D.H., Van Wyngaardt, W., Gerdes, G.H. and Opperman, E. (1991) Laboratory confirmation of African horsesickness in the Western Cape: application of a $F(ab)_2$-based indirect ELISA. *Onderstepoort J. vet. Res.* **58**, 1-3.

Du Plessis, M., Cloete, M., Aitchison, H. and Van Dijk, A.A. (1998) Protein aggregation complicates the development of baculovirus-expressed African horsesickness virus serotype 5 VP2 subunit vaccines. *Onderstepoort J. vet. Res.* **65**, 321-329.

Du Toit, R.M. (1944) The transmission of blue tongue and horsesickness by *Culicoides*. *Onderstepoort J. vet. Sci. Anim. Ind.* **19**, 7-16.

Dufour, B., Moutou, F., Hattenberger, A.M. and Rodhain, F. (2008) Global change: impact, management, risk approach and health measures - the case of Europe. *Rev. Sci. Tech.* **27**, 529-550.

Erasmus, B.J. (1973) Pathogenesis of African horsesickness. In: *Equine Infectious Diseases III*, Ed: H. Gerber, Karger SA, Basel. pp 1-11.

Erasmus, B.J. (1978) A new approach to polyvalent immunization against African horsesickness. In: *Equine Infectious Diseases IV*, Eds: J.T. Bryans and H. Gerber, Veterinary Publications Incorporated, Princeton, New Jersey. pp 401-403.

Erasmus, B.J., Young, E., Pieterse, L.M. and Boshoff, S.T. (1978) The susceptibility of zebra and elephants to African horsesickness virus. In: *Equine Infectious Diseases IV*, Eds: J.T. Bryans and H. Gerber, Veterinary Publications Incorporated, Princeton, New Jersey. pp 409-413.

Fernandez-Pinero, J., Fernandez-Pacheco, P., Rodriguez, B., Sotelo, E., Robles, A., Arias, M. and Sanchez-Vizcaino, J.M. (2008) Rapid and sensitive detection of African horse sickness virus by real-time PCR. *Res. vet. Sci.* **86**, 353-358.

Grubman, M.J. and Lewis, S.A. (1992) Identification and characterization of the structural and nonstructural proteins of African horsesickness virus and determination of the genome coding assignments. *Virol.* **186**, 444-451.

Haig, D.A., McIntosh, B.M., Cumming, R.B. and Hempstead, J.F.D. (1956) An outbreak of horsesickness, complicated by distemper in a pack of foxhounds. *J. S. Afr. vet. med. Ass.* **27**, 245-249.

Hamblin, C., Salt, J.S., Mellor, P.S., Graham, S.D., Smith, P.R. and Wohlsein, P. (1998) Donkeys as reservoirs of African horse sickness virus. *Arch. Virol.* **14**, 37-47.

Hamblin, C., Mellor, P.S., Graham, S.D., Hooghuis, H., Montejano, R.C., Cubillo, M.A. and Boned, J. (1991) Antibodies in horses, mules and donkeys following monovalent vaccination against African horsesickness. *Epidemiol. Infect.* **106**, 365-371.

Hazrati, A. (1967) Identification and typing of horse-sickness virus strains isolated in the recent epizootic of the disease in Morocco, Tunisia and Algeria. *Arch. Inst. Razi.* **19**, 131-143.

Henning, M.W. (1956) African horsesickness, perdesiekte, pestis equorum. In: *Animal Diseases of South Africa,* Central News Agency Ltd., Pretoria. pp 785-808.

Howell, P.G. (1960) The 1960 epizootic of African Horsesickness in the Middle East and S.W. Asia. *J. S. Afr. vet. med. Ass.* **31**, 329-334.

Howell, P.G. (1962) The isolation and identification of further antigenic types of African horsesickness virus. *Onderstepoort J. vet. Res.* **29**, 139-149.

Howell, P.G. (1963) Emerging diseases of animals. II. African horsesickness. *FAO Agric. Stud.* **61**, 71-108.

Koekemoer, J.J. (2008) Serotype-specific detection of African horsesickness virus by real-time PCR and the influence of genetic variations. *J. Virol. Methods* **154**, 104-110.

Koekemoer, J.J., Paweska, J.T., Pretorius, P.J. and Van Dijk, A.A. (2003) VP2 gene phylogenetic characterization of field isolates of African horsesickness virus serotype 7 circulating in South Africa during the time of the 1999 African horsesickness outbreak in the Western Cape. *Virus Res.* **93**, 159-167.

Koekemoer, J.J.O. and Van Dijk, A.A. (2004) African horsesickness virus serotyping and identification of multiple co-infecting serotypes with a single genome segment 2 RT-PCR amplification and reverse line blot hybridization. *J. Virol. Methods* **122**, 49-56.

Lubroth, J. (1988) African horsesickness and the epizootic in Spain 1987. *Equine Pract.* **10**, 26-33.

M'Fadyean, J. (1900) African horsesickness. *J. comp. Pathol. Therapeutics* **13**, 1-20.

MacLachlan, N.J., Balasuriya, U.B., Davis, N.L., Collier, M., Johnston, R.E., Ferraro, G.L. and Guthrie, A.J. (2007) Experiences with new generation vaccines against equine viral arteritis, West Nile disease and African horse sickness. *Vaccine* **25**, 5577-5582.

Martinez-Torrecuadrada, J.L. and Casal, J.I. (1995) Identification of a linear neutralization domain in the protein VP2 of African horse sickness virus. *Virol.* **210**, 391-399.

McIntosh, B.M. (1955) Horsesickness antibodies in the sera of dogs in enzootic areas. *J. S. Afr. vet. med. Ass.* **26**, 269-272.

McIntosh, B.M. (1958) Immunological types of horsesickness virus and their significance in immunization. *Onderstepoort J. vet. Res.* **27**, 465-539.

Meiswinkel, R., Baylis, M. and Labuschagne, K. (2000) Stabling and the protection of horses from *Culicoides bolitinos* (Diptera: Ceratopogonidae), a recently identified vector of African horse sickness. *Bull. Entomol. Res.* 509-515.

Mirchamsy, H. and Taslimi, H. (1964) Attempts to vaccinate foals with living tissue culture adapted horsesickness virus. *Bull. de l'Office Int. des Epizooties* **62**, 911-921.

Piercy, S.E. (1951) Some observations on African horse-sickness including an account of an outbreak among dogs. *East Afr. Agric. J.* **17**, 62-64.

Pitchford, N. and Theiler, A. (1903) Investigations into the nature and causes of horsesickness. *Agric. J. Cape Good Hope* **23**, 153-156.

Quan, M., van, V.M., Howell, P.G., Groenewald, D. and Guthrie, A.J. (2008) Molecular epidemiology of the African horse sickness virus S10 gene. *J. Gen. Virol.* **89**, 1159-1168.

Reid, N.R. (1961) African horse sickness. *Br. vet. J.* **118**, 137-142.

Rodriguez, M., Hooghuis, H. and Castano, M. (1992) African horse sickness in Spain. *Vet. Microbiol.* **33**, 129-142.

Rodriguez-Sanchez, B., Fernandez-Pinero, J., Sailleau, C., Zientara, S., Belak, S., Arias, M. and Sanchez-Vizcaino, J.M. (2008) Novel gel-based and real-time PCR assays for the improved detection of African horse sickness virus. *J. Virol. Methods* **151**, 87-94.

Romito, M., Du Plessis, D.H. and Viljoen, G.J. (1999) Immune responses in a horse inoculated with the VP2 gene of African horsesickness virus. *Onderstepoort J. vet. Res.* **66**, 139-144.

Roy, P., Mertens, P.P. and Casal, I. (1994) African horse sickness virus structure. *Comp. Immunol. Microbiol. Infect. Dis.* **17**, 243-273.

Sailleau, C., Seignot, J., Davoust, B., Cardinale, E., Fall, B., Hamblin, C. and Zientara, S. (2000a) African horse sickness in Senegal: serotype identification and nucleotide sequence determination of segment S10 by RT-PCR. *Vet. Rec.* **146**, 107-108.

Sailleau, C., Hamblin, C., Paweska, J.T. and Zientara, S. (2000b) Identification and differentiation of the nine African horse sickness virus serotypes by RT-PCR amplification of the serotype-specific genome segment 2. *J. Gen. Virol.* **81**, 1-7.

Sailleau, C., Moulay, S., Cruciere, C., Laegreid, W.W. and Zientara, S. (1997) Detection of African horse sickness virus in the blood of experimentally infected horses: comparison of virus isolation and a PCR assay. *Res. vet. Sci.* **62**, 229-232.

Salama, S.A., Dardiri, A.H., Awad, F.I., Soliman, A.M. and Amin, M.M. (1981) Isolation and identification of African horsesickness virus from naturally infected dogs in Upper Egypt. *Can. J. Comp. Med.* **45**, 392-396.

Sellers, R.F., Pedgley, D.E. and Tucker, M.R. (1977) Possible spread of African horse sickness on the wind. *J. Hyg.* **79**, 279-298.

Skowronek, A.J., LaFranco, L., Stone-Marschat, M.A., Burrage, T.G., Rebar, A.H. and Laegreid, W.W. (1995) Clinical pathology and hemostatic abnormalities in experimental African horsesickness. *Vet. Pathol.* **32**, 112-121.

Stone-Marschat, M., Carville, A., Skowronek, A. and Laegreid, W.W. (1994) Detection of African horse sickness virus by reverse transcription-PCR. *J. clin. Microbiol.* **32**, 679-700.

Theiler, A. (1906) Transmission of horse sickness into dogs. *Rep. Govern. Vet. Bacteriol.* 160-162.

Theiler, A. (1920) Paralysis of the oesophagus in the horse as a sequel to horsesickness. *Rep. Dir. Vet. Res.* **7-8**, 339-357.

Theiler, A. (1921) African horse sickness (*pestis equorum*). *Sci. Bull.* **19**, 1-29.

Verwoerd, D.W., Huismans, H. and Erasmus, B.J. (1979) Orbiviruses. In: *Comprehensive Virology*, Eds: H. Fraenkel-Conrat and R.R. Wagner, Plenum Press, London. pp 285-345.

Wilson, W.C. (1994) Development of nested-PCR test based on sequence analysis of epizootic hemorrhagic disease viruses non-structural protein 1 (NS1). *Virus Res.* **31**, 357-365.

Zeleke, A., Sori, T., Powel, K., Gebre-Ab, F. and Endebu, B. (2005) Isolation and identification of circulating serotypes of African horse sickness virus in Ethiopia. *Intern. J. Appl. Res. Vet. Med.* **3**, 40-43.

Zientara, S., Sailleau, C., Moulay, S. and Cruciere, C. (1994) Diagnosis of the African horse sickness virus serotype 4 by a one-tube, one manipulation RT-PCR reaction from infected organs. *J. Virol. Methods* **46**, 179-188.

Zientara, S., Sailleau, C., Plateau, E., Moulay, S., Mertens, P.P. and Cruciere, C. (1998) Molecular epidemiology of African horse sickness virus based on analyses and comparisons of genome segments 7 and 10. *Arch. Virol., Suppl.* **14**, 221-234.

WEST NILE VIRUS ENCEPHALOMYELITIS

M. A. Bourgeois, M. T. Long* and K. K. Seino†

Department of Infectious Diseases and Pathology, College of Veterinary Medicine, University of Florida, PO Box 110880, 2015 SW 16th Ave, Gainesville, Florida 32611-0880; and †Washington State University College of Veterinary Medicine, Pullman, Washington, USA.

Keywords: horse; West Nile virus; encephalitis: encephalomyelitis; vaccination

Summary

Since the introduction of West Nile virus (WNV) into North America, over 25,000 cases of equine neurological disease have been reported. Clinical signs of infection can range from subclinical disease to severe encephalomyelitis (changes in mentation, cranial nerve deficits, spinal cord abnormalities) to death. If disease is suspected, serum and/or CSF fluid should be collected and sent for testing using the IgM capture ELISA. There is currently no effective treatment and infected horses should receive supportive care. Multiple vaccines have been developed for use in the horse and are highly effective at preventing clinical disease, including killed and modified live formulations. Given the recent licensing of a WNV vaccine in Europe, large numbers of horses can be successfully protected against severe, fatal encephalitis in anticipation of new outbreaks in North America, South America and Europe.

Introduction

West Nile virus (WNV) encephalitis is one of the leading causes of equine neurological disease in the USA. Since the introduction of WNV into the USA in 1999, over 25,000 clinical cases of disease have been confirmed in horses (Agaton *et al.* 2002). This disease is devastating to the equine industry not only due to the direct costs of vaccination, diagnosis, treatment, and mortality, but also due to the indirect costs associated with long-term health effects in survivors and loss of valuable blood stock when large cyclical outbreaks occur. Therefore, it is imperative that the clinician gain a solid understanding of WNV in order to understand how to prevent disease and how to effectively recognise and treat cases that may occur.

*Author to whom correspondence should be addressed.

Epidemiology

West Nile virus was first discovered in 1937 in the West Nile province of Uganda. Before 1999, the virus was enzootic to Africa, the Middle East, the Mediterranean, and west/central Asia with periodic incursions into Europe. WNV was first introduced to North America in 1999, when a single point introduction of WNV occurred in New York City (Anon 1999; Lanciotti *et al.* 1999). Since that time, the virus has spread to affect almost the entire western hemisphere, as far north as Canada and as far south as Argentina. WNV is now the most widely distributed Flavivirus, present on all continents except Antarctica (Hayes *et al.* 2005). Although a new introduction to the New World, neuroinvasive WNV has been active in both Eastern and Western Europe, with the latest outbreak in horses occurring in 2008 in Northern Italy.

Ecology and host range

West Nile virus is a seasonal disease, with case occurrence corresponding with peak mosquito vector activity. In northern, temperate climates, peak activity occurs in the summer months (July and August). In tropical and subtropical climates, disease activity is high year-round, although it may fluctuate slightly dependent upon rainfall (Hayes *et al.* 2005). One of the major questions in the ecology of WNV is how the virus survives the winter, especially in Northern latitudes. It is possible that the virus survives in overwintering female mosquitoes, (Anon 1999; Riesen *et al.* 2005; Cupp *et al.* 2007) is transmitted back up north with migratory birds, and/or chronically infects birds or nontraditional reservoir hosts.

West Nile virus is maintained in nature in a bird-mosquito-bird cycle (**Fig 1**). In North America, over

60 species of mosquito have been found to be capable of transmitting WNV, with *Culex* species as the main vector among birds. The specific *Culex* species vary according the region- in the Northeast, the main species is *Culex pipiens*, in the West the main species is *Culex tarsalis*, and in the South the main species are *Culex quinquefasciatus* and *Culex nigripalpus* (Sardelis *et al.* 2001; Tesh *et al.* 2004; Turell *et al.* 2001a,b, 2005; Reisen *et al.* 2005). The *Culex* species of mosquitoes were originally not considered efficient bridge vectors of WNV to mammals, but WNV epidemics are likely driven by shifts in mosquito feeding that occur with dispersal of avian hosts resulting in movement of WNV from bird to man in urban centres (Savage *et al.* 2007). The species that appear to be capable of functioning as bridge vectors include *Aedes* spp., *Anopheles* spp. and *Coquillettidia* spp. (Sardelis *et al.* 2001, 2002; Savage *et al.* 2007).

It was originally thought that *Corvidae* (i.e. crows, blue jays, ravens) served as the major reservoir for the virus. However, while these bird species develop high viraemias, they quickly succumb to clinical disease (Komar *et al.* 2003; Weingartl *et al.* 2004). Therefore while *Corvidae* function as excellent sentinels for monitoring the introduction of WNV into an area, they do not survive long enough to function as effective reservoirs. Instead, it appears that other bird species, including the American robin, Northern cardinal, common grackle and house finch, may actually serve as the reservoir hosts of WNV (Komar *et al.* 2003; Kilpatrick *et al.* 2006a; Savage *et al.* 2007). In addition, there is now evidence that other, 'nontraditional' species may serve as reservoirs for WNV. These include rodents, lagomorphs (notably squirrels and chipmunks) (Platt *et al.* 2007, 2008) and reptiles (including alligators) (Klenk *et al.* 2004; Jacobson *et al.* 2005). Thus, wild rodents and reptiles may serve as WNV reservoirs in nature, altering the traditional view of a bird-mosquito-bird maintenance cycle.

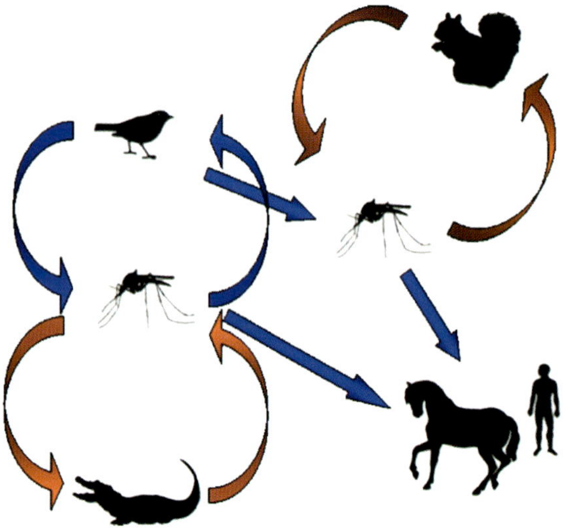

FIGURE 1: Life cycle of West Nile virus.

Molecular epidemiology

West Nile virus is classified as a Flavivirus within the genus *Flaviviridae*. The genera *Flaviviridae* encompasses a wide range of viruses, most of which are spread through mosquitoes and ticks (arthropod-borne diseases). Other, related viruses of veterinary import within this genera include bovine viral diarrhoea and classical swine fever (Pestiviruses), as well as St Louis encephalitis and tick-borne encephalitis (Flaviviruses).

There are 2 distinct phylogenetic lineages of West Nile virus. Lineage 1 viruses, which were introduced into North America, are generally considered more pathogenic while lineage 2 viruses are considered less pathogenic. However both lineage 1 and 2 viruses can result in neuroinvasive disease (Botha *et al.* 2008). Genetic mutations within the viruses are responsible for the differences in virulence and phylogenetic classification, and include alterations in the E protein and nonstructural proteins (Chambers *et al.* 1998; Beasley *et al.* 2005; Botha *et al.* 2008). This can be seen in North America, where a dominant unique phenotype emerged during spread (Beasley *et al.* 2003, 2004a,b; Kilpatrick *et al.* 2006b; Davis *et al.* 2007). Over time mutations of the virus may have resulted in changes in transmission and this is associated with geographic location. An increase in transmission has been predicted in isolates obtained in the northeastern USA since 2002 while a possible decrease in pathogenesis appears to be occurring in Central and South American isolates. Long-term epizootics are likely to continue and occurrence will likely depend upon a culmination of climatic, geographic and host factors, yet to be completely modelled and predicted.

Viral structure and life cycle

West Nile virus is an enveloped, single-stranded positive sense RNA virus, approximately 50 nm in size. The genome of WNV is approximately 11,000 bp in length and codes for 10 viral proteins, including 3 nonstructural (NS) proteins and 7 structural proteins in the order 5'-Capsid-preMembrane-Envelope-NS1-NS2A-NS2B-NS3-NS4A-NS4B-NS5-3'. The nonstructural proteins are largely involved in viral replication, while the structural proteins mainly function in maintenance of the virion and are responsible for the majority of host immunogenicity (**Fig 2**) (reviewed in Lanciotti *et al.* 1999; Brinton 2002).

The first step in viral infection occurs when domain III of the envelope (E) protein binds to as-yet-uncharacterised host cell receptors. Receptor-mediated endocytosis occurs, and the virus enters the host cell within a low pH vesicle. The virus is then released from the vesicle into the cellular cytoplasm as a single strand of positive sense RNA. Translation occurs first, since viral proteins are required for subsequent RNA replication steps. Host cell elongation initiation factors (eIF) bind to the 5' untranslated region (UTR) of the viral genome. The traditional initiation, elongation and termination steps of translation then occur, and form a viral polyprotein coding for 10 proteins (5'-Capsid-preMembrane-Envelope-NS1-NS2A-NS2B-NS3-NS4A-NS4B-NS5-3'). Host cell proteases then cleave the polyprotein, allowing replication to occur. In subsequent translational events, the viral NS2B/NS3 protease carries out the cleavage of the polyprotein.

Replication of viral RNA starts at the 3' UTR of the genome. The viral NS4B/NS5 RNA-dependent-RNA-polymerase (RdRp) binds to conserved stem loop structures of the 3'UTR along with a variety of host cell proteins in an as-yet-uncharacterised event. Other viral proteins involved in this replication complex include NS1 and NS4A. The viral NS3 helicase acts to unwind/stabilise the RNA genome. Replication of a negative-sense RNA strand then occurs in a 5' to 3' direction. These negative sense strands serve as the template for the creation of positive-sense viral RNA genomes. Replication of positive-sense RNA strands occurs when the same viral and host replication complex binds to the 3' end of the negative-sense RNA (5' UTR of the viral genome). There is evidence that only a few negative strands are created, and that multiple replication events occur simultaneously on one of these strands to produce a large amount of positive sense RNA viral genomes. These positive-sense RNA strands then serve 2 functions: as a translational template for the creation of more polyproteins, and as a viral genome that is released from the cell. There is no polyA tail on the viral RNA genome, but a 5' cap is added by the NS5 viral protein.

Viral packaging occurs once enough viral proteins and genomes have been created in the golgi apparatus. The capsid (C) protein is arranged in an icosahedral symmetry around the positive-sense RNA with the assistance of NS2A. prM and E proteins are then arranged around the viral capsid. The prM conformation of the E protein protects the low pH mediated membrane fusion domain of the E protein during transit in a vesicle from the cell. Once released by exocytosis, the prM protein is cleaved to the M (membrane) form. The virus is then ready to bind to and infect new host cells.

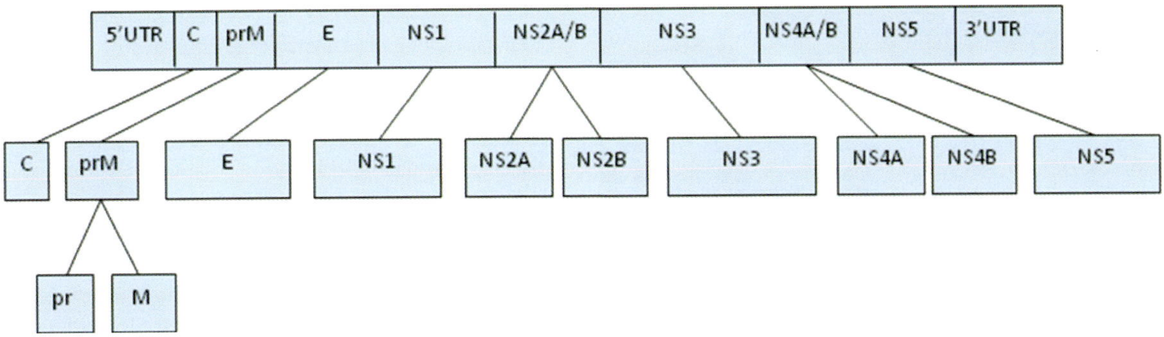

FIGURE 2: Molecular structure of West Nile virus.

Clinical signs

In the horse, the majority of WNV infections are subclinical. It is estimated, based on experimental mosquito challenge and epidemiological analysis, that about 10% of horses naturally exposed to WNV actually develop clinical disease (Bunning *et al.* 2001). Clinical signs usually begin within 9–11 days of infection (Bunning *et al.* 2001; Snook *et al.* 2001; Long *et al.* 2007). Initially, these include the general systemic signs of fever (38.3–39.4°C), anorexia and depression. The onset of neurological disease is usually abrupt and there are changes in behaviour or mentation with an insidious onset of motor deficits (Porter *et al.* 2001; Snook *et al.* 2001). Horses exhibit signs consistent with an encephalomyelitis (diffuse inflammation of the brain and spinal cord disease) exhibited by a combination of mentation and spinal cord abnormalities and defects in cranial nerves (**Fig 3**). Spinal cord abnormalities include a stiff stilted gait (which can be mistaken for lameness), ataxia (involving 2 or more limbs, symmetric or asymmetric), flaccid paralysis (lower motor neuron disease), paresis and recumbency. Muscle fasciculations (most notable around the muzzle but can involve the entire body) are often noted. Cranial nerve abnormalities include weakness of the tongue (CNXII- hypoglossal), muzzle deviation (CNVII-facial), head tilt and/or difficulty balancing (CN-VIII-vestibulocochlear), and difficulty swallowing (CNIX-glossopharyngeal). Changes in mentation include a change *in sensorium* defined as 'a change in animal's normal habits, personality, attitude, reaction to environment' and hyperaesthesia (Mayhew 1989). In addition, changes in behaviour including severe aggression, somnolence and coma may be seen.

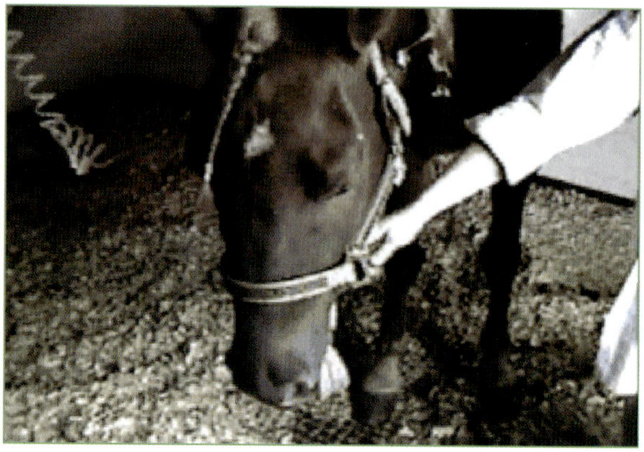

FIGURE 3: Horse with West Nile virus encephalomyelitis exhibiting typical loss of mentation (head position) and left-sided paralysis of the tongue (CN IX and XII).

Approximately 30% of horses with clinical signs of disease die spontaneously or are humanely subjected to euthanasia (this number increases to 100% if the horse is recumbent). The remaining 70% of horses with clinical disease recover within 3–7 days. However, approximately 30% of the horses that recover will recrudesce within 2 weeks. Of the horses that completely recover, 10% will retain long-term complications, including weakness, ataxia, and fatigue (Snook *et al.* 2001; Bunning *et al.* 2002; Long *et al.* 2007).

Clinicopathologically, neuroinvasive flaviviruses cause a polioencephalomyelitis (inflammation of the gray matter) mainly involving the midbrain, hindbrain and spinal cord (Long *et al.* 2007). This is characterised grossly by an increasing number of lesions progressing from the diencephalon through the hindbrain and down to the spinal cord. Spinal cord lesions become progressively worse caudally. Congestion of the meninges and haemorrhagic foci may be seen. Histopathologically, inflammatory lesions characterised by layers of monocellular perivascular cuffing are present. These layers of monocellular cells may also be present in the gray matter (gliosis). These lesions are most severe in the basal ganglia, thalamus, pons, and medulla. Gliosis and monocellular perivascular cuffing are also present in the spinal cord and become worse caudally. Few, if any, lesions are seen in the cerebrum and cerebellum, further emphasising the predilection of this virus for the midbrain, hindbrain and spinal cord (Long *et al.* 2007).

Immune response/pathophysiology

After the bite of an infected mosquito, WNV is inoculated peripherally into the skin and muscle. Dendritic cells take up the virus and transport it to the regional lymph nodes, where an innate and adaptive immune response is initiated (Diamond *et al.* 2003; Samuel and Diamond 2006). This is largely driven by the cytokine expression pattern of the macrophages and dendritic cells, as well as by NK T-cells. These APCs produce IFN-γ which functions to upregulate MHC-I expression, recruit CD8+ T-cells, and enhance NK cell activity. Expression of IL-12 by macrophages and dendritic cells induces the differentiation of T-helper cells into Th1 cells. These cells secrete IL-2 and IFN-γ, which, along with NK T-cell production of IFN-γ, activates and enhances the activity of CD8+ T-cells (Shrestha and Diamond 2004; Shrestha *et al.* 2006).

CD8+ T-cells kill virally infected cells by inducing apoptosis in target cells expressing the proper MHC-I/ PAMP combination (Samuel and Diamond 2006). Apoptosis can be induced by T-cells through 2 pathways: the perforin/granzyme pathway or the Fas/FasL pathway (TNF-α and TGF-β secreted by microglia can also induce the Fas/FasL pathway). Both mechanisms of apoptosis result in the death of an infected cell.

In contrast, expression of IL-4/5/10 by macrophages and dendritic cells drives the differentiation of T-helper cells into Th2 cells. Th2 cells function to stimulate the B-cell response (including B-cell phagocytic activity, antibody isotype switching and somatic hypermutation) and to inhibit the Th1 cell response (thus inhibiting the activity of CD8+ T-cells). B-cells initially produce IgM antibodies to WNV and then undergo an isotype switch to produce IgG (Kesson *et al.* 2002; Diamond *et al.* 2003; Wang and Fikrig 2004; Samuel and Diamond 2006). Antibodies are important in fighting viral infection through multiple mechanisms, including direct viral inhibition (binding to the virus to prevent binding to cell receptors), antibody-dependent cell-mediated cytotoxicity (binding to the virus to enhance Fc receptor recognition from NK cells and phagocytosis of the virus) and complement activation. This host immune response corresponds with a viraemia approximately 2–4 days post infection.

If the host is unable to neutralise the virus, the virus may gain access to the central nervous system through a breach of the blood brain barrier. There are multiple theories as to how this may happen. The first includes disruption of the barrier when endothelial cells are exposed to proinflammatory cytokines released by macrophages and dendritic cells of the innate immune system (Samuel and Diamond 2006). The second theory involves the infection of circulating peripheral mononuclear cells that migrate across the blood brain barrier (Wang and Fikrig 2004; Samuel and Diamond 2006) A third theory includes the use of peripheral nerves such as the olfactory nerve to travel to the CNS (Samuel and Diamond 2006).

Once the virus gains access to the CNS, a combination of the neuronal cell response, innate and adaptive immunity, and the virus life cycle produce neuropathological changes that lead to clinical disease in the horse. The virus initially binds to host T-cell receptors on microglia including TLR-3, RIG-1, MDA-5, and integrins which begins the immunological cascade (Fredericksen *et al.* 2004, 2008; Town *et al.* 2006). Binding to the cell receptors activates a signaling cascade involving transcription factors such as IRF-3, NFk-β, and MAPK, which lead to the production of type I interferons (IFN-α and IFN-β) (Fredericksen *et al.* 2004). These IFNs then bind to cell receptors and induce an antiviral response through secondary signalling, including the JAK/STAT pathway (Samuel and Diamond 2005). For the majority of the time, the antiviral response by microglial cells is beneficial to the host. The type 1 IFNs induce the transcription of 2'5'oligodenylate synthetase which leads to RNAseL production and the degradation of viral RNA, as well the transcription of PKR kinase which leads to the production of eIF-2 and inhibition of viral transcription (Samuel and Diamond 2006; Scherbik *et al.* 2006). Polymorphisms in these genes are associated with susceptibility to WNV in horses (Rios *et al.* 2007).

Neuronal infection by WNV also leads to host cell damage, both directly through the actions of the virus, and indirectly through the host immune response. During infection, neurons express CXCL10 and CCR5- chemokines which drive the recruitment of CD8+ T-cells (Klein *et al.* 2005). This, combined with IFN-γ secreted by NK T-cells and IFN-γ and IL-2 secreted by Th1 cells, functions to recruit CD8+ T-cells to sites of viral replication and upregulate MHC-I expression. CD8+ T-cells, once activated, undergo positive feedback through the self secretion and stimulation of IFN-γ and IL-2. CD8+ T-cells kill virally infected cells by inducing apoptosis in target cells through the Fas/FasL pathways and the perforin/granzyme pathway as mentioned above (Shresth *et al.* 2006). Both mechanisms of apoptosis result in the death of an infected cell and are essential to host survival (Shrestha and Diamond 2004). However, CD8+ T-cell activity has also been found to be detrimental to the host. The activity of CD8+ T cells can lead to direct neuronal damage, decreased survival time with high viral loads, and inflammation (Wang *et al.* 2003). Thus CD8+ T-cells appear to function in both the recovery from and pathology of WNV infection. Since WNV preferentially infects the neuronal cell bodies of the thalamus, midbrain, hindbrain and spinal cord, the gray matter of these regions is most affected leading to virus and immune-induced neuropathology.

Diagnostics

Since no clinical signs are pathognomonic for WNV infection, all horses that are suspected of being infected with WNV should undergo ancillary diagnostic testing to rule out other diseases. This should include complete blood count (CBC) and serum biochemistry as well as a cerebrospinal fluid analysis (CSF). Blood analysis is usually normal, although there may be a lymphopenia, elevated muscle enzymes secondary to trauma and hyponatraemia. Cell and protein counts in the CSF may be elevated, usually consisting of an elevated mononuclear cell population >7 cells/μg, protein concentration >700 mg/l, and mild xanthochromia (Wamsley *et al.* 2002; Porter *et al.* 2003).

Differentials for neurological disease in the horse suspected of WNV infection should include hepatoencephalopathy, rabies, alphavirus infection (EEE, WEE), equine protozoal myeloencephalitis (EPM), leucoencephalomalacia, tremorigenic toxicities, equine herpesvirus-1 (EHV-1), botulism, hypocalcaemia and verminous meningoencephalmyelitis (Long *et al.* 2007). These diseases and metabolic conditions can be ruled out with pertinent testing.

The preferred test developed by the National Veterinary Services Laboratory for the detection of WNV in the horse is the IgM capture enzyme-linked immunosorbent assay (MAC) (Ostlund *et al.* 2000, 2001). This test detects whether the horse has had recent exposure to WNV by testing for the presence of IgM antibodies. High levels of IgM antibodies are quickly formed post exposure to WNV by the horse and last for approximately 4–6 weeks. After this time, circulating levels of IgM WNV antibodies decline rapidly in the horse. Serum and/or CSF should be shipped overnight on ice to a testing laboratory. The test takes approximately 24–48 h to perform and most USA diagnostic laboratories perform this test (Ostlund *et al.* 2000). The antigens are available commercially and allow for development of ELISA testing in new locales upon encroachment. One standard dilution is measured for serum (1:400) and CSF (1:2) and the sensitivity and specificity of this test on serum is 81% and 100%, respectively.

In the unvaccinated horse, the plaque reduction neutralisation test (PRNT) is the gold standard and is used in arbovirus surveillance testing to differentiate between closely related viruses. In totally naïve populations (not previously exposed, not vaccinated), a positive MAC and PRNT is confirmatory for WNV exposure. Otherwise this test can be used to confirm recent WNV infection if there is a 4-fold rise in paired neutralising antibody titres. Horses with high levels of neutralising antibody will have no plaques even at high dilutions of the serum (i.e. 1:320 or lower) due to the antibody binding to and preventing the virus from infecting the cells. Horses with little or no neutralising antibodies will have wells demonstrating a cytopathic effect (plaques) even at low dilutions (i.e. 1:2). In this manner, the titre of the antibody can be determined (the lowest dilution at which there are no viral plaques). If this test is run sequentially (i.e. at 1 and 4 weeks) and there is a 4-fold rise in the antibody titres, then the horse has been exposed to WNV. However, this test has fallen out of favour for diagnosis of WNV infection due to the fact that vaccination produces antibodies that confound the results. Another issue with this test is that it requires the use of live WNV, which is a human pathogen that must only be used in high containment laboratories (Biosafety Level-3). WNV chimera viruses developed as vaccines, are avirulent. Since these also form plaques in cell culture, these viruses offer a safe alternative to the use of virulent WNV (Arroyo *et al.* 2001). In addition to confirmatory diagnostic testing, PRNT formats are important for assessing field and vaccine induced immunity. A microtitre variant of the PRNT has been developed and is used by regulatory and diagnostic laboratories; the test is somewhat faster and requires less virus. Thus this test is used for endpoint titre testing. The microtitre assay has relatively higher titres than those achieved using the PRNT; thus, values must be compared within the range of this test rather than between formats. This test is now mainly used to determine the titre of antibodies to WNV in the subject of interest, especially post vaccination responses. Serum and/or CSF should be sent via overnight mail on ice to a testing laboratory and the test takes 1–2 weeks (Ostlund *et al.* 2000, 2001). There is no ELISA-based format that accurately predicts levels of serum neutralising antibody; a competitive inhibition ELISA is available that detects mainly IgG, and its value is in multispecies, rapid surveillance.

Other methods for confirmation of WNV infection in the horse require *post mortem* testing for the virus in brain and spinal cords and these include virus isolation, and various PCR techniques and immunohistochemistry to detect viral antigens. If these forms of testing are required, whole brains (especially the midbrain and hindbrain) and/or spinal cord should be submitted to a testing laboratory chilled in the proper containers for biocontainment (Tewari *et al.* 2004) Infection in the horse even in severe clinical symptomology is characterised by low virus load; thus *post mortem* confirmation is frequently unsuccessful and frustrating to the practitioner. An understanding of predilection of the virus for certain parts of the brain and spinal cord can enhance detection. Unlike alphavirus infection, this virus can localise focally to the caudate nucleus, the thalamus, the pons/medulla, and the thoracic and lumbar spinal cords. Frequently horse brains in the US are tested by public health laboratories, first for rabies virus, and then the remaining brain tested for arboviruses. Because of the emphasis of diagnosis of rabies virus on hindbrain and cerebellum, the cerebrum is frequently the only site tested for arboviruses. Given the limited virus distribution and the large amount of tissue available, the sensitivity of even the most sensitive tests such as PCR is drastically reduced. Site specific and lesion specific testing of the mid and hindbrain will increase sensitivity of all antigen detection methods.

Treatment

Currently, there is no effective anti-viral treatment for WNV. Treatment should focus on providing supportive care. Horses that present with clinical signs of WNV should be placed on flunixin meglumine- 1.1 mg/kg bwt q. 12 h i.v. This appears to reduce the muscle tremors and fasciculations associated with WNV. There is controversy over the use of corticosteroids in horses affected with WNV due to the possibility of enhancing the viral load both peripherally and in the CNS. However, recumbent horses generally require more aggressive therapy, including corticosteroids, due to the high mortality associated with recumbency. This should include dexamethasone sodium (0.05–0.1 mg/kg bwt q. 24 h i.v.) and mannitol (0.25–2.0 g/kg bwt q. 24 h i.v.). For the short-term relief of anxiety, acepromazine can be used (0.02 mg/kg bwt i.v. or 0.05 mg/kg bwt i.m.). For long-term tranquilisation, detomidine hydrochloride (0.02–0.04 mg/kg bwt i.v. or i.m.) can be used. Therapies that have yet to be tested and proven efficacious include the use of IFN-α, WNV-specific i.v. immunoglobulin and viral inhibitors. Several novel anti-RNA virus compounds are in experimental development and demonstrate promise; the expectation is that these new products will have limited use due to initial expense for the equine owner.

The most exciting interventional therapy is in the administration of WNV specific immunoglobulin after onset of clinical disease. Although initial results with IgG were unrewarding after experimental challenge, recent work with high titre IgG from recovered WNV patients demonstrate increased survival by 30% in a lethal mouse model (Makhoul *et al.* 2009). Further development of nonmouse monoclonal antibodies may further increase efficacy.

Vaccination

Upon encroachment of West Nile virus, a widespread industry response resulted in the development of several different vaccine formulations labeled against viraemia and/or disease due to West Nile virus. Institution of vaccination well before the first equine case would provide protection against loss of susceptible and valuable bloodstock. Four unique formulations are available for prevention of WNV in equids. Comparative efficacy studies indicate that vaccination against WNV is highly effective and WNV should be a core and recommended vaccine for all horses residing or travelling to WNV endemic areas (Seino *et al.* 2007). Early recognition of risk for new encroachment of WNV into new locales should lead to equine vaccination campaigns. In these comparative efficacy studies, 3 available vaccines (inactivated whole virion, canarypox modified live, modified live flavivirus chimera) were tested in a model of grave virulent virus challenge that induces disease and mortality in 100% of nonvaccinated horses. At 28 days post vaccination, all vaccinated horses survived, regardless of product used. Thus, there are several options that can be tailored for any equine management operation, the difference being dictated by the quality of post marketing investigations of specific risk factors such as age, pregnancy status, presence of maternal antibody and time to induction of immunity (for coverage of naïve horses during an outbreak).

Inactivated whole virion/subunit vaccines

Killed and subunit vaccines are often used in veterinary medicine for their safety record (less likely to revert to live virus) and for their potential in over-the-counter marketing. The first licensed vaccine (Innovator)[1], available since 2001, is a killed West Nile vaccine consisting of a formalin-inactivated whole virion. The adjuvant present in this vaccine is MetaStim[1] - a proprietary oil, non-aluminium, dual phase adjuvant (Ng *et al.* 2003; Tesh *et al.* 2004). This vaccine is currently labelled for the control of viraemia of WNV infection in the horse. Efficacy and duration of immunity studies using this vaccine demonstrated that 18 out of 19 vaccinated horses did not develop a detectable viraemia for up to 12 months after vaccination. It should be noted that the duration of protection against WNV clinical disease has yet to be tested in the clinical challenge model (Epp *et al.* 2007). Initial field studies indicate that there is a rapid decrease in the level of antibodies by 5–7 months after vaccination (Davidson *et al.* 2005). Inactivated whole virion vaccines do not actively replicate once administered in the host. Thus multiple vaccinations are required for the naïve equine. As of January 2009, this vaccine became the first WNV vaccine licensed in Europe (Duvaxyn WNV)[1].

A series of 2 vaccinations given 3–6 weeks apart, prior to the period when vectors are active, is recommended in adult horses. In foals, an initial series of 3 immunisations should follow a schedule of vaccination (similar to that for EEE and WEE). Foals born to immunised mares or those that have had WNV infection can start receiving vaccines at age 4–6 months of age. In WNV challenge studies, it appears that 10% of properly immunised horses do not produce neutralising antibodies to WNV and that 2.3–3% of equine WNV cases are seen in the field in fully vaccinated horses (Davidson *et al.* 2005). The duration of immunity from vaccination with the killed, adjuvanted WNV vaccine is unknown. It has been recommended that a booster be given every 4 months in regions where the virus is exceptionally active throughout the year. Logically, the frequency of injection may be minimised to once or twice per year in climates that have short mosquito seasons and limited activity has historically been reported. For adults with an unknown vaccination history and/or no history of vaccination, a 2-dose series of vaccines should be given with the second dose given 4–6 weeks after the first. These horses should be given a booster before the onset of the vector season. In adult horses with a known history of vaccination, one vaccination is required prior to the onset on the vector season (usually in the spring) each year. However, if the horse lives in an area with vector activity year-round (i.e. the southeast USA), 2 (and possibly 3) doses of vaccine are recommended each year- one before the onset of peak vector activity in the spring and a booster in the late summer/autumn.

Modified live vaccines

Modified live virus vaccines are developed due to their ability to mimic natural infection without causing clinical disease, thus inducing long-term immunity to viral pathogens. Two recombinant live vector preparations are licensed for commercial use in horses. The canarypoxvirus vector vCP2017 (CP-WN; Recombitek)[2] was the first licenced in 2004. This vaccine expresses the WNV membrane (prM) and envelope (E) genes under control of and packaged with a carbopol adjuvant, which is a proprietary cross-linking polymer adjuvant that has a depot effect to slow release of antigen. This adjuvant is considered superior to the aluminium-based adjuvants as it is proposed to induce both humoural and T cell responses. After a single dose of CP-WN, 90% of horses demonstrated protection against viraemia (Siger *et al.* 2004). Several post marketing studies have been performed and have demonstrated that for horses previously vaccinated with another product this vaccine has been shown to induce an antibody response; therefore vaccines can be interchanged without primary inoculation. Protection against viraemia was demonstrated with one dose of the vaccine in naïve horses. Ninety percent of vaccinated horses were protected in using the intrathecal challenge model when live virus was administered within 6 weeks of vaccination.

In foals born to both vaccinated and unvaccinated mares, a 3-dose series of vaccines should start with the initial dose at age 5–6 months (in areas with high vector activity, an extra dose at age 3 months for foals born to unvaccinated mares, and the first dose at age 3 months in foals born to vaccinated mares should be given). The second dose should be given 4 weeks after the first and the third dose at 3 months or 12 weeks after the first dose. In adult horses with an unknown vaccination history, a 2-dose series of vaccines should be given 4–6 weeks apart with a booster prior to the onset of peak vector activity. In horses with a history of vaccination, annual boosters should be given before peak vector activity. If living in areas with high mosquito activity year round (endemic for WNV), 2 vaccines should be given: one in the spring and one in the late summer/early autumn.

A nonadjuvanted, single-dose attenuated WNV, live flavivirus chimera (WN-FV) vaccine (PreveNile)[5] became available in 2006 (Arroyo *et al.* 2001). This vaccine expresses the envelope (E) and membrane (prM) of WNV in the yellow fever vaccine 17D (YF17D). The safety, efficacy and duration of immunity of the veterinary chimera (YF-WN) were investigated (Long *et al.* 2007). This vaccine, given at a 20x and100x immunogenicity dosages did not revert to virulence or have a detectable viraemia despite the development of neutralising antibody after vaccination. This vaccine does not contain any adjuvant and is marketed as a single injection product for induction of primary immunity. Efficacy studies have been performed solely using the intrathecal model previous to licensure and the product is currently the only one labeled for a 12 month duration of protection against clinical disease in addition to viraemia. Induction of immunity is quite rapid, and within 10 days, 83% of horses survived intrathecal challenge.

Care must be taken in vaccinating mares with no recent vaccine use in their history (and their foals that are age <6 months). If there is no history of vaccination in the mare or limited use of any arbovirus vaccine in the dam, then both the mare and foal should be considered naïve. Mares should undergo a primary series according to the label, and in areas of high vector activity, revaccination within 6 months is recommended irrespective of vaccine. Foals from naïve mares should be started with vaccination before age 4-6 months if the arbovirus season is active. At present, there is limited information on the protective immunity against challenge in foals aged <5 months. However, foals born to mares that are consistently vaccinated attain high levels of neutralising antibody upon ingestion of colostrum and these are maintained for at least 5–6 months. Thus for previously vaccinated mares, the most efficient way to provide the first 4–6 months of protection to the foal is through maternally derived antibody and a booster immunisation of mares is recommended at 30 days before foaling. For naïve mares, primary immunisation should begin during pregnancy, especially if at risk for disease and these mares should receive a booster injection again when open. For foals born to naïve dams, vaccination should commence at age 3 months and multiple injections are recommended in these foals regardless of product.

One of the first ever DNA vaccines for use in animals has also been developed against WNV and is now available as of 2009 (Innovator DNA)[1]. Early studies investigated this construct in mice and horses using a needle challenge model. Mice were protected against lethality in this model and horses from viraemia (Tesh *et al.* 2002). No post marketing studies are available at this time due to its recent market availability.

Conclusions

West Nile virus has the widest geographic distribution of all Flaviviruses. Given its explosive movement across North America, it is likely this virus will continue to expand and encroach into new areas throughout the world. Due to the fact that WNV mutates, little prediction can be made as to the short and long-term consequences of new WNV encroachment and endemic activity. Yet, given the availability of efficacious vaccines, severe mortality and morbidity can now be avoided. Agricultural policy in nations of high numbers and value of equine populations should reflect preparedness through surveillance and availability of vaccines. The next decade of products will probably provide post exposure mitigation and new methods for vector control.

Manufacturers' addresses

[1]Fort Dodge Animal Health, Overland Park, Kansas, USA.
[2]Merial, Duluth, Georgia, USA.
[3]Intervet, DeSoto, Kansas, USA.

References

Agaton, C., Unneberg, P., Sievertzon, M., Holmberg, A., Ehn, M., Larsson, M., Odeberg, J., Uhlen, M. and Lundeberg, J. (2002) Gene expression analysis by signature pyrosequencing. *Gene* **289**, 31-39.

Anon (1999) Outbreak of West Nile-like viral encephalitis - CDC New York, 1999. *MMWR Morb. Mortal Wkly. Rep.* **48**, 845-849.

Arroyo, J., Miller, C.A., Catalan, J. and Monath, T.P. (2001) Yellow fever vector live-virus vaccines: West Nile virus vaccine development. *Trends Mol. Med.* **7**, 350-354.

Beasley, D.W., Davis, C.T., Estrada-Franco, J., Navarro-Lopez, R., Campomanes-Cortes, A., Tesh, R.B., Weaver, S.C. and Barrett, A.D. (2004a) Genome sequence and attenuating mutations in West Nile virus isolate from Mexico. *Emerg. Infect. Dis.* **10**, 2221-2224.

Beasley, D.W., Davis, C.T., Whiteman, M., Granwehr, B., Kinney, R.M. and Barrett, A.D. (2004b) Molecular determinants of virulence of West Nile virus in North America. *Arch. Virol., Suppl.* **18**, 35-41.

Beasley, D.W., Davis, C.T., Guzman, H., Vanlandingham, D.L., Travassos da Rosa, A.P., Parsons, R.E., Higgs, S., Tesh, R.B. and Barrett, A.D. (2003) Limited evolution of West Nile virus has occurred during its southwesterly spread in the United States. *Virology* **309**, 190-195.

Beasley, D.W., Whiteman, M.C., Zhang, S., Huang, C.Y., Schneider, B.S., Smith, D.R., Gromowski, G.D., Higgs, S., Kinney, R.M. and Barrett, A.D. (2005) Envelope protein glycosylation status influences mouse neuroinvasion phenotype of genetic lineage 1 West Nile virus strains. *J. Virol.* **79**, 8339-8347.

Botha, E.M., Markotter, W., Wolfaardt, M., Paweska, J.T., Swanepoel, R., Palacios, G., Nel, L.H. and Venter, M. (2008) Genetic determinants of virulence in pathogenic lineage 2 West Nile virus strains. *Emerg. Infect. Dis.* **14**, 222-230.

Brinton, M.A. (2002) The molecular biology of West Nile Virus: a new invader of the western hemisphere. *Ann. Rev. Microbiol.* **56**, 371-402.

Bunning, M.L., Bowen, R.A., Cropp, B., Sullivan, K., Davis, B., Komar, N., Godsey, M., Baker, D., Hettler, D., Holmes, D. and Mitchell, C.J. (2001) Experimental infection of horses with West Nile virus and their potential to infect mosquitoes and serve as amplifying hosts. *Ann. N.Y. Acad. Sci.* **951**, 338-339.

Bunning, M.L., Bowen, R.A., Cropp, C.B., Sullivan, K.G., Davis, B.S., Komar, N., Godsey, M.S., Baker, D., Hettler, D.L., Holmes, D.A., Biggerstaff, B.J. and Mitchell, C.J. (2002) Experimental infection of horses with West Nile virus. *Emerg. Infect. Dis.* **8**, 380-386.

Chambers, T.J., Halevy, M., Nestorowicz, A., Rice, C.M. and Lustig, S. (1998) West Nile virus envelope proteins: nucleotide sequence analysis of strains differing in mouse neuroinvasiveness. *J. Gen. Virol.* **79**, 2375-2380.

Cupp, E.W., Hassan, H.K., Yue, Y., Oldland, W.K., Lilley, B.M. and Unnasch, T.R. (2007) West Nile virus infection in mosquitoes in the mid-south USA, 2002-2005. *J. med. Entomol.* **44**, 117-125.

Davidson, A.H., Traub-Dargatz, J.L., Rodeheaver, R.M., Ostlund, E.N., Pedersen, D.D., Moorhead, R.G., Stricklin, J.B., Dewell, R.D., Roach, S.D., Long, R.E., Albers, S.J., Callan, R.J. and Salman, M.D. (2005) Immunologic responses to West Nile virus in vaccinated and clinically affected horses. *J. Am. vet. med. Ass.* **226**, 240-245.

Davis, C.T., Li, L., May, F.J., Bueno, R. Jr, Dennett, J.A., Bala, A.A., Guzman, H., Quiroga-Elizondo, D., Tesh, R.B. and Barrett, A.D. (2007) Genetic stasis of dominant West Nile virus genotype, Houston, Texas. *Emerg. Infect. Dis.* **13**, 601-604.

Diamond, M.S., Shrestha, B., Mehlhop, E., Sitati, E. and Engle, M. (2003) Innate and adaptive immune responses determine protection against disseminated infection by West Nile encephalitis virus. *Viral Immunol.* **16**, 259-78.

Epp, T., Waldner, C. and Townsend, H.G. (2007) A case-control study of factors associated with development of clinical disease due to West Nile virus, Saskatchewan 2003. *Equine vet. J.* **39**, 498-503.

Fredericksen, B.L., Keller, B.C., Fornek, J., Katze, M.G. and Gale, M. Jr. (2008) Establishment and maintenance of the innate antiviral response to West Nile Virus involves both RIG-I and MDA5 signaling through IPS-1. *J. Virol.* **82**, 609-616.

Fredericksen, B.L., Smith, M., Katze, M.G., Shi, P.Y. and Gale, M. Jr. (2004) The host response to West Nile Virus infection limits viral spread through the activation of the interferon regulatory factor 3 pathway. *J. Virol.* **78**, 7737-7747.

Hayes, E.B., Komar, N., Nasci, R.S., Montgomery, S.P., O'Leary, D.R., and Campbell, G.L. (2005) Epidemiology and transmission dynamics of West Nile virus disease. *Emerg. Infect. Dis.* **11**, 1167-1173.

Jacobson, E.R., Ginn, P.E., Troutman, J.M., Farina, L., Stark, L., Klenk, K., Burkhalter, K.L. and Komar, N. (2005) West Nile virus infection in farmed American alligators (*Alligator mississippiensis*) in Florida. *J. Wildl. Dis.* **41**, 96-106.

Kesson, A.M., Cheng, Y. and King, N.J. (2002) Regulation of immune recognition molecules by flavivirus, West Nile. *Viral Immunol.* **15**, 273-283.

Kilpatrick, A.M., Daszak, P., Jones, M.J., Marra, P.P. and Kramer, L.D. (2006a) Host heterogeneity dominates West Nile virus transmission. *Proc. Biol. Sci.* **273**, 2327-2333.

Kilpatrick, A.M., Kramer, L.D., Jones, M.J., Marra, P.P. and Daszak, P. (2006b) West Nile virus epidemics in North America are driven by shifts in mosquito feeding behavior. *PLos. Biol.* **20064**, 606-610.

Klein, R.S., Lin, E., Zhang, B., Luster, A.D., Tollett, J., Samuel, M.A., Engle, M. and Diamond, M.S. (2005) Neuronal CXCL10 directs CD8+ T-cell recruitment and control of West Nile virus encephalitis. *J. Virol.* **79**, 11457-11466.

Klenk, K., Snow, J., Morgan, K., Bowen, R., Stephens, M., Foster, F., Gordy, P., Beckett, S., Komar, N., Gubler, D. and Bunning, M. (2004) Alligators as West Nile virus amplifiers. *Emerg. Infect. Dis.* **10**, 2150-2155.

Komar, N., Langevin, S., Hinten, S., Nemeth, N., Edwards, E., Hettler, D., Davis, B., Bowen, R. and Bunning, M. (2003) Experimental infection of North American birds with the New York 1999 strain of West Nile virus. *Emerg. Infect. Dis.* **9**, 311-322.

Lanciotti, R.S., Roehrig, J.T., Deubel, V., Smith, J., Parker, M., Steele, K., Crise, B., Volpe, K.E., Crabtree, M.B., Scherret, J.H., Hall, R.A., MacKenzie, J.S., Cropp, C.B., Panigrahy, B., Ostlund, E., Schmitt, B., Malkinson, M., Banet, C., Weissman, J., Komar, N., Savage, H.M., Stone, W., McNamara, T. and Gubler, D.J. (1999) Origin of the West Nile virus responsible for an outbreak of encephalitis in the northeastern United States. *Science* **286**, 2333-2337.

Long, M.T., Gibbs, E.P., Mellencamp, M.W., Bowen, R.A., Seino, K.K., Zhang, S., Beachboard, S.E. and Humphrey, P.P. (2007) Efficacy, duration, and onset of immunogenicity of a West Nile virus vaccine, live Flavivirus chimera, in horses with a clinical disease challenge model. *Equine vet. J.* **39**, 491-497.

Makhoul, B., Braun, E, Herskovitz, M, Ramadan, R, Hadad, S. and Norberto, K. (2009) Hyperimmune gammaglobulin for the treatment of West Nile virus encephalitis. *Isr. Med. Assoc. J.* **11**, 151-153.

Mayhew, I.G. (1989) *Large Animal Neurology*, Lea & Febiger.

Minke, J.M., Siger, L., Karaca, K., Austgen, L., Gordy, P., Bowen, R., Renshaw, R.W., Loosmore, S., Audonnet, J.C. and Nordgren, B. (2004) Recombinant canarypoxvirus vaccine carrying the prM/E genes of West Nile virus protects horses against a West Nile virus-mosquito challenge. *Arch. Virol. Suppl.* 221-230.

Ng, T., Hathaway, D., Jennings, N., Champ, D., Chiang, Y.W. and Chu, H.J. (2003) Equine vaccine for West Nile virus. *Dev. Biol. (Basel)* **114**, 221-227.

Ostlund, E.N., J.E. Andresen and M. Andresen (2000) West Nile encephalitis. *Vet. Clin. N. Am.: Equine Pract.* **16**, 427-441.

Ostlund, E.N., Crom, R.L., Pedersen, D.D., Johnson, D.J., Williams, W.O. and Schmitt, B.J. (2001) Equine West Nile encephalitis, United States. *Emerg. Infect. Dis.* **7**, 665-669.

Platt, K.B., Tucker, B.J., Halbur, P.G., Blitvich, B.J., Fabiosa, F.G., Mullin, K., Parikh, G.R., Kitikoon, P., Bartholomay, L.C. and Rowley, W.A. (2008) Fox squirrels (*Sciurus niger*) develop West Nile virus viremias sufficient for infecting select mosquito species. *Vector Borne Zoonotic Dis.* **8**, 225-233.

Platt, K.B., Tucker, B.J., Halbur, P.G., Tiawsirisup, S., Blitvich, B.J., Fabiosa, F.G., Bartholomay, L.C. and Rowley, W.A. (2007) West Nile virus viremia in eastern chipmunks (*Tamias striatus*) sufficient for infecting different mosquitoes. *Emerg. Infect. Dis.* **13**, 831-837.

Porter, M.B., Long, M.T., Getman, L.M., Giguère, S., MacKay, R.J., Lester, G.D., Alleman, A.R., Wamsley, H.L., Franklin, R.P., Jacks, S., Buergelt, C.D. and Detrisac, C.J. (2003) West Nile virus encephalomyelitis in horses: 46 cases (2001). *J. Am. vet. med. Ass.* **222**, 1241-1247.

Reisen, W.K., Fang, Y. and Martinez, V.M. (2005) Avian host and mosquito (*Diptera: Culicidae*) vector competence determine the efficiency of West Nile and St Louis encephalitis virus transmission. *J. Med. Entomol.* **42**, 367-375.

Rios, J.J., Perelygin, A.A., Long, M.T. Lear, T.L., Zharkikh, A. A., Brinton, M.A. and Adelson, D.L. (2007) Characterization of the equine 2'-5' oligoadenylate synthetase 1 (OAS1) and ribonuclease L (RNASEL) innate immunity genes. *BMC Genomics* **8**, 313-327.

Samuel, M.A. and Diamond, M.S. (2005) Alpha/beta interferon protects against lethal West Nile virus infection by restricting cellular tropism and enhancing neuronal survival. *J. Virol.* **79**, 13350-13361.

Samuel, M.A. and Diamond, M.S. (2006) Pathogenesis of West Nile Virus infection: a balance between virulence, innate and adaptive immunity, and viral evasion. *J. Virol.* **80**, 9349-9360.

Sardelis, M.R., Turell, M.J., Dohm, D.J. and O'Guinn, M.L. (2001) Vector competence of selected North American *Culex* and *Coquillettidia* mosquitoes for West Nile virus. *Emerg. Infect. Dis.* **7**, 1018-1022.

Sardelis, M.R., Turell, M.J., O'Guinn, M.L., Andre, R.G. and Roberts, D.R (2002) Vector competence of three North American strains of *Aedes albopictus* for West Nile virus. *J. Am. Mosq. Control Assoc.* **18**, 284-289.

Savage, H.M., Aggarwal, D., Apperson, C.S., Katholi, C.R., Gordon, E., Hassan, H.K., Anderson, M., Charnetzky, D., McMillen, L., Unnasch, E.A. and Unnasch, T.R. (2007) Host choice and West Nile virus infection rates in blood-fed mosquitoes, including members of the *Culex pipiens* complex, from Memphis and Shelby County, Tennessee, 2002-2003. *Vector Borne Zoonotic Dis.* **7**, 365-386.

Scherbik, S.V., Paranjape, J.M., Stockman, B.M., Silverman, R.H. and Brinton, M.A. (2006) RNase L plays a role in the antiviral response to West Nile virus. *J. Virol.* **80**, 2987-2999.

Seino, K.K., Long, M.T., Gibbs, E.P., Bowen, R.A., Beachboard, S.E., Humphrey, P.P., Dixon, M.A. and Bourgeois, M.A. (2007) Comparative efficacies of three commercially available vaccines against West Nile virus (WNV) in a short-duration challenge trial involving an equine WNV encephalitis model. *Clin. Vaccine Immunol.* **14**, 1465-1471.

Shrestha, B. and Diamond, M.S. (2004) Role of CD8+ T cells in control of West Nile virus infection. *J. Virol.* **78**, 8312-8321.

Shrestha, B., Samuel, M.A. and Diamond, M.S. (2006) CD8+ T cells require perforin to clear West Nile virus from infected neurons. *J. Virol.* **80**, 119-129.

Siger, L., Bowen, R.A., Karaca, K., Murray, M.J., Gordy, P.W., Loosmore, S.M., Audonnet, J.C., Nordgren, R.M. and Minke, J.M. (2004) Assessment of the efficacy of a single dose of a recombinant vaccine against West Nile virus in response to natural challenge with West Nile virus-infected mosquitoes in horses. *Am. J. vet. Res.* **65**,1459-1462.

Snook, C.S., Hyman, S.S., Del Piero, F., Palmer, J.E., Ostlund, E.N., Barr, B.S., Desrochers, A.M. and Reilly, L.K. (2001) West Nile virus encephalomyelitis in eight horses. *J. Am. vet. med. Ass.* **218**, 1576-1579.

Tesh, R.B., Arroyo, J., Travassos Da Rosa, A.P., Guzman, H., Xiao, S.Y. and Monath, T.P. (2002) Efficacy of killed virus vaccine, live attenuated chimeric virus vaccine, and passive immunization for prevention of West Nile virus encephalitis in hamster model. *Emerg. Infect. Dis.* **8**, 1392-1397.

Tesh, R.B., Parsons, R., Siirin, M., Randle, Y., Sargent, C., Guzman, H., Wuithiranyagool, T., Higgs, S., Vanlandingham, D.L., Bala, A.A., Haas, K. and Zerinque, B. (2004) Year-round West Nile virus activity, Gulf Coast region, Texas and Louisiana. *Emerg. Infect. Dis.* **10**, 1649-1652.

Tewari, D., Kim, H., Feria, W., Russo, B. and Acland, H. (2004) Detection of West Nile virus using formalin fixed paraffin embedded tissues in crows and horses: quantification of viral transcripts by real-time RT-PCR. *J. Clin. Virol.* **30**, 320-325.

Town, T., Jeng, D., Alexopoulou, L., Tan, J. and Flavell, R.A. (2006) Microglia recognize double-stranded RNA via TLR3. *J. Immunol.* **176**, 3804-3812.

Turell, M.J., O'Guinn, M.L., Dohm, D.J. and Jones, J.W. (2001a) Vector competence of North American mosquitoes (*Diptera: Culicidae*) for West Nile virus. *J. Med. Entomol.* **38**, 130-134.

Turell, M.J., Sardelis, M.R., Dohm, D.J. and O'Guinn, M.L. (2001b) Potential North American vectors of West Nile virus. *Ann. NY Acad. Sci.* **951**, 317-324.

Turell, M.J., Dohm, D.J., Sardelis, M.R., Oguinn, M.L., Andreadis, T.G. and Blow, J.A. (2005) An update on the potential of north American mosquitoes (*Diptera: Culicidae*) to transmit West Nile Virus. *J. Med. Entomol.* **42**, 57-62.

Wamsley, H.L., Alleman, A.R., Porter, M.B. and Long, M.T. (2002) Findings in cerebrospinal fluids of horses infected with West Nile virus: 30 cases (2001). *J. Am. vet. med. Ass.* **221**, 1303-1305.

Wang, T. and Fikrig, E. (2004) Immunity to West Nile virus. *Curr. Opin. Immunol.* **16**, 519-523.

Wang, Y., Lobigs, M., Lee, E. and Mullbacher, A. (2003) CD8+ T cells mediate recovery and immunopathology in West Nile virus encephalitis. *J. Virol.* **77**, 13323-13334.

Weingartl, H.M., Neufeld, J.L., Copps, J. and Marszal, P. (2004) Experimental West Nile virus infection in blue jays (*Cyanocitta cristata*) and crows (*Corvus brachyrhynchos*). *Vet. Pathol.* **41**, 362-370.

ALPHAVIRAL ENCEPHALOMYELITIS (EEE, WEE AND VEE)

R. J. MacKay

Alec P. and Louise P. Courtelis Equine Teaching Hospital, College of Veterinary Medicine, University of Florida, PO Box 100136, Gainesville, Florida 32610, USA.

Keywords: horse; EEE; WEE; VEE; neurological; alphavirus; epizootic

Summary

Beginning in the 19th or 20th century, the New World arboviruses responsible for eastern, western, and Venezuelan equine encephalomyelitis (EEE, WEE and VEE) have reportedly killed many thousands of equids in the North and South American continents. Outbreaks in equids occur after viral amplification in birds (WEE, EEE) or horses (VEE). Horses are dead-end hosts for EEE and WEE viruses. While WEE has almost disappeared from North America, at least 100 cases of EEE are reported annually. Although the major IAB epizootic strain of VEE may be extinct, neurovirulent mutant IE virus has caused recent outbreaks of fatal equine disease in Mexico.

Introduction

The causative agents of eastern, western and Venezuelan equine encephalomyelitis (EEE, WEE and VEE) are New World arboviruses belonging to the genus *Alphavirus* of the family Togaviridae (Calisher 1994; Hahn *et al.* 1999; Booss and Esiri 2003; Gibbs and Long 2007). These diseases affect all common domestic equid species including horses, mules and donkeys. Each of the viruses was first isolated during epizootics in the 1930s (Giltner and Shahan 1933; Meyer 1933; Kubes and Ríos 1939). Alphaviruses are unsegmented single-stranded positive-sense RNA viruses; EEE and WEE genomes are 11–12 kb and infectious virions are spherical enveloped particles 60–70 nm in diameter (Calisher 1994; Weaver *et al.* 1999, 2004). Each of the 3 equine alphaviral encephalitides is among the 13 equine infectious diseases that are notifiable to the OIE (Office International des Épizooties; Anon 2008a).

The WEE virus is thought to be derived from recombination of ancestral EEE-like and Sindbis-like viruses (Calisher 1994). At least 3 genotypic subtypes of WEE have been identified. Two of these are found in both North and South America, suggesting that circulation of viruses between the New World continents is common (Calisher 1994; Weaver *et al.* 1999). There are distinct North American (including the Caribean) and South American antigenic varieties of EEE that diverged from a common ancestor approximately 1000 years ago (Weaver *et al.* 1994). In contrast to the situation with WEE, there is no evidence for movement of EEE virus between North and South America.

The VEE antigenic complex contains 7 viral species and 6 subtypes and 14 varieties (Weaver *et al.* 2004), most of which are maintained continuously in enzootic life cycles in northern South America (**Fig 1**). All known isolates of epizootic subtypes IAB and IC appear to have arisen since the beginning of the 20th century from a single enzootic ID lineage (Weaver *et al.* 1999). There is some evidence that a strain of the enzootic IE subtype isolated from horses during VEE outbreaks in Mexico in the 1990s acquired neuroinvasiveness by a single-base mutation in the gene encoding the E2 viral envelope protein (Brault *et al.* 2002). Venezuelan equine encephalomyelitis virus is also a highly developed biological weapon amenable to use in warfare or terrorism. The current emphasis on biological defence has therefore renewed interest in the virus, both as a naturally emerging pathogen and as a terrorist agent that could be introduced artificially to cause widespread disease (Weaver 2004).

History and distribution

Western equine encephalomyelitis

What was almost certainly the first recorded outbreak of WEE in horses occurred in Kansas, Nebraska,

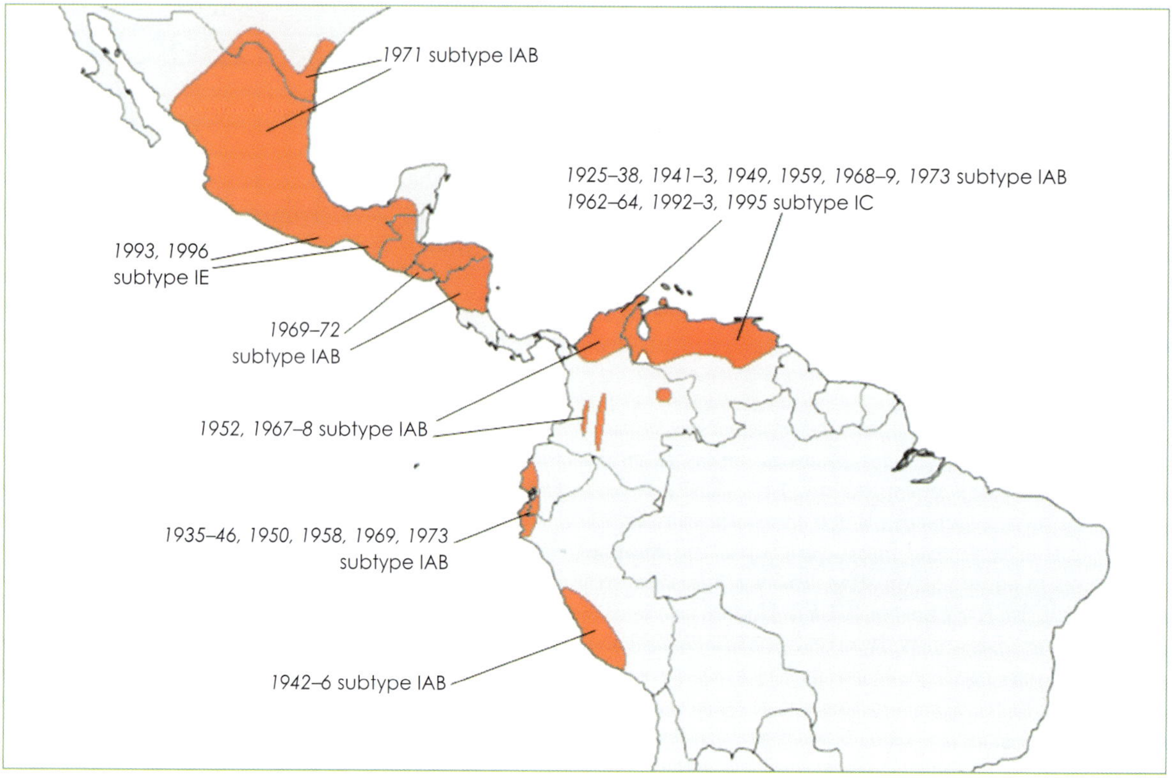

FIGURE 1: Map showing locations of VEE epizootics since the virus was isolated in 1938, along with virus subtypes implicated as the aetiological agents (redrawn from Figure 1 Weaver et al. 2004).

Colorado and Oklahoma during the late summer and early autumn of 1912 when at least 35,000 horses died of the disease (Meyer 1933; Nalca *et al.* 2003). Successive WEE epizootics in California and other western states in 1930, 1931 and 1932 resulted in the deaths of an estimated 9200 horses and mules (approximately 50% of those affected) (Meyer 1932, 1933). Virus was isolated from the brains of 2/9 animals tested. In 1938, WEE was recognised in every state west of the Mississippi river and was estimated by the United States Bureau of Animal Industry to have affected more than 184,000 horses in that year alone (Hagan *et al.* 1981). By the 1970s, WEE had been recorded as far east as Tennessee (Weaver *et al.* 1999). WEE virus also was implicated in outbreaks of fatal equine disease in the early 20th century in Canada and Argentina and epizootics have since been reported in Saskatchewan, Alberta, and Manitoba in western Canada and in Mexico and central and South America (Hanson 1972). Over the last 30 years, the disease has become progressively less prevalent in the USA and is now seldom reported: between 1972 and 1981 there was an annual average of 267 cases of WEE in horses reported by the National Veterinary Services Laboratory in Ames, Iowa (Hagan *et al.* 1981); in 1993 there were 15 cases in 10 states and since 2005 no case has been reported in the USA (Anon 2008b). Surprisingly, however, there was no difference in virulence for mice among 10 WEE isolates obtained during every decade from the 1940s to the 1990s (Forrester *et al.* 2008). There have been isolated cases of encephalomyelitis in Florida horses associated with the Highlands J virus, an eastern member of the WEE virus complex with epidemiological characteristics very similar to those of EEE virus (Karabatsos *et al.* 1988).

Eastern equine encephalomyelitis

An outbreak of what was probably EEE was recorded in August and September of 1831 in Massachusetts (Hanson 1957). Approximately 100 horses were affected and 75 died. Over the subsequent century, there were at least 5 other outbreaks consistent with EEE – in Long Island, New York (1845), North Carolina (1902), New Jersey (1905), Florida (1908), and Maryland, New Jersey and Virginia (1912) (Scott and Weaver 1989). The virus was recovered in 1933 from the brain of a horse in New Jersey that died during an epizootic involving at least 1000 horses in the coastal regions of Delaware, Virginia and Maryland (Giltner and Shahan 1933). During recurrent outbreaks in the same region in 1934–35, the disease was experimentally induced in horses, neutralising antibody was detected in the blood of affected horses, the agents of EEE and WEE were differentiated, and the role of mosquitoes in transmission of the EEE virus was elucidated (Merrill *et al.* 1934, 1936). Epizootics of EEE in North America have since occurred periodically in the coastal areas of the Atlantic, the southeastern USA and Texas. The largest recorded outbreak was in 1947 in southern Louisiana and Texas when 14,344 cases of EEE were recorded resulting in 11,722 deaths (mortality rate of 81%) (Oglesby 1948). Focal outbreaks and sporadic cases have also occurred more or less regularly in Michigan (Ross and Kaneene 1996) and are occasionally reported from other locations in the eastern half of the USA and Canada (Sellers 1989; Nasci *et al.* 1993; Del Piero *et al.* 2001). A single case of EEE in a stallion in California was reported in 2002 (Franklin *et al.* 2002). Although the origin of the infection in this horse was not determined with certainty, incompletely activated EEE vaccine was suspected. Despite the availability of effective vaccines since the late 1930s (Byrne 1972), cases of EEE still occur every year in Florida and other southeastern states. Annual incidence of EEE in the USA over the last 5 years has ranged from 112 (2006) to 732 (2003) (Anon 2008b).

Epizootics of what was probably EEE have been reported in Argentina since 1908 and the first EEE isolate was recovered from a horse in 1930, although it was not identified until 1953 (Scott and Weaver 1989). Since then, reports of EEE in Central and South America have been widespread, extending from Panama south to Argentina (Scott and Weaver 1989). The disease has also caused serious losses in the Caribbean with epizootics documented in the Dominican Republic, Haiti, Jamaica and Trinidad (Hanson 1957).

Venezuelan equine encephalomyelitis

There is no clear evidence of the occurrence of the disease in the 19th century and phylogenetic estimates derived from the DNA sequences of VEE virus strains suggest that epizootic VEE virus probably first evolved early in the 20th century. The history of VEE epizootics can be divided into 5 distinct periods (Weaver *et al.* 2004).

1) *Mid-1920s–1938:* The disease in equids was first recognised and described in Venezuela and Colombia and VEE virus was isolated from a horse brain in 1938 (Kubes and Ríos 1939a).

2) *1938–1969:* At intervals of approximately 10 years, there were large subtype IAB or IC epizootics of VEE in northern South America that usually involved tens of thousands of horses. Many of these outbreaks arose in the desert-like Guajira peninsula of Colombia and Venezuela or in the coastal regions of Peru and spread rapidly and often noncontiguously. One epizootic in central Colombia during 1962–64 was estimated to have killed 100,000 horses (Sellers *et al.* 1965). Also during this period, the VEE virus was associated for the first time with human neurological disease and nonvirulent enzootic varieties of VEE virus were identified.

3) *1969–1973:* An outbreak of VEE caused by subtype IAB began in Peru in the winter of 1969, jumped to central America in June 1969, then spread north into Mexico in 1970. Thousands of horses died on the isthmus of Tehuantepec. The outbreak spread north to the US border in the spring of 1971 and the first case of VEE in a horse in the USA was confirmed on 30th June (Zehmer *et al.* 1974). By the time of the last case on 7th November 1971, more than 1500 horses had died in the southern counties of Texas. Small outbreaks were recorded in Mexico into 1972.

4) *1973–1992:* There was no epizootic activity reported. This led to speculation that subtype IAB VEE virus had become extinct (Walton and Alvarez 1988).

5) *1992 to present:* In Venezuela in 1992, there was a small outbreak (24 cases) of VEE due to subtype IC that spread discontinuously to the rest of the country. In 1995, subtype IC VEE returned in the form of a

massive epizootic involving 95,000 horses in Colombia alone (Navarro *et al.* 2005). Subtype IE was associated for the first time with fatal VEE in small epizootics in Mexico in 1993 (Chiapis, 125 horses) and 1996 (Oaxaca, 32 horses; Oberste *et al.* 1998; Brault *et al.* 1999).

Natural history

EEE and WEE

In North America, the WEE and EEE viruses are maintained between epizootics by low-level cycling between songbirds and ornithophilic mosquitoes in freshwater, forested swamp habitats (Hahn *et al.* 1999; Gibbs and Long 2007). Infected mosquitoes can be found throughout the year in Florida and other southeastern states. The mechanisms of apparent overwintering of virus in temperate states such as Massachusetts and Michigan are not completely understood, but may include: 1) transovarial transmission in mosquitoes or survival of long-lived mosquitoes or other haematophagous insects in warm microclimates; 2) persistent infections in poikolotherms (e.g. snakes); or 3) seasonal reintroduction, perhaps by windblown mosquitoes (Scott and Weaver 1989). Under favourable environmental conditions, the viruses periodically spread outward from focal reservoirs to infect the general wild bird population, where they are propagated and amplified by rapid bird-mosquito-bird transmission. The mosquito vectors involved in maintenance and amplification of WEE and EEE viruses are usually *Culex tarsalis* and *Culiseta melanura*, respectively. Many avian species including migratory songbirds, wading birds and starlings become infected and develop high-order viraemia and high serum titres to EEE or WEE but usually do not become ill. Some introduced species, including pigeons, house sparrows, Chukar partridges and Chinese pheasants, may suffer high morbidity and mortality when infected with EEE virus.

Cases of encephalomyelitis usually begin in susceptible horses 2–3 weeks after virus spreads into birds. Human cases may occur several weeks later. *Culex tarsalis* transfers WEE virus from bird to horse (and human). Different 'bridge' vectors are required for EEE transfer, including *Ochlerotatus* (formerly *Aedes*) *sollicitans*, *Aedes vexans*, *Ochlerotatus Canadensis*, and *Coquillettidia perturbans* (Scott and Weaver 1989). Although mosquito-mediated transmission of EEE between horses has been confirmed in an experimental setting (Sudia *et al.* 1956), viraemia is of relatively low titre, so further infection of feeding mosquitoes with either virus is unlikely and horses are considered 'dead-end' hosts. Both EEE and WEE viruses have been associated with naturally-occurring and experimentally-induced neurological disease in calves, and EEE has been associated with clinical and experimental infections in South American camelids, deer, ratite birds, cats, dogs, mice, foxes and pigs (Sellers 1989; Walton 1992; Farrar *et al.* 2005; Nolen-Walston *et al.* 2007).

Epizootics of EEE and WEE usually last 1–3 months and occur in summer and early fall when warmth and humidity favour breeding, longevity and mobility of mosquito populations (Ross and Kaneene 1996). Outbreaks in Massachusetts and Michigan were most likely during the second consecutive year in which rainfall exceeded the annual mean by more than 20 cm; however, unusually high temperatures did not appear to be a risk factor (Grady *et al.* 1978; Ross and Kaneene 1996). By contrast, it was "exceedingly hot and dry" in the San Joaquin and Sacramento valleys before and at the onset of the extensive California epizootics of WEE in 1930 and 1931 (Meyer 1933). The month of peak incidence of disease onset varies from June in Florida to August or September in northern and western states (Meyer 1933; Wilson *et al.* 1986; Przelomski *et al.* 1988; Sellers 1989). In Florida and some other southeastern states, isolated cases of EEE can be seen at any time of year (Wilson *et al.* 1986; Hahn *et al.* 1999). Standing surface water for mosquito larval development, bush cover for wild hosts, and the immune status of the various hosts also affect the timing and magnitude of equine epizootics. Many of these physical factors are significantly affected by the cultivation, clearing and irrigation of land, and by drainage of swamps. The equine epizootic usually declines with the onset of cool or dry weather unsuitable for mosquito and/or bird activity, and with the depletion of susceptible equine hosts by death or development of immunity among survivors. Many other vertebrate species become infected and seroconvert during an equine epizootic but rarely with serious disease or viraemia sufficient to infect feeding mosquitoes.

The epidemiology of EEE and WEE viruses in South America is poorly understood. Small mammals play a greater role in sylvatic cycles of viral transmission than is the case in North America. *Culex* (*Melanoconion*) subspecies and *Ochlerotatus albifasciatus* appear to be involved in transmission of EEE and WEE, respectively (Calisher 1994; Weaver *et al.* 1994).

VEE

Enzootic VEE viruses are maintained by cycling between mosquitoes and small rodents or birds. The Everglades virus, a subtype II VEE virus found in the Everglades region of Florida, is of this type, cycling between *Culex* (*Melanoconion*) subspecies mosquitoes and wild rodents. Bijou Bridge, a subtype III virus, was isolated in Colorado in the 1970s but has not reappeared (Weaver *et al.* 2004). The epizootic varieties IAB and IC have probably arisen on at least 4 separate occasions by mutation of a single enzootic subtype 1D strain and changes in host range (Weaver *et al.* 1999). The defining characteristic of epizootic VEE varieties is the use of equids as amplification hosts. In both natural and experimental infections, peak viral titres in blood are usually at least an order of magnitude higher than the 10^5 suckling mice LD_{50} doses/ml needed to infect feeding mosquitoes (Weaver *et al.* 2004; Kuno and Chang 2005). Domestic rabbits, goats, dogs and sheep also suffer fatal disease during VEE outbreaks (Weaver *et al.* 2004). There does not appear to be any single 'epizootic' vector mosquito species; during outbreaks, virus may be isolated from mosquitoes of many different species including *Ochlerotatus taeniorhynchus*, *Psorophora confinnis* and *Anopheles aquasalis* (Walton *et al.* 1992; Weaver *et al.* 2004). Epidemiological studies have confirmed that VEE epizootics terminate when susceptible horses are no longer available (Walton *et al.* 1992). The leapfrog spread characteristic of VEE is usually attributed to transport of horses incubating the virus. Movement of infected bats also may contribute to discontinuous spread of virus (Weaver *et al.* 2004). By contrast to the situation with the WEE and EEE viruses, birds do not have an important role in amplification and spread of epizootic VEE virus. It is not yet clear whether neurovirulent subtype IE virus is amplified in horses. Evidence from experimental infections suggests that viral titres in blood of infected horses may be insufficient to infect feeding mosquitoes (Brault *et al.* 2002; Sahu *et al.* 2003)

Outbreaks typically begin in arid areas after a period of unusually high rainfall. In wet seasons, the Guajira desert, with its large population of unvaccinated feral burros, is particularly conducive to amplification of virus and initiation of a VEE epizootic. After VEE spread across Venezuela and into Trinidad during 1936–1938, high-titred formalin-inactivated vaccines were introduced and widely used to protect against VEE (Kuno and Chang 2005). Genotypic analyses of epizootic virus isolates have indicated that most or all of the many outbreaks between 1938 and 1973 began after inoculation of horses with improperly inactivated vaccine (Kinney *et al.* 1992; Weaver *et al.* 2004) and evidence has been offered for a laboratory origin for the subtype IC virus that caused the 1995 outbreak in Colombia and Venezuela (Navarro *et al.* 2005), although the latter interpretation has been disputed (Navarro *et al.* 2005). Since the introduction of attenuated tissue-culture-origin vaccine in 1967, outbreaks have occurred only infrequently. The interepizootic reservoir of epizootic varieties, if any, is not known with certainty. There is some evidence for the persistence, since 1995, of alternative, cryptic transmission cycles involving survival of subtype IC VEE virus through the dry season in infected vertebrates or insect vectors (Navarro *et al.* 2005).

Clinical findings

Clinical signs following infection with each of the viruses are similar although signs of EEE are typically more severe and rapidly progressive than those of VEE and WEE (Giltner and Shahan 1933; Meyer 1933; Oglesby 1948; Miller *et al.* 1973; Walton *et al.* 1992; Ross and Kaneene 1995; Hahn *et al.* 1999; Franklin *et al.* 2002). Infected horses respond in any to all of the following ways following experimental infections (Byrne 1972) (**Fig 2**): 1) Inapparent infection with a very low-grade viraemia and fever about 2 days after inoculation. This presentation corresponds to the initial viraemia following viral proliferation in regional lymph nodes and probably occurs commonly during outbreaks without progression to subsequent stages. 2) Generalised febrile illness (up to 41.7°C), with anorexia, depression, tachycardia and diarrhoea. This stage is associated with viral proliferation in various body organs after spread from regional

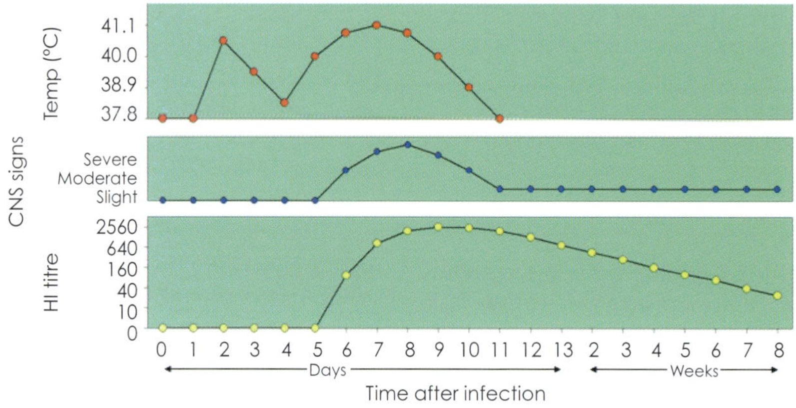

FIGURE 2: Clinical, virological and serological responses of horses to EEE virus. CNS = central nervous system; HI = haemagglutination inhibition. From Byrne (1972).

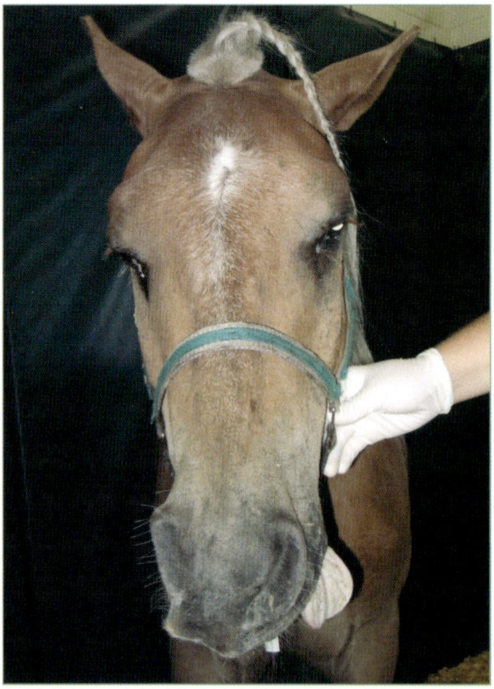

FIGURE 3: This yearling Palamino filly was bought 2 days previously at a public auction in southern Georgia. The vaccination history was not available. Approximately 12 h before the image was recorded, the filly was seen standing in the corner of a paddock, uninterested in herdmates or the hay that was offered. Rectal temperature was 41.2°C. At the time of presentation to the Alec P. and Louise P. Courtelis Equine Teaching Hospital at the University of Florida, the filly was stuporous, its poll was rotated to the left, and there was tongue protrusion and left-sided facial paralysis. The filly's condition continued to deteriorate and she was subjected to euthanasia 8 h after admission.

lymph nodes. 3) Clinical encephalomyelitis, which is the classic form of the disease. Young horses (especially yearlings) are most susceptible: approximately 90% of 95 horses with EEE admitted to the University of Florida (UF) were aged <5 years (Suarez and MacKay 2008). The onset of neurological signs is associated with the second febrile crisis and typically occurs about 5 days after infection (range 2 days to 2 weeks) and most deaths occur 2–3 days later (Byrne 1972; Walton *et al.* 1992). Almost all horses with EEE are febrile at the onset of neurological signs (mean of 40.3°C in horses admitted to UF) although the temperature declines thereafter. The onset of severe neurological signs is

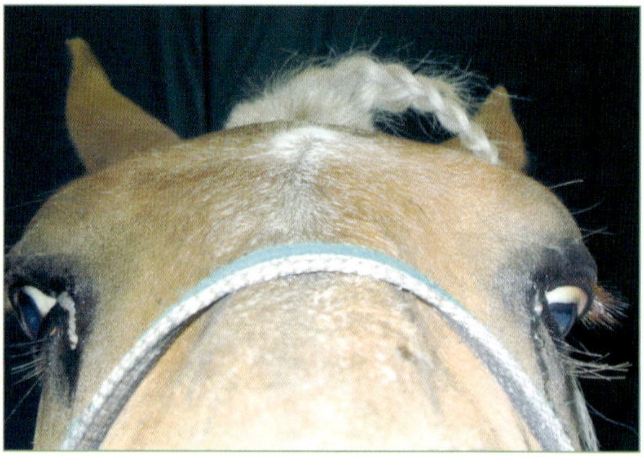

FIGURE 4: Same filly as shown in Figure 3. Note the downward and inward rotation of the left eyeball and the upward and outward rotation of the right eyeball, reflecting asymmetric dysfunction of the central vestibular nuclei and connections.

peracute to acute and progression is rapid. Horses may be found recumbent and comatose or dead. If observed, initial CNS signs are quite variable and referable to diffuse or multifocal cerebral disease; evidence of brainstem and spinal cord involvement quickly become obvious as the illness progresses (**Figs 3–6**). Obtundation is the most common initial clinical sign although owners also report suspected colic as part of the initial presentation. Affected horses often stand apart from pasture mates, have no interest in food, or fail to respond to an owner's call. Further signs of dementia may follow including head-pressing (**Fig 6**), teeth-grinding, hyperaesthesia, irritability, aggression (rarely), leaning against a wall or fence, or compulsive walking, often in a circle (especially around the inside of a stall or small paddock). Several observers have noted a 'peculiar looseness of the lips' as a characteristic early sign (Meyer 1933; Byrne *et al.* 1961). Blindness and lack of a menace response may be noted at this stage. Signs of cranial nerve disease, including abnormal pupillary light reflexes, head tilt (**Figs 4** and **6**), nystagmus, tight circling, facial paralysis, and tongue paralysis and inability to swallow, often occur as the disease advances. Abnormal signs usually present asymmetrically, at least initially. Ataxia and paresis of the trunk and limbs result in a progressively more unsteady gait. Tremors are seen in the anti-gravity muscles of the limbs. Once recumbent (**Fig 7**), affected horses seldom regain their footing and are often noted to make galloping or swimming movements in lateral recumbency (Meyer 1933). Seizures occur in about a third of horses with EEE and may happen at any stage (Suarez and MacKay 2008). Mucopurulent nasal and ocular discharges and abrasions and lacerations of the face and limbs are the most common non-neurological findings; the latter occurs secondary to trauma from falling, seizures or running into objects.

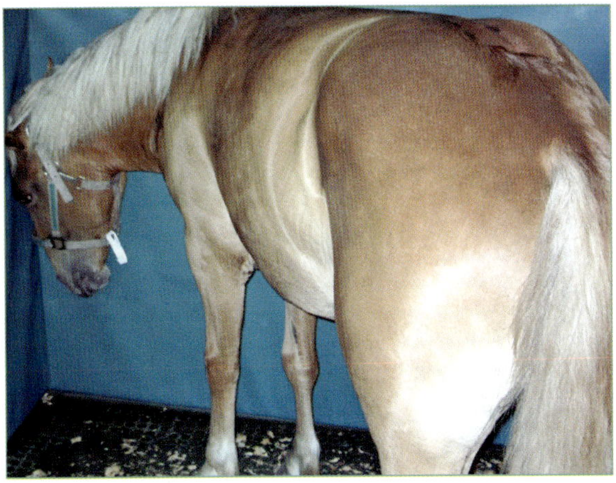

FIGURE 5: Same filly as shown in Figure 3. Between periods of walking in clockwise circles, the filly would press her head into the corner of the stall for periods of 5–10 min.

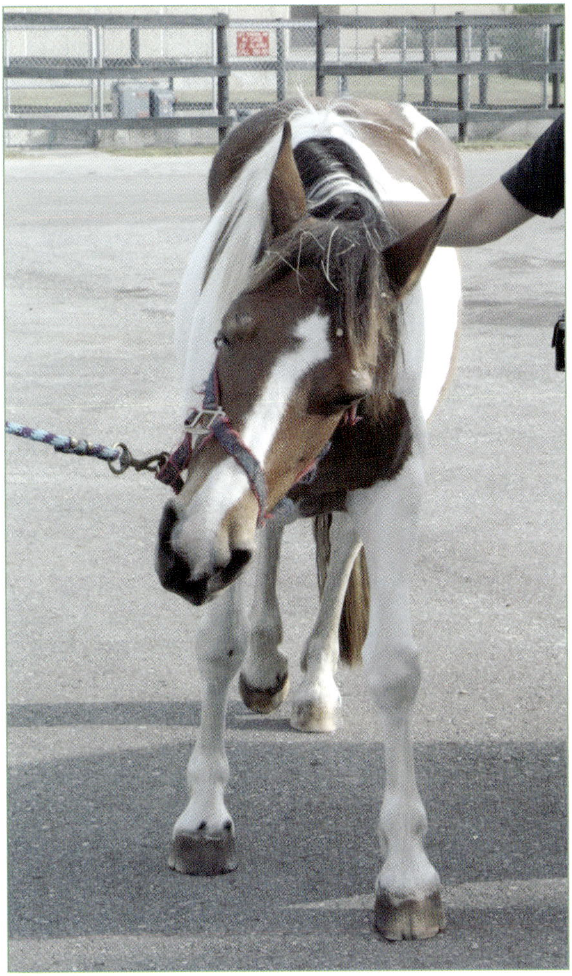

FIGURE 6: This 3-year-old Paint Horse filly was found lethargic and stumbling in her paddock on the morning of presentation. Her last EEE vaccination had been 8 months earlier. At presentation, the filly had a normal temperature of 37.4°C, was moderately obtunded, and had a head tilt to the right. The filly recovered completely over a period of weeks.

Mortality rates are 75–95% for EEE, 19–50% for WEE and 19–83% for VEE (Meyer 1933; Oglesby 1948; Gibbs 1976; Weaver *et al.* 2004). Vaccination within the preceding year was associated with lower risk of death in horses with EEE (Ross and Kaneene 1995). Death, if it occurs, usually is preceded by a period of recumbency during which the horse may be semi-comatose and convulsing. Surviving horses gradually recover over a period of weeks. Many horses with WEE apparently recover completely but it is estimated that two-thirds of horses that survive EEE have residual signs of CNS damage such as central blindness, dullness and diminished learning capacity or signs of cranial nerve dysfunction such as facial paralysis and head tilt (Scott and Weaver 1989). Such horses are often referred to as 'dummies'.

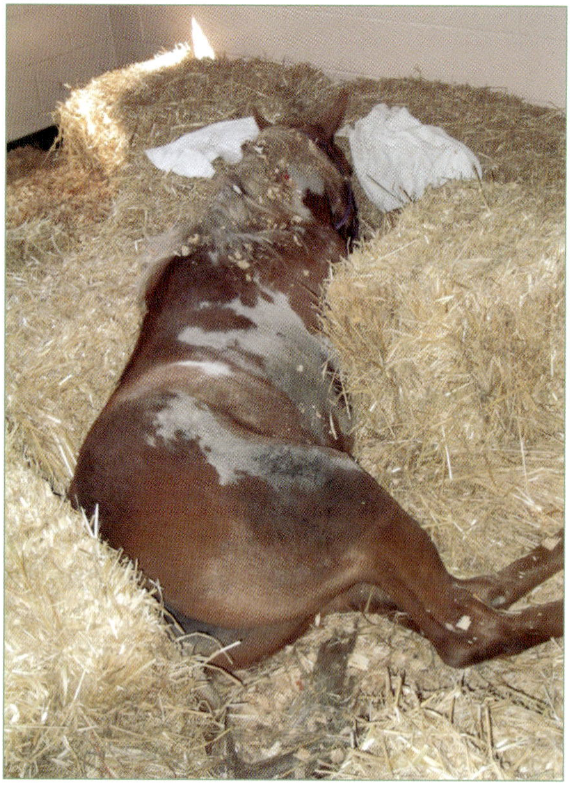

FIGURE 7: This yearling Appaloosa colt had not been vaccinated for EEE. After appearing normal at feeding time the previous evening, he was found recumbent and obtunded the next morning with a rectal temperature of 40.3°C. He was subjected to euthanasia approximately 10 h after admission.

Laboratory findings

Abnormalities seen in haemograms and plasma chemistry panels of horses with alphaviral encephalomyelitis are minor and nonspecific. Horses with EEE may have abnormal white blood cell counts and high fibrinogen concentration. In 73 horses with EEE admitted to UF (Suarez and MacKay 2008), the following haematological abnormalities were noted: leucocytosis, (56%), neutrophilia (60%), hyperfibrinogenaemia (57%), monocytosis (36%), lymphopenia (13%), leucopenia (7%), neutropenia (4%) and lymphocytosis (3%). Slight leucopenia was noted during experimental infections of horses with WEE virus (Meyer 1933). Mild elevations in plasma enzyme activities of affected horses reflect organ damage secondary to anorexia, fever, stress, recumbency and seizures. Hyponatraemia is found in some horses with EEE (Suarez and MacKay); however, its presence does not predict mortality (in contrast with EEE in human patients).

The results of CSF analysis for horses with EEE are quite distinctive. More than 95% of horses with EEE admitted to UF had abnormal CSF cytology (Suarez and MacKay 2008). Among UF cases, 88% of samples had high protein concentrations (mean of all

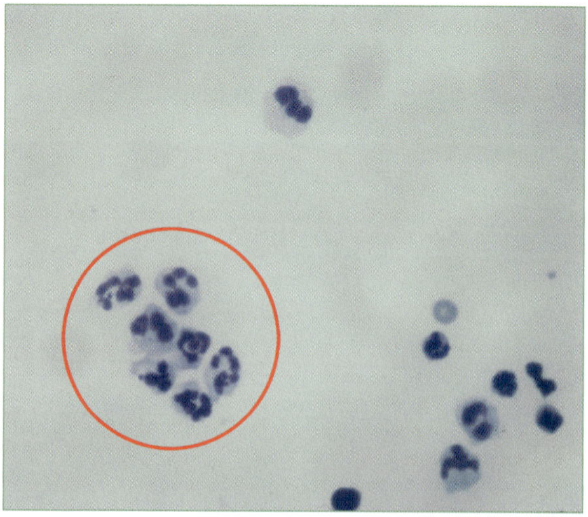

FIGURE 8: Characteristic cytology of CSF collected from a horse with EEE. In the lower left centre of the image [circle], note the clump of neutrophils with hypersegmented and slightly karyorrhectic nuclei (Wright-Giemsa stain, 400x magnification). Courtesy of Joe Mayhew, Massey University, Palmerston North, New Zealand.

samples: 1.39 g/l, range 0.38–5.26 g/l). Nucleated cell counts were high in 87% of samples (mean 2.48 x 10^8 cells/l, range 0–3.1 x 10^9/l; normal range 0–6 x 10^6 cells/l); pleocytosis is characterised by high neutrophil concentrations (mean 46%, range 0–97%) (**Fig 8**). Neutrophils are usually described as nondegenerate. Protein concentration and nucleated cell counts typically are higher in samples obtained from the atlanto-occipital site than they are in samples from lumbosacral taps. In the WEE outbreaks of 1930–32, CSF nucleated cell counts were typically 1.2–3.0 x 10^7/l and most cells were lymphocytes (Meyer 1932).

Diagnosis

A presumptive diagnosis usually is made clinically, especially in areas where these diseases are prevalent during the mosquito season. The finding in a CSF sample of moderate neutrophilic or lymphocytic pleocytosis further supports a diagnosis of alphaviral encephalomyelitis. Haemagglutination-inhibition (HI), complement fixation, fluorescent antibody and virus neutralisation tests have been traditionally been used for serological diagnosis (Scott and Weaver 1989). The MAC-ELISA (IgM capture ELISA) is the method of choice for use in horses with viral encephalomyelitis because it can distinguish between vaccinal (IgG only) and viral infection-induced (IgM and IgG) titres (Calisher *et al.* 1986; Sahu *et al.* 1994). These assays are available at many state diagnostic laboratories and also at the National Veterinary Services Laboratories (NVSL) in Ames, Iowa. In surviving horses, demonstration of a ≥4-fold rise in HI or plaque-reduction neutralising titre between acute and convalescent samples provides additional diagnostic support. It should be noted that positive results in these tests could simply reflect subclinical infection with either virus. Virus can be isolated from fresh or frozen brain in tissue culture or mice and can be detected in histological sections by immunohistochemistry or PCR techniques (Del Piero *et al.* 2001). Differential diagnoses include hepatoencephalopathy, idiopathic hypermmonaemia, heavy metal or other toxicosis, rabies, other viral encephalomyelitis (West Nile, Borna disease, equine herpesvirus-1, Aujesky's disease, Louping Ill), equine protozoal myeloencephalitis, trypanosomal (South America), verminous, or bacterial meningoencephalomyelitis, space-occupying lesion within the calvarium (e.g. cholesterol granuloma, neoplasia, brain abscess), brain infarct, brain trauma, and leucoencephalomalacia.

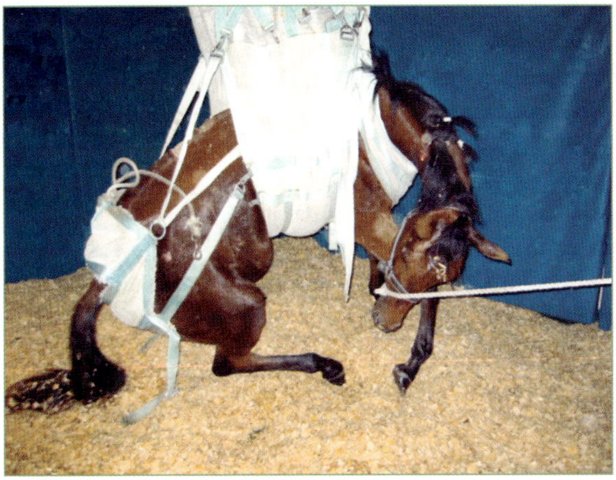

FIGURE 9: Attempted slinging of a yearling Thoroughbred colt demonstrating the futility of this procedure in horses with EEE that are recumbent.

Treatment

Treatment is largely supportive and, in the case of EEE, usually ineffective. Any adult horse with EEE that is unable to stand should be subjected to euthanasia. Such horses certainly should not be subjected to slinging (**Fig 9**). Hyperthermia is known to exacerbate brain injury and must be treated vigorously with cold water or alcohol baths until rectal temperature is <38.9°C. Convulsions can be controlled with diazepam, xylazine or barbiturates (pentobarbital or phenobarbital).

In addition to receiving excellent general nursing care, all horses should be treated for brain oedema and inflammation, although only horses whose signs are mainly cerebral are likely to respond. Drugs used for this purpose include dimethyl sulphoxide, 1 g/kg bwt as a 10% solution i.v. or intragastric, flunixin meglumine (or equivalent NSAID) i.m., i.v., or *per os* at 1.1 mg/kg bwt every 12 h for 3 days, dexamethasone (or equivalent corticosteroid) i.m. or i.v. at 0.05–0.1 mg/kg bwt daily for several days for 3 days then tapered, and mannitol (i.v. at 0.25–1 g/kg bwt as a 20% solution) or hypertonic saline (e.g. 7.2% saline i.v. at 2 ml/kg bwt 4–6 times during the first day). A lengthy course of dexamethasone appears to be an important determinant of neurological recovery

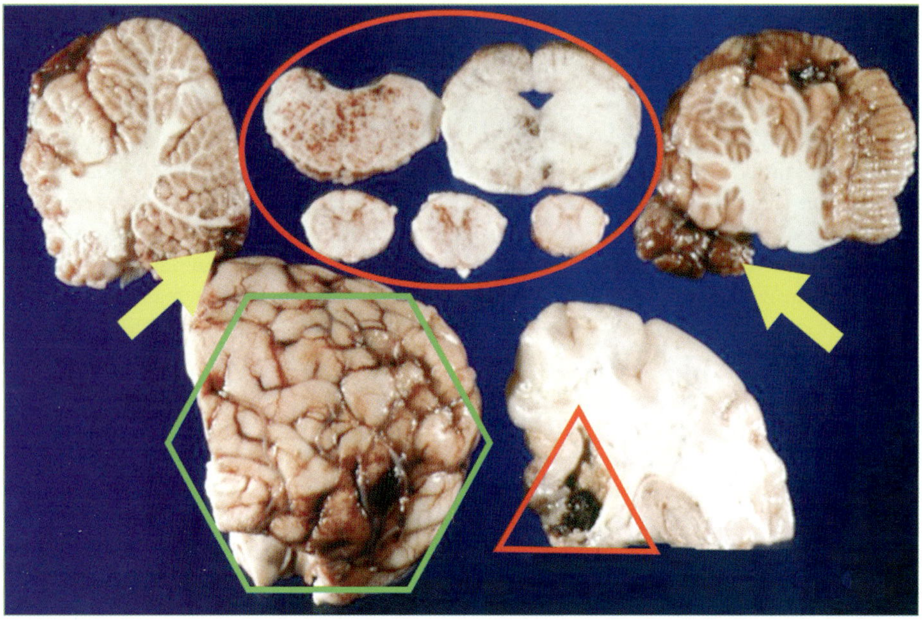

FIGURE 10: Sections of the brain of a horse that died with EEE. Note the extensive petechial and ecchymotic haemorrhages on cross-sections of the brainstem and spinal cord (red oval, upper centre), injury to the cerebellar vermis (yellow arrows) associated with hernia through the foramen magnum, flattening of cerebral gyri reflecting cerebral oedema and pressure lesion from occipital lobe herniation (green hexagon, bottom left), and intraventricular haemorrhage (red triangle, bottom right). Courtesy of Joe Mayhew, Massey University, Palmerston North, New Zealand.

in surviving cases. Treatment should be titrated to minimise neurological signs but generally must be tapered over several weeks. Complete recovery, if it occurs, may take several months.

Treatment with serum from horses hyperimmunised against WEE virus was thought to reduce mortality modestly during the 1930–32 outbreak; however, these claims were not tested scientifically (Meyer 1933). Furthermore, administration of large quantities of hyperimmune serum to experimentally-infected horses by investigators at Lederle Laboratories was reported to have no beneficial effect (Lyon 1939).

Adjuvant antiviral therapy with interferon (IFN) α or β has salutary effects in some experimental models of alphaviral encephalitis and could be tried in valuable horses (Julander *et al.* 2007). A reasonable dosage is $3–15 \times 10^6$ iu IFN-β1a i.m. or i.v. (Avonex 30 µg)[1] given 3 times weekly. The guanosine analogue ribavirin has *in vitro* activity against encephalitic alphaviruses (Briolant *et al.* 2004) and holds some potential as future therapy for EEE in man and perhaps horses.

EEE, WEE and VEE in man

All 3 viruses infect man causing subclinical, febrile or neurological disease (Calisher 1994; Weaver *et al.* 2004). Since 1964, there have been 640 cases of human WEE reported in the USA, with an average of 27 cases/year in the period up to 1987 (Anon 2008c). Since 1988, there have only been 5 cases of WEE reported. By contrast, the 254 human cases of EEE reported in the USA since 1964 have occurred at a fairly steady rate of 6 cases/year (range 0–21) (Anon 2008c). Epidemics of VEE are closely associated with equine epizootics; thus, during the 1962–64 epizootic in central Colombia which killed about 100,000 horses, 200,000 human subjects were infected, of whom 0.5% died. Although usually considered to be relatively nonpathogenic, the enzootic Everglades subtype II strain has caused human encephalitis in Florida. No cases of human disease were recorded during the VEE subtype IE equine epizootics in Mexico in 1993 and 1996 (Weaver 2004).

Between 5 and 8 days after being bitten by an infected mosquito, there is abrupt onset of clinical signs that include malaise, fever, chills, and severe retro-orbital or occipital headache. Myalgia typically centres in the thighs and lumbar region of the back. There is leucopenia, tachycardia and fever, frequently accompanied by nausea, vomiting and diarrhoea. Signs and symptoms of central nervous system involvement include convulsions, somnolence, confusion and photophobia. Encephalitis occurs most commonly among infants and the elderly. Cases of human encephalitis typically occur days to weeks after the onset of equine epizootics. Risk factors for development of EEE or WEE include age (young or old), rural location, length of residence and male gender (Calisher 1994). Short-term human mortality rates of EEE, WEE and VEE are 74%, 4% and <1%, respectively. Most survivors of EEE suffer long-term neurological impairment.

Post mortem findings

There is congestion of most organs and a slate-grey discolouration, often with petechial haemorrhage, of the brain and spinal cord, especially obvious on section of formalin-fixed tissue (Larsell *et al.* 1934; Hahn *et al.* 1999; Del Piero *et al.* 2001). Often there is brain swelling and evidence of occipital subtentorial herniation, with brainstem compression (**Fig 10**). Histologically, there is evidence of acute to subacute and multifocal to diffuse meningoencephalomyelitis. There is predominant involvement of grey matter, with diffuse neuronal degeneration, gliosis, perivascular and neuroparenchymal infiltrates, and meningitis. Neutrophils are prominent in acute EEE, whereas lymphocytes predominate in older lesions. On occasion, eosinophils may predominate in EEE. Lymphocytes usually are the primary inflammatory cell in WEE lesions (Larsell *et al.* 1934). Previous therapy with potent anti-inflammatory agents, particularly corticosteroids, may suppress the inflammatory-cell infiltrates, which then appear very mild.

Bronchopneumonia is found in about 20% of fatal cases of EEE, probably secondary to pharyngeal paresis and aspiration of particulate material (Suarez and MacKay 2008). Up to 10% of horses with EEE have histological evidence of myocardial necrosis, likely a sign of brain-heart syndrome (Hahn *et al.* 1999). Myonecrosis and mononuclear infiltration were found in the small intestine of a foal with EEE (Poonacha *et al.* 1998).

Because high infection rates in man have been documented following exposure to aerosols from infected laboratory animals or from laboratory accidents (or, potentially, equine carcases), necropsies of horses with suspected VEE should only be performed by personnel who possess demonstrable immunity in the form of neutralising antibody (Rusnak *et al.* 2004). All laboratory manipulations must be carried out within certified biological safety cabinets following containment level 3 procedures.

Control

Active immunisation through use of formalinised vaccines derived from infected horse or guinea pig brain was first demonstrated in 1934 (Shahan and Giltner 1934). Propagation of virus in chick embryos in 1935 allowed large-scale production of formalin-inactivated vaccines for horses (Beard *et al.* 1938). In 1966, vaccine production was shifted to chick embryo tissue culture (Gutekunst 1969). Inactivated tissue culture-origin vaccines are still the only commercial method of immunisation of horses against EEE and WEE. These inactivated vaccines are also used routinely to protect ratites from EEE and WEE and South American camelids from EEE (Nolen-Watson *et al.* 2007). The attenuated, tissue-culture-origin vaccine, TC-83, derived from a Trinidad VEE virus isolate, which was originally developed to protect military personnel, provides durable immunity against VEE and was effective in minimising the incursion of VEE into the USA in 1971 (Zehmer *et al.* 1974) and in limiting the 1993 and 1996 outbreaks in Mexico. Although TC-83 is no longer licensed for use in horses in the USA, a formalin-inactivated vaccine containing the TC-83 vaccine strain is available and often is included with EEE and WEE in trivalent products (Barber *et al.* 1978). For any of the formalin-inactivated alphavirus vaccines, adult horses should be given an initial 2 inoculations 3–4 weeks apart at least a month before the anticipated risk period or before the onset of vector mosquito activity, and then revaccinated at intervals reflecting the likely risk. Vaccination should begin in January or February in Florida to May or June in parts of Canada and the northern USA. Clinical evidence suggests <6 months of protection following vaccination against EEE or WEE, so revaccination at least once during the mosquito season is necessary in areas with warm climates and long mosquito seasons. Vaccinated mares should receive a booster dose 4–6 weeks before foaling to provide colostral antibody for newborn foals.

According to recently updated AAEP guidelines (Anon 2008d), foals of vaccinated dams in high-risk areas should be vaccinated beginning at age 2–3 months. Two additional inoculations are then given at approximately 4 week intervals and a booster at age 10–12 months, before the onset of mosquito season. It will be important to validate this method of vaccination because of concerns that early frequent vaccinations may suppress immune responses to EEE (Gibbs and Wilson 1988). Until this issue has been resolved, the author will continue to recommend that the initial inoculation be given to foals in high-risk areas no earlier than age 4 months (as for foals in moderate-risk areas). The updated AAEP guidelines recommend that, in moderate-risk temperate areas, foals should receive an initial inoculation at age 4–6 months (vaccinated mare) or 3–4 months (unvaccinated mare), then a second inoculation 4–6 weeks later and a booster at age 10–12 months.

Routine surveillance of the virus pool by serum antibody testing of sentinel chickens and virus detection in trapped mosquitoes by health authorities often provides early warning of an impending outbreak and allows time for vaccination of susceptible horses. General mosquito control (removal of standing water, spraying by local authorities) will reduce risk of EEE and VEE in horses (Ross and Kaneene 1995). Because of the role of horses in amplification and transmission of VEE virus, quarantine of infected and exposed horses with area-wide and international restrictions on horse movement is an integral part of the management of VEE epizootics (Walton and Alvarez 1988).

Manufacturer's address

[1]Biogen IDEC, Cambridge, Massachusetts, USA.

References

Anon (2008a) *Animal Diseases Data: OIE-listed Diseases.* http://www.oie.int/eng/maladies.

Anon (2008b) *Disease Maps 2008.* U.S. Department of the Interior/U.S. Geological Survey. http://diseasemaps.usgs.gov/.

Anon (2008c) CDC. Division of vector-borne infectious diseases: Arboviruses. http://www.cdc.gov/ncidod/dvbid/Arbor/

Anon (2008d) *American Association of Equine Practitioners Guidelines for the Vaccination of Horses. Eastern/Western Equine Encephalomyelitis.* http://www.aaep.org/ eee_wee.htm.

Barber, T., Walton, T. and Lewis, K. (1978) Efficacy of trivalent inactivated encephalomyelitis virus vaccine in horses. *Am. J. vet. Res.* **39**, 621-625.

Beard, J.W., Finkelstein, H., Sealy, W.C. and Wyckoff, R.W.G. (1938) Immunization against equine encephalomyelitis with chick embryo vaccines. *Science* **87**, 490-490.

Booss, J. and Esiri, M.M. (2003) The arboviruses. In: *Viral Encephalitis in Humans*, ASM Press, Washington DC.

Briolant, S., Garin, D., Scaramozzino, N., Jouan, A. and Crance, J.M. (2004) *In vitro* inhibition of Chikungunya and Semliki Forest viruses replication by antiviral compounds: synergistic effect of interferon-alpha and ribavirin combination. *Antiviral Res.* **61**, 111-117.

Brault, A., Powers, A., Holmes, E., Woelk, C. and Weaver, S. (2002) Positively charged amino acid substitutions in the E2 envelope glycoprotein are associated with the emergence of Venezuelan equine encephalitis virus. *J. Virol.* **76**, 1718-1730.

Brault, A.C., Powers, A.M., Chavez, C.L.V., Lopez, R.N., Cachon, M.F., Gutierrez, L.F.L., Kang, W.L., Tesh, R.B., Shope, R.E. and Weaver, S.C. (1999) Genetic and antigenic diversity among eastern equine encephalitis viruses from North, Central, and South America. *Am. J. Trop. Med. Hyg.* **61**, 579-586.

Byrne, R.J. (1972) The control of eastern and western arboviral encephalomyelitis of horses. In: *Third International Conference on Equine Infectious Diseases*, Karger, Basel. pp 115-123.

Byrne, R.J., Scanlon, J.E., Locke, L.N., Hetrick, F.M. and Hastings, J.W. (1961) Observations on eastern equine encephalitis in Maryland in 1959. *J. Am. vet. med. Ass.* **139**, 661-664.

Calisher, C.H. (1994) Medically important arboviruses of the United States and Canada. *Clin. Microbiol. Rev.* **7**, 89-116.

Calisher, C.H., Mahmud, M., Elkafrawi, A.O., Emerson, J.K. and Muth, D.J. (1986) Rapid and specific serodiagnosis of western equine encephalitis-virus infection in horses. *Am. J. vet. Res.* **47**, 1296-1299.

Del Piero, F., Wilkins, P.A., Dubovi, E.J., Biolatti, B. and Cantile, C. (2001) Clinical, pathologic, immunohistochemical, and virologic findings of eastern equine encephalomyelitis in two horses. *Vet. Pathol.* **38**, 451-456.

Farrar, M., Miller, D., Baldwin, C., Stiver, S. and Hall, C. (2005) Eastern equine encephalitis in dogs. *J. vet. diag. Invest.* **17**, 614-617.

Forrester, N., Kenney, J., Deardorff, E., Wang, E. and Weaver, S. (2008) Western equine encephalitis submergence: Lack of evidence for a decline in virus virulence. *Virol.* **380**, 170-172.

Franklin, R., Kinde, H., Jay, M., Kramer, L., Green, E., Chiles, R., Ostlund, E., Husted, S., Smith, J. and Parker, M. (2002) Eastern equine encephalomyelitis virus infection in a horse from California. *Emerg. Infect. Dis.* **8**, 283-288.

Gibbs, E.P.J. (1976) Equine viral encephalitis. *Equine vet. J.* **8**, 66-71.

Gibbs, E.P.J. and Wilson, J.H. (1988) Studies on passive immunity and the vaccination of foals against eastern equine encephalitis in Florida. In: *Equine Infectious Diseases V: Proceedings of the Fifth International Conference,* Ed: D.G. Powell, University Press of Kentucky, Lexington. pp 201-205.

Gibbs, E.P.J. and Long, M.T. (2007) Equine alphaviruses. In: *Equine Infectious Diseases*, Eds: D.C. Sellon and M.T. Long, W.B. Saunders, St Louis.

Giltner, L. and Shahan, M. (1933) The 1933 outbreak of infectious equine encephalomyelitis. *North Am. Vet.* **14**, 25-27.

Grady, G.F., Maxfield, H.K., Hildreth, S.W., Timperi, R.J., Gilfillan, R.F., Rosenau, B.J., Francy, D.B., Calisher, C.H., Marcus, L.C. and Madoff, M.A. (1978) Eastern equine encephalitis in Massachusetts, 1957-1976 – prospective study centered upon analyses of mosquitos. *Am. J. Epidemiol.* **107**, 170-178.

Gutekunst, D.E. (1969) Immunity to bivalent tissue culture origin equine encephalomyelitis vaccine. *J. Am. vet. med. Ass.* **155**, 368-374.

Hagan, W.A.T., Bruner, D.W. and Timoney, J.F. (1981) *Hagan and Bruner's Microbiology and Infectious Diseases of Domestic Animals*, 7th edn., Cornell University Press, Ithaca.

Hahn, C.N., Mayhew, I.G. and MacKay, R.J. (1999) The nervous system. In: *Equine Medicine and Surgery*, 5th edn., Eds: P.C. Colahan, I.G. Mayhew, A.M. Merritt and J. Moore, Mosby, St Louis.

Hanson, R.P. (1957) An epizootic of equine encephalomyelitis that occurred in Massachusetts in 1831. *Am. J. Trop. Med. Hyg.* **6**, 858-862.

Hanson, R.P. (1972) Virology and epidemiology of eastern and western arboviral encephalomyelitis of horses. In: *Third International Conference on Equine Infectious Diseases*, Karger, Basel. pp 100-114.

Julander, J.G., Siddharthan, V., Blatt, L.M., Schafer, K., Sidwell, R.W. and Morrey, J.D. (2007) Effect of exogenous interferon and an interferon inducer on western equine encephalitis virus disease in a hamster model. *Virology* **360**, 454-460.

Karabatsos, N., Lewis, A., Calisher, C., Hunt, A. and Roehrig, J. (1988) Identification of Highlands J virus from a Florida horse. *Am. J. Trop. Med. Hyg.* **39**, 603-606.

Kinney, R.M., Tsuchiya, K.R., Sneider, J.M. and Trent, D.W. (1992) Molecular evidence for the origin of the widespread Venezuelan equine encephalitis epizootic of 1969 to 1972. *J. Gen. Virol.* **73**, 3301-3305.

Kubes, V. and Ríos, F. (1939) The causative agent of infectious equine encephalomyelitis in Venezuela. *Science* **90**, 20-21.

Kuno, G. and Chang, G. (2005) Biological transmission of arboviruses: reexamination of and new insights into components, mechanisms, and unique traits as well as their evolutionary trends. *Clin. Microbiol. Rev.* **18**, 608-637.

Larsell, O., Haring, C.M. and Meyer, K.F. (1934) Histological changes in the central nervous system following equine encephalomyelitis. *Am. J. Pathol.* **10**, 361-374.

Lyon, B.M. (1939) Present status of equine encephalomyelitis and its control. *Cornell Vet.* **29**, 198-216.

Miller, L.D., Pearson, J.E. and Muhm, R.L. (1973) A comparison of clinical manifestations and pathology of the equine encephalidites: VEE, WEE, EEE. In: *Proceedings of the Annual Meeting of the U.S. Animal Health Association* **75**, 629-631.

Merrill, M.H. (1936) Quantitative studies on the neutralization of equine encephalomyelitis virus by immune serum I. Combination of virus and antibody *in vitro*. *J. Immunol.* **30**, 185-192.

Merrill, M.H., Lacaillade, C.W. and TenBroeck, C. (1934) Mosquito transmission of equine encephalomyelitis. *Science* **80**, 251-252.

Meyer, K. (1933) Equine encephalomyelitis. *N. Am. Vet.* **14**, 30-48.

Meyer, K.F. (1932) A summary of recent studies on equine encephalomyel(i)tis. *Ann. Intern. Med.* **6**, 645-654.

Nalca, A., Fellows, P.F. and Whitehouse, C.A. (2003) Vaccines and animal models for arboviral encephalitides. *Antiviral Res.* **60**, 153-174.

Nasci, R.S., Berry, R.L., Restifo, R.A., Parsons, M.A., Smith, G.C. and Martin, D.A. (1993) Eastern equine encephalitis virus in Ohio during 1991. *J. Med. Entomol.* **30**, 217-222.

Navarro, J.C., Medina, G., Vasquez, C., Coffey, L.L., Wang, E.Y., Suarez, A., Biord, H., Salas, M. and Weaver, S.C. (2005) Postepizootic persistence of Venezuelan equine encephalitis virus, Venezuela. *Emerg. Infect. Dis.* **11**, 1907-1915.

Nolen-Walston, R., Bedenice, D., Rodriguez, C., Rushton, S., Bright, A., Fecteau, M.E., Short, D., Majdalany, R., Tewari, D., Pedersen, D., Kiupel, M., Maes, R. and Del Piero, F. (2007) Eastern equine encephalitis in 9 South American camelids. *J. vet. Intern. Med.* **21**, 846-852.

Oglesby, W.T. (1948) 1947 outbreak of infectious equine encephalomyelitis in Louisiana. *J. Am. vet. med. Ass.* **113**, 267-270.

Oberste, M.S., Fraire, M., Navarro, R., Zepeda, C., Zarate, M.L., Ludwig, G.V., Kondig, J.F., Weaver, S.C., Smith, J.F. and Rico-Hesse, R. (1998) Association of Venezuelan equine encephalitis virus subtype IE with two equine epizootics in Mexico. *Am. J. Trop. Med. Hyg.* **59**, 100-107.

Poonacha, K., Gregory, C. and Vickers, M. (1998) Intestinal lesions in a horse associated with eastern equine encephalomyelitis virus infection. *Vet. Pathol.* **35**, 535-538.

Przelomski, M., O'Rourke, E., Grady, G., Berardi, V. and Markley, H. (1988) Eastern equine encephalitis in Massachusetts: a report of 16 cases, 1970-1984. *Neurology* **38**, 736-739.

Ross, W.A. and Kaneene, J.B. (1995) A case-control study of an outbreak of eastern equine encephalomyelitis in Michigan (USA) equine herds in 1991. *Prev. vet. Med.* **24**, 157-170.

Ross, W.A. and Kaneene, J.B. (1996) Evaluation of outbreaks of disease attributable to eastern equine encephalitis virus in horses. *J. Am. vet. med. Ass.* **208**, 1988-1997.

Rusnak, J.M., Kortepeter, M.G., Hawley, R.J., Boudreau, E., Aldis, J. and Pittman, P.R. (2004) Management guidelines for laboratory exposures to agents of bioterrorism. *J. Occup. environ. Med.* **46**, 791-800.

Sahu, S.P., Alstad, A.D., Pedersen, D.D. and Pearson, J.E. (1994) Diagnosis of eastern equine encephalomyelitis virus infection in horses by immunoglobulin M and G capture enzyme-linked immunosorbent assay. *J. vet. diag. Invest.* **6**, 34-38.

Sahu, S.P., Pedersen, D.D., Jenny, A.L., Schmitt, B.J. and Alstad, A.D. (2003) Pathogenicity of a Venezuelan equine encephalomyelitis serotype IE virus isolate for ponies. *Am. J. Trop. Med. Hyg.* **68**, 485-494.

Scott, T.W. and Weaver, S.C. (1989) Eastern equine encephalomyelitis virus - epidemiology and evolution of mosquito transmission. *Adv. Virus Res.* **37**, 277-328.

Sellers, R., Bergold, G., Suarez, O. and Morales, A. (1965) Investigations during Venezuelan equine encephalitis outbreaks in Venezuela 1962-1964. *Am. J. Trop. Med Hyg.* **14**, 460-469.

Sellers, R.F. (1989) Eastern equine encephalitis in Quebec and Connecticut, 1972 – Introduction by infected mosquitos on the wind. *Can. J. vet. Res.* **53**, 76-79.

Shahan, M.S. and Giltner, L.T. (1934) Some aspects of infection and immunity in equine encephalomyelitis. *J. Am. vet. med. Ass.* **84**, 928-934.

Suarez-Mier, G. and MacKay, R.J. (2008) Alphaviral encephalomyelitis (EEE, WEE, and VEE). In: *Current Therapy in Equine Medicine*, 6th edn., Eds: N.E. Robinson and K.A. Sprayberry, W.B. Saunders, Philadelphia. pp 618-621.

Sudia, W.D., Stamm, D.D., Chamberlain, R.W. and Kissling, R.E. (1956) Transmission of eastern equine encephalitis to horses by *Aedes sollicitans* mosquitoes. *Am. J. Trop. Med. Hyg.* **5**, 802-808.

Walton, T. (1992) Arboviral encephalomyelitides of livestock in the western hemisphere. *J. Am. vet. med. Ass.* **200**, 1385-1389.

Walton, T. and Alvarez, O., Jr. (1988) Venezuelan equine encephalomyelitis. In: *Epidemiology and Ecology*, Ed: T. Monath, CRC Press, Boca Raton. pp 203-231.

Walton, T., Holbrook, F., Bolivar-Raya, R., Ferrer-Romero, J. and Ortega, M. (1992) Venezuelan equine encephalomyelitis and African horse sickness. Current status and review. *Ann. N.Y. Acad. Sci.* **653**, 217-227.

Weaver, S., Ferro, C., Barrera, R., Boshell, J. and Navarro, J. (2004) Venezuelan equine encephalitis. *Ann. Rev. Entomol.* **49**, 141-174.

Weaver, S.C., Hagenbaugh, A., Bellew, L.A., Gousset, L., Mallampalli, V., Holland, J.J. and Scott, T.W. (1994) Evolution of alphaviruses in the eastern equine encephalomyelitis complex. *J. Virol.* **68**, 158-169.

Weaver, S.C., Powers, A.M., Brault, A.C. and Barrett, A.D.T. (1999) Molecular epidemiological studies of veterinary arboviral encephalitides. *Vet. J.* **157**, 123-138.

Wilson, J.H., Rubin, H.L., Lane, T.J. and Gibbs, E.P.J. (1986) A survey of eastern equine encephalomyelitis in Florida horses – prevalence, economic impact, and management practices, 1982-1983. *Prev. vet. Med.* **4**, 261-271.

Zehmer, R.B., Dean, P.B., Sudia, W.D., Calisher, C.H., Sather, G.E. and Parker, R.L. (1974) Venezuelan equine encephalitis epidemic in Texas, 1971. *Health Services Report* **89**, 278-282.

JAPANESE ENCEPHALITIS

J. R. Gilkerson* and P. M. Ellis†

Equine Infectious Disease Laboratory, Faculty of Veterinary Science, The University of Melbourne, Australia; and †PO Box 236, Yarra Glen, Victoria 3775, Australia.

Keywords: horse; Japanese encephalitis; JEV; arbovirus; flavivirus

Summary

Japanese encephalitis (JE) is an arbovirus disease of birds and mosquitoes that spills over to cause disease of incidental hosts such as horses and man when climatic conditions favour expansion of the insect vector population. The natural reservoir hosts of JE virus are ardeid water birds and groundwater breeding *Culex* species of mosquito. Horses with JE may show clinical signs of encephalitis and central nervous system disease such as ataxia, blindness, collapse and death. JEV is an important cause of epidemic encephalitis in unvaccinated human subjects, but widespread vaccination programmes in horses have reduced the likelihood and severity of equine disease outbreaks.

Aetiology

Japanese encephalitis virus (JEV) is a mosquito-borne virus of the *Flavivirus* genus of the family *Flaviviridae* and is serologically grouped with a number of other flaviviruses including West Nile virus, St Louis encephalitis virus, Kunjin virus and Murray Valley encephalitis virus. Japanese encephalitis (JE) is an acute arboviral disease of man, swine, horses and other domestic species (Geering *et al.* 1995). Man and horses are considered dead-end or incidental hosts as viraemia in these species is considered insufficient to re-infect a mosquito host and thus perpetuate the cycle of infection. Most JEV infections are asymptomatic and the ratio of symptomatic to asymptomatic infections in human subjects range from 1:25 to 1:1000 depending upon host factors, exposure to mosquitoes and virus virulence (Solomon and Winter 2004). Antibodies to JEV have been reported in a wide range of vertebrate species (Burke and Leake 1988), but significant disease associated with JEV infection has only been reported in pigs and horses.

The JE serological group includes viruses that are found on all continents except Antarctica. JEV is found in eastern, southern and south-eastern parts of Asia, as well as in Papua New Guinea and the Torres Strait (Mackenzie *et al.* 2002). Epidemics of JE in people occur in the temperate regions of Asia, such as Japan, China, Korea, Sri Lanka and India, and JE is endemic in tropical regions of Asia such as Malaysia, southern Thailand, Vietnam and Indonesia (Weaver *et al.* 1999). Human cases of JE have been reported in Australia in 1995 on the island of Badu in the Torres Strait and in the far north of the Australian mainland (Hanna *et al.* 1996, 1999). No horses developed clinical disease in this outbreak, although 70% (7/10) of the horses tested on Badu had antibodies to JEV.

Members of the family *Flaviviridae* are enveloped, single stranded positive sense RNA viruses. The envelope surrounds the nucleocapsid and is composed of a lipid bilayer with 2 or more species of envelope (E) glycoproteins. The genome of JEV is a positive sense, single-stranded RNA molecule approximately 11 kb in length (Thiel *et al.* 1990). Genomic sequencing of JEV isolates from different geographical areas has identified at least 4 genotypes, with some degree of overlap in their geographical range and capacity to cause epidemics of JE (Chen *et al.* 1990, 1992; Tsuchie *et al.* 1997; Williams *et al.* 2000).

Epidemiology

Japanese encephalitis virus is maintained in nature in a bird/mosquito cycle with virus replication occurring in both the avian and arthropod hosts (Scherer *et al.* 1959, 1959). Ground water breeding *Culex* species of mosquitoes are the insect vector

*Author to whom correspondence should be addressed.

responsible for transmission of JEV between vertebrate hosts. The principal mosquito vector for human and animal infection is *Culex tritaeniorhynchus*, which is a night time biting mosquito that feeds preferentially on birds and large mammals, but only infrequently on human sujects. JEV has been isolated from other species of mosquitoes, particularly in tropical regions, and these species may be locally important in the epidemiology of JE (Halstead and Jacobson 2003). JE occurs primarily in rural areas in Asia where competent vector species of mosquito are able to proliferate in areas with high populations of wading birds and ducks (Burke and Leake 1988). Ardeid bird species such black crowned night herons (*Nycticorax nycticorax*), plumed egrets (*Egretta intermedia*) and great egrets (*Egretta alba*) have been shown to be important avian host species (Buescher *et al.* 1959; Scherer *et al.* 1959; Burke and Leake 1988). Pigs play an important role in the epidemiology of JE as an amplifier host species. Nearly all pigs that become infected develop a viraemia sufficient to infect subsequent biting mosquitoes (Scherer *et al.* 1959), while the high rate of population turnover in farmed pigs provides a constant supply of susceptible animals. Human and equine disease occur as a result of spillover of JE infection from the natural sylvatic maintenance cycle.

Disease

Japanese encephalitis virus is an important cause of human epidemic viral encephalitis, with 30,000–50,000 reported cases of JE each year, mostly in children aged <10 years, with a case fatality rate of 5–50% (Solomon and Vaughn 2002; Halstead and Jacobson 2003). Clinical signs of human JE are typically encephalopathic in nature, with seizures occurring commonly, especially in children (Gould and Solomon 2008). JEV also causes encephalitis in horses and reproductive losses in pigs.

Horses and pigs are important vertebrate hosts of JEV (Halstead and Jacobson 2003). Pigs are important amplifying hosts, while horses (and humans) are dead-end or incidental hosts. Adult, nonpregnant pigs show few clinical signs of infection with JEV; however, infection of pregnant sows may be vertically transmitted to the fetuses, resulting in abortion, or birth of mummified or weak piglets (Burns 1950). During times of peak virus transmission up to one third of pregnant sows may lose their litters (Takashima *et al.* 1988), but these losses have been ameliorated by the widespread use of JE vaccination (Fujisaki *et al.* 1975). Vaccination of pigs has been shown to have a favourable impact on the prevalence of human JE (Igarashi 2002).

In man, clinical illness may follow a moderate incubation period of 6–16 days. Disease may manifest as periods of headache and fever, followed by signs of encephalitis, including muscular rigidity, cranial nerve palsy, coarse tremors and involuntary movements, and convulsions. Convulsions are frequent in children but occur in <10% of adult patients (Gubler *et al.* 2007). The exact mechanism for virus transport across the blood-brain barrier is unknown, but is likely to occur by invasion across the cerebral capillaries. Gross *post mortem* examinations of the brains of human patients who died from JE showed vascular congestion. On haematoxylin and eosin staining of brain tissue there was significant peri-vascular cuffing, often by polymorphonuclear cells, and infiltration of cells into the brain parenchyma, neuronophagia and formation of glial nodules in the cerebral cortex, thalamus and brainstem (Johnson *et al.* 1985).

Prior to the introduction of routine JE vaccination of horses in Japan, outbreaks of equine encephalitis tended to coincide with the seasonal epidemics of human JE. The incidence of encephalitis in horses was 10–50 per 100,000 horses and the case-fatality rate approximately 50% (Matsuda 1962). Horses may show variable clinical signs of JEV infection, ranging from transient fever, lethargy and ataxia, to hyperexcitability, central CNS signs, blindness, profuse sweating, collapse and death. There are no characteristic gross lesions in the brain of encephalitic horses. A diffuse nonsuppurative encephalomyelitis with phagocytic destruction of nerve cells, focal gliosis, perivascular cuffing and engorged blood vessels containing many mononuclear cells has been reported (Burns *et al.* 1949; Miyake 1964). Recent reports of equine JE are uncommon (Lam *et al.* 2005), as most 'at-risk' horse populations in Asian countries are vaccinated. Despite the paucity of recent equine cases of JE a recent serological study in Japan found that the annual equine infection rates varied between 15 and 67% of surveyed horses in the absence of clinical disease (Konishi *et al.* 2004).

Control

Control of JE in horses is focused on prevention of disease by vaccination in endemic areas (Goto 1976). There are no antiviral therapies for human JE, and although control of JE based on mosquito control and reducing human exposure to mosquitoes may have contributed to reduced disease prevalence, these strategies do not offer a long-term solution. Immunisation is the single most important control measure in some endemically affected countries (Anon 2006). There are currently 3 types of vaccine used to control human JE: a mouse-brain derived inactivated vaccine, a cell-culture derived inactivated vaccine and a cell culture derived live attenuated vaccine. A formalin inactivated cell-culture vaccine based on the Beijing P-3 strain is available for horses and is widely used in Asian countries such as Japan, Hong Kong, Macau, Malaysia and Singapore where mass vaccination is used to protect the health of thoroughbred racehorse populations, many of which are imported from countries in which JE does not occur (Ellis *et al.* 2000).

Diagnosis

Specimens should be collected from animals in the acute stages of disease, or from animals that have been dead for less than 12 h (Geering *et al.* 1995). Definitive diagnosis of JE depends on isolation of the virus from brain tissue of affected horses. As the virus is difficult to isolate, clinical, pathological and serological findings are also useful in establishing a diagnosis. Tissue samples are inoculated onto cell culture monolayers, or intracerebrally into suckling mice (Anon 2008). Unfortunately, the isolation rate is low, due to instability of the virus and the presence of antibody in affected animals (Anon 2008), but nucleic acid detection techniques, such as reverse-transcription polymerase chain reaction (RT-PCR) have been developed (Tanaka 1993; Williams *et al.* 2001; Lian *et al.* 2002).

Serological diagnosis is complicated by the high proportion of inapparent JE infections of horses in endemic areas. Serological confirmation of JE requires an increased JE specific antibody titre between acute and convalescent samples collected 14–28 days apart. A number of serological tests are described in the OIE Manual of Diagnostic Tests and Vaccines for Terrestrial Animals (Anon 2008).

References

Anon (2006) Japanese encephalitis vaccines. *Wkly. Epidemiol. Rec.* **81**, 331-340.

Anon (2008) *Manual of Diagnostic Tests and Vaccines for Terrestrial Animals 2008: Japanese Encephalitis.* World Organisation for Animal Health, Paris.

Buescher, E.L., Scherer, W.F., Rosenberg, M.Z., Kutner, L.J. and Mc, C.H. (1959) Immunologic studies of Japanese encephalitis virus in Japan. IV. Maternal antibody in birds. *J. Immunol.* **83**, 614-619.

Burke, D.S. and Leake, C. (1988) Japanese encephalitis. In: *The Arboviruses: Epidemiology and Ecology*, Ed: T. Monath, CRC, Boca Raton. pp 63-92.

Burns, K.F. (1950) Congenital Japanese B encephalitis infection of swine. *Proc. Soc. expt. biol. Med.* **75**, 621-625.

Burns, K.F., Tigertt, W.D. and Matumoto, M. (1949) Japanese equine encephalomyelitis; 1947 epizootic; serological and etiological studies. *Am. J. Hyg.* **50**, 27-45.

Chen, W.R., Rico-Hesse, R. and Tesh, R.B. (1992) A new genotype of Japanese encephalitis virus from Indonesia. *Am. J. trop. Med. Hyg.* **47**, 61-69.

Chen, W.R., Tesh, R.B. and Rico-Hesse, R. (1990) Genetic variation of Japanese encephalitis virus in nature. *J. Gen. Virol.* **71**, 2915-2922.

Ellis, P.M., Daniels, P.W. and Banks, D.J. (2000) Japanese encephalitis. *Vet. Clin. N. Am.: Equine Pract.* **16**, 565-578, x-xi.

Fujisaki, Y., Sugimori, T., Morimoto, T., Miura, Y. and Kawakami, Y. (1975) Immunization of pigs with the attenuated S- strain of Japanese encephalitis virus. *Natl. Inst. Anim. Health. Q. (Tokyo)* **15**, 55-60.

Geering, W., Forman, A. and Nunn, M. (1995) Exotic diseases of animals: a field guide for Australian veterinarians, Australian Government Publishing Service, Canberra.

Goto, H. (1976) Efficacy of Japanese encephalitis vaccine in horses. *Equine vet. J.* **8**, 126-127.

Gould, E.A. and Solomon, T. (2008) Pathogenic flaviviruses. *Lancet* **371**, 500-509.

Gubler, D.J., Kuno, G. and Markoff, L. (2007) Flaviviruses. In: *Field's Virology*, Eds: D. Knipe and P. Howley, Lippincott Williams & Wilkins, Philadelphia. pp 1154-1252.

Halstead, S.B. and Jacobson, J. (2003) Japanese encephalitis. *Adv. Virus. Res.* **61**, 103-138.

Hanna, J.N., Ritchie, S.A., Phillips, D.A., Lee, J.M., Hills, S.L., van den Hurk, A.F., Pyke, A.T., Johansen, C.A. and Mackenzie, J.S. (1999) Japanese encephalitis in north Queensland, Australia, 1998. *Med. J. Aust.* **170**, 533-536.

Hanna, J.N., Ritchie, S.A., Phillips, D.A., Shield, J., Bailey, M.C., Mackenzie, J.S., Poidinger, M., McCall, B.J. and Mills, P.J. (1996) An outbreak of Japanese encephalitis in the Torres Strait, Australia, 1995. *Med. J. Aust.* **165**, 256-260.

Igarashi, A. (2002) Control of Japanese encephalitis in Japan: immunization of humans and animals, and vector control. *Curr. Top. Microbiol. Immunol.* **267**, 139-152.

Johnson, R.T., Burke, D.S., Elwell, M., Leake, C.J., Nisalak, A., Hoke, C.H. and Lorsomrudee, W. (1985) Japanese encephalitis: immunocytochemical studies of viral antigen and inflammatory cells in fatal cases. *Ann. Neurol.* **18**, 567-573.

Konishi, E., Shoda, M. and Kondo, T. (2004) Prevalence of antibody to Japanese encephalitis virus nonstructural 1 protein among racehorses in Japan: indication of natural infection and need for continuous vaccination. *Vaccine* **22**, 1097-1103.

Lam, K.H., Ellis, T.M., Williams, D.T., Lunt, R.A., Daniels, P.W., Watkins, K.L. and Riggs, C.M. (2005) Japanese encephalitis in a racing Thoroughbred gelding in Hong Kong. *Vet. Rec.* **157**, 168-173.

Lian, W.C., Liau, M.Y. and Mao, C.L. (2002) Diagnosis and genetic analysis of Japanese encephalitis virus infected in horses. *J. Vet. Med. B. Infect. Dis. Vet. Public Health* **49**, 361-365.

Mackenzie, J.S., Barrett, A.D. and Deubel, V. (2002) The Japanese encephalitis serological group of flaviviruses: a brief introduction to the group. *Curr. Top. Microbiol. Immunol.* **267**, 1-10.

Matsuda, S. (1962) An epidemiological study of Japanese B encephalitis with special reference to the effectiveness of the vaccination. *Bull. Inst. Public Health* **11**, 173-190.

Miyake, M. (1964) The pathology of Japanese encephalitis. A Review. *Bull. World Health Organ.* **30**, 153-160.

Scherer, W.F., Buescher, E.L. and McClure, H.E. (1959) Ecologic studies of Japanese encephalitis virus in Japan. V. Avian factors. *Am. J. trop. Med. Hyg.* **8**, 689-697.

Scherer, W.F., Moyer, J.T., Izumi, T., Gresser, I. and McCown, J. (1959) Ecologic studies of Japanese encephalitis virus in Japan. VI. Swine infection. *Am. J. trop. Med. Hyg.* **8**, 698-706.

Scherer, W.F., Buescher, E.L., Flemings, M.B., Noguchi, A. and Scanlon, J. (1959) Ecologic studies of Japanese encephalitis virus in Japan. III. Mosquito factors. Zootropism and vertical flight of *Culex tritaeniorhynchus* with observations on variations in collections from animal-baited traps in different habitats. *Am. J. trop. Med. Hyg.* **8**, 665-677.

Solomon, T. and Vaughn, D.W. (2002) Pathogenesis and clinical features of Japanese encephalitis and West Nile virus infections. *Curr. Top. Microbiol. Immunol.* **267**, 171-194.

Solomon, T. and Winter, P.M. (2004) Neurovirulence and host factors in *flavivirus* encephalitis--evidence from clinical epidemiology. *Arch. Virol. Suppl.* **18**, 161-170.

Takashima, I., Watanabe, T., Ouchi, N. and Hashimoto, N. (1988) Ecological studies of Japanese encephalitis virus in Hokkaido: interepidemic outbreaks of swine abortion and evidence for the virus to overwinter locally. *Am. J. trop. Med. Hyg.* **38**, 420-427.

Tanaka, M. (1993) Rapid identification of *flavivirus* using the polymerase chain reaction. *J. Virol. Methods* **41**, 311-322.

Thiel, H.-J., Collett, M., Gould, E., Heinz, F., Hiughton, M., Meyers, G., Purcell, R. and Rice, C. (1990) Family *Flaviviridae*. In: *Virus Taxonomy. Classification and Nomenclature of Viruses. The Eighth Report of the International Committee on the Taxonomy of Viruses*, Eds: C. Fauquet, M. Mayo, J. Maniloff, U. Desselberger and L. Ball, Elsevier Academic Press, Oxford. p 1259.

Tsuchie, H., Oda, K., Vythilingam, I., Thayan, R., Vijayamalar, B., Sinniah, M., Singh, J., Wada, T., Tanaka, H., Kurimura, T. and Igarashi, A. (1997) Genotypes of Japanese encephalitis virus isolated in three states in Malaysia. *Am. J. trop. Med. Hyg.* **56**, 153-158.

Weaver, S.C., Powers, A.M., Brault, A.C. and Barrett, A.D. (1999) Molecular epidemiological studies of veterinary arboviral encephalitides. *Vet. J.* **157**, 123-138.

Williams, D.T., Wang, L.F., Daniels, P.W. and Mackenzie, J.S. (2000) Molecular characterization of the first Australian isolate of Japanese encephalitis virus, the FU strain. *J. gen. Virol.* **81**, 2471-2480.

Williams, D.T., Daniels, P.W., Lunt, R.A., Wang, L.F., Newberry, K.M. and Mackenzie, J.S. (2001) Experimental infections of pigs with Japanese encephalitis virus and closely related Australian flaviviruses. *Am. J. trop. Med. Hyg.* **65**, 379-387.

EQUINE BORNA DISEASE

C. Herden and J. A. Richt*

*Institute of Pathology, University of Veterinary Medicine Hannover, Bünteweg 17, 30559 Hanover, Germany; and *Department of Diagnostic Medicine/Pathobiology, College of Veterinary Medicine, K224B Mosier Hall, Manhattan, Kansas 66506-5601, USA.*

Keywords: horse; Borna disease; CNS; equine; natural infection; meningoencephalitis

Summary

Borna disease (BD) is an endemic neurological disorder predominantly affecting horses and sheep, caused by the neurotropic Borna disease virus (BDV). In the last 20 years, substantial progress has been made in BDV research and basic understanding of its molecular features, its mechanism of persistence, its immunopathogenesis and epidemiology has been attained. However, our knowledge is still incomplete as shown by the recent discovery that psittacine birds harbor an avian BDV. Recent advances on the aetiology and natural distribution of BD, underlying pathogenesis, clinical signs, gross and histopathological lesions and diagnostic possibilities are summarised in this review.

Introduction

Borna disease (BD) is an endemic, sporadically occurring, usually fatal disorder caused by the highly neurotropic Borna disease virus (BDV) (Heinig 1969; Danner 1982; Rott and Becht 1995; Staeheli 2002; Richt *et al.* 2007). The name originated from a devastating epidemic among horses of a cavalry regiment in the years 1894 through 1896 near the town of Borna in Saxony/Germany. BD has been reported for over 200 years and formerly used synonyms were 'hot-headed disease' or 'epidemic encephalomyelitis', reflecting the restriction of the disease to the central nervous system (CNS). The characteristic neurological signs are immunopathological in nature (not caused by the virus itself), resulting in a nonpurulent meningopolioencephalitis (Narayan *et al.* 1983a,b; Richt *et al.* 1989, 1994; Hallensleben *et al.* 1998; Hausmann *et al.* 2001; Stitz *et al.* 2002). Several lines of evidence indicate a T-cell-mediated delayed type hypersensitivity reaction as the basic phenomenon. BD is characterised by a persistent, noncytopathic infection which is achieved by a multitude of viral strategies, e.g. direct modification of the viral genome, tight regulation of replication and protein synthesis and by interaction with host cell factors (Planz *et al.* 2001a; Tomonaga *et al.* 2002; Bourtelee *et al.* 2005; Schneider 2005; de la Torre 2006; Schneider *et al.* 2007).

Borna disease predominantly affects horses and sheep but other equids, farm animals, zoo animals or companion animals occasionally are diagnosed with natural BD (reviewed by Rott and Becht 1995; Dürrwald and Ludwig 1997; Staeheli *et al.* 2000; Richt *et al.* 2007). Recently, infection of psittacine birds with a novel BDV-like agent named avian BDV associated with proventricular dilatation disease was reported (Honkavouri *et al.* 2008; Kistler *et al.* 2008; Gancz *et al.* 2009; Rinder *et al.* 2009).

The zoonotic capacity of BDV, namely its association with human psychiatric diseases, is still controversial. The existence of BDV-specific serum antibodies in psychiatric patients is widely accepted (Rott *et al.* 1985; Van de Woude *et al.* 1990; Richt *et al.* 1997; Billich *et al.* 2002; Schwemmle and Billich 2004), whereas the presence of BDV-specific nucleic acids in blood of such patients is yet debated due to the perception that sample contamination might be an issue (Richt *et al.* 1997; Lieb and Staeheli 2001; Schwemmle 2001; Wolff *et al.* 2006; Dürrwald *et al.* 2007).

Clinically manifest BD has been described in endemic areas of Germany, Switzerland, Liechtenstein and Austria (Herzog *et al.* 1994,

*Author to whom correspondence should be addressed. Dr Herden's present address: Institute of Veterinary Pathology, Justus-Liebig-University Gießen, Frankfurter Str. 96, D-35392 Gießen, Germany.

Weissenböck *et al.* 1998a; Caplazi *et al.* 1999; Dürrwald *et al.* 2006). The presence of natural BD outside the European endemic areas, the possible association of BDV infections with other clinical symptoms and the presence of virus-specific antibodies and/or nucleic acids in animals from several countries (reviewed by Staeheli *et al.* 2000; Richt and Rott 2001; Dürrwald *et al.* 2006; Richt *et al.* 2007) is still discussed controversially. Thus, there are many open questions and our knowledge on the epidemiology of BD, the survival strategies of the causative agent BDV, and BDV-associated disorders is still incomplete.

Aetiology

The proof for a viral aetiology of BD had already been described in 1927 by Zwick *et al.* (1927) when the disease was reproduced with bacteria-free filtrates of brain homogenates from affected horses. During the last 20 years, substantial progress regarding the molecular characterisation of BDV, the viral replication strategies and persistence mechanisms has been attained (Lipkin *et al.* 1990; Van de Woude *et al.* 1990; Richt *et al.* 1991; Briese *et al.* 1994; Cubitt *et al.* 1994a,b; Tomonaga *et al.* 2002; de la Torre 2006; Schneider *et al.* 2007). With the advent of a reverse genetics system to produce infectious BDV cDNA clones, detailed molecular analysis of the viral genome organisation, the corresponding gene products and the control of genome expression were made possible (Perez *et al.* 2003; Schneider 2005; de la Torre 2006; Ackermann *et al.* 2007a,b; Schneider *et al.* 2007).

The organisation of the BDV genome and unique features such as the nuclear site of BDV replication and transcription, termination site read-through, RNA-splicing, and overlapping open reading frames (ORF) and transcription units led to the classification as the new family *Bornaviridae* in the order Mononegavirales (Briese *et al.* 1994; Cubitt *et al.* 1994a,b; Schneemann *et al.* 1995; Pringle 1996; de la Torre 2002, 2006; Tomonaga *et al.* 2002; Poenisch *et al.* 2008a). BDV is an enveloped virus with a nonsegmented, negative-sense, single-stranded (ss) condensed RNA genome of 8.9 kb. BDV particles are spherical, enveloped, and approximately 130 nm in diameter, with spikes of 7 nm in length and a nucleocapsid that is 4 nm in diameter (Kohno *et al.* 1999).

The complete sequence of the genome from several BDV isolates has been determined (Briese *et al.* 1994; Cubitt *et al.* 1994a; Nowotny *et al.* 2000; Pleschka *et al.* 2001; Kolodziejek *et al.* 2005) and revealed a high degree of genetic stability and homology among wild-type and experimentally host-adapted viruses (Binz *et al.* 1994; Herzog *et al.* 1997; Staeheli *et al.* 2000; Pleschka *et al.* 2001). Phylogenetic analysis of wild-type and laboratory strains indicate distinct virus clusters with a high homology corresponding to geographical endemic areas in Central Europe (Kolodziejek *et al.* 2005). BDV isolates from the same geographical area exhibited a clearly higher degree of identity to each other than to BDV isolates from other regions, independent of host species and year of isolation (Kolodziejek *et al.* 2005). All field and laboratory strains, as well as the vaccine strain, clearly segregated from the recently described and highly divergent BDV strain No/98, which originated from Styria in Austria where Borna disease is not endemic. The high genome conservation was interpreted as adaptation to the noncytopathic life cycle of BDV and might imply that BDV adapts easily to various animal species without the necessity of significant genetic change. Recently, it was shown that amino acid changes in the viral polymerase which improve enzymatic activity are essential for the adaptation of BDV from rats to mice (Ackermann *et al.* 2007a,b). Additionally, mutations in equine field isolates occur at random that lead to exchanges in antigenic epitopes of the viral nucleoprotein, which might mask the diagnosis of a natural BDV infection (Richt *et al.* 1997; Herden *et al.* 1999).

Interestingly, the novel avian BDV sequences shared less than 70% sequence identity to any of the previously identified mammalian BDV isolates (Honkavouri *et al.* 2008; Kistler *et al.* 2008; Rinder *et al* 2009). So far, a sequence divergence of >15% has only been described for the equine BDV strain No/98 from Austria (Nowotny *et al.* 2000).

On the complementary positive-strand viral RNA (cRNA) 6 ORFs have been identified that are located in 3 transcription units. ORF I is located in the first monocistronic transcription unit at the 5'-end of the cRNA, and encodes the BDV nucleoprotein, BDV-N. The second bicistronic transcription unit contains ORF II coding for the phosphoprotein (BDV-P) and ORFx1 encoding the small protein BDV-p10 or BDV-X. RNA-

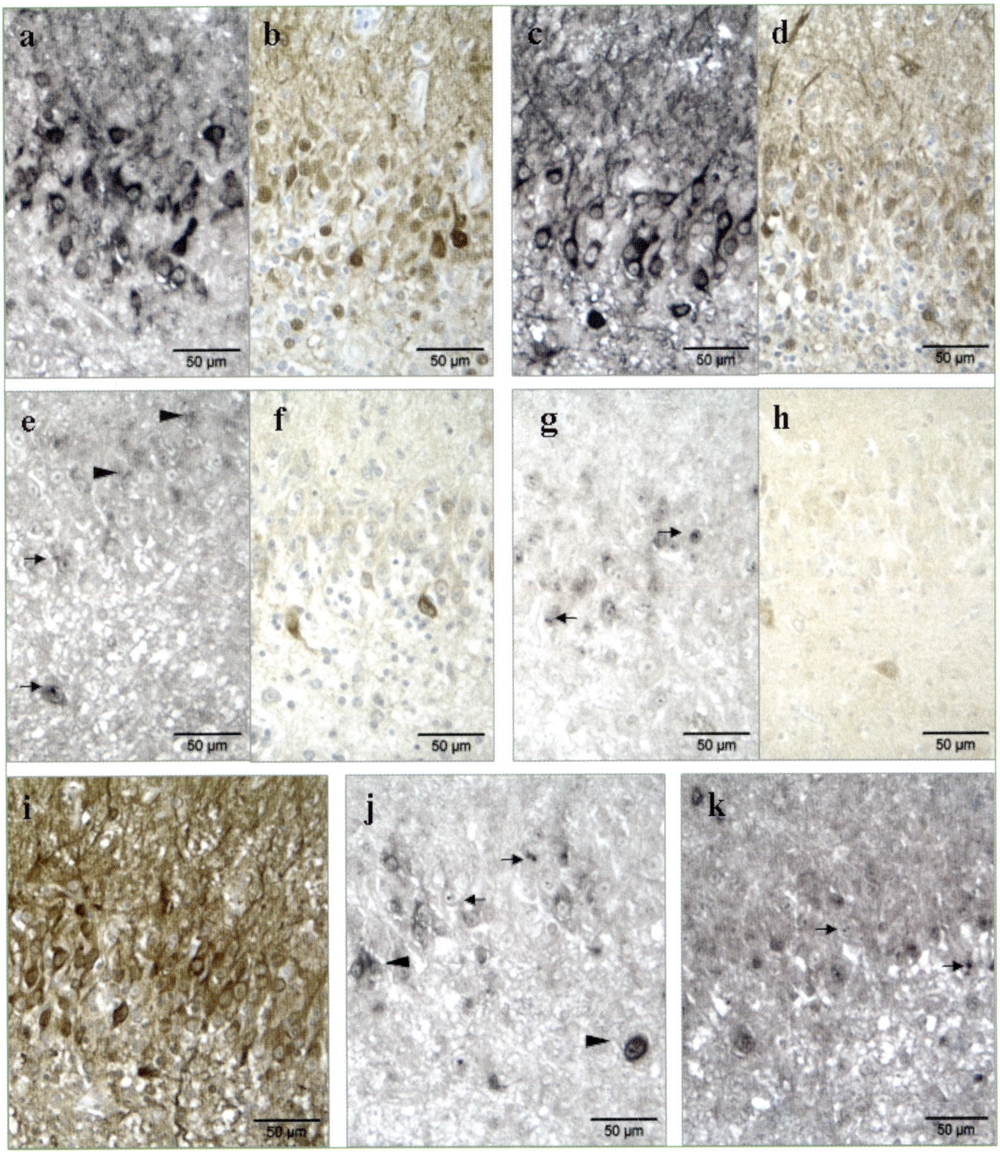

FIGURE 1: Demonstration of BDV-specific RNAs and proteins in a horse with typical BD by in situ hybridisation and immunohistology. a, c, e, g, j, k) Demonstration of BDV-specific RNAs. b, d, f, h, i) Demonstration of BDV-specific proteins. a) Detection and distribution of BDV-N-specific mRNA, mainly in the cytoplasm and processes of neurons. b) Widespread detection of the BDV-N using the monoclonal antibody Bo 18. BDV-N is present in the cytoplasm and nuclei of infected neurons and in the neuropil. c) Detection and distribution of BDV-P-specific mRNA, mainly in the cytoplasm and processes of neurons. d) Widespread detection of the BDV-P using a polyclonal, monospecific antibody. BDV-P is present in the cytoplasm and few nuclei of neurons and in the neuropil. e) Demonstration of BDV-M-specific mRNA in the cytoplasm (arrowheads) and few nuclei; note dot-like signal (arrows) in some neurons. f) Detection of the BDV-M using a polyclonal, monospecific antibody. BDV-M is present mainly in the cytoplasm of some neurons. g) Demonstration of BDV-GP-specific mRNA, mainly in the nuclei of cells; note the dot-like appearance (arrows) in some neurons. h) Detection of the BDV-GP using a monospecific, polyclonal antibody. BDV-GP is present only in the cytoplasm of a few neurons. i) Detection of BDV-X using a polyclonal antibody. BDV-X is present mainly in the cytoplasm of neurons and in the neuropil. j) Demonstration of BDV-L-specific mRNA in the cytoplasm (arrowheads) and nuclei as dot-like signal (arrows) in some neurons. k) Demonstration of BDV-genomic RNA in the nuclei of neurons as dot-like signal (arrows). Bar: 50 µm.

transcripts originating from the third transcriptional contain up to 3 introns and depending on whether intron 1 and/or intron 2 is spliced, the respective mature mRNA can code for BDV-M from the ORF III, BDV-GP from ORF IV or BDV-L from the ORF V located at the 3' end of the cRNA (Schneemann *et al.* 1995; Walker *et al.* 2000; Cubitt *et al.* 2001; de la Torre 2002; Tomonaga *et al.* 2002; Schneider 2005). In horses, all virus-specific proteins except for the viral polymerase (due to the lack of suitable antibodies) have been detected (**Figs 1b, d, f, h, i**). Recent evidence indicates that BDV-N, BDV-P together with BDV-L are part of the ribonucleoprotein complex (RNP) and are therefore, the functional BDV replication complex with BDV-X as the regulator (Wolff *et al.* 2000; Perez *et al.* 2003; Schneider *et al.* 2003; Schneider 2005; de la Torre 2006; Poenisch *et al.* 2008b). BDV-RNPs are infectious after transfection into susceptible cell lines (Cubitt and de la Torre 1994). As shown in a BDV minireplicon model, the activity of the BDV polymerase depends on the ratios of the viral proteins BDV-N, BDV-P and BDV-X. BDV-P is a central regulatory element of BDV replication (Schneider 2005). BDV replication and transcription in the nucleus of cells enables the virus to employ the cellular splicing machinery to process primary transcripts and to regulate expression of viral gene products (Cubitt *et al.* 1994b; Jehle *et al.* 2000; de la Torre 2002; Tomonaga *et al.* 2002), e.g. to control synthesis of BDV-M, BDV-GP and BDV-L. This is particularly important to avoid detection by the antiviral immune response of the host.

The matrix protein and the glycoprotein are major components of the viral envelope. The BDV-M is a nonglycosylated matrix protein similar to that in other viruses of the order *Mononegavirales* (Kraus *et al.* 2001). Recent evidence indicates that BDV-M also interacts with the BDV-RNP, and therefore is most likely to be involved in viral replication control similar to the matrixprotein of *Filo-* and *Rhabdoviridae* (Chase *et al.* 2006). BDV possesses a single surface glycoprotein, BDV-GP (Gonzales-Dunia *et al.* 1997; Schneider *et al.* 1997; Richt *et al.* 1998), which is post-translationally modified by N-glycosylation and cleavage into 2 fragments (GP-N, GP-C) by a subtilisin-like protease; this cleavage event is a prerequisite for the invasion of BDV into cells. The restricted and regulated expression of the BDV-glycoprotein represents an important step to achieve viral persistence in the infected host (Richt *et al.* 1998; de la Torre 2002; Werner-Keišs *et al.* 2008).

Control and regulation of BDV replication is furthermore achieved by a tightly regulated co-expression of the viral genome (vRNA) and its replicative intermediate, the viral antigenome (cRNA), as shown by high ratios of genomic: antigenomic RNA in infected rat brain tissues (Porombka *et al.* 2008a). Furthermore, BDV restricts its propagation efficacy by defined 3'- and 5'-terminal trimming of genomic and antigenomic RNA-molecules (Rosario *et al.* 2005, Schneider 2005; de la Torre 2006; Schneider *et al.* 2007). The 5'-trimming strategy eliminates triphosphate groups in order to circumvent a host antiviral IFN-response (Schneider *et al.* 2007; Habjan *et al.* 2008). Recently, interactions of BDV or defined BDV proteins with host cell proteins or signalling cascades have been described (e.g. neurotrophin signalling, Raf/ MEK/ERK-pathway, inhibition of nitric oxide synthase gene expression, activation of NFκB, induction of the antiviral IFN-response; Planz *et al.* 2001a; Bourtelee *et al.* 2005, Gonzales-Dunia *et al.* 2005; Unterstab *et al.* 2005, Peng *et al.* 2007). For example, BDV seems to manipulate the neurotrophin pathways to increase viral synthesis (reviewed by Gonzales-Dunia *et al.* 2005).

In summary, the control mechanisms and cellular interactions of BDV known so far nicely illustrate the complexity of the viral strategies to induce a persistent noncytopathic infection *in vitro* and *in vivo*. These strategies might also explain the low BDV replication rate and the difficulty to detect mature virus particles in infected material.

Epidemiology

Horses and sheep represent the main natural hosts but it is well-known that other equids, farm animals such as cattle or goats, rabbits, lynx, zoo animals (alpacas, sloth, vari monkeys, hippopotamus) or various companion animals can occasionally be infected with BDV and develop clinical BD (Heinig 1969; Danner 1982; Caplazi *et al.* 1994; Lundgren *et al.* 1995; Rott and Becht 1995; Dürrwald and Ludwig 1997; Jaunin *et al.* 1998; Weissenböck *et al.* 1998a; Degiorgis *et al.* 2000; Staeheli *et al.* 2000). This is in line with data of experimental BDV infections where the virus had been successfully transmitted to various animal species ranging from chickens to nonhuman primates (reviewed by Heinig 1969; Rott and Becht 1995).

Recently, a BDV-like agent has been detected in psittacine birds (Honkavouri *et al.* 2008; Kistler *et al.* 2008; Gancz *et al.* 2009; Rinder *et al.* 2009) in animals suffering from a disease named 'proventricular dilatation disease' (PDD). The question of whether BDV can infect humans and might be involved in certain human psychiatric diseases is still not resolved (Richt *et al.* 1997; Lieb and Staeheli 2001; Schwemmle 2001; Wolff *et al.* 2006; Dürrwald *et al.* 2007). At present, it is widely accepted that BDV-specific antibodies might occur in serum of psychiatric patients (Billich *et al.* 2002; Schwemmle and Billich 2004), whereas presence of BDV-specific nucleic acids in the blood of such patients is yet debated. The relatively high sequence similarities of so-called 'human' BDV sequences with BDV laboratory strains and field BDV isolates handled in the respective laboratories reporting human BDV sequences, indicates to some authors (Richt *et al.* 1997; Schwemmle *et al.* 1999; Dürrwald *et al.* 2007) that sample cross-contamination might be responsible for reports of 'human' BDV sequences.

Clinically manifest equine BD occurs in different endemic areas of southern Germany, Switzerland, Liechtenstein and Austria (Herzog *et al.* 1994; Weissenböck *et al.* 1998b; Caplazi *et al.* 1999), interestingly all German speaking areas in Central Europe. A more widespread distribution or disease pattern is supported by the presence of natural BD outside the above described endemic areas, the possible association of BDV infections with other clinical symptoms and the presence of virus-specific antibodies and/or nucleic acids in animals from different continents (reviewed by Ludwig and Bode 2000; Staeheli *et al.* 2000; Dürrwald *et al.* 2006; Richt *et al.* 2007). However, many of these results are still controversial and are questioned by the possibility of laboratory artifacts and cross-contaminations; therefore, additional epidemiological studies are urgently needed.

The incidence of BD in endemic areas is relatively low; fewer than 100 horses or sheep are identified per year, most often as single cases (Herzog *et al.* 1994; Staeheli *et al.* 2000; Dürrwald *et al.* 2006). Importantly, BDV infection of susceptible hosts does not always result in clinical disease.

Extensive studies of the BDV seroprevalence in horses are only available from Germany. A seasonal accumulation of cases in spring and early summer and secular dynamics are observed (reviewed by Dürrwald *et al.* 2006). These epidemiological data imply a natural reservoir for BDV. Often, BDV infections in horses (and sheep) appear to be inapparent (Herzog *et al.* 1994; Müller-Doblies *et al.* 2004; Richt *et al.* 2007) since the average seroprevalence of BDV-specific antibodies in clinically healthy German horses is approximately 11.5% (Herzog *et al.* 1994). In endemic regions, BDV seroprevalence is significantly higher (22.5%) and increases up to 50% in stables with BD (Grabner *et al.* 2002). Repeated outbreaks of BD within the same premises are also possible (Grabner *et al.* 2002; Richt *et al.* 2007). There is no satisfactory explanation for the discrepancy between the high BDV seroprevalence and the low BD-incidence but clearly indicates that not all infected hosts develop disease. Other parameters such as age, immune status and genetic background of the host, virulence of the virus and dose of infection seem to play a critical role.

There is evidence that open nerve endings in the nasal and pharyngeal mucosa are the route of entry in natural transmission. In rats, BDV can be shed in nasal and lacrimal secretions as well as urine and saliva (Morales *et al.* 1988; Sauder and Staeheli 2003). For natural transmission, a rodent reservoir has been postulated, possibly consisting of several species with a habitat restricted to the endemic areas in Central Europe. Recently, BDV antigen and BDV-specific RNA have been found in shrews in an endemic area in Switzerland (Hilbe *et al.* 2006); this finding supports the concept of a natural rodent reservoir of BDV. It seems that BDV-infected horses do not to play a major role in virus transmission (Richt *et al.* 1993; Schmidt *et al.* 1999; Staeheli *et al.* 2000; Dürrwald *et al.* 2006). For natural BDV infection, the infectious dose is unknown. In experimental intracerebral BDV infections of rats, transmission is possible with a minimum infectious dose of 10^4 ID_{50} of a rat-adapted virus.

Typically, natural BDV infection in horses leads to death 1–4 weeks after onset of signs in >80% of animals (Schmidt 1952; Grabner and Fischer 1991; Dürrwald and Ludwig 1997; Uhlig and Kinne 1998; Grabner *et al.* 2002; Richt *et al.* 2007). In cattle and sheep, death occurred after 1–6 weeks or 1–3 weeks in >50% of animals, respectively (Bode *et al.* 1994a; Richt *et al.* 1997).

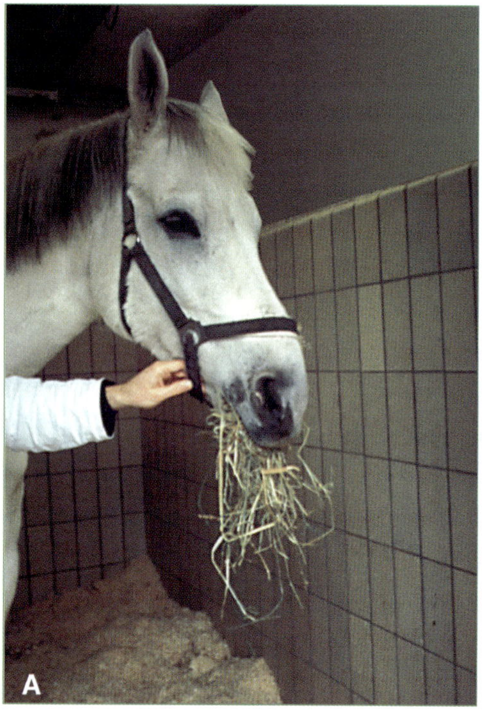

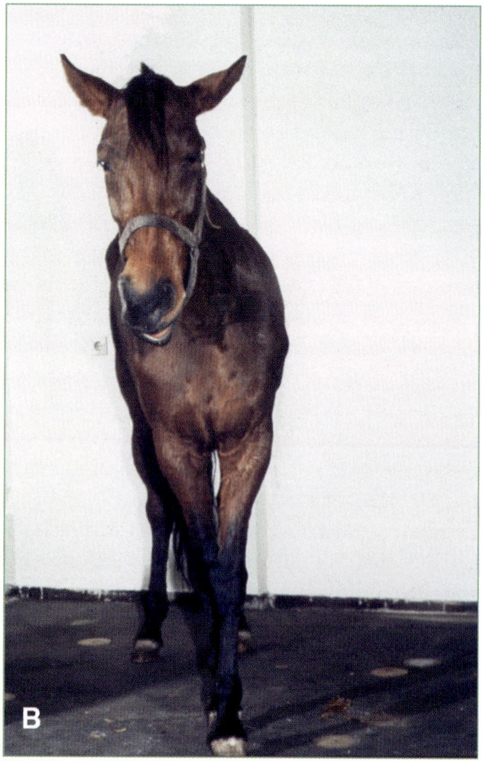

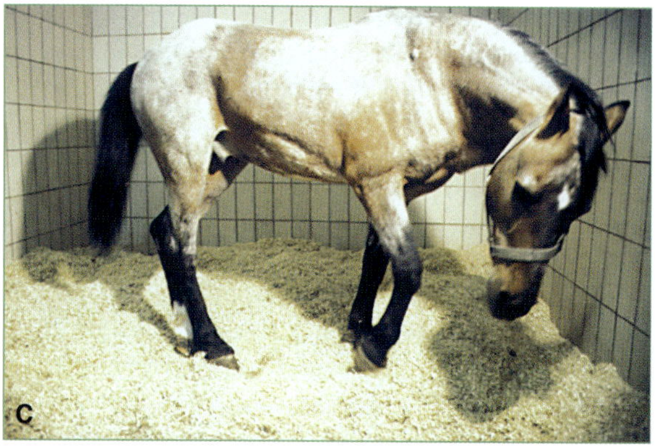

FIGURE 2: Clinical signs of equine Borna Disease (reproduced with permission from Richt et al. 2007). A) Early stage of BD. The BDV-infected horse displays somnolence and eating arrest with chewing movements ('Pfeifenrauchen' or 'pipe smoking'). B) More advanced stage of BD. The BDV-infected horse shows abnormal posture as sign of disturbed proprioception and paralysis of the facial nerve. C) Final stage of BD. The BDV-infected horse exhibits neurogenic torticollis and compulsive circular walking.

Clinical findings

In horses, natural BDV infection can run an inapparent, peracute, acute or subacute course. Rarely, clinical recovery or relapses are observed (reviewed by Grabner and Fischer 1991; Dürrwald and Ludwig 1997; Richt *et al.* 2007). The incubation period for natural BD might range from 2 to several months (Schmidt 1952). Recent experimental intracerebral infection of 3 ponies with various doses of BDV resulted in an incubation period of 15–26 days (Katz *et al.* 1998).

Clinical signs of BD in horses may vary depending on the area of the brain affected by inflammatory lesions and might change during the course of the disease (Zwick 1939; Ludwig *et al.* 1985; Grabner and Fischer 1991; Dürrwald and Ludwig 1997; Richt *et al.* 2007). Typically, simultaneous or consecutive changes in psyche, sensorium, sensibility, motility and in the autonomous nervous system are noted (**Fig 2**). In the early stages, alterations in behaviour and consciousness are characteristic and these signs progressively worsen. Slow motion eating, eating arrest with chewing movements (**Fig 2A**, called 'Pfeifenrauchen', 'pipe smoking'), recurrent fever, lethargy, somnolence, stupor, hyperexcitability, fearfulness and aggressiveness have been described in variable degrees. The latter could be due to inflammatory lesions in the limbic system, e.g. in the hippocampus (Grabner and Fischer 1991; Bilzer *et al.* 1996; Herden *et al.* 1999; Grabner *et al.* 2002). Hypokinesia, postural unawareness or hyporeflexia, head tilt and hypoaesthesia with disturbances in proprioceptive sensory functions are signs of more advanced stages of BD (**Fig 2B**). Horses may also exhibit ataxia and imbalance. In final stages of BD, a neurogenic torticollis, compulsive circular walking, slight head tremor followed by convulsions, head pressing due to a high cerebrospinal fluid (CSF) pressure and coma are characteristic (**Fig 2C**). Blindness can also occur. Furthermore, cranial nerve dysfunctions as a consequence of the inflammation could result in various signs, e.g. dysphagia, salivation, decreased tongue tension, trismus, facial nerve paresis, nystagmus, strabismus or miosis (Grabner *et al.* 2002; Richt *et al.* 2007). Diffuse mental or gait disturbances, recurrent colic, emaciation, chronic lameness and behavioural abnormalities such as 'head shaking' have also been described (Bode *et al.* 1994b; Berg *et al.* 1999; Ludwig and Bode 2000; Dieckhöfer 2008) but were not observed by others.

In sheep, clinical signs are comparable to the equine disease, but often disturbances in behaviour and movement predominate (Caplazi *et al.* 1999). In addition, mild or inapparent courses might occur. The role of the novel avian BDV for the pathogenesis of PDD in psittacine birds, a disease leading to gastrointestinal dysfunction, wasting and neurological signs, has to be investigated further (Honkavouri *et al.* 2008; Kistler *et al.* 2008). Recent experimental infections provide first evidence for an association of the avian BDV and PDD (Gancz *et al.* 2009)

Pathogenesis

The pathogenesis of BD was predominantly analysed using experimental studies in rodent models, e.g. Lewis rats and mice (Narayan *et al.* 1983a,b; Herzog *et al.* 1984; Deschl *et al.* 1990; Richt *et al.* 1994; Hallensleben *et al.* 1998; Hausmann *et al.* 1999, 2005; Herden *et al.* 2000; Freude *et al.* 2002; Pletnikov *et al.* 2002a,b). The availability of genetically altered animals in particular has opened many new avenues to study the neuropathogenesis of BD.

Generally, the virus enters the brain via retrograde intra-axonal transport. In the CNS, it replicates in brain cells, preferentially neurons of the limbic system. Neurons seem to offer the virus the optimal milieu for persistent replication, although astrocytes, oligodendrocytes or ependymal cells are also infected by BDV (Carbone *et al.* 1991; Richt *et al.* 1991; Rott and Becht 1995; Porombka *et al.* 2008b). Intra-axonal transport of BDV supports evasion from recognition by the hosts' immune system. Details on the mechanisms of how BDV infects neighbouring cells and spread within the brain are still missing. Recent data on the expression of the BDV glycoprotein as part of the viral envelope indicate that at least trans-neuronal transmission events probably occur via enveloped virus particles (Bajramovic *et al.* 2003; Werner-Keišs *et al.* 2008).

In adult rats, BDV is strictly neurotropic and persists only in the CNS. This strict neurotropism of BDV is also a feature of equine BDV infection. Viral antigen and infectious BDV is also regularly present in the retina in most of the affected horses (Herden *et al.* 1999). In rats, the occurrence of clinical signs correlates with the appearance of inflammatory lesions in the brain. The inflammatory reaction consists of mononuclear cells, and is located predominantly in the cerebral cortex, thalamus, hippocampus and amygdala (Narayan *et al.* 1983a,b, Deschl *et al.* 1990; Herden *et al.* 2000). Interestingly, late after infection, the inflammation decreases despite the presence of viral antigen and infectious virus (Narayan *et al.* 1983a,b; Deschl *et al.* 1990; Herden *et al.* 2000). This might be due to a switch of a Th1- to a Th2-immune response (Hatalski *et al.* 1998). A long lasting activation of astrocytes and microglial cells is found regularly. Microglial activation precedes astroglial reaction but seems to depend on persistent infection of neurons and activation of astrocytes (Herden *et al.* 2005; Ovanesov *et al.* 2008). There are a few reports of chronic BDV infections in the horse, which show few inflammatory CNS infiltrates and also a severe gliosis (Algermissen *et al.* 2007). In immunologically immature, neonatal rats infected with BDV, infectious virus is not only present in the CNS but nearly in every parenchymal organ (Herzog *et al.* 1984). These animals develop a tolerated, persistent BDV infection and shed virus in various secretions and excretions and, therefore, are virus carriers (Herzog *et al.* 1984; Morales *et al.* 1988). Such animals might play a role as a natural reservoir for virus transmission to other rodents or other BDV-susceptible animal species.

Clinical BD is caused by a virus-induced immunopathological reaction (reviewed by Stitz *et al.* 2002). Thus, infection of adult immunocompetent rats results in encephalitis and disease, whereas infection of newborn, athymic or immunosuppressed rats neither leads to encephalitis nor disease, despite persistently high levels of virus in the CNS (Herzog *et al.* 1984; Narayan *et al.* 1983a,b; Richt *et al.* 1989, 1994; Stitz *et al.* 1989, 1991). Persistently infected newborn rats, develop no overt clinical disease; however, 'luxury functions' of the CNS are affected and disturbances in cognitive, emotional functions and social behaviour are reported (Rubin *et al.* 1999; Sauder *et al.* 2000; Pletnikov *et al.* 2002a; Lancaster *et al.* 2007). In addition, learning deficits and elevated cytokine or chemokine expression even in the absence of inflammation and degeneration of post natally developing areas of the brain occur. For the induction of BD in immunosuppressed virus carriers, only adoptive transfer of immune cells derived from BDV-infected animals but not transfer of BDV-specific antibodies was effective (Narayan *et al.* 1983a,b), confirming a cell-mediated immunopathological basis of BD.

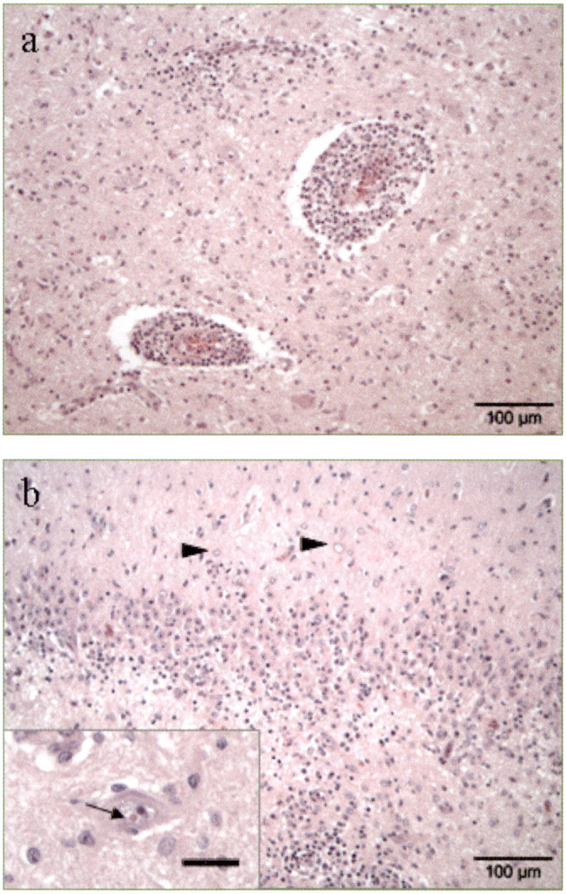

FIGURE 3: Histopathological lesions in a horse with typical BD a) Severe perivascular and moderate parenchymal mononuclear immune cell infiltrates in the CNS. b) Moderate to severe parenchymal immune cell infiltrates with astroglial activation (arrowhead) in a more advanced stage of BD. Insert: Intranuclear 'Joest-Degen' inclusion body (arrow). Bar: a, b: 100 µm, Insert: 25 µm.

Borna disease virus infections of neonatal mice results in a nonpurulent meningoencephalitis with a typical neurological disorder. In contrast, adult BDV-infected mice show neither obvious clinical signs nor significant inflammatory alterations in the brain (Rubin *et al.* 1993; Hallensleben *et al.* 1998). The reason for the age-dependent course of experimental BDV infection in rats and mice remains unclear but could be related to the time point of antigen priming in the periphery (Hausmann *et al.* 2005). The clinical signs of neonatal BDV-infected mice range from ataxia to paralysis of the hindlimbs, in combination with pre-sensitising events even epileptic seizures might occur (Hallensleben *et al.* 1998; Freude *et al.* 2002; Kramer *et al.* 2008). The incidence and severity of clinical disease vary considerably between different mouse strains despite comparable distribution of the virus. This was shown to be related to the MHC-haplotype and the recognition of the epitope TELEISSI within BDV-N (Schamel *et al.* 2001). Interestingly, overexpression of IL-12 or TNF results in clinical signs even in mice with less susceptible genetic background (Freude *et al.* 2002; Hofer *et al.* 2004; Kramer *et al.* 2004, 2008).

In BD, T-cells play a crucial role for the immunopathogenesis of BD (reviewed by Stitz *et al.* 2002); the disease most likely represents a delayed type hypersensitivity reaction. The role of virus-specific T-cells was demonstrated by passive transfer of *in vitro* established BDV-specific CD4+ T-cells into immunosuppressed virus carriers. The recipients consistently developed clinical signs of acute BD (Richt *et al.* 1989, 1994). There is evidence in rats and in mice that CD8+ T-cells are also involved in pathological alterations (Hausmann *et al.* 1999; Planz and Stitz 1999; Planz *et al.* 2001b; Schamel *et al.* 2001). The major viral antigen for BDV-specific CD8+ and CD4+ T-cells is the BDV-N (Richt *et al.* 1989, 1994; Hausmann *et al.* 1999; Planz and Stitz 1999; Planz *et al.* 2001b; Schamel *et al.* 2001). Recently, it was shown that virus-specific CD8+ T-cells can recognise viral antigen expressed as transgene on resident brain cells, indicating a role of neurons and astrocytes for virus recognition (Baur *et al.* 2008). Nevertheless, there is no lysis of BDV-infected neurons in the CNS of mice or rats indicating that cytokines and other inflammatory mediators are critical for disease induction. Neuronal dysfunctions also result from disruption of synaptic plasticity (Gonzales-Dunia *et al.* 2005). The composition of infiltrating immune cells and the increased expressions of MHC class I- and class II-antigens in naturally infected horse brains are similar to rats infected with BDV (Bilzer *et al.* 1995; Caplazi and Ehrensperger 1998; Herden *et al.* 1999); therefore, a similar pathogenesis in naturally infected equids and rats is assumed.

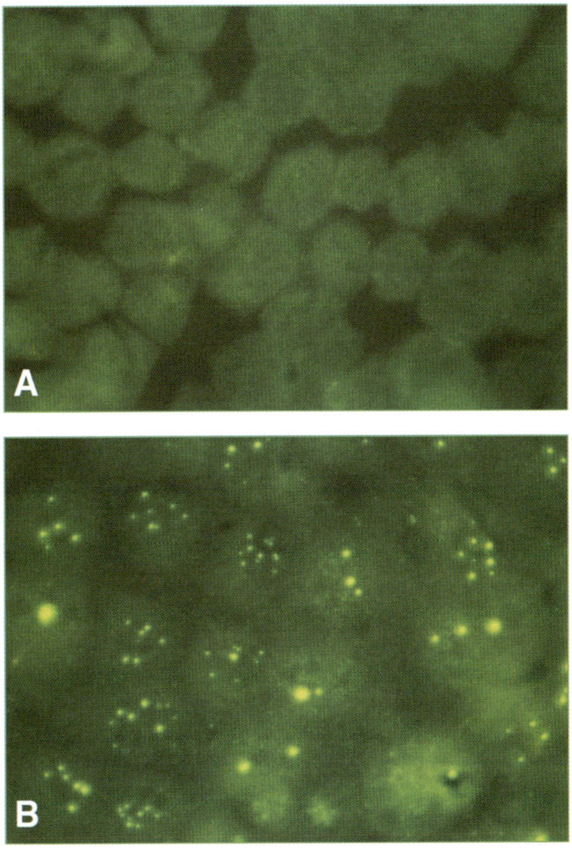

FIGURE 4: Indirect immunofluorescence assay for the detection of BDV-specific antibodies using Madin-Darby Canine Kidney (MDCK) cells (reproduced with permission from Richt et al. 2007). A) BDV-positive serum incubated with mock-infected MDCK cells. b) BDV-positive serum incubated with persistently BDV-infected MDCK cells. Note the typical granular reaction in the nuclei of cells.

Gross and histopathological findings

Gross findings in horses consist of leptomeningeal hyperaemia, brain oedema or *hydrocephalus internus* in later disease stages (Zwick *et al.* 1927; Zwick 1939; Heinig 1969; Katz *et al.* 1998). In all mammalian species, histopathological changes associated with BDV infection are quite comparable. Lesions are mainly restricted to the gray matter areas of the CNS, spinal cord and retina. Typically, a severe nonpurulent poliomeningoencephalomyelitis with massive perivascular and parenchymal infiltrations, is present (**Fig 3**), predominantly in the olfactory bulb, basal cortex, caudate nucleus, thalamus, hippocampus and periventricular areas of the medulla oblongata. The inflammatory infiltrate consists of macrophages, T-cells (CD4+ and CD8+) and, in later stages of infection, plasma cells (Deschl *et al.* 1990; Bilzer *et al.* 1996; Caplazi and Ehrensperger 1998; Herden et al. 1999). In horses, degeneration of neurons and neuronophagia might occur accompanied by severe astrogliosis. Intranuclear eosinophilic, so called 'Joest-Degen' inclusion bodies might be present in neurons (**Fig 3b**); they are regarded as pathognomonic for BD. Severe alterations in the retina have not been observed in horses yet, but degeneration of retinal neurons resulting in blindness has recently been described (Bilzer *et al.* 1996; Herden *et al.* 1999; Dietzel *et al.* 2007). In cases without alterations of the retina, blindness might result from severe inflammation in the optic region of the thalamus. BDV-infected rats and rabbits typically develop a nonpurulent chorioretinitis with degeneration of rods and cones leading to blindness (Krey *et al.* 1979; Narayan *et al.* 1983a,b).

Diagnosis

Ante mortem diagnosis

A clinical diagnosis of BD must remain tentative until verified using confirmatory tests. Neurological signs might exhibit a complex pattern depending on the brain areas affected and CNS-infections with a multitude of pathogens may result in similar signs. Differential diagnosis of BD includes infections with equine herpesviruses, rabies virus, alphaviruses or flaviviruses (equine encephalitides, looping ill, West Nile virus). Various bacterial diseases, e.g. botulism, bacterial meningitis, and parasitic diseases, e.g verminous myeloencephaliti and equine protozoal myeloencephalitis might also cause similar clinical signs.

Because of the lack of specificity of clinical signs, equine BD must be confirmed by the demonstration of BDV-specific antibodies in the serum and/or CSF (Grabner and Fischer 1991; Grabner *et al.* 2002) and/or BDV, BDV-specific antigens or RNA in the CNS post mortem. BDV-specific antibody tests can be performed using western blot (WB) analysis (Herzog *et al.* 1994, 2008), enzyme-linked immunosorbent assay (ELISA; Bode *et al.* 2001) or an indirect immunofluorescence assay (IFA; **Fig 4**; Herzog and Rott 1980; Grabner *et al.* 2002; Herzog *et al.* 2008). The IFA using BDV-infected and control cells is acknowledged to be the most reliable method for the detection of BDV-specific antibodies with a high sensitivity and specificity (Herzog *et al.* 2008).

Serum antibody titres range between 1:5 to 1:1280, and between 1:2 and 1:1280 in the CSF, but titres do not correlate with clinical signs or the outcome of infection (Herzog *et al.* 1994; Grabner *et al.* 2002). In acute BD, CSF pleocytosis and BDV-specific antibodies are regularly found. BDV-specific antibodies can be lacking in peracute BD, at the beginning of acute BD or after pretreatment with corticosteroids (Grabner *et al.* 2002). In clinically healthy horses, BDV-specific antibodies may be found in the serum, but not in the CSF, indicating inapparent or cleared infections (Herzog *et al.* 1994; Grabner *et al.* 2002).

The detection of BDV-specific RNA in peripheral blood mononuclear cells, the demonstration of BDV antigen in plasma of leucocytes or circulating immune complexes have been proposed as alternative means of an *ante mortem* diagnosis of BD (Nakamura *et al.* 1995; Bode *et al.* 2001; Dieckhöfer 2008). However, the presence of BDV RNA or BDV antigens in peripheral blood could not be confirmed by others (Grabner *et al.* 2002; Wolff *et al.* 2006; Herzog *et al.* 2008).

In summary, *ante mortem* diagnosis of BD can be regarded as positive, when animals show neurological signs and antibodies are detectable in serum and/or CSF accompanied by a CSF pleocytosis. Alternatively, seroconversion can be documented by a significant increase of antibody titres at different collection times during the course of the disease. If other methods than detection of BDV-specific antibodies by IFA are used for the ante mortem diagnosis of BD, a *post mortem* investigation is indispensable to exclude false positive *intra vitam* results (Herzog *et al.* 2008).

Post mortem diagnosis

The *post mortem* diagnosis of natural BD requires histopathology, detection of viral proteins and RNA and, if possible, infectious virus. Histopathologically, as described above, a nonpurulent meningoencephalitis is present (**Fig 3**). Demonstration of viral proteins by various monoclonal or polyclonal antibodies is possible by immunohistochemistry (IHC; **Figs 1b**, **d**, **f**, **h**, **i**) or WB analysis (Bilzer *et al.* 1996; Herden *et al.* 1999; Grabner *et al.* 2002). Comparative studies indicate that all 3 methods (histopathology, IHC, WB) as well as nested RT-PCR give identical diagnostic results in acute cases of BD (Herden *et al.* 1999; Grabner *et al.* 2002). The isolation of infectious BDV and the demonstration of virus-specific RNA by *in situ* hybridisation (**Figs 1a**, **c**, **e**, **h**, **j**, **k**) can support a *post mortem* diagnosis. These latter methods are less suitable when the material is in an advanced state of decomposition. In this case, IHC and WB are preferred (Herden *et al.* 1999).

Concluding remarks

In the last 20 years, substantial progress in BD research has been achieved regarding the molecular characterisation of the causative agent, the Borna disease virus, the underlying immunopathogenesis, the mechanism of viral persistence and the natural distribution of BD. However, some of the findings, especially in regards to the worldwide epidemiology of BD in various warm-blooded animals and man, are still controversial. Therefore, further investigations will improve our understanding of the complexity of the disease mechanisms, BDV-associated disorders and the epidemiology of Borna disease in animals and man.

Acknowledgement

The authors are grateful to Sibylle Herzog for critical reading the manuscript, to Wolfgang Baumgärtner,

Wolfgang Garten and Arthur Grabner for their generous support and to Dorothee Algermissen for help with the figures.

References

Ackermann, A., Kugel, D., Schneider, U. and Staeheli, P. (2007a) Enhanced polymerase activity confers replication competence of Borna disease virus in mice. *J. Gen. Virol.* **88**, 3130-3132.

Ackermann, A., Staeheli, P. and Schneider, U. (2007b) Adaptation of borna disease virus to new host species attributed to altered regulation of viral polymerase activity. *J. Virol.* **81**, 7933-7940.

Algermissen, D., Porombka, D., Schaudien, D., Kramer, K., Baumgärtner, W. and Herden, C. (2007) Expression profile of Borna disease virus specific proteins and RNAs in naturally infected horses. In: *25th Meeting of the European Society of Veterinary Pathologists.*

Baur, K., Rauer, M., Richter, K., Pagenstecher, A., Götz, J., Hausmann, J. and Staeheli, P. (2008) Antiviral CD8 T cells recognize Borna disease virus antigen transgenically expressed in either neurons or astrocytes. *J. Virol.* **82**, 3099-3108.

Bajramovic, J.J., Munter, S., Syan, S., Nehrbass, U., Brahic, M. and Gonzalez-Dunia, D. (2003) Borna disease virus glycoprotein is required for viral dissemination in neurons. *J. Virol.* **77**, 12222-12231.

Berg, A.L., Dörries, R. and Berg, M. (1999) Borna disease virus infection in racing horses with behavioural and movement disorders. *Arch. Virol.* **144**, 547-559.

Billich, C., Sauder, C., Frank, R., Herzog, S., Bechter, K., Takahashi, K., Peters, H., Staeheli, P. and Schwemmle, M. (2002) High-avidity human serum antibodies recognizing linear epitopes of Borna disease virus proteins. *Biol. Psychiatry* **51**, 979-987.

Bilzer, T., Planz, O., Lipkin, W.I. and Stitz, L. (1995) Presence of CD4+ and CD8+ T cells and expression of MHC class I and MHC class II antigen in horses with Borna disease virus-induced encephalitis. *Brain Pathol.* **5**, 223-230.

Bilzer, T., Grabner, A. and Stitz, L. (1996) Immunpathologie der Borna-Krankheit beim Pferd: klinische, virologische und neuropathologische Befunde. *Tierärztl. Prax.* **24**, 567-576.

Binz, T., Lebelt, J., Niemann, H. and Hagenau, K. (1994) Sequence analysis of the p24 gene of Borna disease virus in naturally infected horse, donkey and sheep. *Virus Res.* **34**, 281-289.

Bode, L., Dürrwald, R. and Ludwig, H. (1994a) Borna virus infection in cattle associated with fatal neurological disease. *Vet. Rec.* **135**, 283-284.

Bode, L., Dürrwald R., Koeppel P. and Ludwig, H. (1994b) Neue Aspekte der equinen Borna-Virus-Infektion mit und ohne Krankheit. *Prakt. Tierarzt* **75**, 1065-1068.

Bode, L., Reckwald, P., Severus, W.E., Stoyloff, R., Ferszt, R., Dietrich, D.E. and Ludwig, H. (2001) Borna disease virus-specific circulating immune complexes, antigenemia, and free antibodies- the key marker triplet determining infection and prevailing in severe mood disorders. *Mol. Psychiatry* **6**, 481-491.

Bourteele, S., Österle, K., Pleschka, S., Unterstab, G., Ehrhardt, C., Wolff, T., Ludwig, S. and Planz, O. (2005) Constitutive activation of the transcription factor NF-kappaB results in impaired borna disease virus replication. *J. Virol.* **79**, 6043-6051.

Briese, T., Schneemann, A., Lewis, A.J., Park, Y.S., Kim, S., Ludwig, H. and Lipkin, W.I. (1994) Genomic organization of Borna disease virus. *Proc. Natl. Acad. Sci. USA* **91**, 4362-4366.

Caplazi, P. and Ehrensperger, F. (1998) Spontaneous Borna disease in sheep and horses: immunophenotyping of inflammatory cells and detection of MHC-I and MHC-II antigen expression in Borna encephalitis lesions. *Vet. Immunol. Immunopathol.* **61**, 203-220.

Caplazi, P., Waldvogel, A., Stitz, L., Braun, U. and Ehrensperger, F. (1994) Borna disease in naturally infected cattle. *J. comp. Pathol.* **111**, 65-72.

Caplazi, P., Melzer, K., Goetzmann, R., Rohner-Cotti, A., Bracher, V., Zlinszky, K. and Ehrensperger, F. (1999) Die Bornasche Krankheit in der Schweiz und im Fürstentum Liechtenstein. *Schweiz. Arch. Tierheilk.* **141**, 521-527.

Carbone, K.M., Moench, T.R. and Lipkin, W.I. (1991) Borna disease virus replicates in astrocytes, Schwann-cells and ependymal cells in persistently infected rats: localization of viral mRNA by *in situ* hybridisation. *J. Neuropathol. Exp. Neurol.* **50**, 205-214.

Chase, G., Mayer, D., Hildebrand, A., Frank, R., Hayashi, Y., Tomonaga, K. and Schwemmle, M. (2006) Borna disease virus matrix protein is an integral component of the viral ribonucleoprotein complex that does not interfere with polymerase activity. *J. Virol.* **81**, 743-749.

Cubitt, B. and de la Torre, J.C. (1994) Borna disease virus (BDV), a nonsegmented RNA virus, replicates in the nuclei of infected cells where infectious BDV ribonucleoproteins are present. *J. Virol.* **68**, 1371-1381.

Cubitt, B., Ly, C. and de la Torre, J.C. (2001) Identification and characterization of a new intron in Borna disease virus. *J. Gen. Virol.* **82**, 641-646.

Cubitt, B., Oldstone, C. and de la Torre, J.C. (1994a) Sequence and genome organization of Borna disease virus. *J. Virol.* **68**, 1382-1396.

Cubitt, B., Oldstone, C., Valcarcel, J. and de la Torre, J.C. (1994b) RNA splicing contributes to the generation of mature mRNA of Borna disease virus, a non-segmented negative -strand RNA virus. *Virus Res.* **34**, 69-79.

Danner, K. (1982) *Borna-Virus und Borna-Infekionen*, Enke Copythek, Stuttgart.

Degiorgis, M.P., Berg, A.L., Hard, A.F., Segerstad, C., Morner, T., Johansson, M. and Berg, M. (2000) Borna disease in a free-ranging lynx (*Lynx lynx*). *J. clin. Microbiol.* **38**, 3087-3091.

De la Torre, J.C. (2002) Molecular biology of Borna disease virus and persistence. *Front Biosci.* **7**, d569-579.

De la Torre, J.C. (2006) Reverse-genetic approaches to the study of Borna disease. *Nature Rev. Microbiol.* **4**, 777-783.

Deschl, U., Stitz, L., Herzog, S., Frese, K. and Rott R. (1990) Determination of immune cells and expression of major histocompability complex class II antigen in encephalitic lesions of experimental Borna disease. *Acta Neuropathol.* **81**, 41-50.

Dieckhöfer, R. (2008) Infections in horses: Diagnosis and therapy. *APMIS Suppl.* **124**, 40-43.

Dietzel, J., Kuhrt, H., Stahl, T., Kacza, J., Seeger, J., Weber, M., Uhlig, A., Reichenbach, A., Grosche, A. and Pannicke, T. (2007) Morphometric analysis of the retina from horses infected with the Borna disease virus. *Vet. Pathol.* **44**, 57-63.

Dürrwald, R. and Ludwig, H. (1997) Borna disease virus (BDV), a (zoonotic?) worldwide pathogen: a review of the history of the disease and the virus infection with comprehensive bibliography. *J. vet. Med. B* **44**, 147-184.

Dürrwald, R., Kolodziejek, J., Muluneh, A., Herzog, S. and Nowotny, N. (2006) Epidemiological pattern of classical Borna disease and regional genetic clustering of Borna disease virus point towards the existence of to-date unknown endemic reservoir host populations. *Microbes Infect.* **8**, 917-929.

Dürrwald, R., Kolodziejek, J., Herzog, S. and Nowotny, N. (2007) Meta-analysis of putative human bornavirus sequences fails to provide evidence implicating Borna disease virus in mental illness. *Rev. Med. Virol.* **17**, 181-203.

Freude, S., Hausmann, J., Hofer, M., Pham-Mitchell, N., Campbell, I.L., Staeheli, P. and Pagenstecher, A. (2002) Borna disease virus accelerates inflammation and disease associated with transgenic expression of interleukin-12 in the central nervous system. *J. Virol.* **76**, 12223-12232.

Gonzalez-Dunia, D., Cubitt, B., Grasser, F.A. and de la Torre, J.C. (1997) Characterization of Borna disease virus p56 protein, a surface glycoprotein involved in virus entry. *J. Virol.* **71**, 3208-3218.

Gonzales-Dunia, D., Volmer, R., Mayer, D. and Schwemmle, M. (2005) Borna disease virus interference with neuronal plasticity. *Virus Res.* **111**, 224-234.

Grabner, A. and Fischer, A. (1991) Symptomatologie und Diagnostik der Borna-Enzephalitis des Pferdes: Eine Fallanalyse der letzten 13 Jahre. *Tierärztl. Prax.* **19**, 68-73.

Grabner, A., Herzog, S., Lange-Herbst, H. and Frese, K. (2002) Die intra-vitam-Diagnose der Bornaschen Krankheit bei Equiden. *Pferdeheilkunde* **18**, 579-586.

Habjan, M., Andersson, I., Klingström, J., Schümann, M., Martin A., Zimmermann, P., Wagner, V., Pichlmair, A., Schneider, U., Mühlberger, E., Mirazimi, A. and Weber, F. (2008) Processing of genome 5' termini as a strategy of negative-strand RNA viruses to avoid RIG-I-dependent interferon induction. *Plos One*, **3**, e2032. doi:10.1371/journal.pone.0002032.

Hallensleben, W., Schwemmle, M., Hausmann, J., Stitz, L., Volk, B., Pagenstecher, A. and Staeheli, P. (1998) Borna disease virus–induced neurological disorder in mice: infection of neonates results in immunopathology. *J. Virol.* **72**, 4379-4386.

Hatalski, C.G., Hickey, W.F. and Lipkin, W.I. (1998) Evolution of the immune response in the central nervous system following infection with Borna disease virus. *J. Neuroimmunol.* **90**, 137-142.

Hausmann, J., Schamel, K. and Staeheli, P. (2001) CD8(+) T lymphocytes mediate Borna disease virus-induced immunopathology independently of perforin. *J. Virol.* **75**, 10460-10466.

Hausmann, J., Pagenstecher, A., Baur, K., Richter, K., Rziha, H.J. and Staeheli, P. (2005) CD8 T cells require gamma interferon to clear borna disease virus from the brain and prevent immune system-mediated neuronal damage. *J. Virol.* **79**, 13509-13518.

Hausmann, J., Hallensleben, W., De la Torre, J.C., Pagenstecher, A., Zimmermann, C., Pircher, H. and Staeheli, P. (1999) T cell ignorance in mice to Borna disease virus can be overcome by peripheral expression of the viral nucleoprotein. *Proc. Natl. Acad. Sci. USA* **96**, 9769-9774.

Heinig, A. (1969) Die Bornasche Krankheit der Pferde und Schafe. In: *Handbuch der Virusinfektionen bei Tieren*, Ed: Röhrer, H., Fischer, Jena. p 83-148.

Herden, C., Herzog, S., Wehner, T., Zink, C., Richt, J.A. and Frese, K. (1999) Comparison of different methods of diagnosing Borna disease in horses *post mortem*. In: *Equine Infectious Diseases VIII*. Eds: U. Wernery, J. Wade, J.A. Mumford and O.R. Kaaden, R&W Publications, Newmarket. pp 286-290.

Herden, C., Herzog, S., Richt, J.A., Nesseler A., Christ, M., Failing, K. and Frese, K. (2000) Distribution of Borna disease virus in the brain of rats infected with an obesity-inducing virus strain. *Brain Pathol* **10**, 39-48.

Herden, C., Schluesener, H.J. and Richt, J.A. (2005) Expression of allograft inflammatory factor-1 and haeme oxygenase-1 in brains of rats infected with the neurotropic Borna disease virus. *Neuropathol. Appl. Neurobiol.* **31**, 512-521.

Herzog, S. and Rott, R. (1980) Replication of Borna disease virus in cell cultures. *Med. Microbiol. Immunol.* **168**, 153-158.

Herzog, S., Frese, K., Richt, J.A. and Rott, R. (1994) Ein Beitrag zur Epizootiologie der Bornaschen Krankheit beim Pferd. *Wien. Tierärztl. Monatsschr.* **81**, 374-379.

Herzog, S., Kompter, C., Frese, K. and Rott, R. (1984) Replication of Borna disease virus in rats: age-dependent differences in tissue distribution. *Med. Microbiol. Immunol.* **173**, 171-177.

Herzog, S., Pfeuffer, I., Haberzettl, K., Feldmann, H., Frese, K., Bechter, K. and Richt, J.A. (1997) Molecular characterization of Borna disease virus from naturally infected animals and possible links to human disorders. *Arch. Virol. Suppl.* **13**, 183-190.

Herzog, S., Herden, C., Frese, K., Lange-Herbst, H. and Grabner, A. (2008) Borna disease of horses: contradictory results between antemortem and postmortem investigations. *Pferdeheilkunde* **24**, 766-774.

Hilbe, M., Herrsche, R., Kolodziejek, J., Nowotny, N., Zlinszky, K. and Ehrensperger, F. (2006) Shrews as reservoir hosts of borna disease virus. *Emerg. Infect. Dis.* **12**, 675-677.

Hofer, M., Hausmann, J., Staeheli, P. and Pagenstecher, A. (2004) Cerebral expression of interleukin-12 induces neurological disease via differential pathways and recruits antigen-specific T cells in virus-infected mice. *Am. J. Pathol.* **165**, 949-958.

Honkavouri, K. S., Shivaprasad, H.L., Williams, B.L., Quan, P., Hornig, M., Street, C., Palacious, G., Huchison, S.K., Franca, M., Egholm, M., Briese, T. and Lipkin, W. (2008) Novel Borna disease virus in psittacine birds with proventricular dilatation disease. *Emerg. Inf. Dis.* **14**, 1883-1886.

Jaunin, V.B., Fatzer, R., Melzer, K., Gonin Jmaa, D., Caplazi, P. and Ehrensperger, F. (1998) A case of Borna disease in a cat. *Eur. J. Vet. Path.* **4**, 33-35.

Jehle, C., Lipkin, W.I., Staeheli, P., Marion, R.M. and Schwemmle, M. (2000) Authentic Borna disease virus transcripts are spliced less efficiently than cDNA-derived viral RNAs. *J. Gen. Virol.* **81**, 1947-1954.

Katz, J.B., Alstad, D., Jenny, A.L., Carbone, K.M., Rubin, S.A. and Waltrip II, R.W. (1998) Clinical, serologic, and histopathologic characterization of experimental Borna disease in ponies. *J. vet. diagn. Invest.* **10**, 338-343.

Kistler, A.L., Gancz, A., Clubb, S., Skewes-Cox, P., Fischer, K., Sorber, K., Chiu, C.Y., Lublin, A., Mechani, S., Farnoushi, Y.,

Greninger, A., Wen, C.C., Karlene, S.B., Ganem, D. and DeRisi, J.L. (2008) Recovery of divergent avian bornaviruses from cases of proventricular dilatation disease: identification of a candidate etiologic agent. *Virology J.* **5**, 88, doi:10.1186/1743-422X-5-88.

Kohno, T., Goto, T., Takasaki, T., Morita, C., Nakaya, T., Ikuta, K., Kurane, I., Sano, K. and Nakai, M. (1999) Fine structure and morphogenesis of Borna disease virus. *J. Virol.* **73**, 760-766.

Kolodziejek, J., Dürrwald, R., Herzog, S., Ehrensperger, F., Lussy, H., and Nowotny N. (2005) Genetic clustering of Borna disease virus natural animal isolates, laboratory and vaccine strains strongly reflects their regional geographical origin. *J. Gen. Virol.* **86**, 385-398.

Kramer, K., Schaudien, S., Eisel, U., Baumgärtner, W. and Herden, C. (2008) Epileptic seizures in TNF-transgenic mice infected with the neurotropic Borna disease virus are associated with altered prodynorphin mRNA levels in the brain. *Acta Neuropathol. Berl.* **116**, 349.

Kramer, K., Schaudien, D., Marchetti, L., Eisel, U., Richt, J.A., Baumgärtner, W. and Herden, C. (2004) Effect of TNFα-overexpression in the CNS of mice infected with the neurotropic Borna disease virus. *Acta Neuropathol. Berl.* **108**, 364.

Kraus, I., Eickmann, M., Kiermayer, S., Scheffczik, H., Fluess, M., Richt, J.A. and Garten, W. (2001) Open reading frame III of Borna disease virus encodes a nonglycosylated matrix protein. *J. Virol.* **75**, 12098-12104.

Krey, H.F., Ludwig, H. and Boschek, C.B. (1979) Multifocal retinopathy in Borna disease virus infected rabbits. *Am. J. Ophthalmol.* **87**, 157-164.

Lancaster, K., Dietz, D.M., Moran, T.H. and Pletnikov, M.V. (2007) Abnormal social behaviors in young and adult rats neonatally infected with Borna disease virus. *Behav. Brain Res.* **176**, 141-148.

Lieb, K. and Staeheli, P. (2001) Borna disease virus – does it infect humans and cause psychiatric disorders? *J. clin. Virol.* **21**, 119-127.

Lipkin, W.I., Travis, G.H., Carbone, K.M. and Wilson, M.C. (1990) Isolation and characterization of Borna disease agent cDNA clones. *Proc. Natl. Acad. Sci. USA* **87**, 4184-4188.

Ludwig, H. and Bode, L. (2000) Borna disease virus: new aspects on infection, disease, diagnosis and epidemiology. *Rev. sci. tech. Off. int. Epiz.* **19**, 259-288.

Ludwig, H., Kraft ,W., Kao, M., Gosztonyi, G., Dahme, F. and Krey, H. (1985) Borna-Virus-Infektion (Borna-Krankheit) bei natürlich und experimentell infizierten Tieren: Ihre Bedeutung für Forschung und Praxis. *Tierärztl. Praxis* **13**, 421-453.

Lundgren, A.L., Zimmermann, W., Bode, L., Czech, G., Gosztonyi, G., Lindberg, R. and Ludwig, H. (1995) Staggering disease in cats: isolation and characterization of the feline Borna disease virus. *J. Gen. Virol.* **76**, 2215-2222.

Morales, J.A., Herzog, S., Kompter, C., Frese, K. and Rott, R. (1988) Axonal transport of Borna disease virus along olfactory pathways in spontaneously and experimentally infected rats. *Med. Microbiol. Immunol.* **177**, 51-68.

Müller-Doblies, D., Baumann, S., Grob, P., Hulsmeier, A., Müller-Doblies, U., Brunker, P., Ehrensperger, F., Staeheli, P., Ackermann, M. and Suter, M. (2004) The humoral and cellular immune response of sheep against Borna disease virus in endemic and non-endemic areas. *Schw. Arch. Tierheilk.* **146**, 159-172.

Nakamura, Y., Kishi, M., Nakaya, T., Asahi, S., Tanak, H., Sentsui, H., Ikeda, K. and Ikuta, K. (1995) Demonstration of Borna disease virus RNA in peripheral blood mononuclear cells from healthy horses in Japan: *Vaccine* **13**, 1076-1079.

Narayan, O., Herzog, S., Frese, K., Scheefers, R. and Rott, R. (1983a) Behavioural disease in rats caused by an immunopathological response to persistent Borna virus in the brain. *Science* **220**, 1401-1403.

Narayan, O., Herzog, S., Frese, K., Scheefers, R. and Rott, R. (1983b) Pathogenesis of Borna disease in rats: immunemediated viral opthalmoencephalopathy causing blindness and behavioural abnormalities. *J. Infect. Dis.* **148**, 305-315.

Nowotny, N., Kolodziejek, J., Jehle, C.O., Suchy, A., Staeheli, P. and Schwemmle, M. (2000) Isolation and characterization of a new subtype of Borna disease virus. *J. Virol.* **74**, 5655-5658.

Ovanesov, M.V., Ayhan, Y., Wolbert, C., Moldovan, K., Sauder, C. and Pletnikov, M.V. (2008) Astrocytes play a key role in activation of microglia by persistent Borna disease virus infection. *J. Neuroinflamm.* **5**, 50.

Peng, G., Zhang, F., Zhang, Q., Wu, K. and Wu, J. (2007) Borna disease virus P protein inhibits nitric oxide synthase gene expression in astrocytes. *Virol.* **366**, 446-452.

Perez, M., Sanchez, A., Cubitt, B., Rosario, D. and de la Torre, J.C. (2003) A reverse genetics system for Borna disease virus. *J. Gen. Virol.* **84**, 3099-3104.

Planz, O. and Stitz, L. (1999) Borna disease virus nucleoprotein (p40) is a major target for CD8(+)-T-cell-mediated immune response. *J. Virol.* **73**, 1715-1728.

Planz, O., Pleschka, S. and Ludwig, S. (2001a) MEK-specific inhibitor U0126 blocks spread of Borna disease virus in cultured cells. *J. Virol.* **75**, 4871-4877.

Planz, O., Dumrese, T., Hulpusch, S., Schirle, M., Stevanovic, S. and Stitz, L. (2001b) A naturally processed rat major histocompatibility complex class I-associated viral peptide as target structure of borna disease virus-specific CD8+ T cells. *J. Biol. Chem.* **276**, 13689-13694.

Pleschka, S., Staeheli, P., Kolodziejek, J., Richt, J.A., Nowotny, N. and Schwemmle, M. (2001) Conservation of coding potential and terminal sequences in four different isolates of Borna disease virus. *J. Gen. Virol.* **82**, 2681-2690.

Pletnikov, M.V., Rubin, S.A., Vogel, M.W., Moran, T.H. and Carbone, K.M. (2002a) Effects of genetic background on neonatal Borna disease virus infection-induced neurodevelopmental damage. I. Brain pathology and behavioural deficits. *Brain Res.* **944**, 97-107.

Pletnikov, M.V., Rubin, S.A., Vogel, M.W., Moran, T.H. and Carbone, K.M. (2002b) Effects of genetic background on neonatal Borna disease virus infection-induced neurodevelopmental damage. II. Neurochemical alterations and responses to pharmacological treatments. *Brain Res.* **944**, 108-23.

Poenisch, M., Staeheli, P. and Schneider, U. (2008a) Viral accessory protein X stimulates the assembly of functional Borna disease virus polymerase complex. *J. Gen. Virol.* **89**, 1442-1445.

Poenisch, M., Wille, S., Staeheli, P. and Schneider, U. (2008b) Polymerase read through at the first transcription termination site contributes to regulation of Borna disease virus gene expression. *J. Virol.* **82**, 9537-9545.

Porombka, D., Baumgärtner, W., Eickmann, M. and Herden, C.

(2008a) Implications for a regulated replication of Borna disease virus in brains of experimentally infected Lewis rats. *Virus Genes* **36**, 415-420.

Porombka, D., Baumgärtner, W. and Herden, C. (2008b): A rapid method for gene expression analysis of Borna disease virus in neurons and astrocytes using laser microdissection and real-time RT-PCR. *J. Virol. Meth.* **148**, 58-65.

Pringle, C.R. (1996) Virus Taxonomy 1996 – A bulletin from the Xth International Congress of Virology in Jerusalem. *Arch. Virol.* **141**, 2251-2256.

Richt, J.A. and Rott, R. (2001) Borna disease virus: a mystery as emerging zoonotic pathogen. *Vet. J.* **161**, 24-40.

Richt, J.A., Stitz, L., Wekerle, H. and Rott, R. (1989) Borna disease, a progressive meningoencephalitis as a model for CD4+ T-cell mediated immunopathology in the brain. *J. expt. Med.* **170**, 1045-1050.

Richt, J.A., Herzog, S., Haberzettl K. and Rott, R. (1993) Demonstration of Borna disease virus–specific RNA in secretions of naturally infected horses by the polymerase chain reaction. *Med. Microbiol. Immunol.* **182**, 293-304.

Richt, J.A., Grabner, A., Herzog, S., Garten, W. and Herden, C. (2007) Borna disease in Equines. In: *Equine Infectious Diseases.* Eds: D.C. Sellon and M.T. Long, Saunders Elsevier, St Louis. pp 201-216.

Richt, J.A., van de Woude, S.A., Zink, M.C., Narayan, O. and Clements, J.E. (1991) Analysis of Borna disease virus-specific RNAs in infected cells and tissues. *J. Gen. Virol.* **72**, 2251-2255.

Richt, J.A., Pfeuffer, I., Christ, M., Frese, K., Bechter, K. and Herzog, S. (1997) Borna disease virus infection in animals and humans. *Emerg. Infect. Dis.* **3**, 343-352.

Richt, J.A., Schmeel, A., Frese, K., Carbone, K.M., Narayan, O. and Rott, R. (1994) Borna disease virus specific T-cells protect against or cause immunopathological Borna disease. *J. expt. Med.* **179**, 1467-1473.

Richt, J.A., Fürbringer, T., Koch, A., Pfeuffer, I., Herden, C., Bause-Niedrig, I. and Garten, W. (1998) Processing of the Borna disease virus glycoprotein gp94 by the subtilisin-like endoprotease furin. *J. Virol.* **72**, 4528-4533.

Rosario, D., Perez, M. and de la Torre, J.C. (2005) Functional characterization of the genomic promoter of Borna disease virus (BDV): implications of 3′-terminal sequence heterogenicity for BDV persistence. *J. Virol.* **79**, 6544-6550.

Rott, R. and Becht, H. (1995) Natural and experimental Borna disease in animals. In: *Borna disease.* Eds: H. Koprowski and W.I. Lipkin, Springer, Berlin. pp 17-30.

Rott, R., Herzog, S., Fleischer, B., Wunokur, A., Amsterdam, J., Dyson, W. and Koprowski, H. (1985) Detection of serum antibodies to Borna disease virus in patients with psychiatric disorders. *Science* **228**, 1755-1756.

Rubin, S.A., Waltrip, R.W. 2nd, Bautista, J.R. and Carbone, K.M. (1993) Borna disease virus in mice: host-specific differences in disease expression. *J. Virol.* **67**, 548-552.

Rubin, S.A., Sylves, P., Vogel, M., Pletnikov, M.V., Moran, T.H., Schwartz, G.J. and Carbone, K.M. (1999) Borna disease virus-induced hippocampal dentate gyrus damage is associated with spatial learning and memory deficits. *Brain Res. Bull.* **48**, 23-30.

Sauder, C. and Staeheli, P. (2003) Rat model of Borna disease virus transmission: epidemiological implications. *J. Virol.* **77**, 12886-12890.

Sauder, C., Hallensleben, W., Pagenstecher, A., Schneckenburger, S., Biro, L., Pertlik, D., Hausmann, J., Suter, M. and Staeheli, P. (2000) Chemokine gene expression in astrocytes of Borna disease virus-infected rats and mice in the absence of inflammation. *J. Virol.* **74**, 9267-9280.

Schamel, K., Staeheli, P. and Hausmann, J. (2001) Identification of the immunodominant H-2Kk-restricted cytotoxic T-cell epitope in the Borna disease virus nucleoprotein. *J. Virol.* **75**, 8579-8588.

Schmidt, J. (1952) Die Bornakrankheit des Pferdes: 55 Jahre Forschung und Lehre. *Arch. Exp. Veterinärmed.* **6**, 177-187.

Schmidt, P., Herzog, S., Frese, K., Grabner, A., Hafner, A., Herden, C. and Schmahl, W. (1999) Pathological and virologiral studies of Borna disease in horses. In: *Equine Infectious Diseases VIII.* Eds: U. Wernery, J. Wade, J.A. Mumford and O.R. Kaaden, R&W Publications, Newmarket. pp 493-494.

Schneemann, A., Schneider, P.A., Lamb, R.A. and Lipkin, W.I. (1995) The remarkable coding strategy of Borna disease virus: a new member of the nonsegmented negative strand RNA viruses. *Virology* **210**, 1-8.

Schneider, P.A., Hatalski, C.G., Lewis, A.J. and Lipkin, W.I. (1997) Biochemical and functional analysis of the Borna disease virus G protein. *J. Virol.* **71**, 331-336.

Schneider, U. (2005) Novel insights into the regulation of the viral polymerase complex of neurotropic Borna disease. *Virus Res.* **111**, 148-160.

Schneider, U., Naegele, M., Staeheli, P. and Schwemmle, M. (2003) Active borna disease virus polymerase complex requires a distinct nucleoprotein-to-phosphoprotein ratio but no viral X protein. *J. Virol.* **77**, 11781-1179.

Schneider, U., Martin, A., Schwemmle, M. and Staeheli, P. (2007) Genome trimming by Borna disease virus: viral replication control or escape from the cellular surveillance? *Cell. Mol. Life Sci.* **64**, 1038-1042.

Schwemmle, M. (2001) Borna disease virus infection in psychiatric patients: are we on the right track? *Lancet Infect. Dis.* **1**, 46-52.

Schwemmle, M. and Billich, C. (2004) The use of peptide arrays for the characterization of monospecific antibody repertoires from polyclonal sera of psychiatric patients suspected of infection by Borna disease virus. *Mol. Divers.* **8**, 247-250.

Schwemmle, M., Jehle, C., Formella, S. and Staeheli, P. (1999) Sequence similarity between human bornavirus isolates and laboratory strains question human origin. *Lancet* **354**, 1973-1974.

Staeheli, P. (2002) Bornaviruses. *Virus Res.* **82**, 55-59.

Staeheli, P., Sauder, C., Hausmann, J., Ehrensperger, F. and Schwemmle, M. (2000) Epidemiology of Borna disease virus. *J. Gen. Virol.* **81**, 2123-2135.

Stitz, L., Schilken, D. and Frese, K. (1991) Atypical dissemination of highly neurotropic Borna disease virus during persistent infection of cyclosporine A-treated, immunodepressed rats. *J. Virol.* **65**, 457-460.

Stitz, L, Bilzer, T. and Planz, O. (2002) The immunopathogenesis of Borna disease virus infection. *Front Biosci.* **7**, d541-555.

Stitz, L., Soeder, D., Deschl, U., Frese, K. and Rott, R. (1989) Inhibition of immune-mediated meningoencephalitis in persistently Borna disease virus-infected rats by cyclosporine A. *J. Immunol.* **143**, 4250-4256.

Tomonaga, K., Kobayashi, T. and Ikuta, K. (2002) Molecular and cellular biology of Borna disease virus infection. *Microbes Infect.* **4**, 491-500.

Uhlig, A. and Kinne, J. (1998) Neurologische Befunde bei Pferden mit Bornascher Krankheit. *Prakt. Tierärztl. Coll. Vet. XXVIII*, 33-39.

Unterstab, G., Ludwig, S., Anton, A., Planz, O., Dauber, B., Krappmann, D., Heins, G., Ehrhardt, C. and Wolff, T. (2005) Viral targeting of the interferon-β-inducing Traf family member–associated NFκB activator (TANK)–binding kinase. *Proc. Natl. Acad. Sci. USA* **102**, 13640-13645.

Van de Woude, S., Richt, J.A., Zink, M.C., Rott, R., Narayan, O. and Clements, J.E. (1990) A Borna virus cDNA encoding a protein recognized by antibodies in humans with behavioural disease. *Science* **250**, 1278-1281.

Walker, M.P., Jordan, I., Briese, T., Fischer, N. and Lipkin, W.I. (2000) Expression and characterization of the Borna disease virus polymerase. *J. Virol.* **74**, 4425-4428.

Weissenböck, H., Nowotny, N., Caplazi, P., Kolodziejek, J., and Ehrensperger, F. (1998a) Borna disease in a dog with lethal Meningoencephalitis. *J. clin. Microbiol.* **36**, 2127-2130.

Weissenböck, H., Suchy, A., Caplazi, P., Herzog, S. and Nowotny, N. (1998b) Borna disease in Austrian horses. *Vet. Rec.* **143**, 21-22.

Werner-Keišs, N., Garten, W., Richt, J.A., Porombka, D., Algermissen, D., Herzog, S., Baumgärtner, W. and Herden, C (2008) Restricted expression of Borna disease virus glycoprotein in brains of experimentally infected Lewis rats. *Neuropathol. Appl. Neurobiol.* **34**, 590-602.

Wolff, T., Pfleger, R., Wehner, T., Reinhardt, J. and Richt, J.A. (2000) A short leucine rich sequence in the Borna disease virus p10 protein mediates association with the viral phospho- and nucleoproteins. *J. Gen. Virol.* **81**, 939-947.

Wolff, T., Heins, G., Pauli, G., Burger, R. and Kurth, R. (2006) Failure to detect Borna disease virus antigen and RNA in human blood. *J. clin. Virol.* **36**, 309-311.

Zwick, W. (1939) Bornasche Krankheit und Enzephalomyelitis der Tiere. In: *Handbuch der Viruskrankheiten*, Vol. 2, Eds: E. Gildenmeister E. Haagen and O. Waldmann, Fischer, Jena, pp 254-356.

Zwick, W., Seifried, O. and Witte, J. (1927) Experimentelle Untersuchungen über die seuchenhafte Gehirn- und Rückenmarksentzündung der Pferde (Bornasche Krankheit). *Z. Infkrkh. Haustiere* **30**, 42-136.

EQUINE RABIES

D. L. Horton* and A. R. Fooks

Rabies and Wildlife Zoonoses Group, Virology Department, Veterinary Laboratories Agency Weybridge, New Haw, Addlestone, Surrey KT15 3NB, UK.

Keywords: horse; rabies; lyssavirus; encephalitis; zoonosis

Summary

Rabies is a fatal zoonotic disease, with a virtually global distribution and wide host range. Important reservoir species include dogs, foxes, skunks and bats. Cases in horses are rare and sporadic, most often caused by bites or scratches from rabid wildlife or domestic animals that are often not witnessed. Rabies virus then travels up the peripheral nerves to the central nervous system, causing acute encephalitis that invariably ends in coma and death. A variable incubation period and multiple, nonspecific signs mean the disease is difficult to diagnose *ante mortem*. Although untreatable once clinical signs develop, rabies in horses is preventable with appropriate vaccination.

Virus

Rabies is caused by classical rabies virus, one of 7 genotypes of lyssavirus in the family Rhabdoviridae. Lyssaviruses are neurotropic enveloped viruses with a single stranded negative sense RNA genome. The glycoprotein is the sole viral surface protein and induces neutralising antibodies, which are considered the main protective mechanism against the virus (Dietzschold *et al.* 1992; Hooper *et al.* 1998). All lyssaviruses are capable of causing fatal disease clinically similar to rabies but only classical rabies has been associated with deaths in horses (Green 1997).

Pathogenesis and clinical signs

Rabies virus is most commonly transmitted in saliva via bites or scratches from infected animals. Rarely, transmission has been reported by contamination of mucous membranes but not through intact skin. Viral replication can occur at the site of inoculation, but is not essential before virus gains entry to the neurons via the neuromuscular junction (Shankar *et al.* 1991). Virus moves up the peripheral nerves into the central nervous system (CNS) by fast axonal transport at 50–100 mm per day (Tsiang 1993), is then distributed widely within the CNS (Tirawatnpong *et al.* 1989) and subsequently disseminates to multiple organs including sensory nerve endings in the nasal and oral cavities, adrenal glands, kidney, cardiac muscle, hair follicles, and the salivary glands. Histopathological changes within the CNS are often limited but include varying degrees of inflammation and classic cytoplasmic inclusion bodies known as Negri bodies in neurons. The degree of inflammation varies depending on the viral isolate, host and individual (Hicks *et al.* 2009).

The incubation period is commonly 1–2 months but can vary from one week to several years (Johnson *et al.* 2008). A specific incubation period for equine rabies has not been well documented, as exposure to the virus is rarely witnessed. One experimental study in horses showed a mean incubation period of 12.3 days (Hudson *et al.* 1996) but the dose and route of inoculation, site and severity of the wound, and pathogenicity of the viral strain will all have an effect on the incubation period (Warrell and Warrell 2004).

Clinical signs in horses do not appear to adhere strictly to the classic 'furious' or 'dumb' manifestations of disease, characterised by hyperactivity or paralysis respectively. Instead there is a wide spectrum of signs, which overlap (Green 1997) (**Table 1**). Although previous reports suggest a predominance of aggressive signs (Barnard 1979), the most common presenting signs in a case series of naturally infected North American horses were ataxia and paresis (43%), lameness (29%), recumbency (14%), pharyngeal paralysis (10%) and

*Author to whom correspondence should be addressed.

colic (10%) (Green *et al.* 1992). In 21 experimentally infected horses the most common signs were muzzle tremors (81%), lethargy (71%), ataxia (71%) and pharyngeal paralysis (71%) (Hudson *et al.* 1996). It is not infrequent for horses to present just with choke due to the pharyngeal paralysis. Death occurs within 7 days from the onset of clinical signs (Green *et al.* 1992; Hudson *et al.* 1996).

Diagnosis

The wide range of clinical signs and frequent absence of relevant history make clinical diagnosis difficult. In over 20 confirmed naturally occurring cases in North America, none had visible bite wounds (Green *et al.* 1992). Laboratory confirmation *ante mortem* is also challenging as CSF may be normal, although detection of viral RNA in saliva and skin biopsies are currently used to aid human rabies diagnosis *ante mortem* (Nagaraj *et al.* 2006; Dacheux *et al.* 2008). A rising serum antibody titre can also be used to indicate exposure.

Most cases in horses are only confirmed *post mortem* using CNS samples, primarily brainstem, cerebellum, hippocampus and medulla (Warrell and Warrell 2004; Carrieri *et al.* 2006). Direct fluorescent antibody testing (FAT) of fixed brain smears will detect viral antigen, and confirmation of diagnosis can be made by inoculation of tissue culture, inoculation of mice (Bourhy *et al.* 1989) or molecular tests. Although molecular tests only prove evidence of viral genomic material and not viable virus, they have the advantages that they are very sensitive and specific and allow genetic typing of any virus detected. The most recent developments of real-time quantitative polymerase chain reaction (real-time PCR) not only allow rapid diagnosis but also differentiation between genotypes of lyssavirus (Wakeley *et al.* 2005).

TABLE 1 : Signs of rabies in the horse (Barnard 1979; Green *et al.* 1992; O'Toole *et al.* 1993; Hudson *et al.* 1996; Green 1997; Sabeta and Randles 2005)

Pyrexia
Muzzle tremors
Lethargy
Ataxia and paresis (Typically ascending)
Hyperaesthesia
Pharyngeal paresis/paralysis
Lameness
Recumbency
Tail, perineal and anal sphincter hypotonia
Aggression
Tenesmus
Biting
Convulsions
Colic
Head tilt
Circling
Hypersalivation
Abnormal vocalisation

Epidemiology

Classical rabies virus is maintained in endemic cycles in a variety of mammals worldwide (including dogs, racoons, foxes, skunks) and in both terrestrial animals and bats in the Americas. Several countries such as the UK, Australia and much of Western Europe are free from disease. Cases in horses are rare, usually sporadic consequences of 'spill-over' infections where an infected animal transmits the disease to a different species. Therefore the risk of rabies to horses depends upon the occurrence of infected reservoir species. Of the 7259 rabies cases reported in the USA in 2007, only 42 were in horses or donkeys, similar to the average of 52 cases per year over the preceding 4 years (Krebs *et al.* 2005; Blanton *et al.* 2007, 2008). Although the specific vector species is not known in many cases of equine rabies, the elimination of canine and rise in wildlife rabies in North America (Rupprecht *et al.* 2006; Blanton *et al.* 2008; Velasco-Villa *et al.* 2008) suggest that rabid wildlife pose the largest threat to horses in the USA. In South America vampire bats play a significant role, infecting horses when taking a blood meal (Mayen 2003). In many parts of the world, dog rabies remains a problem and therefore represents a threat to horses and other equids (Anon 2009a).

There are no recorded cases of lyssaviruses other than classical rabies virus causing disease in horses, but the potential for exposure reinforces the benefits of molecular diagnosis and testing of suspect rabies cases.

Prevention

Despite current interest in experimental human therapy (Willoughby *et al.* 2005), there are still no effective treatments and therefore control depends crucially on prevention of the disease developing. Immediate thorough wound cleaning is the most simple and effective preventive measure after potential exposure (Anon 2009b) but this is rarely applicable for horses if a bite is not witnessed. Vaccination with modern tissue culture based vaccines is safe and effective for preventing disease (Green 1997; Muirhead *et al.* 2008). Although rabies in horses is rare, vaccination is generally recommended where possible in endemic countries. The difficulties in clinical diagnosis, combined with close contact between people and horses make vaccination also justified to reduce the risk to man. This is particularly important for animals with exposure to large numbers of people, such as those in petting zoos or riding stables (Feder *et al.* 1998).

Rabies cases have been reported in vaccinated horses (Green *et al.* 1992; Wilson and Clark 2001) and although this does not necessarily indicate vaccine failure it means rabies should be included in the differential diagnosis for neurological conditions in rabies endemic countries, even in vaccinated horses (Green 1997). Although vaccinating horses will prevent disease, it has been shown repeatedly that the best way to reduce spill-over infections in man and domestic animals is to control or eliminate disease in the reservoir species (Rupprecht *et al.* 2006).

It is recommended that vaccinated horses exposed to a confirmed rabid animal be immediately revaccinated and then observed for 45 days for development of clinical signs of rabies. If horses are unvaccinated, it is recommended that they are subjected to euthanasia immediately (Anon 2009c). Full public health interventions are usually necessary for the handlers of horses that are diagnosed with rabies.

Acknowledgements

Department for the Environment, Food and Rural Affairs (Defra) grant SEV3500 and Cambridge Infectious Diseases Consortium.

References

Anon (2009a) http://apps.who.int/globalatlas/default.asp, RabNet, accessed 23rd July 2009.

Anon (2009b) Current WHO guide for Rabies Pre and Post-exposure prophylaxis in humans. http://www.who.int/rabies/PEProphylaxisguideline.pdf, World Health Organisation, accessed 4th February 2009.

Anon (2009c) *American Association of Equine Practitioners: Rabies Guidelines.* www/aaep.org/rabies.htm, accessed 23rd July 2009.

Barnard, B.J. (1979) [Symptoms of rabies in pets and domestic animals in South Africa and South West Africa (author's translation)]. *J. S. Afr. vet. Ass.* **50**, 109-111.

Blanton, J.D., Hanlon, C.A. and Rupprecht, C.E. (2007) Rabies surveillance in the United States during 2006. *J. Am. vet. med. Ass.* **231**, 540-556.

Blanton, J.D., Palmer, D., Christian, K.A. and Rupprecht, C.E. (2008) Rabies surveillance in the United States during 2007. *J. Am. vet. med. Ass.* **233**, 884-897.

Bourhy, H., Rollin, P.E., Vincent, J. and Sureau, P. (1989) Comparative field evaluation of the fluorescent-antibody test, virus isolation from tissue culture, and enzyme immunodiagnosis for rapid laboratory diagnosis of rabies. *J. clin. Microbiol.* **27**, 519-523.

Carrieri, M.L., Peixoto, Z.M., Paciencia, M.L., Kotait, I. and Germano, P.M. (2006) Laboratory diagnosis of equine rabies and its implications for human postexposure prophylaxis. *J. Virol. Methods* **138**, 1-9.

Dacheux, L., Reynes, J.M., Buchy, P., Sivuth, O., Diop, B.M., Rousset, D., Rathat, C., Jolly, N., Dufourcq, J.B., Nareth, C., Diop, S., Iehle, C., Rajerison, R., Sadorge, C. and Bourhy, H. (2008) A reliable diagnosis of human rabies based on analysis of skin biopsy specimens. *Clin. Infect. Dis.* **47**, 1410-1417.

Dietzschold, B., Kao, M., Zheng, Y.M., Chen, Z.Y., Maul, G., Fu, Z.F., Rupprecht, C.E. and Koprowski, H. (1992) Delineation of putative mechanisms involved in antibody-mediated clearance of rabies virus from the central nervous system. *Proc. Natl. Acad. Sci. USA* **89**, 7252-7256.

Feder, H.M., Nelson, R.S., Cartter, M.L. and Sadre, I. (1998) Rabies prophylaxis following the feeding of a rabid pony. *Clin. Pediatr.* **37**, 477-481.

Green, S.L. (1997) Rabies. *Vet. Clin. N. Am.: Equine Pract.* **13**, 1-11.

Green, S.L., Smith, L.L., Vernau, W. and Beacock, S.M. (1992) Rabies in horses: 21 cases (1970-1990). *J. Am. vet. med. Ass.* **200**, 1133-1137.

Hicks, D.J., Nunez, A., Healy, D.M., Brookes, S.M., Johnson, N. and Fooks, A.R. (2009) Comparative pathological study of the murine brain after experimental infection with classical rabies virus and European bat lyssaviruses. *J. comp. Pathol.* **140**, 113-126.

Hooper, D.C., Morimoto, K., Bette, M., Weihe, E., Koprowski, H. and Dietzschold, B. (1998) Collaboration of antibody and inflammation in clearance of rabies virus from the central nervous system. *J. Virol.* **72**, 3711-3719.

Hudson, L.C., Weinstock, D., Jordan, T. and Bold-Fletcher, N.O. (1996) Clinical presentation of experimentally induced rabies in horses. *Zentralbl. Veterinarmed. B* **43**, 277-285.

Johnson, N., Fooks, A. and McColl, K. (2008) Human rabies case with long incubation, Australia. *Emerg. Infect. Dis.* **14**, 1950-1951.

Krebs, J.W., Mandel, E.J., Swerdlow, D.L. and Rupprecht, C.E. (2005) Rabies surveillance in the United States during 2004. *J. Am. vet. med. Ass.* **227**, 1912-1925.

Mayen, F. (2003) Haematophagous bats in Brazil, their role in rabies transmission, impact on public health, livestock industry and alternatives to an indiscriminate reduction of bat population. *J. vet. med. B. Infect. Dis. Vet. Public. Health.* **50**, 469-472.

Muirhead, T.L., McClure, J.T., Wichtel, J.J., Stryhn, H., Frederick Markham, R.J., McFarlane, D. and Lunn, D.P. (2008) The effect of age on serum antibody titers after rabies and influenza vaccination in healthy horses. *J. vet. intern. Med.* **22**, 654-661.

Nagaraj, T., Vasanth, J.P., Desai, A., Kamat, A., Madhusudana, S.N. and Ravi, V. (2006) *Ante mortem* diagnosis of human rabies using saliva samples: comparison of real time and conventional RT-PCR techniques. *J. clin. Virol.* **36**, 17-23.

O'Toole, D., Mills, K., Ellis, J., Welch, V. and Fillerup, M. (1993) Poliomyelomalacia and ganglioneuritis in a horse with paralytic rabies. *J. vet. diagn. Invest.* **5**, 94-97.

Rupprecht, C.E., Willoughby, R. and Slate, D. (2006) Current and future trends in the prevention, treatment and control of rabies. *Expert Rev. Anti. Infect. Ther.* **4**, 1021-1038.

Sabeta, C.T. and Randles, J.L. (2005) Importation of canid rabies in a horse relocated from Zimbabwe to South Africa. *Onderstepoort. J. vet. Res.* **72**, 95-100.

Shankar, V., Dietzschold, B. and Koprowski, H. (1991) Direct entry of rabies virus into the central nervous system without prior local replication. *J. Virol.* **65**, 2736-2738.

Tirawatnpong, S., Hemachudha, T., Manutsathit, S., Shuangshoti, S., Phanthumchinda, K. and Phanuphak, P. (1989) Regional distribution of rabies viral antigen in central nervous system of human encephalitic and paralytic rabies. *J. Neurol. Sci.* **92**, 91-99.

Tsiang, H. (1993) Pathophysiology of rabies virus infection of the nervous system. *Adv. Virus. Res.* **42**, 375-412.

Velasco-Villa, A., Reeder, S.A., Orciari, L.A., Yager, P.A., Franka, R., Blanton, J.D., Zuckero, L., Hunt, P., Oertli, E.H., Robinson, L.E. and Rupprecht, C.E. (2008) Enzootic rabies elimination from dogs and reemergence in wild terrestrial carnivores, United States. *Emerg. Infect. Dis.* **14**, 1849-1854.

Wakeley, P.R., Johnson, N., McElhinney, L.M., Marston, D., Sawyer, J. and Fooks, A.R. (2005) Development of a real-time, TaqMan reverse transcription-PCR assay for detection and differentiation of lyssavirus genotypes 1, 5, and 6. *J. clin. Microbiol.* **43**, 2786-2792.

Warrell, M.J. and Warrell, D.A. (2004) Rabies and other lyssavirus diseases. *Lancet* **363**, 959-969.

Willoughby, R.E., Jr., Tieves, K.S., Hoffman, G.M., Ghanayem, N.S., Amlie-Lefond, C.M., Schwabe, M.J., Chusid, M.J. and Rupprecht, C.E. (2005) Survival after treatment of rabies with induction of coma. *N. Engl. J. Med.* **352**, 2508-2514.

Wilson, P.J. and Clark, K.A. (2001) Postexposure rabies prophylaxis protocol for domestic animals and epidemiologic characteristics of rabies vaccination failures in Texas: 1995-1999. *J. Am. vet. med. Ass.* **218**, 522-525.

EQUINE ENCEPHALOSIS

A. J. Guthrie*, A. D. Pardini and P. G. Howell

Equine Research Centre, Faculty of Veterinary Science, University of Pretoria, Onderstepoort 0110, Republic of South Africa.

Keywords: horse; equine encephalosis virus; equine ephemeral fever

Summary

Equine encephalosis (EE) is usually a mild or subclinical orbivirus infection of horses. Equine encephalosis virus is transmitted by species of *Culicoides*, which are endemic to the temperate regions of Africa and as a result, the epidemiology has much in common with African horse sickness. This paper reviews the aetiology, clinical signs, pathology, epidemiology, diagnosis and control of EE.

Introduction

The disease referred to as 'equine ephemeral fever' by Sir Arnold Theiler in the early 1900s (Theiler 1909, 1910) is probably the first description of equine encephalosis (EE). EE is usually a mild or subclinical orbivirus infection of horses. The virus is transmitted by species of *Culicoides*, which are endemic to the temperate regions of Africa and as a result, the epidemiology has much in common with African horse sickness (AHS).

In March 1967 a virus, subsequently named equine encephalosis virus (EEV) was isolated from the blood and tissues of a 13-year-old Thoroughbred mare that was subjected to euthanasia after showing a peracute nervous derangement. Two other mares on the same stud became ill during the following few days. One of these died, while the second recovered after a convalescence of 14 days. The virus was also recovered from blood samples taken from horses that had exhibited no clinical signs of disease except for a fever. EEV was also recovered from the organs of horses that had died in other parts of the country (Erasmus *et al.* 1970).

Seroconversion to EEV of between 30% (Howell *et al.* 2002) and 84% (Howell *et al.* 2008) has been demonstrated in horses in South Africa without neurological signs or other clinical manifestations of the disease previously described, including acute cardiac failure, ataxia, liver dysfunction, abortion and death (Erasmus *et al.* 1970). This suggests that the recovery of virus from blood or organ samples must be interpreted with caution. Attempts to induce the disease experimentally (Theiler 1909; Erasmus *et al.* 1970; Dardiri *et al.* 1975; Erasmus *et al.* 1978) have failed to reproduce the clinical signs described as EE (Erasmus *et al.* 1970) in all but one horse that developed neurological signs 3 days after the end of the pyrexia (10 days post challenge).

Aetiology

Equine encephalosis virus is classified as an *Orbivirus* in the family *Reoviridae* and the morphological and physiochemical characteristics conform to the criteria associated with this genus. Seven valid serotypes have been described (Howell *et al.* 2002) and there is negligible cross reactivity between heterologous antigens and antisera (Erasmus *et al.* 1978; Gerdes and Pieterse 1993; Howell *et al.* 2002). Using electron microscopy negatively stained virus particles closely resemble those of AHS and bluetongue (BT) (Lecatsas *et al.* 1973). The capsid is composed of 32 morphological subunits, as described for bluetongue virus (BTV) (Els and Verwoerd 1969) and represents a subviral particle. The complete virion has an outer diffuse polypeptide layer and has a diameter of 73 nm (Lecatsas *et al.* 1973).

Polyacrylamide gel electrophoresis (PAGE) has confirmed that the genome is composed of

*Author to whom correspondence should be addressed. Present address: Equine Research Centre, Faculty of Veterinary Science, University of Pretoria, Private Bag X04, Onderstepoort 0110, Republic of South Africa. Dr Pardini's present address: PO Box 25294, Monument Park 0105, Republic of South Africa. Prof. Howell's present address: 384 Amberglen, PO Box X004, Howick 3290, Republic of South Africa.

10 segments, which showed some differences from the separation profiles of BTV and AHSV (Viljoen and Huismans 1989). Separation of 7 structural proteins on SDS-PAGE gels showed that the molecular weight varied from 36–120 kD with 4 major and 3 minor protein components. These fractionation patterns closely resemble those of BTV and AHSV (Viljoen and Huismans 1989). Hybridisation techniques have been used to show that segment 2 encodes for the serotype specific antigen. Segment 10 sequence data have been compared with those of BTV and AHS (van Niekerk *et al.* 2003; Quan *et al.* 2008).

Clinical signs

The incubation period of the disease is 3–5 days. In excess of 90% of animals show either no obvious signs of infection or develop only very mild clinical signs. Initially most affected horses show either a slightly elevated rectal temperature (39°C) for one or 2 days or a high fever (40–41°C) for 1–5 days. Fever may be accompanied by varying degrees of listlessness and inappetance. There may be an increase in pulse and respiratory rate, and, in some animals, a slight reddish brown discolouration of the mucous membranes as a result of congestion and mild icterus. Occasionally, varying degrees of swelling of the eyelids and supraorbital fossae may be observed (**Fig 1**). Central nervous system involvement, respiratory distress, abortion and acute heart failure have been observed in individual animals from which equine encephalosis has been isolated (Erasmus *et al.* 1978); however, until such observations can be reproduced experimentally, their significance remains questionable.

Pathology

Post mortem examination of horse carcasses from which EEV has been isolated, have revealed varying degrees of lung oedema and hydropericardium, slight mild hepatomegaly and splenomegaly, petechiae in serosal surfaces (particularly of the intestines), hyperaemia of the glandular part of the stomach, and congestion and oedema of the brain. In cases with liver involvement, histopathological examination revealed diffuse, cloudy swelling and hydropic fatty degeneration of the liver. In the first described case, nervous signs were accompanied by congestion

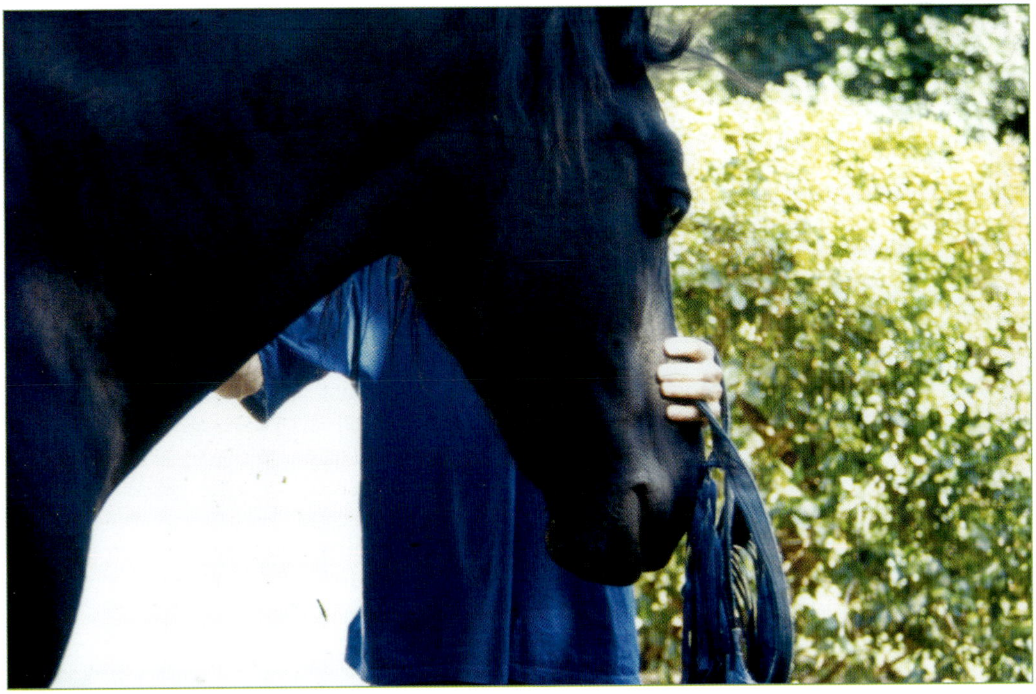

FIGURE 1: Swelling of supraorbital fossa and of lips associated with infection with equine encephalosis virus in a horse. © A.J. Guthrie.

and oedema of the brain, particularly in the periventricular areas in the midbrain and thalamus (Erasmus *et al.* 1970). Significantly, no evidence of viral encephalitis were observed histologically, the disease was thus termed 'encephalosis'. Although leucoencephalomalacia is the most useful diagnostic lesion for fumonisin toxicity in horses, cerebral oedema alone has been described in experimental fumonisin intoxication in horses (Smith *et al.* 2002).

In 2007 a total of 18 horses died on the Cape Peninsula in South Africa and EEV was isolated from all cases (Anon 2007). Whilst a severe alveolar oedema with accumulation of foam in the trachea was present in all cases that died, the intermuscular oedema, hydrothorax, hydropericardium and ascites usually present in AHS cases were not observed in any of these cases. Subsequent investigations revealed that there was widespread circulation of EEV serotypes 1 and 4 in the area at the time and all cases that showed severe clinical signs, or that died, were receiving diets with a maize inclusion rate of at least 10%. Unfortunately, none of the feed was subjected to analysis for mycotoxins. Two of the horses that died in this outbreak showed neurological signs similar to those reported in the horse Cascara in 1967 (Erasmus *et al.* 1970). Furthermore, a mycotoxin binding agent (Mycosorb)[1], was used in some of the cases showing severe clinical signs and this, in conjunction with removal of all concentrate feed resulted in a dramatic improvement in these cases. EEV has also recently been implicated as the cause of pyrexia in approximately 150 of 800 horses in Israel (Anon 2009).

Epidemiology

Equine encephalosis and AHS have similar natural hosts, vectors and environmental conditions under which transmission occurs. No vaccine has been developed for EEV, with the result that the prevalence of natural infection whether determined by seroconversion or by recovery of virus, is not influenced by vaccination. EEV of various serotypes has been recovered from horses of all breeds and ages, and horses are the only species in which clinical signs have been recorded. The majority of the 59 isolates of EEV that were recovered from horses over 14 years were obtained incidentally (Paweska *et al.* 1999). Neutralising antibody to a single or multiple serotypes of EEV has been detected in 20–84% of yearlings prior to the age of 18 months and mares at stud (Howell *et al.* 2002, 2008). A survey using a group specific indirect enzyme linked immunosorbent assay (ELISA) on a random sample of 604 equine sera collected over 14 years revealed a mean seroprevalence of 74%, which appeared to be uniformly high throughout South Africa (Paweska *et al.* 1999).

In Africa, due to its resistance to clinical disease, the donkey is an ideal sentinel to determine the prevalence and distribution of both EEV and AHS through the detection of both group and serotype specific antibody. A study over 12 years using a group reactive ELISA showed that 49.3% of a sample of almost 5000 donkeys of all ages were positive for antibody to EEV (Venter *et al.* 1999a; Lord *et al.* 2002). In a similar survey of healthy donkeys in Zimbabwe, an overall seroprevalence of 85% was found throughout the country. When compared with the prevalence of antibody to AHS, EE appears to have a wider distribution in the donkey population (Lord *et al.* 2002). Zebra have been shown to be susceptible to the virus (Williams *et al.* 1993; Barnard 1997) with neutralising antibody to all serotypes being identified. Seroprevalence increased from 18% in 6-month-old zebra foals to 60% in yearlings, with EEV serotype 1 having the highest prevalence (Barnard 1997).

The transmission of EEV has a seasonal cycle in the temperate regions of southern Africa and virus may be recovered from equids between December and July. Vector activity is terminated by the onset of winter and low precipitation (Paweska *et al.* 1999). The distribution of EEV appears to be determined by the distribution and abundance of competent vectors. Serotype 1 of EEV was first recovered from a pool of processed *Culicoides* in 1969 (Theodoridis *et al.* 1979). Subsequently, experimental feeding of wild caught *Culicoides* including *C. imicola* and *C. bolitinos* on infected blood, through a chicken skin membrane, has shown that serotype 1 will replicate in the surviving engorged females (Venter *et al.* 1999b, 2002). Completion of the biological transmission cycle and the minimal infective dose required to infect equids has not been established. Other species of wild caught *Culicoides* have not been examined in sufficient numbers to establish their competence as vectors.

A study of the prevalence of serotype specific antibody in groups of resident brood mares on stud farms in the major Thoroughbred horse breeding areas of South Africa, (Howell *et al.* 2002) revealed that 56.9% of the mares were positive for neutralising antibody to one or multiple serotypes of EEV. Between 19.2 and 43.6% of the animals were previously infected with only a single serotype, while the percentage of mares showing evidence of previous infection with more than one serotype varied from 3.3–33.8% on individual farms. Individual serotypes are responsible for localised foci of seroconversion with an unpredictable seasonal and year-to-year distribution. Prior to 1990 and more recently, serotype 1 appears to have been the predominant serotype, followed by serotypes 6 and 7, while antibody to the remaining serotypes are only occasionally identified. Antibody to serotype 2, which appears to have been the predominant serotype in 1967 (Erasmus *et al.* 1970), was identified in only 8 of 518 mares sampled between 1995 and 1998 (Howell *et al.* 2002) and 5 of 2992 Thoroughbred yearlings sampled between 1999 and 2004 (Howell *et al.* 2008).

Diagnosis

Infection with EEV is usually subclinical and the majority of infections are confirmed by seroconversion. In animals showing a febrile reaction or clinical signs a diagnosis can be made by isolation of the virus from blood or from tissues (spleen, thymus, liver, lung and brain). Early confluent monolayers of BHK21/C13 cells can be used for virus isolation. Alternatively, intracerebellar inoculation of 3–5-day-old suckling mice may be used to recover EEV. Antisera produced in sheep have given unequivocal specificity in the routine identification and classification of all field isolates recovered to date. The first or second passage in tissue culture or the harvested suckling mouse brain can be subject to an antigen capture ELISA to confirm the presence of EEV. This ELISA is based on the procedures previously described for AHS (Hamblin *et al.* 1992) as modified by Crafford (Crafford 2001; Crafford *et al.* 2003). To date, no polymerase chain reaction based assays for the detection of EEV nucleic acid have been described.

A single dilution indirect group reactive ELISA has been described (Williams 1987; Williams *et al.* 1993) and can be used in seroepidemiological surveys to detect antibody in various equid species. This assay is more reliable for the detection of IgG in equine sera than the complement fixation (CF) or agar gel immunodiffusion (AGID) tests. A competitive ELISA for the detection of antibody against EEV has subsequently been developed (Crafford 2001). This assay can be used to determine end-point titres in individual serum samples. Both of these ELISAs are specific and no cross reactions have been identified between sera to other orbiviruses.

Confirmation of the diagnosis of a suspected case of EE is essential, primarily to distinguish the infection from mild forms of AHS as well as other febrile or vector borne diseases encountered in an endemic region. Currently this may be achieved by the recovery and identification of the responsible virus in blood samples from febrile horses, or the demonstration of seroconversion in paired sera.

Fever and the mild, nonspecific signs of illness evident in a large proportion of horses infected with EEV are features of many other infectious diseases of horses in the endemic regions. In animals manifesting fever, listlessness, inappetence and reddish brown mucous membranes, piroplasmosis should be considered. Those animals with swelling of the eyelids may be confused with horses suffering from AHS. However, the mortality rate of AHS in naïve unvaccinated animals is usually much higher (approximately 90%).

The signs of frenzy, convulsions and uncontrolled running into walls or objects observed in the case described as EE (Erasmus *et al.* 1970) have been reported in horses suffering from leucoencephalomalacia (*Fusarium moniliforme* poisoning) and chronic seneciosis. Similar clinical signs have been described in rabies, eastern, western and Venezuelan encephalomyelitis, and Borna disease, and these conditions should be included as possible differential diagnoses. Ataxia, particularly of the hind quarters, should be differentiated from similar signs that have been reported following equine herpesvirus 1 and *Trypanosoma equiperdum* infections, Haloxon/carbon disulphide poisoning, in wobblers, and in horses suffering from thrombo embolism of a branch of the external or internal iliac artery.

Control

As infection with EE is usually subclinical no vaccine has been developed and no control measures are usually implemented in endemic areas. The stabling of horses from an hour or 2 before sunset until an hour or 2 after sunrise the next day (the period when *Culicoides* midges are particularly active) is a useful control method. If it is practical, stables should be screened against flying insects, and no lights that could attract insects should be left burning at night in or in close proximity to the stables. Insect repellents can be sprayed on horses and on plastic mesh screens placed over the entrances to stables. If horses cannot be stabled at night, sheep or cattle should be allowed to graze in the same paddocks as the horses to act as a decoy for the midges. Affected animals should be treated symptomatically. Nonsteroidal anti-inflammatory drugs can be used to combat the fever.

Conclusions

'Equine encephalosis' is unfortunately a misnomer for this disease since organic disease, dysfunction or degenerative lesions of the brain are not features of the infection. The name 'equine ephemeral fever' that Sir Arnold Theiler proposed for the disease he described in 1910 is probably more accurate. Despite numerous attempts, experimental challenge with EEV has only resulted in the development of subclinical or mild disease in infected animals. The neurological signs described in the first case described as EE (Erasmus *et al.* 1970) bear a strong resemblance with those described in association with fumonisin intoxication in horses. During the 2007 outbreak of EE on the Cape Peninsula in South Africa an association between animals receiving diets with high maize inclusion rates and severe clinical signs was established. This association warrants further investigation but suggests that there may be a synergism between EEV and as yet unidentified factors, possibly mycotoxins, associated with maize in rations.

Manufacturer's address

[1]Alltech (PTY) Ltd., Stellenbosch, South Africa.

Acknowledgements

Various colleagues, including Dr Baltus Erasmus, Dr Truuske Gerdes and Mr Rudi Meiswinkel, for fruitful discussions on equine encephalosis.

References

Anon (2007) Equine encephalosis - South Africa (Western Cape). ProMED-mail 2007; 9 Sep:20070509.1495. Accessed 2nd November 2008.

Anon (2009) Equine encephalosis - Israel: 2008. ProMED-mail 2009; 1 Apr:20090401.1254. Accessed 2nd April 2009.

Barnard, B.J.H. (1997) Antibodies against some viruses of domestic animals in southern African wild animals. *Onderstepoort J. vet. Res.* **64**, 95-110.

Crafford, J.E. (2001) *Development and Validation of Enzyme Linked Immunosorbent Assays for Detection of Equine Encephalosis Virus Antibody and Antigen,* MSc Thesis, University of Pretoria. pp 1-88.

Crafford, J.E., Guthrie, A.J., Van Vuuren, M., Mertens, P.P., Burroughs, J.N., Howell, P.G. and Hamblin, C. (2003) A group-specific, indirect sandwich ELISA for the detection of equine encephalosis virus antigen. *J. Virol. Methods* **112**, 129-135.

Dardiri, A.H., Kopec, J.D. and Colgrove, G.S. (1975) Certain biological properties of equine encephalosis virus. *Abs. Ann. Mtg. Am. Soc. Microbiol.* **75**, 218.

Els, H.J. and Verwoerd, D.W. (1969) Morphology of bluetongue virus. *Virol.* **38**, 213-219.

Erasmus, B.J., Boshoff, S.T. and Pieterse, L.M. (1978) The isolation and characterization of equine encephalosis and serologically related orbiviruses from horses. In: *Equine Infectious Diseases IV*, Eds: J.T. Bryans and H. Gerber, Veterinary Publications Incorporated, Princeton. pp 447-450.

Erasmus, B.J., Adelaar, T.F., Smit, J.D., Lecatsas, G. and Toms, T. (1970) The isolation and characterization of equine encephalosis virus. *Bull. OIE* **74**, 781-789.

Gerdes, G.H. and Pieterse, L.M. (1993) The isolation and identification of Potchefstroom virus: A new member of the equine encephalosis group of orbiviruses. *J. S. Afr. vet. Ass.* **64**, 131-132.

Hamblin, C., Anderson, E.C., Mellor, P.S., Graham, S.D., Mertens, P.P.C. and Burroughs, J.N. (1992) The detection of African horse sickness virus antigens and antibodies in young *equidae*. *Epidemiol. Infect.* **108**, 193-201.

Howell, P.G., Nurton, J.P., Nel, D., Lourens, C.W. and Guthrie, A.J. (2008) Prevalence of serotype specific antibody to equine encephalosis virus in Thoroughbred yearlings in South Africa (1999-2004). *Onderstepoort J. vet. Res.* **75**, 153-161.

Howell, P.G., Groenewald, D.M., Visage, C.W., Bosman, A., Coetzer, J.A.W. and Guthrie, A.J. (2002) The classification of seven serotypes of equine encephalosis virus and the prevalence of homologous antibody in horses in South Africa. *Onderstepoort J. vet. Res.* **69**, 79-93.

Lecatsas, G., Erasmus, B.J. and Els, H.J. (1973) Electron microscope studies on equine encephalosis virus. *Onderstepoort J. vet. Res.* **40**, 53-58.

Lord, C.C., Venter, G.J., Mellor, P.S., Paweska, J.T. and Woolhouse, M.E. (2002) Transmission patterns of African horse sickness and equine encephalosis viruses in South African donkeys. *Epidemiol. Infect.* **128**, 265-275.

Paweska, J.T., Gerdes, G.H., Woods, P.S.A. and Williams, R. (1999) Equine encephalosis in Southern Africa: Current situation. In: *Equine Infectious Diseases VIII*. Eds: U. Wernery, J.F. Wade, J.A. Mumford and O.R. Kaaden, R & W Publications Ltd, Newmarket. pp 303-305.

Smith, G.W., Constable, P.D., Foreman, J.H., Eppley, R.M., Waggoner, A.L., Tumbleson, M.E. and Haschek, W.M. (2002) Cardiovascular changes associated with intravenous administration of fumonisin B1 in horses. *Am. J. Vet. Res.* **63**, 538-545.

Theiler, A. (1909) Investigations into South African diseases. (g) Fever reactions in horses simulating horse-sickness. *Rep. Govern. vet. Bacteriol.* 114-126.

Theiler, A. (1910) Notes on a fever in horses simulating horse-sickness. *Transvaal Agric. J.* **8**, 581-586.

Theodoridis, A., Nevill, E.M., Els, H.J. and Boshoff, S.T. (1979) Viruses isolated from *Culicoides* midges in South Africa during unsuccessful attempts to isolate bovine ephemeral fever virus. *Onderstepoort J. vet. Res.* **46**, 191-198.

Venter, G.J., Paweska, J.T., Williams, R. and Nevill, E.M. (1999a) Prevalence of antibodies against African horse sickness and equine encephalosis viruses in donkeys in southern Africa. In: *Equine Infectious Diseases VIII.* Eds: U. Wernery, J.F. Wade, J.A. Mumford and O.R. Kaaden, R & W Publications Ltd, Newmarket. pp 299-302.

Venter, G.J., Groenewald, D.M., Paweska, J.T., Venter, E.H. and Howell, P.G. (1999b) Vector competence of selected South African *Culicoides* species for the Bryanston serotype of equine encephalosis virus. *Med. Vet. Entomol.* 393-400.

Venter, G.J., Groenewald, D., Venter, E., Hermanides, K.G. and Howell, P.G. (2002) A comparison of the vector competence of the biting midges, *Culicoides (Avaritia) bolitinos* and *C. (A.) imicola*, for the Bryanston serotype of equine encephalosis virus. *Med. Vet. Entomol.* **16**, 372-377.

Viljoen, G.J. and Huismans, H. (1989) The characterization of equine encephalosis virus and the development of genomic probes. *J. Gen. Virol.* **70**, 2007-2015.

Williams, R. (1987) A single dilution enzyme-linked immunosorbent assay for the quantitative detection of antibodies to African horsesickness virus. *Onderstepoort J. vet. Res.* **54**, 67-70.

Williams, R., Du Plessis, D.H. and Van Wyngaardt, W. (1993) Group-reactive ELISAs for detecting antibodies to African horsesickness and equine encephalosis viruses in horses, donkey, and zebra sera. *J. vet. diagn. Invest.* **5**, 3-7.

VESICULAR STOMATITIS VIRUS INFECTION IN HORSES

J. L. Traub-Dargatz* and B. McCluskey†

Animal Population Health Institute, College of Veterinary Medicine and Biomedical Sciences, Colorado State University, Fort Collins, Colorado 80523-1678; and †The Veterinary Services Regional offices, 2150 Centre Ave. Bldg B., Fort Collins, Colorado 80526, USA.

Keywords: horse; ulcerative stomatitis; coronitis; VSV

Summary

Vesicular stomatitis virus (VSV) infection occurs in equids in the western hemisphere leading to vesicular lesions that rapidly progress to ulcerative stomatitis and other lesions such as coronitis and crusting dermatitis of the muzzle and nares. Outbreaks of VSV occur periodically in livestock during the summer and autumn in the western USA. This is a reportable event and, if VSV is confirmed, leads to movement restrictions that have economic impact for the animal industry. Treatment is symptomatic and there is currently no vaccine available in the USA for prevention of the disease. Avoiding exposure to insects that can spread the disease and inspection of livestock entering events during outbreak years are the primary means of control.

Clinical signs

The primary clinical disease sign of vesicular stomatitis virus (VSV) infection in horses is ulcerative stomatitis. Although the disease starts with the formation of vesicles in the oral cavity and on the mucocutaneous junction of the lips, the condition has usually progressed to the ulcerative phase by the time the disease is recognised by the owner or manager of the horse (Knight and Messer 1983; Reif 1994; McCluskey and Mumford 2000). The first clinical sign in horses that is generally recognised by the owner or manager is excessive salivation and discomfort when prehending and masticating feed. The onset of signs is often quite rapid; for example, the history might be that the horse appeared fine last night but this morning he is slobbering and/or having some difficulty eating.

There are usually multiple oral lesions occurring most commonly on the tongue but they can also occur on the gingival and mucocutaneous junction of the lips (**Figs 1** and **2**). If the lesions occur on the lips these maybe readily visible to the equine owner or manager but those in the oral cavity will not be seen unless a thorough examination is performed by parting the lips and viewing the dorsal surface of the tongue and the gingival surfaces. It is important to wear gloves when performing the oral examination because VSV is a zoonotic agent and in order to reduce the risk of spreading the virus to other livestock (**Fig 3**).

Horses infected with VSV can also develop dermatitis on the skin of the muzzle with associated swelling of the muzzle and lips (**Figs 4** and **5**). Vesicular stomatitis virus infection can also result in

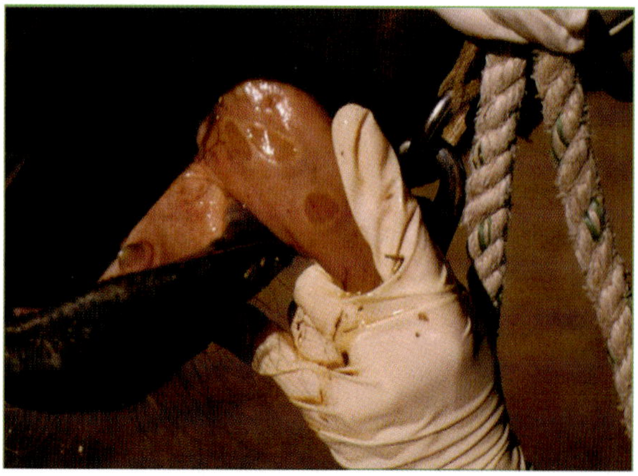

FIGURE 1: Vesicle formation on the surface of the tongue. It is rare to find these vesicles as they have typically ruptured prior to examination.

*Author to whom correspondence should be addressed.

lesions on the mammary gland or teats of mares, external genitalia and/or on the coronary band leading to lameness (Knight and Messer 1983; Reif 1994) (**Fig 6**). Lesions in these locations are less common than those in the oral cavity and on the lips and muzzle.

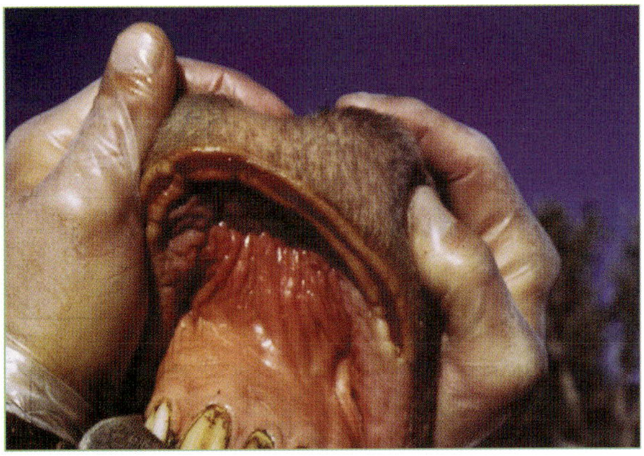

FIGURE 2: Ulceration of the mucocutaneous junction of the oral cavity is a common finding. These lesions often result in ptyalism and anorexia.

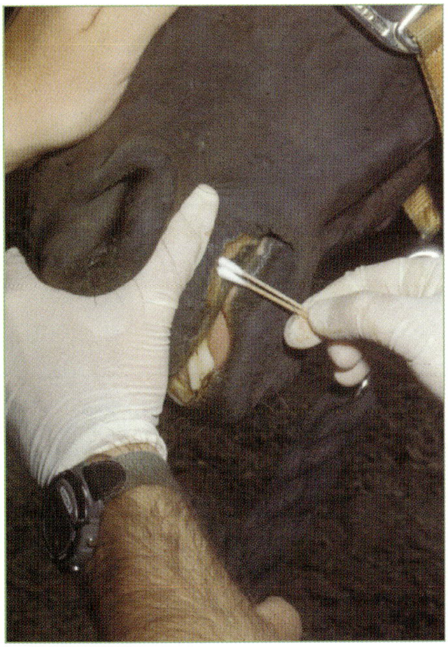

FIGURE 3: General infectious disease barrier practices (e.g. examination gloves) should be employed to reduce risk of spreading the virus between examined animals and also to reduce risk to the examiner as VSV has zoonotic potential albeit low risk.

Horses with VSV infection are usually afebrile at the time of initial examination. Subclinical infections can occur. Horses and cattle aged <1 year appear less

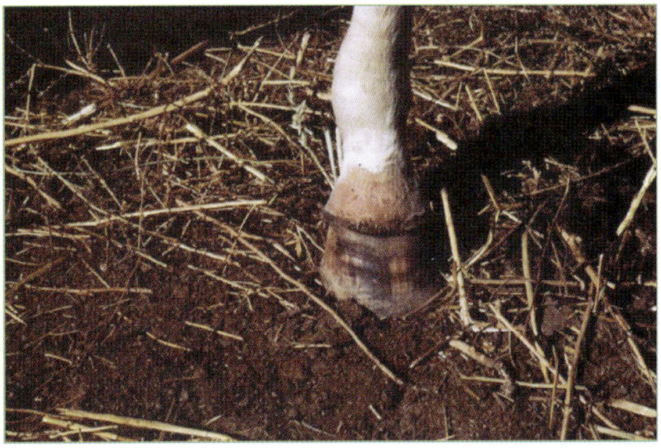

FIGURE 4: Coronitis, resulting in mild to severe lameness, can be a clinical finding in horses.

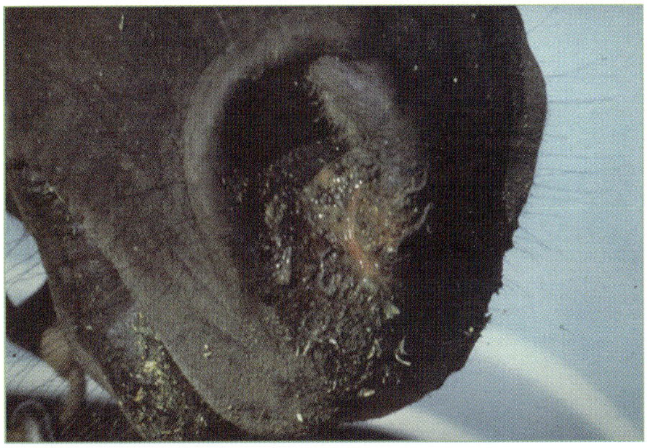

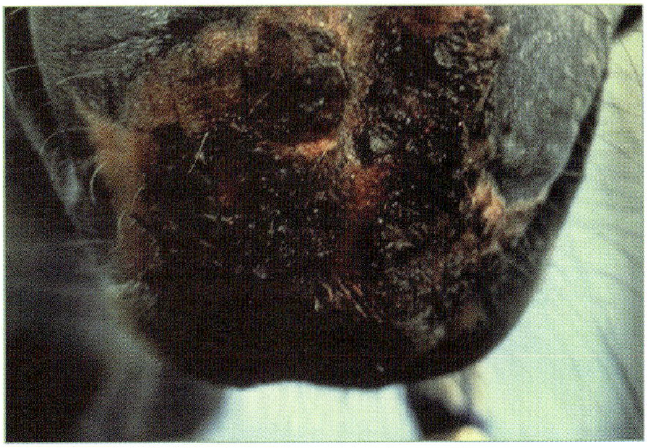

FIGURES 5 and 6: Crusting dermatitis of the muzzle and nares may be observed and may include swelling and mild exudate. These lesions are generally believed to be the result of attraction of insects to these particular sites.

TABLE 1: Noninfectious causes of stomatitis

Agent/cause	Clinical signs similar to VS	Other clinical aspects	Method of diagnosis
Use of bedding derived from wood shavings of the *Simaroubaceae* family (e.g. Amargo, Bitterwood, Marupa, Quassia).	Outbreaks of bullous lesions on lingual surface, with dry cracked areas around nose, lips and anus.	Other signs include jaundice, haematuria and anorexia.	Epidemiological investigation for risk factors for outbreak of stomatitis with bedding type being identified as a potential risk factor and subsequent testing of the bedding for compounds quassin and neoquassin.
Physical trauma from course forage or presence of plant awns in forage.	Oral ulcers and erosions.		Awns or fine hair like plant material noted grossly in ulcerative lesions in oral cavity or through microscopic examination.
Canthardin or blister beetle toxicity.	Vesicles on mucosal surfaces in oral cavity.	Shock, inflammation of gastrointestinal and urinary tracts, myocardial failure, hypocalcaemia and death.	Clinical signs, history of consumption of hay that when examined may contain parts of beetle bodies, testing of urine and stomach contents for canthardin.
Nonsteroidal drug administration such as phenylbutazone or flunixin meglumine.	Single or multiple oral ulcers.	Azotaemia, colic due to gastric or colonic lesions, hypoproteinaemia, ventral oedema, anorexia.	History of oral administration of nonsteroidal drug especially at high doses or for prolonged periods.
Pemphigus foliaceous	Vesicles and pustules on epithelium of head and limbs.	Skin as well as oral lesions.	Histological examination of biopsy of lesion.
Equine exfoliative eosinophilic dermatitis.	Oral ulcers	Scaling and crusting lesions on skin of face or coronary band.	Histological examination of biopsy of lesion.
Photosensitisation	Erythema, oedema and vesicle formation on white skinned areas especially if occurs around the head.	Usually no oral lesions	No oral lesions, potentially history of consumption of plants that lead to photosensitisation.
Dental eruption or retained deciduous cheek teeth.	Ulceration at the base or gingival surface of the tooth that is erupting from the gum or in gum area near retained deciduous cheek tooth. There is occasionally excess salivation and difficulty chewing associated with retained deciduous teeth.		On oral examination with this condition the ulcerative process is often a single lesion and occurs in only a limited area of the dental problem.

susceptible to clinical disease when compared to animals aged >1 year. The clinical and subclinical attack rate on infected premises varies greatly with one report suggesting that horses at pasture are at higher risk of clinical disease, perhaps related to mucosal abrasion associated with consumption of rough forage causing an entry point for the virus (B. McCluskey, unpublished observation).

Vesicular stomatitis is a disease of horses as well as other livestock that is endemic only in the western hemisphere. Infections occur seasonally every year in areas of Mexico and Central and South America. Clinical disease is seen sporadically in the western USA. From 1995 through 2005, outbreaks of VSV have occurred in 1995, 1997, 1998, 2004 and 2005 (Bridges *et al.* 1997; McCluskey *et al.* 1999). In the USA, most commonly the disease is first recognised in early summer and ends in the fall after the first frost. In some outbreak years the disease persists into the winter and early spring and may represent spread through direct animal to animal contact verses through insect vector transmission.

Oral vesicular lesions or ulcers are not uncommon in horses and there are multiple differential diagnoses that need to be considered in addition to VSV infection. The differentials for oral ulceration beyond VSV include noninfectious causes of stomatitis and other infectious causes of stomatitis. The noninfectious causes of stomatitis in equids include plant related toxicoses and trauma, insect or drug related toxicoses, and dermatological related conditions (McCluskey and Mumford 2000) (**Table 1**).

There is limited experimental and epidemiological evidence for other infectious causes of stomatitis other than VSV infection; however, the literature does contain field based reports of other viral agents being identified from horses with ulcerative or erosive oral lesions including equine viral arteritis, equine herpesvirus, Jamestown Canyon virus (JCV), caliciviruses and equine adenovirus. In 1997, a horse with classic clinical signs of VSV infection was examined by a Federal Animal Veterinary Diagnostician, the workup for VSV infection was negative but based on examination of tissue collected from oral lesions a diagnosis of JCV was made (Sahu *et al.* 1999) This report was the first to identify lesions similar to VSV infection being associated with JCV infection. An additional differential is *Gastrophilus nasalis* (bots) larvae that can burrow in the spaces around the teeth and cause gingival irritation and necrosis around the base of the teeth (Sellon *et al.* 2007). There are also recognised outbreaks of ulcerative stomatitis in the USA and New Zealand in which an aetiological agent is never found (McCluskey and Mumford 2000). The lesions are indistinguishable from VSV infection and occur in multiple animals on a premises or limited geographic area. In some instances the disease appears to spread with horse movement between premises thus implicating a contagious disease agent and yet none is identified. In New Zealand the outbreak of ulcerative stomatitis that occurred in 1998 was eventually termed Balclutha horse syndrome, after the location where the disease was recognised (O'Neil 2008).

Important clinical work up includes determining the history regarding the duration and type of clinical signs, the progression of disease in the individual animal, the number of animals affected on a given premises or limited geographic region along with the number and location of ulcerative oral lesions. In VSV infection in horses there are usually multiple lesions with at least some of the lesions on the tongue. There is also often a history of additional cases in the geographic area although all outbreaks of VSV have to start with a first case.

Epidemiology/causative agent

Vesicular stomatitis is the disease caused by the VSV. There are 2 serotypes of VSV, Indiana and New Jersey. Vesciular stomatitis is endemic in Mexico, Central and northern South America, and Ossabaw Island in Georgia USA. In the US (excluding Ossabaw Island) the disease occurs sporadically. Outbreaks in the USA have a seasonal pattern with most occurring initially during the early summer and ending with the first frost although during some outbreaks cases are identified into winter and early spring. There have been 5 outbreaks of VSV that occurred from 1995–2005, and depending on the given year, these occurred in livestock in the states of Arizona, Colorado, Idaho, Montana, Nebraska, New Mexico, Texas, Utah and/or Wyoming (Anon (2007). New Mexico and Colorado had VS cases in each of the 5 outbreaks occurring from 1995–2005 (Anon 2007). The outbreak that occurred in 2005 was the largest in the decade 1995–2005 based on both the number of premises affected and the number of states with premises impacted, 445 premises and 9 states in all (Anon 2007).

Epidemiological data including seasonality and geographic area for disease occurrence suggest that an insect vector plays a role in the transmission of VSV. Many insect species have been proposed as potential vectors of VSV. *Simulium* spp. (black flies) and *Lutzymoia* spp. (sand flies) can acquire VSV through a blood meal, support biological reproduction of the virus in the gut and transmit the virus to new hosts (**Fig 7**) (Cupp *et al.* 1992; Comer *et al.* 1993) In endemic areas for VS, rodents are thought to be the reservoir host. No mechanism for persistence or latency has been determined for VSV.

The VSV is also thought to be transmitted by direct contact with lesions on infected animals, through contaminated fomites or saliva of infected animals. Transmission may be more efficient if the mucous membranes are traumatised because of consumption of rough forage. Mechanical transmission of VSV can occur through contact with insect vectors such as nonhaematophagous flies.

Diagnosis

Vesicular stomatitis due to infection with VSV can not be definitively diagnosed based on clinical signs and history alone. Laboratory testing is necessary to confirm VSV infection as the cause of the clinical disease. In most states in the USA there is mandatory reporting of the occurrence of vesicular or ulcerative stomatitis or coronitis in livestock as it is considered a potential foreign animal disease (FAD). The report of a potential FAD (vesicular or ulcerative disease) by the private veterinarian who examines the animal initiates standardised investigation procedures by animal health officials. Early and frequent discussion between private veterinary practitioners and animal health officials are encouraged in order to avoid delays in response to an FAD.

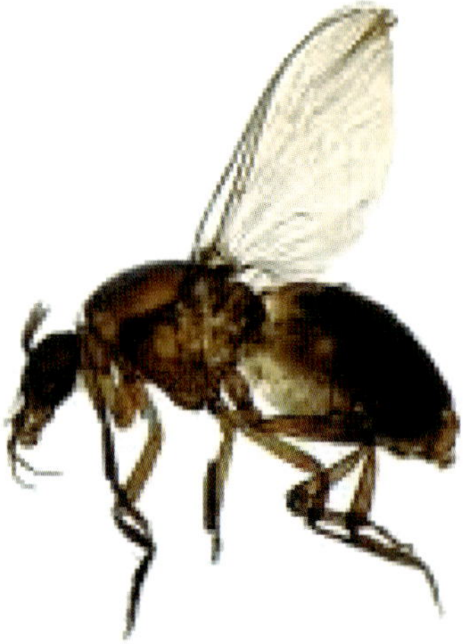

FIGURE 7: Black flies, Simulidae spp. and Sand flies, Lutzyomia spp. (not pictured) are proven arthropod vectors of vesicular stomatitis viruses. Many other arthropods are proposed to be either biological or mechanical vectors of the virus.

Diagnosis of VSV infection can be made through serological testing, virus isolation or detection of genetic material by molecular techniques. All investigative procedures conducted by the Foreign Animal Disease Diagnostician (FADD) are done at no charge to the owner or private veterinary practitioner. The FADD will collect appropriate samples and submit them for testing.

Several serological tests are available for detection of serum antibodies to VSV. The competitive enzyme-linked immunosorbent assay (cELISA) is often used as the screening test (Schmitt 2000). A capture ELISA test that detects IgM class antibodies (mcELISA) facilitates detection of recent exposure to VSV (Vernon and Webb 1985). There is also a complement fixation test (CFT), with samples with detectable antibody at greater than 1:40 dilution considered positive. The current serological diagnostic testing scheme employed during VS outbreaks in the USA is to screen samples with the cELISA for both serotypes of VSV then confirm any cELISA positive sample by the CFT and virus neutralisation test. Swabs or tissue from fresh lesions are ideal for virus isolation. VSV is easily propagated on various cell lines but testing of clinical equine cases often results in negative findings on virus isolation. This may be the result of detection of disease in horses occurring after active virus infection has occurred. The detection of genomic sequences of VSV maybe used to identify the presence of virus in tissue or swab samples. Various polymerase chain reaction (PCR) tests to detect VSV in biological samples has been used on a research basis (McCluskey 2007).

Treatment

There is no specific treatment for VS in horses. The disease is typically short lived and self limiting. Supportive care with provision of palatable soft feed is adequate in most horses with VS. If dehydration occurs then i.v. fluid treatment maybe required. Rinsing of oral ulcerative lesions with mild antiseptic solutions may reduce the occurrence of secondary bacterial infections in the lesions. Since VSV can infect man care should be taken to wear eye protection and use barrier precautions when treating ulcerative lesions in affected horses.

Implementation of biosecurity practices to limit spread of the virus is indicated. Wearing of disposable examination gloves when working with affected horses followed by hand washing is indicated. Restriction of movement of affected horses and herd mates is important in control of spread of the disease and mandatory quarantine will be placed on confirmed affected premises by animal health officials.

Prevention

There are currently no licensed commercially available vaccines for the control of VSV infections in the USA. Stopping movement of livestock from premises with confirmed VSV infection is routine in the western states in order to control spread of the virus through direct contact. There have been retrospective studies that suggest that protecting horses from insect exposure during outbreaks of VS may reduce the risk of clinical disease (Duarte *et al.* 2008). Options to reduce risk of inesct exposure include housing horses in the evening and regular application of insect repellants to the horse including to the inner surface of the pinna of the ear (location where blackflies may feed). During years when outbreaks of VS occur, requirements for a certificate of veterinary inspection and examination of horses entering equine events or new entries to a premises may reduce the risk of introduction of VSV into a facility.

References

Anon (2007) USDA:APHIS:VS:CEAH, Equine 2005 Part II: Changes in the U.S. Equine Industry, 1998-2005. #N452.037, http://nahms. aphis.usda.gov, Accessed 22nd July 2008.

Bridges, V.E., McCluskey, B.J., Salman, M.D., Hurd, H.S. and Dick, J. (1997) Review of the 1995 vesicular stomatitis outbreak in the western United States. *J. Am. vet. med. Ass.* **211**, 556-560.

Comer, J.A., Kavanaugh, D.M., Stallknecht, D.E., Ware, G.O., Corn, J.L. and Nettles, V.F. (1993) Effect of forest type on the distribution of *Lutzomyia shannoni* (Diptera: Psychodidae) and vesicular stomatitis virus on Ossabaw Island, Georgia. *J. med. Entomol.* **30**, 555-560.

Cupp, E.W., Mare, C.J. and Cupp, M.S. (1992) Biological transmission of vesicular stomatitis virus (New Jersey) by *Simulium vittatum* (Diptera: *Simuliidae*). *J. med. Entomol.* **29**, 137-140.

Duarte, P.C., Morley, P.S., Traub-Dargatz, J.L. and Creekmore, L.H. (2008) Factors associated with vesicular stomatitis in animals in the western United States. *J. Am. vet. med. Ass.* **232**, 249-256.

Knight, A.P. and Messer, N.T. (1983) Vesicular stomatitis. *Comp. cont. Educ. pract. vet.* **5**, 517-522.

McCluskey, B.J. (2007) Vesicular stomatitis. In: *Equine Infectious Diseases,* Eds: D.C. Sellon and M.T. Long, Saunders Elsevier, St Louis. pp 219-232.

McCluskey, B.J. and Mumford, E.L. (2000) Vesicular stomatitis and other erosive and ulcerative diseases of horses. *Vet. Clin. N. Am: Equine Pract.* **16**, 457-469.

McCluskey, B.J., Hurd, H.S. and Mumford, E.L. (1999) Review of the 1997 outbreak of vesicular stomatitis in the western United States. *J. Am. vet. med. Ass.* **215**, 1259-1262.

O'Neil, B. (1998) Balclutha horse syndrome. Promed Web site Available at http://www.promedmail.org/pls/otn/ f?p=2400: 1202:3644491752354723::NO::F2400_P1202_CHECK_DISPLAY, F2400_P1202_PUB_MAIL_ID:X,6136, Archive number 19980319. 0523, Accessed 22nd July 2008.

Reif, J.S. (1994) Vesicular stomatitis, In: *Handbook of Zoonoses*, Ed: G. Beran, CRC Press, Boca Raton.

Sahu, S.P., Landgraf, J., Wineland, N., Pedersen, D., Alstad, D. and Gustafson, G. (1999) Isolation of Jamestown Canyon virus (California virus group) from vesicular lesions of a horse. *J. vet. diag. Invest.* **12**, 80-83.

Schmitt, B. (2000) Vesicular stomatitis, In: *OIE Manual of Standards for Diagnostic Test and Vaccines*, 4th edn. pp 93-99.

Sellon, D.C. (2007) Miscellaneous parasitic diseases. In: *Equine Infectious Diseases,* Eds: D.C. Sellon and M.T. Long, Saunders Elsevier, St Louis. 473-480.

Vernon, S.D. and Webb, P.A. (1985) Recent vesicular stomatitis virus infection detected by immunoglobulin M antibody capture enzyme-linked immunosorbent assay. *J. Clin. Microbiol.* **22**, 582-586.

ROTAVIRUS

N. M. Slovis

Hagyard Equine Medical Institute, Lexington, Kentucky, USA.

Keywords: horse; equine rotavirus; colic; diarrhoea; disinfection

Summary

Viral gastroenteritis is an important cause of disease among foals worldwide. Since their identification as an equine pathogen in 1975, rotaviruses have been found to be the most important cause of gastroenteritis in equine neonates and foals worldwide.

Transmission occurs directly by animal to animal and indirectly through personnel and fomites. Clearly infected foals shed virus in high concentration at the onset of disease and continue for an average of 3 days after return of normal faeces. Routine diagnosis is universally based on identification of rotavirus in faeces or suspensions of rectal swabs. The cornerstone of therapy for rotavirus-induced diarrhoea is replacement of fluids and electrolytes lost during infection.

Introduction

Viral gastroenteritis is an important cause of disease among foals. Since their identification as an equine pathogen in 1975 (Flewett *et al.* 1980), rotaviruses have been found to be the most important cause of gastroenteritis in equine neonates and foals worldwide (Dwyer *et al.* 1990; Browning *et al.* 1996; Powell *et al.* 1997).

Description of virus

Rotavirus is a genus within the family Reoviridae (Bellamy *et al.* 1990). By electron microscopy, the viruses are noted to be about 70–80 nm in size and look like wheels (rota is derived from the latin word 'wheel') with short spokes radiating from a wide central hub. Rotaviruses are all double stranded, ribonucleic acid (RNA), nonenveloped viruses. Rotavirus is subdivided into several groups (A–G) based on differences in the group specific inner capsid protein, VP6. There are 3 rotavirus groups (A, B and C) that cause human disease (Estes and Cohen 1989) compared to only one group that affects the equine species (Group A). Equine rotavirus can be further subdivided using neutralising antibodies to the VP4 and VP7 outer capsid proteins into P (proteinase sensitive, VP4 positive) and G (Glycoprotein, VP-7 positive) serotypes (Wilson *et al.* 2009). Five P serotypes (P1, P6, P7, P12 and P18) and 8 G serotypes (G1, G3, G5, G8, G10, G13, G14 and G16) have been identified in horses (Wilson *et al.* 2009). The most prevalent equine rotavirus isolated from most parts of the world are of the P12 and G3 serotype in the serogroup A (Powell *et al.* 1997).

Epidemiology

As determined by antibody prevalence studies of more than 400 adult horses in Kentucky, Japan and Argentina, almost all of the horses were exposed to rotavirus (Dwyer 2007). However, equine rotavirus only affects foals clinically, and is considered species specific. These studies were conducted in concentrated horse breeding regions, and therefore the true seroprevalence in adult horses in other regions of the world may be less. In man, the antibody prevalence in serum throughout the world indicates that almost all children are infected with rotavirus within their first 3 years (Yolken *et al.* 1978; Urasawa *et al.* 1984). The exposure rate in equine foals is currently unknown.

The basic questions of epidemiology for rotavirus disease – explanations for the age of susceptibility and reservoir host – remain largely unsolved. Foals are most susceptible to viral diarrhoeas during the neonatal, perinatal and suckling periods by virtue of being immunological naïve. Clinical disease has been reported only among foals aged <6 months and most often among foals aged <3 months (Browning *et al.* 1996; Powell *et al.* 1997; Dwyer 2007). However, clinical disease, sometimes severe can occur in foals aged <1 month. The onset of maximum susceptibility is probably correlated with the decline of acquired maternal antibodies. Serum immunoglobulin G (IgG) of maternal origin tends to disappear between ages 3 and 4 months. However, there is no clear correlation between decline of maternally acquired serum antibodies and onset of susceptibility. Despite acquiring appropriate maternal antibodies severe rotavirus disease is not uncommon in newborn foals and those aged <1 month.

The mode of transmission of rotavirus infection is assumed to be primarily faecal-oral route with an incubation period of 1–2 days (Conner and Darlington 1980; Connor 1983; Dwyer 2007). Transmission occurs directly by animal to animal, and indirectly through personnel and fomites. Clearly infected foals shed virus in high concentration at the onset of disease and continue for an average of 3 days after return of normal faeces (Dwyer 2007). In our hospital population the average duration of diarrhoea in infected foals is 3–5 days.

Rotavirus outbreaks have been demonstrated in central Kentucky foaling barns that had no animal traffic for months before the arrival of newborn foals. As soon as the newborn foals arrive severe gastroenteritis secondary to rotavirus can be diagnosed. The reservoir for the persistence of rotavirus in the herd is unknown. Studies of more than 400 adult horses in Kentucky, Japan and Argentina revealed a seroprevalence rate in broodmares approaching 100% (Dwyer 2007). It is possible that healthy adult horses shed the virus chronically in low numbers. This has been determined to be the case for cattle and swine (Banfield *et al.* 1982; Goto *et al.* 1986). Older immune foals have been documented in our clinic to be shedding rotavirus sub-clinically. This could also lead to the contamination of the environment. The minimal infectious dose for the foal is currently unknown, but volunteer studies have indicated that the human infectious dose may be >1 plaque forming unit (Ward *et al.* 1986). Rotavirus virus can remain viable for up to 9 months at room temperature (Conner and Darlington 1980). It is therefore plausible that inappropriate cleaning and disinfecting of the premises permitted a build up of the infective dose in the environment and that problems arose when the dose of virus exceeded the protective capacity of colostral antibodies.

Pathogenesis

Rotavirus replicates in mature villous epithelial cells that line the small intestine. Rotavirus outer capsid protein vp4 (cleaved in the presence of trypsin) attaches to glycolipids on the host cell surface and enters the cytoplasm by direct plasma membrane penetration (Offit and Clark 2000). This results in blunting of the villi and subsequent villous atrophy. The loss of the villi results in the loss of important disaccharidases, especially lactase. Lactase is responsible for the digestion of disaccharides (lactose) to monosaccharides (glucose and galactose). Lactose remains in the gastrointestinal tract and is readily fermented in the large colon into the following volatile fatty acids: acetate, butyrate and propionate. This fermentation cycle results in a hyperosmotic solution leading to acute diarrhoea. Rotavirus-induced lactase deficiency may last up to 10–14 days (Hyams *et al.* 1981). Subsequent to the villous atrophy, malabsorption and maldigestion of nutrients will also potentiate the diarrhoea. Intestinal crypt cells are not affected and therefore can replicate and eventually replace the villi brush border destroyed by the virus resulting in a self limiting disease. Chronic diarrhoea is not typical of rotavirus infection. If chronic diarrhoea is noted then a secondary intestinal pathogen should be investigated.

Clinical manifestations

Clinical signs of rotaviral diarrhoea are similar to those of other infectious diarrhoeas, with a wide range

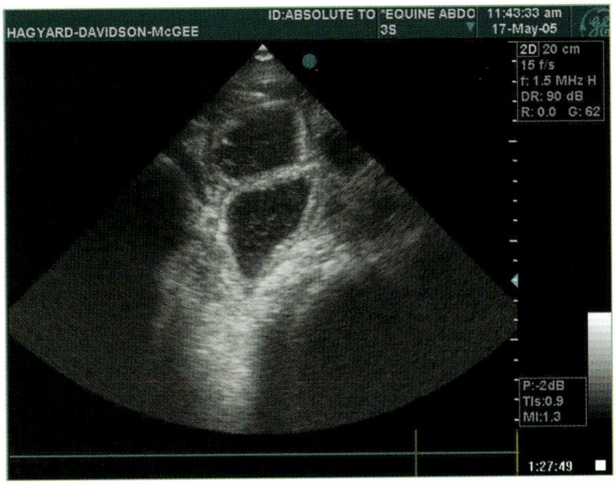

FIGURE 1: Ultrasonographic examination of the abdomen revealing marked distention of the small intestine with poor motility.

from mild diarrhoea to severe watery diarrhoea and dehydration. A foal of any age can be affected, with the younger foal usually being more severely affected. Fevers may or may not be present. Marked bloating maybe noted with an ileus resulting in gastric reflux. The colic signs can be mild to severe depending on the amount of colonic bloating (secondary to fermentation of disaccharides in the hindgut). Colic signs can mimic a surgical lesion therefore appropriate diagnostics (abdominal ultrasound, faecal rotavirus testing etc.) should be pursued before an exploratory celiotomy is warranted.

Abdominal ultrasonography may reveal distended small intestine 2–3 cm in diameter with evidence of poor motility (**Fig 1**). Motility will be present but decreased unlike a small intestinal volvulus in which the small intestine would typically be markedly distended with no evidence of motility. Rarely would the small intestine have serosal oedema (>3 mm thickness). Colonic sonographic findings would include marked fluid distention of the caecum and colon with poor motility.

Electrolyte imbalances may include hyponatraemia, hypochloraemia, hypokalaemia and

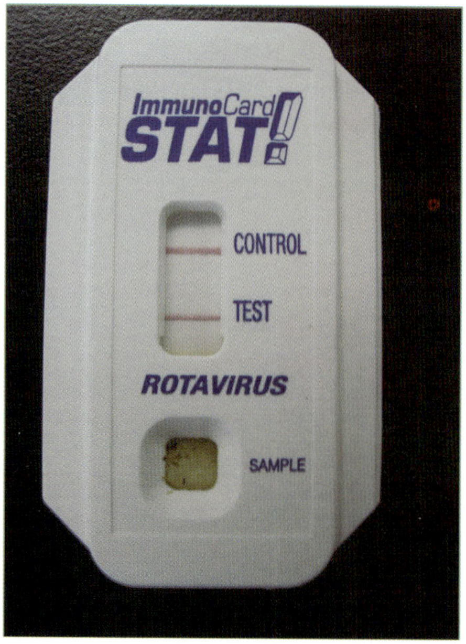

FIGURE 2: Enzyme Linked immunosorbent assay (Immunocard) for the detection of rotavirus. This can be used as a stall side kit with test results in 10–15 min.

metabolic acidosis with a haemogram that is often normal or haemoconcentrated.

Some clinicians have suggested an association between gastroduodenal ulcer syndrome/stenosis and rotavirus, although more studies are needed.

Mortality is relatively low in rotavirus infections. Morbidity, however, can approach 100% in outbreak situations (Conner and Darlington 1980; Dwyer *et al.* 1990). Foals aged <2 weeks are more at risk of death secondary to metabolic derangements and dehydration. The infection produces little inflammatory response of the surrounding tissue; therefore there are no pathognomic lesions noted on histopathology.

Diagnosis

Although rotavirus is by far the most common cause of severe dehydrating diarrhoea in foals, there are no pathognomonic clinical manifestations. Routine diagnosis is universally based on identification of rotavirus in faeces or suspensions of rectal swabs.

The original 'gold standard' test of electron microscopy is not routinely available and has almost been completely replaced by an enzyme linked immunosorbent assay (ELISA). The ELISA (Immunocard Stat)[1] is based on capture antibodies that are primarily directed against the core protein VP6 (antigenically conserved among group A rotavirus strains) (**Fig 2**). Since equine rotavirus is among the group A strains, the use of human test kits would be appropriate for testing equine faeces. The sensitivity of ELISA is equal to that of electron microscopy in both human and bovine patients (Brandt *et al.* 1981; Rubenstein *et al.* 1982; Maes *et al.* 2003). These assays yield results within 10 min. Serology for diagnostic purposes in foals is unreliable (Dwyer 2007). A Rotavirus faecal PCR assay[2] has recently been developed for genes specific to the VP4 and VP7 outer capsid proteins.

Latex agglutination kits have been produced to deliver rapid results within minutes of testing. These tests have a high degree of specificity but somewhat less sensitivity than alternative methods (Sanders *et al.* 1986).

For patients with severe watery diarrhoea, a single negative test result will not be conclusive of the absence of rotavirus infection. Therefore it has been recommended by some authors (Dwyer 2007) that a minimum of 3 negative tests would be warranted to be confident in stating that a foal does not have rotavirus.

Treatment

The cornerstone of therapy for rotavirus-induced diarrhoea is replacement of fluids and electrolytes lost during infection. Isotonic fluid therapy to correct electrolyte imbalances is especially important in young foals and those that are significantly dehydrated.

The initial formulation of a fluid plan should be based on careful clinical examination of the patient and laboratory parameters (**Table 1**).

It is important to bear in mind that many other factors including the disease process in question may affect many of the laboratory parameters.

The initial fluid plan is often formulated based on many subjective factors. However, the keyword is 'initial'; after fluid therapy has started the foal should be reassessed and the plan restructured if required. Blood work may also be repeated after initial fluids have been administered.

The 'rough guide' to fluid therapy

- Water deficit (l) = percentage dehydration x bodyweight (kg). Thus a 10% dehydrated 50 kg foal will have a fluid deficit of 5 l.
  - Foals that present with severe diarrhoea may require 1.5–3 x maintenance fluid requirements.
- Maintenance fluid requirement of a newborn foal is 80–120 ml/kg bwt/day.
  - Maintenance for a foal aged >1 month is 45–60 ml/kg bwt/day.
- Young foals that present without significant reported or detected acid-base or electrolyte abnormalities and mild to moderate dehydration (5–10%) will usually receive an initial 1 l of crystalloid fluid such as lactated Ringers' or normosol, over 1 h and then be reassessed.
- Any neonatal foal that is not nursing should receive fluid therapy. A 'wait and see' policy will not work!
- The initial fluid replacement will in many cases improve attitude and appetence. A foal that may not have been nursing on arrival may start to do so leading to correction of some of its fluid deficit. Most foals if still nursing will not require having its entire deficit replaced by i.v. fluids. In fact doing so may lead to overhydration, which, in compromised foals, could result in generalised oedema.
- Normal saline (0.9% NaCl) is indicated for hyperkalaemia, hyponatraemia, hypochloraemia and metabolic alkalosis. It is not usually used as a maintenance fluid.
- Dextrose (5%) is often added to other fluid types and such fluids should be used in cases of hypoglycaemia or hyperkalaemia.
- Hypertonic saline (7% NaCl) can be used in cases of hypovolaemic/hypotensive shock at a dose of 2–4 ml/kg bwt. However, it must be rapidly followed by either oral administration of fluids or combined oral and i.v. fluid administration. The administration of hypertonic saline should be carefully considered in neonates as many of the contraindications for its use such as seizures, hypernatraemia, hypokalaemia, renal failure and thrombocytopenia may be encountered. It should be considered for situations where rapid stabilisation of the cardiovascular system is required and where failure to do so is likely to result in death.
- Colloids are substances with a large molecular weight that remain restricted to the plasma compartment after administration. Plasma and Hetastarch (10 ml/kg bwt i.v.) are the most frequently administered colloids in equine medicine. Plasma has the added benefit of providing immunoglobulins.

TABLE 1: Factors used to determine dehydration

Dehydration (%)	Skin tent (seconds)	Mucous membrane moisture	Capillary refill time (s)	Packed cell volume (%)	Total protein (g/l)
5	2–3	Moist	1–2	32–40	65–70
10	3–5	Sticky	2–4	36–48	70–75
15	>5	Dry	>4	>48	>75

- When considering a fluid plan the type of disease process involved and the continued losses should be taken into account. The most important example of such in neonates is the foal with severe diarrhoea. Commonly these foals cannot tolerate oral administration of fluids and have high fluid losses.

Administration of bicarbonate:

1) Severe diarrhoea results in metabolic acidosis form a loss of bicarbonate ions and lactic acidosis as a result of poor perfusion. Bicarbonate therapy is indicated when pH<7.2 or the base deficit is >10 mEq/l.
2) Calculation of bicarbonate deficit: bodyweight (kg) x 0.6 (ECF) x deficit (normal = 25 mEq/l)
3) Calculation of the base deficit should be part of the daily laboratory assessment of critically ill foals and foals with diarrhoea. In less than ideal situations where daily measurement is not possible due to a lack of laboratory facilities or a remote location, a significant base deficit should be suspected in foals that are hyperventilating. However, bicarbonate administration should be based on the calculated deficit as overzealous administration can lead to metabolic alkalosis.
4) Commercially available preparations are hypertonic (5% $NaHCO_3$, 8.4% $NaHCO_3$) and must be diluted prior to administration. To make isotonic $NaHCO_3$ (1.3%) add 260 ml of 5% $NaHCO_3$ or 154 ml of 8.4% $NaHCO_3$ to 1 l of sterile water. If adding bicarbonate to other fluids carefully calculate the mEqs of sodium that will be in the final mixture as it is easy to induce hypernatraemia, which may prove difficult to correct.
5) TCO_2 may be used to estimate HCO_3. Generally, HCO_3 is 1–2 mEq/l<TCO_2.
6) Do not use bicarbonate in solutions containing calcium because an insoluble calcium carbonate precipitate will form.
7) Administer 25–33% of the calculated deficit over 30 min, then re-evaluate or administer the remainder slowly over 12–24 h. If respiratory compromise is present, administer 25–33% over a period of 50 min.
8) Monitor blood gases if you administer >1–2 mEq/kg bwt over a short period.

TABLE 2: Administration rates of partial parenteral feed to provide total energy requirement (TER)

% TER	ml/day	ml/h
33%	1200	50
66%	2400	100
100%	3600	150

Severely affected foals with ileus and bloating usually require feed restriction and partial parenteral (PN) feeding. Foals with severe lactose intolerance may require feed restriction for 2–5 days. A 'home made' partial parenteral solution ideal for gastroenteritis can be compounded from 50% dextrose (1000 ml), 20% lipid (500 ml) and 10% amino acids (2000 ml).

Strict aseptic technique is required during preparation. Dextrose and amino acids are mixed first, followed by the lipid to minimise lipid demulsification. A batch is split in half and divided between 2 separate fluid bags. The first bag is used immediately while the other can be refrigerated for 48 h. The total energy requirement (TER) of a sick 50 kg foal is estimated to be 200–300 kJ/kg bwt/day. The rates of administration for this solution are shown in **Table 2**.

The protocol the author prefers for the administration of PN is to start at 33% of TER for the first 6 h, followed by an increase of 33% over a further 8 h and, if 100% TER is desired, then increase of 33% over a further 8 h so that the desired rate is achieved within 24 h. Blood glucose measurements should be performed every 4–6 h and be within the reference range of 0.8–1.8 g/l. If values fall outside this range adjustments in the rate or percentage of dextrose content can be made. A measurement of serum triglycerides and ammonia is especially important in foals that are endotoxaemic and should be checked daily for the first 2 days to assess tolerance of amino acid and lipid component. Parenteral nutrition should not be withdrawn quickly, but should be tapered over 24–36 h.

Foals that are bloated may be administered neostigmine at a dose of 1–2 mg subcutaneously every 1–2 h for 2–3 doses and then 4x daily thereafter. There may be a transient increase in colic signs following administration of neostigmine.

It is not uncommon for foals to present with severe colic signs secondary to rotavirus diarrhoea.

Pain may be controlled with nonsteroidal anti-inflammatory medications such as flunixin meglumine (1.1 mg/kg bwt i.v. q. 12–24 h) or butorphanol (0.02–0.04 mg/kg bwt i.v. q. 4–6 h).

Some clinicians have associated an increase risk of perforating stomach ulcers, duodenal ulceration and stricture in foals that had rotavirus diarrhoea. Prophylactic treatment with proton pump inhibitors such as omeprazole (1–4 mg/kg bwt *per os* s.i.d.) is usually implemented. Other antiulcer medications including i.v. H2 blockers such as ranitidine (1.4 mg/kg bwt i.v. q. 8 h) may be used in foals that cannot tolerate enteral medications. Sucralfate (20 mg/kg *per os* t.i.d. to q.i.d.) can also be used with other gastroprotectants to aid in the prevention of GI ulceration.

Nitazoxanide (Navigator)[2], an FDA approved EPM treatment in the USA, has recently been shown to significantly reduce the duration of rotavirus in hospitalised human paediatric patients (Rossignol *et al.* 2006). Nitazoxanide, a nitrothiazolide, successfully treats infestation by internal parasites and is approved in the USA and UK to treat cryptosporidiosis and giardiasis in man. *In vitro* studies have shown that nitazoxanide inhibits replication of a broad range of viruses including rotavirus, hepatitis B and C. Nitazoxanide (7.5 mg/kg bwt *per os* b.i.d.) given to human pediatric patients (5 months to 7 years: Median age was 11 months) in a randomised double-blind, placebo controlled clinical trial showed that times from first dose to reduction of illness were significantly less for nitazoxanide treated patients than for patients in the placebo group. No significant adverse events were noted. Preliminary findings suggest that tizoxanide (active metabolite of nitazoxanide) has a selective effect on the syntheses of rotavirus structural proteins. In our clinic we have used nitazoxanide at a dose of 25 mg/kg bwt *per os* s.i.d. as an adjunctive treatment for foals with rotavirus. We have treated over 100 foals with nitazoxanide at farms where an outbreak of rotavirus was actively occurring. Subjectively, the patients that received nitazoxanide had a quicker resolution of illness. No adverse affects were noted. It is not known if prophylactic treatment with nitazoxanide could help prevent the 'spread' of rotavirus. Clinical trials in the horse need to be conducted in a larger number of patients to confirm that nitazoxanide is efficacious in the management of rotavirus.

Prevention

Rotavirus has been demonstrated to be one of the most common causes for diarrhoea in foals around the world. Even though mortality is relatively low the morbidity can be high. The prevalence of rotavirus morbidity indicates that an effective vaccine against rotavirus disease would be cost effective. Since 1996, the Equine Rotavirus Vaccine[3] has had a conditional US Department of Agriculture license. The vaccine contains an inactivated strain of the serogroup A serotype P12, G3 equine rotavirus (metabolisable oil in water adjuvant) (Powell *et al.* 1997) that is indicated for the administration to pregnant mares in endemic areas to aid in the prevention of diarrhoea in their foals. Foal vaccination is not indicated because currently there are no data to suggest that vaccination of the newborn foal with an inactivated rotavirus vaccine elicits an appropriate immune response (Wilson *et al.* 2009). The label recommendation requires a 3-dose series of the vaccine to be administered to mares during each pregnancy at 8, 9 and 10 months of gestation. This protocol has been shown to induce significant increases in serum concentrations of neutralising antibodies in vaccinated mares and in the concentrations of antibodies of the IgG, but not IgA subclass in the colostrum and milk (Powell *et al.* 1997). Passive transfer of rotavirus specific antibody of the IgG subclass persisted for up to age 90 days, which was considered significantly higher than that measured in serum of foals born to unvaccinated mares (Powell *et al.* 1997). A field study showed this vaccine to be safe when administered to pregnant mares and provided circumstantial evidence of at least partial efficacy. An approximately 2-fold higher incidence of rotaviral diarrhoea was found in foals from unvaccinated mares compared with the vaccinated mares, but the difference was not significant. The foals that had absorbed colostrum from vaccinated mares were also noted to have a reduction in severity of clinical signs (Powell *et al.* 1997; Barrandeguy *et al.* 1998). The major correlate for protection against rotaviral infection appears to be mucosal immunity, predominantly mucosal IgA, in the GI tract. Current studies have concluded that the inactivated vaccine available is unlikely to provide foals with intestinal protection in the form of IgA. Therefore these foals must rely on the transudation of maternally derived IgG from serum into the intestine to prevent or overcome infection and diarrhoea. Consequently it is not surprising that current protocols may not provide complete protection. The vaccine has been safely used in thousands of mares in Kentucky, Florida, Newmarket (UK) and Ireland. Even though the conditional licensed vaccine available in the USA contains only the P12, G3 serotype of the A serogroup, it appears to reduce the incidence and severity of rotaviral diarrhoea (Wilson *et al.* 2009).

If a farm has an outbreak of rotaviral diarrhoea in their foaling units, then mares that are expected to foal should have access to deliver their newborns elsewhere. In central Kentucky we have been able to stop rotaviral diarrhoea in young foals by foaling outside in paddocks or round pens. This outside delivery is continued until the foaling barn has been thoroughly cleaned and disinfected.

Disinfecting equipment

Rotavirus is a nonenveloped virus that is naturally very resistant to disinfectants. The phenol disinfectants (Tek-Trol[4] and One Stroke Environ[5]), however, are the only commercially available disinfectants to be recognised by the US Environmental Protection Agency to be virucidal against equine rotavirus tested in a 10% organic material and 1000 ppm water hardness (calcium carbonate). Oxidising agents such as Virkon S[5] as a 1% solution was determined in the presence of 400 ppm water hardness and 5% organic material to be effective against bovine rotavirus. It can therefore be inferred that these oxidising agents may be efficacious as a disinfectant against equine rotavirus, but further studies would be warranted. Bleach is not considered efficacious against rotavirus. Pressure washing should not be used in a barn or stable with potential rotavirus infection because of the risk of aerosolisation of pathogens into the rafters. Improper stall cleaning techniques can result in rotavirus surviving for months in the environment (Dwyer 2007). Therefore manure and bedding from stalls of affected foals should be considered infectious and not be spread out on the pastures. The bedding should be disposed of away from horses or composted. Rotaviruses are excreted from diarrhoeic foals in large quantities (1011 particles/g) (Dwyer 2007), which can easily contaminate not only the environment but the hands of caregivers. Hand hygiene (wearing gloves and washing hands) is critical for disease prevention.

Manufacturers' addresses

[1]Meridian Bioscience, Inc., Cincinnati, Ohio, USA.
[2]Idexx Laboratories, Westbrook, Maine, USA.
[3]Fort Dodge Animal Health, Fort Dodge, Iowa, USA.
[4]Tek-Trol Bio-Tek Industries Inc, Atlanta, Georgia, USA.
[5]Steris corporation, St Louis, Missouri, USA.

References

Banfield, D.A., Stotz, I. and Moore, R. (1982) Shedding of rotavirus in feces of sows before and after farrowing. *J. clin. Microbiol.* **16**, 186-190.

Barrandeguy, M., Parreno, V., Marmol, M., Pont, L.F., Rivas, C., Valle, C. and Fernandez, F. (1998) Prevention of rotavirus diarrhoea in foals by parenteral vaccination of the mares: field trial. *Dev. Biol. Stand.* **92**, 253-257.

Bellamy, R. and Both, G. (1990) Molecular biology of rotaviruses. *Adv. Virus Res.* **38**, 1-43.

Brandt, C.D., Kim, H.W. and Rodriguez, W.J. (1981) Comparison of Direct electron microscopy, immune electron microscopy and rotavirus enzyme-linked immunosorbent assay for detection of gastroenteritis viruses in children. *J. clin. Microbiol.* **13**, 976-981.

Browning, G.F. (1996) Equine rotavirus infections. In: *Virus Infections of Equines*, Ed: M.J. Studdert, Elsevier, Amersterdam. pp 127-135.

Conner, M.E. (1983) Detection of rotavirus in horses with and without diarrhoea with electron microscopy and rotazyme test. *Cornell Vet.* **73**, 280-287.

Conner, M.E. and Darlington, R.W. (1980) Rotavirus infection in foals. *Am. J. vet. Res.* **41**, 1699-1703.

Dwyer, R.M., Powell, D.G. and Roberts, A. (1990) A study of the etiology and control of infectious diarrhoea among foals in central Kentucky. *Proc. Am. Ass. equine Practnrs.* **36**, 335-337.

Dwyer, R.M. (2007) Equine rotavirus. In: *Equine Infectious Diseases*, Eds: D. Sellon and M. Long, Elsevier, St Louis. pp 181-183.

Estes, M. and Cohen, J. (1989) Rotavirus gene structure and function. *Microbiol. Rev.* **53**, 410-449.

Flewett, T.H., Bryden, A.S. and Davies, H. (1980) Virus diarrhoea in foals and other animals. *Vet. Rec.* **96**, 477.

Goto, Y., Kurogi, H. and Inaba, Y. (1986) Sequential isolation of rotavirus from individual calves. *Vet. Microbiol.* **11**, 177-184.

Hyams, J., Krause, P. and Gleason, P. (1981) Lactose malabsorption following rotavirus infection in young children. *J. pediatric.* **99**, 916-918.

Maes, R.K., Grooms, D.L., Wise, A.G., Han, C., Ciesicki, V., Hanson, L., Vickers, M.L., Kanitz, C. and Holland, R. (2003) Evaluation of a human group A rotavirus assay for on-site detection of bovine rotavirus. *J. clin. Microbiol.* **41**, 290-294.

Offit, P.A. and Clark, H.R. (2000) Rotavirus. In: *Principles and Practice of Infectious Disease,* 5th edn.. Eds: G.L. Mandell, J.E. Bennett and R. Dolin, Churchill-Livingstone, Philadelphia. pp 1696-1701.

Powell, D.G., Dwyer, R.M., Traub-Dargatz, J.L. Fulker, R.H., Whalen, J.W. Jr, Srinivasappa, J., Acree, W.M. and Chu, H.J.

(1997) Field study of the safety, immunogenicity, and efficacy of an inactivated equine rotavirus vaccine. *J. Am. vet. med. Ass.* **211**, 193-198.

Rossignol, J.F., Abu-Zekry, M., Hussein, A. and Santoro, M.G. (2006) Effect of nitazoxanide for treatment of severe rotavirus diarrhoea: Randomised double-blind placebo-controlled trial. *Lancet* **368**, 124-129.

Rubenstein, A.S. and Miller, M.F. (1982) Comparison of enzyme immunoassay with electron microscopy procedures for detecting rotavirus. *J. clin. Microbiol.* **15**, 938-944.

Sanders, R.C., Campbell, A.D. and Jenkins, A.F. (1986) Routine detection of human rotavirus by latex agglutination: Comparison with latex agglutination, electron microscopy and polyacrylamide gel electrophoresis. *J. Virol Methods.* **13**, 285-290.

Urasawa, S., Urasawa, T., Taniguchi, K. and Chiba, S. (1984) Serotype determination of human rotavirus isolates and antibody prevalence of pediatric population in Hokkaido. *Japan Arch. Virol.* **81**, 1-12.

Ward, R., Bernstein, D. and Young, E. (1986) Human Rotavirus studies in volunteers: Determination of Infectious dose and serological response to infection. *J. Infect. Dis.* **154**, 871-880

Wilson, W.D., East, N., Rowe, J.D. and Cortese, V.S. (2009) Use of biologics in the prevention of infectious diseases. In: *Large Animal Internal Medicine*, Ed: B.P. Smith, Mosby, St Louis. p 1586.

Yolken, R., Wyatt, R., Zissis, G., Brandt, C.D., Rodriguez, W.J., Kim, H.W., Parrott, R.H., Urrutia, J.J., Mata, L., Greenberg, H.B., Kapikian, A.Z. and Chanock, R.M. (1978) Epidemiology of human rotavirus types 1 and 2 as studied by enzyme-linked immunosorbent assay. *New Engl. J. Med.* **299**, 1156-1161.

HENDRA VIRUS

J. R. Gilkerson

Equine Infectious Disease Laboratory, Faculty of Veterinary Science, The University of Melbourne, Australia.

Keywords: horse; Hendra virus; henipavirus; bat; flying fox; zoonosis

Summary

Hendra virus is a serious, but extremely uncommon, virus infection of horses with significant zoonotic potential. The reservoir hosts of Hendra virus are several Australian flying fox (fructivorous bat) species and to date disease has only been reported on the east coast of Australia. While the most common clinical signs reported in affected horses are acute respiratory distress and sudden death, in a recent outbreak the index and several subsequent cases showed signs of central nervous system disease. It is not currently known how Hendra virus is transmitted from bats to horses, or from horses to man and no vaccine is available.

Aetiology

Hendra virus, then referred to as equine morbillivirus, was first recognised in 1994 as a cause of severe acute respiratory disease of horses with high mortality (Murray *et al.* 1995a,b). Since then, a further 8 outbreaks have been reported, in 5 of which only a single horse was affected. Hendra virus is a serious zoonotic pathogen and has been responsible for the death of 3 of the 6 known human cases. Hendra virus is closely related to Nipah virus, a cause of respiratory disease and encephalitis in pigs and man, and these 2 viruses together form the genus *Henipavirus* in the *Paramyxovirinae* sub-family of the family *Paramyxyoviridae* (Fauquet *et al.* 2005). Members of the *Henipavirus* genus are enveloped, single stranded, negative sense RNA viruses.

Epidemiology

Sero-surveillance studies and subsequent virological investigations of bats on the east coast of Australia showed that flying foxes, fruit bats of the genus *Pteropus* in the order Chiroptera, are the natural reservoir host of Hendra virus (Young *et al.* 1996; Halpin *et al.* 2000). Serological evidence of Hendra infection has been demonstrated in all 4 species of flying fox found on the Australian mainland and seroprevalence increases with age (Field *et al.* 2001, 2007). The natural distribution of these flying foxes extends the length of the east coast and across the top end of Australia to Western Australia. A number of domestic and wildlife species were tested in these studies, but only bats were seropositive (Field *et al.* 2007).

Some crucial aspects of Hendra virus epidemiology are not currently known, or are poorly understood. What is understood is that Hendra is a bat virus and that the virus circulates within bat populations, generally with no disease manifestations (Daniels *et al.* 2007). Hendra virus has been detected in fetal and neonatal lung and from uterine fluid and renal tissue of adult bats (Halpin *et al.* 2000; Williamson *et al.* 2000; Daniels *et al.* 2007). What is not currently understood is precisely how Hendra virus jumps species from bats to horses. It is also not known how Hendra virus is transmitted from horses to man, or indeed if infection of horses is necessary for human infection to occur, although all human cases to date have been linked to horse infections (**Table 1**). It is not fully understood how Hendra virus is transmitted among horses, nor whether the spread is direct or indirect, but as the 2 largest outbreaks involved housed horses it is not likely that bats played a role in transmission after the index case. Horse to horse transmission has been demonstrated experimentally, (Williamson *et al.* 1998), but this was not a reliable feature of the experiment and it is unclear how experimental challenge relates to transmission of infection in the field situation.

It is important to remember that while Hendra virus disease is extremely uncommon in horses and man, the consequences of infection in these species are dire. The case fatality rate for known cases of Hendra infection in people is 50% and 75% of horses with confirmed Hendra infection die or are subjected to euthanasia on humane grounds.

Disease

In the first recognised outbreak of Hendra virus infection of horses the primary presenting illness was acute respiratory disease characterised by high fever (up to 41°C) and severe dyspnoea. Severe respiratory distress and sudden death were the hallmarks of the first outbreak. Death occurred in the majority of affected horses within 36 h of the onset of clinical signs (Murray 1996). Hendra virus has a definite tropism for vascular endothelium, particularly the arterial endothelium (Hooper *et al.* 2001) and this explains many of the *post mortem* findings such as foam filled airways, dilated pulmonary lymphatics, severe pulmonary oedema and congestion (Daniels *et al.* 2007). In 2008 a second large outbreak of Hendra virus infection occurred in a different suburb of Brisbane, involving 5 horses in residence at a veterinary clinic. The presenting signs in this outbreak were predominantly neurological, which was not consistent with previous Hendra cases, and included depression, anorexia, ataxia with rapid deterioration resulting in euthanasia. Four of the 5 affected horses in this outbreak were subjected to euthanasia for humane reasons, with one horse recovering from the disease. This recovered horse was subjected to euthanasia for reasons of public health and safety.

Experimental studies of Hendra virus infection have, to date, not established the titre or duration of Hendra virus shedding in secretions and excretions of horses, although these experiments are being conducted currently (D. Middleton, personal communication). Concern related to possible within horse persistence of the virus comes from the fact that the first human patient known to have been infected by the virus died from viral encephalitis around 18 months after the initial infection event.

Control

There is currently no human or equine vaccine available to protect against Hendra virus infection or disease, although there is experimental evidence of protection of cats to Hendra challenge after vaccination with a Nipah virus vaccine (Mungall *et al.* 2006). Given the extremely high case-fatality rate of Hendra virus disease in horses and man extreme care should be exercised if this disease is suspected. Development of an efficacious vaccine that provides protection for people and horses against Hendra virus should be a high priority, although the small size of the likely market makes this challenging commercially.

TABLE 1: Hendra virus outbreaks 1994–2008

		Horses			Man	
Date	Location	Infected	Died+	Recovered*	Infected	Died
August 1994	Mackay, Queensland	2	2	0	1	1
September 1994	Brisbane, Queensland	20	13	7	2	1
January 1999	Cairns, Queensland	1	1	0		
November 2004	Cairns, Queensland	1	1	0	1	0
December 2004	Townsville, Queensland	1	1	0		
June 2006	Peachester, Queensland	1	1	0		
October 2006	Murwillambah, New South Wales	1	1	0		
July 2008	Brisbane, Queensland	5	4	1	2	1
July 2008	Proserpine, Queensland	3	3	0		
Total		35	27	8	6	3

+ Died or subjected to euthanasia for humane reasons. * All recovered horses were subsequently subjected to euthanasia for public health reasons.

Diagnosis

No rapid, horse-side test exists for the diagnosis of Hendra virus infection in the field. There is considerable need for the development of such a test to enable practitioners to employ appropriate personal protective equipment should they be called to deal with a suspected Hendra case. Quantitative RT-PCR assays provide rapid results for practitioners and minimise potential exposure of the laboratory worker to infectious material. Virus isolation in cell culture is possible but must be performed under appropriate biosecurity level 4 conditions in specialised laboratories due to the risk to human health posed by this virus. Serological assays to detect Hendra antibodies have been developed. A rapid ELISA-based serological screening test is available, but specificity is not high. Any positive, or suspect positive serum samples are then sent to a high security, BSL-4 level laboratory for testing by virus neutralisation assay.

References

Daniels, P.W., Halpin, K., Hyatt, A. and Middleton, D. (2007) Infection and disease in reservoir and spillover hosts: determinants of pathogen emergence. *Curr. Top. Microbiol. Immunol.* **315**, 113-131.

Fauquet, C., Mayo, M.A., Maniloff, J., Desselberger, U. and Ball, L.A. (2005) *VIIIth Report of the International Committee on Taxonomy of Viruses*, Elsevier, Philadelphia. p 1162.

Field, H., Young, P., Yob, J.M., Mills, J., Hall, L. and Mackenzie, J. (2001) The natural history of Hendra and Nipah viruses. *Microbes. Infect.* **3**, 307-314.

Field, H.E., Mackenzie, J.S. and Daszak, P. (2007) Henipaviruses: emerging paramyxoviruses associated with fruit bats. *Curr. Top. Microbiol. Immunol.* **315**, 133-159.

Halpin, K., Young, P.L., Field, H.E. and Mackenzie, J.S. (2000) Isolation of Hendra virus from pteropid bats: a natural reservoir of Hendra virus. *J. Gen. Virol.* **81**, 1927-1932.

Hooper, P., Zaki, S., Daniels, P. and Middleton, D. (2001) Comparative pathology of the diseases caused by Hendra and Nipah viruses. *Microbes. Infect.* **3**, 315-322.

Mungall, B.A., Middleton, D., Crameri, G., Bingham, J., Halpin, K., Russell, G., Green, D., McEachern, J., Pritchard, L.I., Eaton, B.T., Wang, L.F., Bossart, K.N. and Broder, C.C. (2006) Feline model of acute nipah virus infection and protection with a soluble glycoprotein-based subunit vaccine. *J. Virol.* **80**, 12293-12302.

Murray, K., Rogers, R., Selvey, L., Selleck, P., Hyatt, A., Gould, A., Gleeson, L., Hooper, P. and Westbury, H. (1995a) A novel morbillivirus pneumonia of horses and its transmission to humans. *Emerg. Infect. Dis.* **1**, 31-33.

Murray, K., Selleck, P., Hooper, P., Hyatt, A., Gould, A., Gleeson, L., Westbury, H., Hiley, L., Selvey, L., Rodwell, B. *et al.* (1995b) A morbillivirus that caused fatal disease in horses and humans. *Science* **268**, 94-97.

Murray, P.K. (1996) The evolving story of the equine morbillivirus. *Aust. vet. J.* **74**, 214.

Williamson, M.M., Hooper, P.T., Selleck, P.W., Gleeson, L.J., Daniels, P.W., Westbury, H.A. and Murray, P.K. (1998) Transmission studies of Hendra virus (equine morbillivirus) in fruit bats, horses and cats. *Aust. vet. J.* **76**, 813-818.

Williamson, M.M., Hooper, P.T., Selleck, P.W., Westbury, H.A. and Slocombe, R.F. (2000) Experimental hendra virus infection in pregnant guinea-pigs and fruit bats (*Pteropus poliocephalus*). *J. Comp. Pathol.* **122**, 201-207.

Young, P.L., Halpin, K., Selleck, P.W., Field, H., Gravel, J.L., Kelly, M.A. and Mackenzie, J.S. (1996) Serologic evidence for the presence in *Pteropus* bats of a paramyxovirus related to equine morbillivirus. *Emerg. Infect. Dis.* **2**, 239-240.

GETAH VIRUS INFECTION

T. S. Mair* and P. J. Timoney†

Bell Equine Veterinary Clinic, Mereworth, Maidstone, Kent ME18 5GS; and †Gluck Equine Research Center, University of Kentucky, Lexington, Kentucky 40546-0099, USA.

Keywords: horse; Getah virus; arbovirus; Semliki Forest viruses

Summary

Getah virus is an arbovirus that was first isolated from mosquitoes in Malaysia in 1955. Outbreaks of infection by Getah virus have been recorded in horses in Japan and India. Infection can occur in a wide range of vertebrates, and the virus is probably maintained in a mosquito-pig-mosquito cycle. Clinical disease in horses is generally mild, characterised by pyrexia, oedema of the limbs, urticaria and a stiff gait. An inactivated whole-virus vaccine is available in Japan.

Introduction

Getah virus is an arbovirus that was first isolated from mosquitoes (*Culex gelidus*) in Malaysia in 1955 (Berge 1975). However, it was not until 1978 that the virus was shown to be responsible for a mild disease among racehorses in Japan (Kamada *et al.* 1980; Sentsui and Kono 1980a; Timoney 2004). Subsequent outbreaks of Getah virus infection have been documented in racehorses in Japan in the 1970s and 1980s (Sentsui and Kono 1985) and among breeding horses in India in 1990 (Brown and Timoney 1998). Infection with the virus also occurs in other domestic animals, including pigs where it has been associated with illness and death in young piglets aged up to 18 days. Serological evidence of infection has been found in a large number of vertebrate species (mammals, birds and reptiles) in which the infection appears to be subclinical (Doherty *et al.* 1966). There is no evidence that the virus can infect man (Fukunaga *et al.* 2000).

Aetiology

Getah virus is a positive-stranded RNA virus belonging to the genus *Alphavirus* of the family *Togaviridae* (Calisher *et al.* 1980; Timoney 2004). It is classified in the Semliki Forest complex along with Semliki Forest, Bebaru, Ross River, Chikungunya, O'nyong-nyong, Una and Mayaro viruses (van Regenmortel *et al.* 2000). Several subtypes of Getah virus are recognised, including Sagiyama, Ross River and Bebaru viruses (Calisher and Walton 1996).

Getah virus possesses haemagglutinating and complement fixing antigens, which have been used to develop diagnostic tests for the virus. These tests in addition to the neutralisation test have been used to investigate antigenic relationships between different strains and subtypes of virus (Fukunaga *et al.* 2000).

Epidemiology

Getah virus is transmitted by mosquitoes, and is widely distributed in southeast Australasia and surrounding countries, including Australia, Borneo, Cambodia, China, Indonesia, Japan, Korea, Malaysia, Mongolia, the Philippines, Russia, Thailand, Sarawak, Siberia, Sri Lanka and Vietnam (Calisher and Walton 1996; Fukunaga *et al.* 2000; Timoney 2004). Natural infection in wildlife is believed to be subclinical (Fukunaga *et al.* 2000). In tropical areas of Asia, pigs appear to be important in maintaining a reservoir of infection via a mosquito-pig-mosquito cycle (Chanas *et al.* 1977). Pigs, and possibly other vertebrates, may play an important role as amplifying hosts for the virus (Fukunaga *et al.* 2000).

Serological surveys of horses in Japan have shown that the virus is widespread in this country, with seropositive rates up to 93% (Imagawa *et al.* 1981; Sentsui and Kono 1980b; Brown and Timoney 1998; Sugiura and Shimada 1999). The highest rates of seropositivity occurred in older horses in the cooler regions of northern Japan. Seroprevalence was reported as 17% in India and 25% in Hong Kong (Kamada *et al.* 1991; Shortridge *et al.* 1994). Many

*Author to whom correspondence should be addressed.

cases of Getah virus infection in horses are subclinical (Fukunaga *et al.* 2000).

The principal vectors for the transmission of Getah virus to horses are mosquitoes (species of *Culex* or *Aedes*) (Calisher and Walton 1996; Fukunaga *et al.* 2000), although horse to horse transmission could also occur (Sentsui and Kono 1980a). High levels of virus can be found in nasal secretions of horses experimentally infected by Getah virus by the nasal route (Kamada *et al.* 1991), thereby permitting horse to horse spread in animals in close contact. Nonvector spread of the virus was believed to have contributed to the outbreak of Getah virus in India in 1990 (Brown and Timoney 1998).

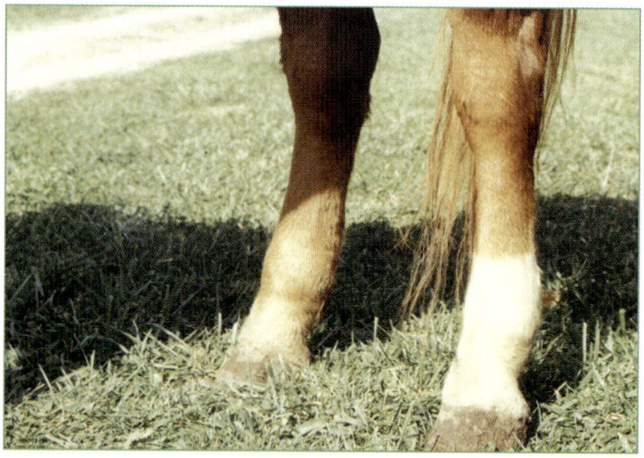

FIGURE 1: Lower limb oedema due to Getah virus infection.

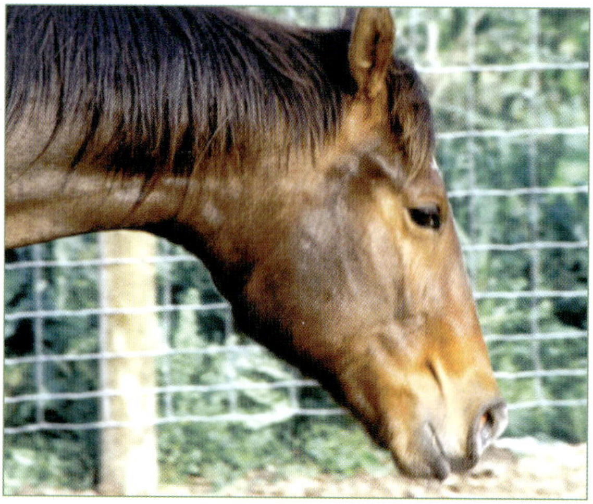

FIGURE 2: Submandibular lymphadenopathy associated with Getah virus infection.

Clinical signs

Clinical infection caused by Getah virus has been observed almost exclusively in the horse. Outbreaks of the disease in horses have been sporadic, and have not been associated with any mortality (Fukunaga *et al.* 2000). The morbidity rate in one outbreak of infection in racehorses was 38% (Kamada *et al.* 1980; Sentsui and Kono 1980a), with slow and irregular spread of infection.

The clinical signs associated with Getah virus infection in horses vary depending on the strain of virus and viral dose (Timoney 2004). Some infections only produce a febrile response with associated inappetence and depression (Sentsui and Kono 1980a). The febrile stage lasts 1–4 days. Other signs seen in infected horses include lower limb oedema (**Fig 1**), swelling of the submandibular lymph nodes (**Fig 2**), urticaria (especially on the neck, shoulders and hind quarters) (**Fig 3**) and a stiff gait (Kamada *et al.* 1980; Sentsui and Kono 1980a; Fukunaga *et al.* 1981a; Brown and Timoney 1998). Mild colic, icterus and scrotal oedema have also been reported (Timoney 2004). Limb oedema and urticaria usually appear several days after the onset of pyrexia. Mild anaemia and a transient lymphopenia may be present (Fukunaga *et al.* 2000). Serum alkaline phosphatase can be elevated during the acute phase of the infection, whereas serum lactic dehydrogenase and glutamine pyruvic transaminase rise during convalescence (Calisher and Walton 1996). Most affected horses make a full clinical recovery within one week, although a small number may require up to 2 weeks to recover (Timoney 2004). Abortion is not a feature of the disease, and foals born to mares that

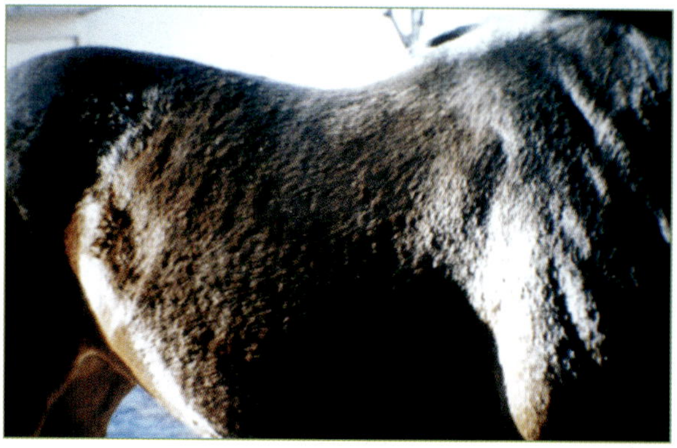

FIGURE 3: Urticaria due to Getah virus infection.

have had the disease during gestation are normal (Brown and Timoney 1998). In experimental infections, the clinical signs are similar, but infected horses also commonly develop a serous nasal discharge (Kamada *et al.* 1991).

Diagnosis

In view of its clinical similarity to a range of other infectious and noninfectious equine diseases, a provisional clinical diagnosis must be confirmed through laboratory examination. Included in a differential diagnosis of Getah virus infection are equine viral arteritis, equine rhinopneumonitis, equine encephalosis, equine influenza, equine infectious anaemia, African horse sickness fever, *purpura haemorrhagica* and hoary alyssum toxicosis. Virus isolation or demonstration of viral nucleic acid by reverse-transcription polymerase chain reaction may be performed on nasal swabs, unclotted blood or saliva of acutely infected animals (Kamada *et al.* 1980; Sentsui *et al.* 1980; Fukunaga *et al.* 1981a). The virus can be cultivated in a range of equine and nonequine cell culture systems, especially Vero and RK-13 cell lines, as well as in suckling mice inoculated by the intracerebral route. Highest rates of virus isolation have been achieved from plasma (Fukunaga *et al.* 1981b). Detection of Getah virus is optimal where specimens are collected as early as possible after the onset of fever.

Serum antibodies to Getah virus can be detected by haemagglutination inhibition, complement fixation, enzyme-linked immunosorbent assay (ELISA) and neutralisation tests (Kamada *et al.* 1980; Sentsui and Kono 1980; Sentsui and Kono 1985; Brown and Timoney 1998). If possible, paired samples taken during the acute and convalescent stages of the disease should be assayed. The neutralisation test is considered the most specific test at differentiating Getah virus infection from other antigenically related alphaviruses (Chanas *et al.* 1977).

Control

Control of Getah virus in endemic areas relies on control of the mosquito vector (Fukunaga *et al.* 2000; Timoney 2004). This can be achieved by eliminating or reducing mosquito breeding sites, and use of larvicides and adulticides. The risk of exposure of horses to virus-infected mosquitoes can be reduced by housing them during dusk and at night.

An inactivated whole-virus vaccine is available in Japan. Horses receive an annual booster dose of the vaccine in May or June, prior to the onset of the mosquito season. No epidemics of Getah virus infection have been recorded in horses in Japan since the current vaccination programme was implemented in 1979 (Timoney 2004).

References

Berge, T.O. (1975) International catalogue of arboviruses, including certain other viruses of vertebrates. In: *DHEW Publication No (CDC) 78-8301. US Department of Health, Education and Welfare*, Public Health Service, Washington DC. p 278.

Brown, C.M. and Timoney, P.J. (1998) Getah virus infection in Indian horses. *Trop. Anim. Hlth. Prod.* **30**, 241-252.

Calisher, C.H. and Walton, T.E. (1996) Getah virus infections. In: *Virus Infections of Equines,* Ed: M.K. Studdert, Elsevier, Amsterdam. pp 157-165.

Calisher, C.H., Shope, R.E., Brandt, W., Casals, J., Karabatsos, N., Murphy, F.A., Tesh, R.B. and Wiebe, M.E. (1980) Proposed antigenic classification of registered arboviruses: Togavitidae, alphavirus. *Intervirol.* **14**, 229-232.

Chanas, A.C., Johnson, K.B. and Simpson, D.I.H. (1977) A comparative study of related alphaviruses – a naturally occurring model of antigenic variation in the Getah sub-group. *J. Gen. Virol.* **35**, 455-462.

Doherty, R.L., Gorman, B.M., Whitebread, R.H. and Carley, J.G. (1966) Studies of arthropod-borne virus infections in Queensland: V. Survey of antibodies to Group A arboviruses in man and other animals. *J. expt. Biol. Sci.* **44**, 365-378.

Fukunaga, Y., Kumanomido, T. and Kamada, M. (2000) Getah virus as an equine pathogen. *Vet. Clin. N. Am.: Equine Pract.* **16**, 605-617.

Fukunaga, Y., Ando, Y., Kamada, M., Imagawa, H., Wada, R., Kumanomido, T., Akiyama, Y., Watanabe, O., Niwa, K., Takenaga, S., Shibata, M. and Yamamoto, T. (1981a) An outbreak of Getah virus infection in horses – clinical and epizootological aspects at the Miho Training Center in 1978. *Bulletin of the Equine Research Institute* **18**, 94-102.

Fukunaga, Y., Kumanomido, T., Imagawa, H., Ando, Y., Kamada, M., Wada, R. and Akiyama, Y. (1981b) Isolation of picornavirus from horses associated with Getah virus infection. *Jap. J. vet. Sci.* **43**, 569-572.

Imagawa, H., Ando, Y., Kamada, M., Sugiura, T., Kumanomido, T., Fukunaga, Y., Wada, R., Hirasawa, K. and Akiyama, Y. (1981) Sero-epizootogical survey of Getah virus infection in light horses in Japan. *Jap. J. vet. Sci.* **43**, 797-802.

Kamada, M., Ando, Y., Fukunaga, Y., Kumanomido, T., Imagawa, H., Wada, R. and Akiyama, Y. (1980) Equine Getah virus infection: Isolation of the virus from racehorses during a enzootic in Japan. *Am. J. Trop. Med. Hyg.* **29**, 984-988.

Kamada, M., Kumanomido, T., Wada, R., Fukunaga, Y., Imagawa, H. and Sugiura, T. (1991) Intranasal infection of Getah virus in experimental horses. *J. vet. Med. Sci.* **53**, 855-858.

Sentsui, H. and Kono, Y. (1980a) An epidemic of Getah virus infection among racehorses: Isolation of the virus. *Res. vet. Sci.* **29**, 157-161.

Sentsui, H. and Kono, Y. (1980b) Survey of antibody to Getah virus in horses in Japan. *Natl. Inst. anim. Health Q.* **20**, 39-43.

Sentsui, H. and Kono, Y. (1985) Reappearance of Getah virus infection among horses in Japan. *Jap. J. vet. Sci.* **47**, 333-335.

Shortridge, K.F., Mason, D.K., Watkins, K.L. and Aaskov, J.G. (1994) Serological evidence for the transmission of Getah virus in Hong Kong. *Vet. Rec.* **134**, 527-528.

Sugiura, T. and Shimada, K. (1999) Seroepizootological survey of Japanese encephalitis virus and Getah virus in regional horse race tracks from 1991 to 1997 in Japan. *J. vet. Med. Sci.* **61**, 877-881.

Timoney, P.J. (2004) Getah virus infection. In: *Infectious Diseases of Livestock*, 2nd edn., Eds: J.A.W. Coetzer and R.C. Tustin, Oxford University Press, Cape Town. pp 1023-1026.

Van Regenmortel, M.H.V., Fauquet, C.M., Bishop, D.H.L., Carstens, E.B., Estes, M.K., Lemon, S.M., Maniloff, J., Mayo, M.A., McGeoch, D.J., Pringle, C.R. and Wickner, R.B. (2000) Virus taxonomy: Classification and nomenclature of viruses. In: *7th Report of the International Committee on Taxonomy of Viruses,* Academic Press, San Diego. pp 884-887.

ROSS RIVER VIRUS

T. S. Mair* and P. J. Timoney†

Bell Equine Veterinary Clinic, Mereworth, Maidstone, Kent ME18 5GS; and †Gluck Equine Research Center, University of Kentucky, Lexington, Kentucky 40546-0099, USA.

Keywords: horse; Ross River virus; Alphavirus; mosquito-borne; horse; zoonosis

Summary

Ross River virus is an arthropod-borne virus (arbovirus) and the cause of the most common mosquito-borne human disease in Australia, being frequently associated with a debilitating polyarthritis. Serological evidence would indicate that subclinical infections with the virus are widespread in horses in many areas of the country. Clinical disease can occur in horses, with affected animals displaying any or all of the following signs: pyrexia, inappetence, lameness, stiffness, swollen joints, reluctance to move, ataxia, mild colic and poor performance. Persistence of certain clinical signs such as limb soreness and impaired performance for months or even years has also been reported in a small percentage of cases. The horse is considered a possible amplifying host for the virus, with the ability to develop a high-titred viraemia and infect various mosquito species.

Introduction

Ross River virus is closely related to Getah virus in terms of its taxonomic classification, ecology and the nature of the clinical disease it can cause in horses. In contrast to Getah virus, however, Ross River virus is also an important human pathogen (Russell 2002). It is an arthropod-borne virus or arbovirus that can be transmitted by a wide range of mosquito species and which is endemic in Australia, in Papua-New Guinea and certain islands in the South Pacific (Spradbrow 1972; Russell 1994, 1996, 2002; Azuolas 1998). Disease caused by Ross River virus is the most common arboviral infection of man in Australia. It is a nonfatal disease that is characterised principally by a debilitating polyarthritis syndrome (Fraser 1986; Russell 1994). Joint pain, limb soreness and locomotor difficulties can persist for several months even years in a percentage of affected individuals (Boughton 1996). Whereas infection with Ross River virus is commonly encountered in horses in many areas of Australia, especially in the northern tropical regions where there is year-round virus activity (Russell 2002), the overall clinical attack rate would appear to be low (Azuolas 1998).

Aetiology

Ross River virus is a single-stranded, positive sense RNA virus with quasi-species structure belonging to the genus *Alphavirus*, family *Togaviridae*. It is classified in the Semliki Forest complex along with Semliki Forest, Bebaru, Getah, Chikungunya, O'nyong-nyong, Una and Mayaro viruses and belongs to the Getah virus serogroup of agents (van Regenmortel *et al.* 2000). Considerable sequence homology exists between the genomes of Ross River and Getah viruses (Strauss and Strauss 1994), with evidence of geographic variability among isolates of Ross River virus (Lindsay *et al.* 1993). Ross River virus is primarily a mosquito-borne infection and an important human pathogen.

Epidemiology

As previously indicated, Ross River virus is arthropod-borne, and infection principally results from the bite of an infected mosquito (Russell 1994, 1996 and 2002). Different mosquito species are involved as vectors in various regions of Australia or wherever the virus is found. The species vary depending on different climatic and environmental conditions, with mosquitoes belonging to the genera *Culex*, *Aedes* (*Ochlerotatus*), *Anopheles*, *Coquillettidia* and *Mansonia* implicated in transmission under field or experimental circumstances (Aaskov 1997; Russell

*Author to whom correspondence should be addressed.

2002). Notwithstanding the wide range of mosquito species that can serve as potential vectors of Ross River virus, only a small number are of primary importance in transmission in coastal or inland, urban or rural settings. Principal vectors in costal situations are the northern saltmarsh mosquito, *Ae. vigilax* and the southern saltmarsh mosquito, *Ae. camptorhynchus*, whereas in inland areas, *Cx. annulirostris* is the major vector. Similar to Getah virus, and many other arboviruses, Ross River virus is maintained in a mosquito-vertebrate-mosquito host cycle. Vertical transmission of the virus has been confirmed in species of culicine mosquitoes (Dhileepan *et al.* 1996).

The natural vertebrate hosts of Ross River virus are considered to be nonmigratory native macropodids e.g. kangaroos and wallabies. Other marsupials may also serve as possible reservoir hosts (Russell 2002). Kangaroos and wallabies are assumed to be the most important amplifying hosts. In the area around Brisbane, marsupials (brushtail possums and Macropods), flying foxes and horses were identified as the most important host species (Kay *et al.* 2007). In the latter study, mosquitoes collected in the Brisbane area were analysed for host blood meals. The most commonly identified blood meal was dog blood (average of 37.4% of all identified blood meals), followed by bird (18.4%), horse (16.8%), brushtail possum (13.3%), human (11.6%), cat (1.7%), flying fox (0.7%) and macropod (0.2%). Since horses infected with Ross River virus may develop high-level viraemias of up to $10^{6.3}$ suckling mouse intracerebral LD_{50}/ml (Kay *et al.* 1987), they serve as an important source of infection for mosquitoes and may well play a role in disseminating and perhaps maintaining the virus in certain areas/regions of the country. There is some evidence to suggest that horses may not necessarily be efficient amplifying hosts (Kay *et al.* 1987). The prevalence of Ross River virus infection in horses is high in endemic areas of Australia. In Queensland (an area believed to have year-round mosquito activity), the seropositivity rate was approximately 80%, compared to 50% in the region of the Gippsland Lakes in southern Australia (an area with seasonal mosquito activity) (Azuolas 1998). In a serological survey of vertebrate sera (1706 samples) obtained from 5 animal species in the area around Brisbane, sera from dogs and horses were most commonly found positive for antibodies to Ross River virus, with antibodies present in 22.5% and 25.5% of samples, respectively.

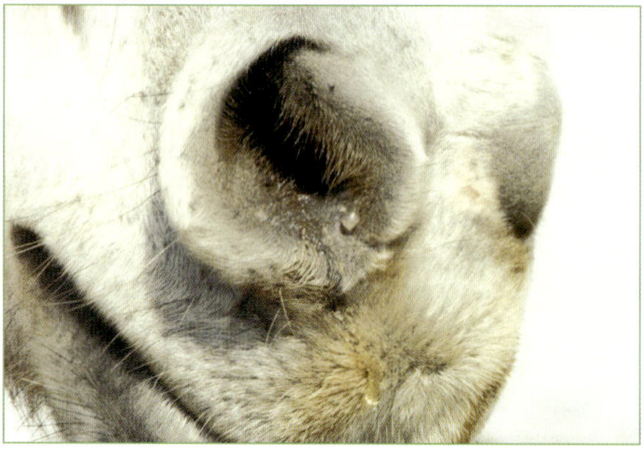

FIGURE 1: Serous nasal discharge associated with Ross River virus infection.

Clinical signs

Ross River virus causes a nonfatal infection in horses. Although seroconversion to Ross River virus is common, the majority of horses infected with the virus develop minimal, if any, signs of disease (Kay *et al.* 1987; Azuolas 1998; Azuolas *et al.* 2003; El-Hage *et al.* 2008). Experimental infection of horses with Ross River virus has failed to result in the development of disease. No clinical signs were reported in either of 2 experimental studies comprising a total of 14 horses (Gard *et al.* 1977). Accepting that variation in pathogenicity probably exists among Ross River virus genotypes (Fraser 1986; Russell 1994), it may be that many virus strains cause only subclinical or inapparent infection. Nonetheless, infection with this virus is considered responsible for musculoskeletal disease in performance horses that has occurred for many years in many riverland and northern regions of Australia (El-Hage *et al.* 2008), notwithstanding the lack of laboratory confirmation of the disease. Clinical signs associated with Ross River virus infection in horses include pyrexia, inappetence, serous nasal discharge (**Fig 1**), lethargy (**Fig 2**), submaxillary lymphadenopathy, distal limb swelling, lameness, stiffness, swollen joints (**Fig 3**), ataxia, reluctance to move, petechial haemorrhages on the gingival mucous membranes and mild colic (Pascoe *et al.* 1978; Azuolas 1998; Azuolas *et al.* 2003; El Hage *et al.*

2008). Persistence of certain clinical signs, especially limb soreness and poor performance are believed to occur in a small percentage of affected horses (El-Hage *et al.* 2008). While seroconversion to Ross River virus is quite common in horses, to date there have been few reports of clinical disease associated with seroconversion or virus isolation (Gard *et al.* 1977; Pascoe *et al.* 1978; Azuolas 1998; Azuolas *et al.* 2003; Studdert *et al.* 2003). In a recent report, Ross River virus was believed to be the cause of acute illness in 4 horses around the Bellarine peninsula in south-west Victoria, Australia, that were naturally exposed to the virus (El-Hage *et al.* 2008). The clinical signs exhibited by the affected individuals included petechial haemorrhages, lymphadenopathy, distal limb swelling and reluctance to move. Fibrinogen levels were also elevated in 3 of the 4 horses. Whilst no virus was isolated, serological testing revealed increased IgM titres to the virus in all the horses, confirming recent infection. The outbreak occurred at a time when a known Ross River virus vector, the mosquito *Aedes camptorhynchus* was recorded in very high numbers in the region. Based on the serological finding of IgM antibodies, there is every reason to relate the clinical signs observed in these 4 horses to recent infection with Ross River virus. The signs displayed were consistent with those identified with this virus infection in humans in whom there is targeting of synovial and musculoskeletal tissues. 'Poor performance' is a frequently reported outcome in horses suspected of being infected with Ross River virus (Azuolas 1998).

Diagnosis

No matter how suggestive the clinical signs exhibited by an affected horse(s) are of infection with Ross River virus, laboratory confirmation of a provisional clinical diagnosis of the disease is essential. Diagnosis is based on detection of the virus in serum or heparinised blood by virus isolation in cell culture or intracerebral inoculation of suckling mice, or by reverse transcription-polymerase chain reaction assay of blood or synovial fluid (Azuolas *et al.* 2003; Studdert *et al.* 2003). To optimise the chances of virus isolation, specimens should be collected as early as possible after the onset of clinical signs. Recent exposure to and infection with Ross River virus can also be established by demonstration of a detectable IgM antibody response in a single serum sample or in the acute sample, where paired blood samples taken 2–3 weeks apart are collected from suspect cases of the disease (Azuolas *et al.* 2003). An IgM antibody response is generally detectable by Day 7–10 after exposure, peaks within 2–3 weeks before declining rapidly and disappearing as IgG antibody levels increase and eventually replace IgM antibodies in the circulation (Azuolas *et al.* 2003).

Treatment

Treatment of horses with suspected Ross River virus infection is supportive and symptomatic, with an emphasis on the use of analgesics and nonsteroidal anti-inflammatory drugs to mitigate the muscle soreness, stiffness in gait and swollen joints.

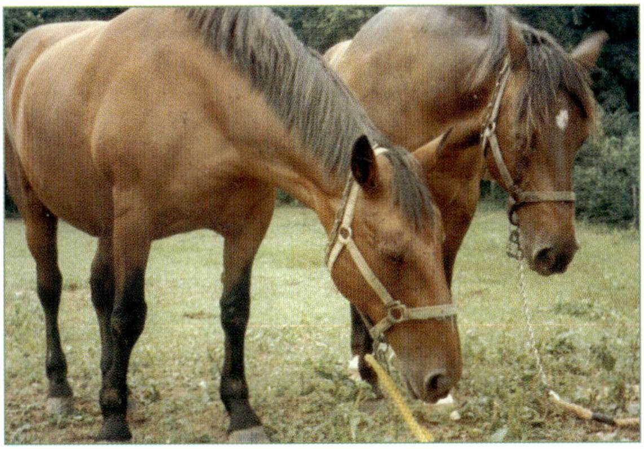

FIGURE 2: Depression, lethargy and inappetence are common clinical signs associated with Ross River virus infection.

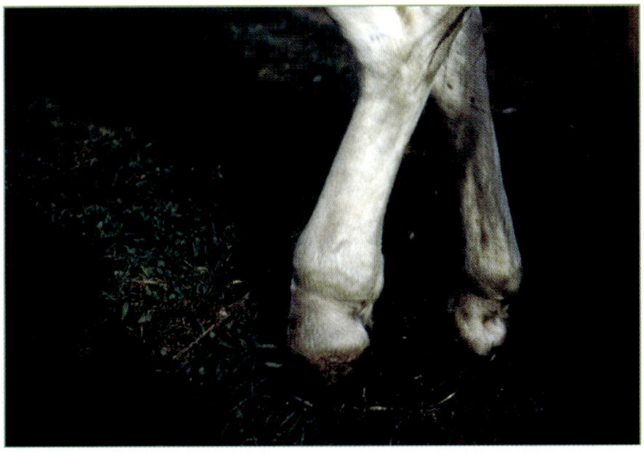

FIGURE 3: Limb oedema and swollen joints associated with Ross River virus infection.

Prevention

There is no vaccine currently available against Ross River virus infection in horses. Preventing exposure of horses to the virus is dependent primarily on controlling the vector (mosquito) population through reduction of breeding sites and use of larvicides, as well as the natural vertebrate hosts of the virus. The use of topical insect repellents is recommended on horses at risk of infection.

References

Aaskov, J. (1997) Towards prevention of epidemic polyarthritis. *Arbovirus Res. Aust.* **7**, 1-4.

Azuolas, J.K. (1998) Ross River virus disease of horses. *Aust. Equine Vet.* **16**, 56-58.

Azuolas, J.K., Wishart, E., Bibby, S. and Ainsworth, C. (2003) Isolation of Ross River virus from mosquitoes and from horses with signs of musculo-skeletal disease. *Aust. vet. J.* **81**, 344–347.

Boughton, C.R. (1996) *Australian Arboviruses of Medical Importance,* Royal Australian College of General Practitioners, Sydney.

Dhileepan, K., Azuolas, J.K. and Gibson, C.A. (1996) Evidence of vertical transmission of Ross River and Sindbis viruses (*Togaviridae*: alphaviruses) by mosquitoes (*Dyptera: Culicidae*) in southeastern Australia. *J. Med. Entomol.* **33**, 180-182.

El-Hage, C.M., McCluskey, M.J. and Azuolas, J.K. (2008) Disease suspected to be caused by Ross River virus infection of horses. *Aust. vet. J.* **86**, 367–370.

Fraser, J.R. (1986) Epidemic polyarthritis and Ross River virus disease. *Clin. Rheum. Dis.* **12**, 369-388.

Gard, G.P., Marshal, I.D., Walker, K.H., Ackland, H. and De Sarem, W.G. (1977) Association of Australian arboviruses with nervous disease in horses. *Aust. vet. J.* **53**, 61-66.

Kay, B.H., Pollit, C.C., Fanning, I.D. and Hall, R.A. (1987) The experimental infection of horses with Murray Valley encephalitis and Ross River viruses. *Aust. vet. J.* **64**, 52-55.

Kay, B.H., Boyd, A.M., Ryan, P.A. and Hall, R.A. (2007) Mosquito feeding patterns and natural infection of vertebrates with Ross River and Barmaf Forest viruses in Brisbane, Australia. *Am. J. Trop. Med. Hyg.* **76**, 417-423.

Lindsay, M.D., Coelen, R.J. and MacKenzie, J.S. (1993) Genetic heterogeneity among isolates of Ross River virus from different geographical regions. *J. Virol.* **67**, 3576-3585.

Pascoe, R.R., St George, T.D. and Cybinski, D.H. (1978) The isolation of a Ross River virus from a horse. *Aust. vet. J.* **54**, 600.

Russell, R.C. (1996) *A Colour Photo Atlas of Mosquitoes of Southeastern Australia,* Department of Medical Entomology, University of Sydney and Westmead Hospital. pp 43-153.

Russell, R.C. (1994) Ross River virus: disease trends and vector ecology in Australia. *Bull. Soc. Vector Ecol.* **19**, 73-81.

Russell, R.C. (2002) Ross River virus: ecology and distribution. *Annu. Rev. Entomol.* **47**, 1-31.

Spradbrow, P.B. (1972) Arbovirus infections of domestic animals of Australia. *Aust. vet. J.* **48**, 181-185.

Strauss, J.H. and Strauss, E.G. (1994) The alphaviruses: gene expression, replication and evolution. *Microbiol. Rev.* **58**, 491-562.

Studdert, M.J., Azuolas, J.K., Vasey, J.R., Hall, R.A., Ficorilli, N. and Huang, J.-A. (2003) Polymerase chain reaction tests for the identification of Ross River, Kunjin and Murray Valley encephalitis infections in horses. *Aust. vet. J.* **81**, 76-80.

Van Regenmortel, M.H.V., Fauquet, C.M., Bishop, D.H.L., Carstens, E.B., Estes, M.K., Lemon, S.M., Maniloff, J., Mayo, M.A., McGeoch, D.J., Pringle, C.R. and Wickner, R.B. (2000) Virus taxonomy: Classification and nomenclature of viruses. In: *7th Report of the International Committee on Taxonomy of Viruses,* Academic Press, San Diego. pp 884-887.

AUJESKY'S DISEASE (PSEUDORABIES) IN THE HORSE

T. S. Mair* and G. R. Pearson†

Bell Equine Veterinary Clinic, Mereworth, Maidstone, Kent ME18 5GS; and †Department of Clinical Veterinary Science, School of Veterinary Science, Bristol University, Langford House, Langford, Bristol BS40 5DU, UK.

Keywords: horse; pseudorabies; suid heperpesvirus-1; Aujesky's disease

Summary

Pseudorabies, caused by suid (porcine) herpesvirus-1, is an acute, contagious disease affecting primarily pigs, but transmission to other species including horses can occur. Pseudorabies has been reported around the world, although it has been eradicated from many countries, including the UK. The pig is the natural host of suid herpesvirus-1, and other species, including horses, are generally infected as a result of close contact with pigs (aerosol spread). Species other than pigs are considered to be dead-end hosts, and they invariably die as a result of acute neurological disease. Natural pseudorabies infections in horses have been rarely reported. Severe neurological signs develop over a period of 1–3 days, followed by death.

Introduction

Pseudorabies (also known as Aujesky's disease, Herpesvirus suis disease, infectious bulbar paralysis, mad itch), caused by suid (porcine) herpesvirus-1, is an acute, contagious disease affecting primarily pigs, but transmission to other species including cattle, sheep, goats, dogs, cats and horses can occur. Since its recognition as a disease entity by Aujesky in 1902, the disease has become of major economic importance. The name pseudorabies was given to the disease because of its similarity to bovine clinical rabies. Pseudorabies has been reported around the world, including Britain, Ireland, continental Europe, North Africa, Asia, South America, New Zealand and the USA, however since the 1980s the disease has been eradicated from many countries. Infection results in neurological signs in piglets, respiratory disease and poor growth performance in fattening pigs, and reproductive failure in sows (Van Oirschot 2004). Older pigs usually survive the acute infection, but carry the virus in a latent form for their entire lives.

Aetiology

Suid herpesvirus-1 has the broadest range of the animal herpesviruses (Crandell 1985). Natural infections of pseudorabies have been observed in pigs, cattle, sheep, goats, horses, dogs, cats, rodents, mink and wild animals. Human infections have been reported, but currently pseudorabies is not considered to be a public health threat. Replication of the virus with cytopathological changes occurs in cell cultures derived from a wide variety of animal species. The virus survives 2–7 weeks in the environment, and up to 5 weeks in meat.

Epidemiology

The pig is the natural host of suid herpesvirus-1. Pigs generally become infected by the nasal route, and the virus is most commonly spread by aerosols. Infection is by consumption of contaminated food or milk, but spread via semen (especially by artificial insemination) and unwashed embryos is also possible. The brown rat may be important in disease transmission from farm to farm (Timoney *et al.* 1988). Other species, including horses are generally infected as a result of close contact with pigs (aerosol spread). Species other than pigs are considered to be dead-end hosts, and they invariably die as a result of acute neurological disease (Van Oirschot 2004).

*Author to whom correspondence should be addressed.

Pathogenesis and clinical signs

The respiratory tract is the natural route of infection in pigs. The primary site of viral replication is the nasopharyngeal region and respiratory tract. The virus enters the olfactory nerves and travels along the glossopharyngeal nerve to the medulla, or to the pons and medulla by way of the trigeminal nerve.

In a natural infection in pigs, the incubation period is 1 week and the disease lasts 2–8 days. Recovered pigs may become latent carriers that actively shed the virus during periods of stress. Infected pigs aged <1 month of age usually die of neurological disease, whereas growing and finishing pigs usually exhibit respiratory disease, and sows abort (Inch 1998). In suckling pigs, the morbidity is high, and mortality can reach 80–100%, but mortality falls to <5% in pigs aged >4 months. In cattle, intense pruritus of some portion of the skin is the principle manifestation ('mad itch'), and generally appears on one of the flanks or the hind legs (Timoney *et al.* 1988). If the part is accessible, the animal licks at it incessantly until the skin becomes abraded and reddened. Intense pruritus is also commonly seen in dogs and cats, in addition to bulbar and pharyngeal paralysis.

Horses do not appear to be particularly susceptible to natural infection with suid herpesvirus-1, and they have been reported to often remain unaffected on farms where other livestock, dogs and cats are dying of the disease (Crandwell 1985). Natural pseudorabies infections in horses have been rarely reported. Van den Ingh *et al.* (1990) described one case in a horse that was pastured next to a maize field that had been manured with pig slurry; a strong wind blew manure into the pasture. Another natural infection in a horse was reported by Kimman *et al.* (1991). This horse originated from a farm where breeding sows, fattening pigs, cattle, ponies and horses were housed in the same barn. In species other than the pig, including the horse, the incubation period following infection is up to one week. Severe neurological signs develop over a period of 1–3 days, followed by death. Clinical signs include anorexia, depression, fever, muscle tremors, hyperexcitability, chewing, hypersalivation, severe pruritus (resulting in self-mutilation), head pressing, nystagmus, iridocyclitis, blindness, ataxia, recumbency and paralysis.

Experimental infection of 2 ponies by instillation of virus into the conjunctiva and nostrils resulted in the development of fever after 7 days (Kimman *et al.* 1991). They subsequently started to show behavioural changes, and developed severe neurological signs 9 days after infection. One pony became excited and one became depressed. One pony died on the ninth day after inoculation and the other was subjected to euthanasia on the tenth day. Both ponies had a significant increase in serum antibody titre against the virus.

Diagnosis

Analysis of cerebrospinal fluid reveals nonsuppurative meningitis. *Post mortem* examination shows nonsuppurative meningoencephalitis with perivascular cuffing (**Fig 1**), focal and diffuse gliosis, neuronal necrosis and focal malacia. Intranuclear inclusion bodies may be seen in intact and necrotic neurons and swollen astrocytes. A definitive diagnosis is made by virus isolation or the demonstration of suid herpesvirus-1 antigen in neurons by immunohistochemistry or the fluorescent antibody technique. A variety of serological assays can be used to demonstrate specific suid herpesvirus-1 antibody, including serum neutralisation, agar-gel immunodiffusion test, microimmunodiffusion test, enzyme-linked immunosorbent assay, indirect solid-phase microradioimmunoassay, modified direct complement-fixation test, countercurrent immunoelectrophoresis and the indirect haemagglutination test.

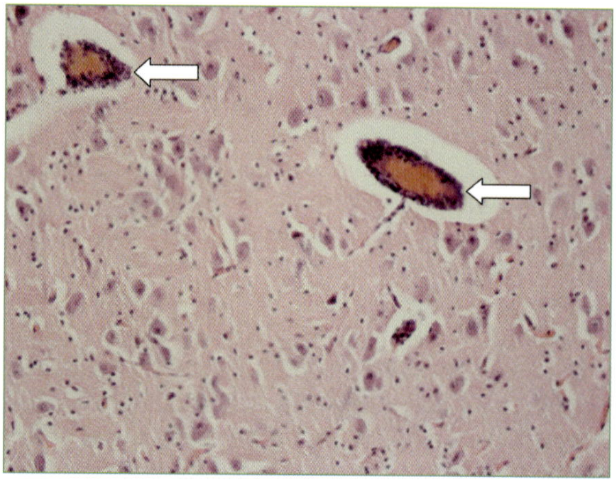

FIGURE 1: Photomicrograph of pig brain infected by Aujesky's disease. Perivascular cuffing (arrows). Haematoxylin and eosin.

Acknowledgement

We thank Dr T.D.G. Bryson, Veterinary Sciences Division, Stormont, Belfast, Northern Ireland for kindly supplying the histological section of Aujesky's disease.

References

Crandwell, R.A. (1985) Selected animal herpesviruses: new concepts and technologies. *Adv. vet. sci. comp. Med.* **29**, 281-327.

Inch, C. (1998) An overview of pseudorabies (Aujesky's disease) and vesicular stomatitis from the Canadian Animal Health Network. *Can. vet. J.* **39**, 23-32.

Kimman, T.G., Binkhorst, G.J., Van den Ingh, T.S., Pol, J.M., Gielkens, A.L. and Roelvink, M.E. (1991) Aujesky's disease in horses fulfils Koch's postulates. *Vet. Rec.* **128**, 103-106.

Timoney, J.F., Gillespie, J.H., Scott, F.W. and Barlough, J.E. (1988) Pseudorabies. In: *Hagan and Bruner's Microbiology and Infectious Diseases of Domestic Animals,* 8th edn., Comstock Publishing Associates, Ithaca. pp 615-622.

Van den Ingh, Binkhorst, G.J., Kimman, T.G., Vreeswijk, J., Pol, J.M.A. and Van Oirschot, J.T. (1990) Aujesky's disease in a horse. *J. vet. Med. B.* **37**, 532-538.

Van Oirschot, J.T. (2004) Pseudorabies. In: *Infectious Diseases of Livestock,* 2nd edn., Eds: J.A.W. Coetzer and R.C. Tustin, Oxford University Press, Cape Town. pp 909-922.

LOUPING ILL IN HORSES

T. S. Mair* and G. R. Pearson†

Bell Equine Veterinary Clinic, Mereworth, Maidstone, Kent ME18 5GS; and †Department of Clinical Veterinary Science, School of Veterinary Science, Bristol University, Langford House, Langford, Bristol BS40 5DU, UK.

Keywords: horse; louping ill; flavivirus; sheep; *Ixodes ricinus*; encephalomyelitis

Summary

Louping ill is an acute encephalitis caused by a tick-borne flavivirus. The disease is seen in certain areas of England, Scotland, Wales and Ireland, and affects mainly sheep, but can rarely affect horses. The natural vector of the virus is the castor bean tick (sheep tick) (*Ixodes ricinus*). Common clinical signs include inappetence, pyrexia, ataxia, gait abnormalities, muscle tremors of the neck and facial areas, altered head carriage, opisthotonus, depression and avoidance of bright light. Abnormal behaviour, including constant exaggerated chewing, is common. Severely affected cases become recumbent and may die or require euthanasia, but the majority of affected horses recover following symptomatic and supportive therapy.

Introduction

Louping ill (also known as infectious encephalomyelitis of sheep) is an acute encephalitis caused by a tick-borne flavivirus. It gets its name from the peculiar leaping gait of the ataxic animals. The disease is seen in moorland areas of England, Scotland, Wales and Ireland, and affects mainly sheep, although it is recognised less commonly in cattle. Infection in other domestic species, including the horse, is rare. There are closely related (possibly identical) viruses that cause encephalomyelitis of sheep in Norway, Spain, Turkey and Bulgaria (Swanepoel and Laurenson 2004). The disease is not known to occur in the southern hemisphere.

Aetiology and epidemiology

Louping ill virus belongs to the Russian spring-summer encephalitis (RSSE) complex of flaviviruses. The natural vector of the virus is the castor bean tick (sheep tick) (*Ixodes ricinus*) (McLeod and Gordon 1932). The larval tick, feeding on infected sheep, conveys the infection to new hosts when it next feeds as a nymph; or if the tick becomes infected as a nymph, it conveys the disease to a new host as an adult (Timoney *et al.* 1988). The disease is prevalent in the early summer, subsides during midsummer, and reappears in early autumn. These periods correspond to the seasons of tick activity in the area. Within endemic areas, isolation of virus and serological assays demonstrate that louping ill virus infection occurs in sheep, cattle, horses, pigs, deer, dogs and man (Swanepoel and Laurenson 2004; Hyde

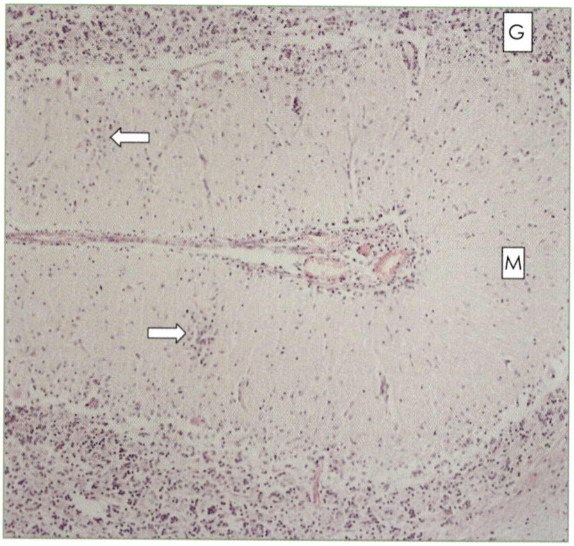

FIGURE 1: Photomicrograph of cerebellum, sheep brain affected by louping ill encephalitis. There is a reduced number of Purkinje cells between the molecular (M) and granular cell (G) layers. Gliosis of the molecular layer (arrows). Haematoxylin and eosin.

*Author to whom correspondence should be addressed.

et al. 2007). However, clinical disease, associated with acute encephalitis (**Fig 1**), is most common in sheep.

A serological survey of horses in Ireland revealed positive antibody titres in 10.6% of 601 mixed breed horses but only 0.7% in 302 Thoroughbred horses (Timoney 1976). This difference was believed to be due to differences in exposure to *Ixodes ricinus*. A limited serological survey carried out in the county of Devon in southwest England revealed positive antibody titres in 5 of 68 horses (Hyde *et al.* 2007); 2 of these 5 positive horses had a history of previous neurological disease.

Clinical signs

In sheep, the incubation period is generally 2–5 days. Typically, there is a biphasic fever with hyperpnoea, serous nasal discharge, and depression. Specific neurological signs develop with the second phase of fever, and include nystagmus, head tilt, twitching and licking of the lips, mild tremors of the head and forequarters, and hyperaesthesia. The trembling worsens and the animal develops involuntary jerking movements and stamping of the limbs. Cerebellar ataxia develops, with torticollis and a high-stepping gait. The animal becomes paretic, and more depressed. Recumbency usually ensues with worsening dyspnoea and death in 9–14 days. Animals that do not die are frequently left with permanent neurological dysfunction.

The disease resembles human poliomyelitis in that it always begins as a generalised infection, which may or may not be followed by an invasion of the central nervous system. If only generalised or viraemic changes occur, the death rate is practically nil (Timoney *et al.* 1988). In the highly infected areas of the British Isles sheep aged >1 year seldom develop the disease; they are immune as a result of unrecognised infections. The clinical disease is most commonly seen in lambs (Timoney *et al.* 1988).

There have only been a limited number of documented cases of louping ill in horses (Fletcher 1937; Timoney *et al.* 1974, 1976; Hyde *et al.* 2007), but the clinical signs broadly resemble those seen in sheep. There does not appear to be any breed, sex or age predisposition. Common clinical signs include inappetence, pyrexia, ataxia, gait abnormalities, muscle tremors of the neck and facial areas, altered head carriage, opisthotonus, depression and avoidance of bright light. Abnormal behaviour, including constant exaggerated chewing, is common. Severely affected cases become recumbent and may die or require euthanasia, but the majority of affected horses recover following symptomatic and supportive therapy. One case described by Fletcher (1937) made an uneventful recovery after an illness of 12 days. The death rates in other affected outbreaks were 2/4 (Timoney *et al.* 1976), and 1/7 (Hyde *et al.* 2007). Some recovered cases are described as having altered demeanour and behaviour patterns (Hyde *et al.* 2007).

Following experimental infection of ponies, a febrile reaction was noted 3–4 days after infection (Timoney 1980). No gross behavioural changes were observed in any animal. Every pony was viraemic for 6–7 days after inoculation, with maximal titres of virus present on Days 1 and 3. Decline and cessation of viraemia was associated with the appearance and rapid increase in titres of circulating antibodies. The results of this study confirmed the susceptibility of horses to the louping ill virus. Moreover, most of the ponies developed viraemia of sufficient intensity for 2–3 days after challenge potentially to infect *Ixodes ricinus* nymphs.

Diagnosis

The diagnosis is achieved by the recognition of suspicious clinical signs in a horse living within an endemic area for louping ill virus. Serological assays include the serum neutralisation assay, complement fixation assay and haemagglutination inhibition test (Reid and Doherty 1971; Timoney *et al.* 1976). The microscopical lesions of fatally ill animals are typical viral encephalomyelitis and meningitis; there are no typical gross lesions. Histological lesions in the central nervous system include neuronal degeneration (particularly the Purkinje cells of the cerebellum), focal gliosis and perivascular lymphoid infiltration (**Fig 1**). The presence of louping ill virus should be established in neurological tissues obtained *post mortem* by standard virus isolation, immunohistochemistry or reverse transcriptase PCR.

Public health risk

Human infection with louping ill was first reported in 1934 (Davidson *et al.* 1991). Four clinical syndromes are seen, an influenza-like illness, a bi-phase encephalitis, a poliomyelitis-like illness and a haemorrhagic fever. Certain occupational groups, e.g. laboratory personnel working with the virus and those who kill infected sheep, are at increased risk of acquiring louping ill infection.

Acknowledgement

We thank Dr T.D.G. Bryson, Veterinary Sciences Division, Stormont, Belfast, Northern Ireland for kindly supplying the histological section of louping ill.

References

Davidson, M.M., Williams, H. and Macleod, J.A. (1991) Louping ill in man: a forgotten disease. *J. Infect.* **23**, 241-249.

Hyde, J., Nettleton, P., Marriott, L. and Willoughby, K (2007) Louping ill in horses. *Vet. Rec.* **160**, 532.

McLeod, J. and Gordon, W.S. (1932) Studies in louping ill (an encephalomyelitis of sheep). II. Transmission by the sheep tick *Ixodes ricinus*. *J. comp. Pathol. Ther.* **43**, 253-256.

Marriott, L., Willoughby, K., Chianini, F., Dagleish, M.P., Scholes, S., Robinson, A.C., Gould, E.A. and Nettleton, P.F. (2006) Detection of louping ill virus in clinical specimens from mammals and birds using TaqMan RT-PCR. *J. Virol. Meth.* **137**, 21-28.

Reid, H.W. and Doherty, P.C. (1971) Experimental louping ill in sheep and lambs. 1. Viraemia and antibody response. *J. comp. Pathol.* **81**, 291-298

Swanpoel, R. and Laurenson, M.K. (2004) Louping Ill. In: *Infectious Diseases of Livestock*, 2nd edn., Eds: J.A.W. Coetzer and R.C. Tustin, Oxford University Press, Cape Town. pp 995-1003.

Timoney, P.J. (1976) Louping ill: a serological survey of horses in Ireland. *Vet. Rec.* **98**, 303.

Timoney, P.J. (1980) Susceptibility of the horse to experimental inoculation with louping ill virus. *J. comp. Pathol.* **90**, 73-86.

Timoney, P.J., Donnelly, W.J., Clements, L.O. and Fenlon, M. (1976) Encephalitis caused by louping ill virus in a group of horses in Ireland. *Equine vet. J.* **8**, 113-117.

Timoney, J.F., Gillespie, J.H., Scott, F.W. and Barlough, J.E. (1988) Louping ill. In: *Hagan and Bruner's Microbiology and Infectious Diseases of Domestic Animals,* 8th edn., Comstock Publishing Associates, Ithaca. pp 770-772.

HORSEPOX

T. S. Mair* and D. Scott†

Bell Equine Veterinary Clinic, Mereworth, Maidstone, Kent ME18 5GS, UK; and †College of Veterinary Medicine, Cornell University, Ithaca, New York, USA.

Keywords: horse; horsepox; grease; vaccinia; Uasin Gishu; molluscum contagiosum

Summary

Classical horsepox is considered to occur only in Europe. The disease is transmitted by direct contact with an infected host or with contaminated grooming equipment. Two main forms of classical horsepox are recognised: the buccal form and the 'grease' form. A poxvirus infection of horses (Uasin Gishu) is also recognised in Africa, and poxvirus infection has been linked with a disease resembling molluscum contagiosum in North America.

Introduction

The poxviruses are a large group of DNA viruses that include Orthopoxvirus (cowpox and vaccinia), Capripoxvirus (sheep-pox, goatpox, bovine lumpy skin disease), Suipoxvirus (swinepox), Parapoxvirus (pseudo-cowpox, bovine papular stomatitis, contagious viral pustular dermatitis) and Molluscipoxvirus (molluscum contagiosum) (Scott and Miller 2003). Horsepox is a rare dermatological viral disease that can have several forms, but that is classically characterised by lesions in and around the mouth or on the legs. The horsepox virus is an epitheliotrophic, unclassified DNA poxvirus, similar to vaccinia virus and cowpox virus; indeed it is possible that horsepox and vaccinia are the same virus. There are few well-documented reports of poxvirus infection in horses, and classical horsepox is considered to occur only in Europe. However, a poxvirus infection of horses (Uasin Gishu) is also recognised in Africa, and poxvirus infection has been linked with a disease resembling molluscum contagiosum in North America.

In the past in Europe, when vaccination against smallpox was being carried out, horses could become infected by vaccinia virus from recently vaccinated human subjects (De Jong 1917; Munz and Dumbell 2004). The disease is currently much less common in Europe than it was in the first half of the 20th century (Timoney *et al.* 1988) following the eradication of smallpox.

The virus gains access to the body by the respiratory tract or via the skin (Timoney *et al.* 1988). A viraemia disseminates the virus back to the skin and other target organs. The virus causes degenerative changes in the epithelium as a result of virus replication and results in the development of vesicular lesions. Degenerative changes in the dermis or subcutis may result from ischaemia secondary to vascular damage. The virus also causes epithelial hyperplasia by stimulating host cell DNA synthesis before the onset of cytoplasmic virus-related DNA replication. Two poxviruses antigenically similar to vaccinia were isolated from horses with natural infections in Kenya (Kaminjolo *et al.* 1974).

Skin lesions typically begin as erythematous macules, which then become papular and then vesicular (Scott and Miller 2003). The vesicular stage is well-developed in some pox infections, but transient or nonexistent in others. Vesicles develop into umbilicated pustules with a depressed centre and a raised erythematous border. This lesion is the so-called pock. The pustules rupture and form a crust. Healed lesions may leave a scar.

Clinical features

Horsepox may affect horses of any age. The disease is transmitted by direct contact with an infected host or with contaminated grooming equipment.

Two main forms of classical horsepox are recognised: the buccal form and the 'grease' form. In the buccal form (which is considered to be the more

*Author to whom correspondence should be addressed.

important), multiple small pox-like lesions develop on the inside of the lips and the opposing surfaces of the gums, on the frenulum of the tongue, and on the inside of the cheeks. The lesions begin as papules, change to vesicles and then become pustules. The animal may have a fever, and young horses may become systemically sick and die (Timoney *et al.* 1988). Affected animals are often inappetent, and saliva drools from the corners of the mouth. The horse may play and dip its mouth in water. Lesions may also develop on the skin of the lips, eyelids, face, trunk and in the nasal passages (Jayo *et al.* 1986). Virus isolated from lesions of horses will infect cattle, and virus from cattle will also infect horses (Timoney *et al.* 1988).

In the 'grease heel' form (also known as 'grease' or 'greasy heel'), papular eruptions develop on the flexor surface of the pastern region. The papules change to vesicles, then to pustules, which finally dry up and form crusts. There may be associated pain and lameness, but affected horses are not systemically ill.

In Africa, a verrucose or papillomatous type of horsepox called Uasin Gishu disease has been recognised (Daubney 1934; Kaminjolo *et al.* 1974a,b; Kaminjolo and Winquist 1975). The virus(es) causing this condition are not well-determined, but it is possible that it is another manifestation of vaccinia infection (Scott and Miller 2003). The lesions can be generalised but occur mainly on the neck, face, back, flank and hindquarters. Early lesions are small nodules covered by tufts of hair, which are covered by powdery white scab-like material. These scabs detach leaving bleeding patches. When the affected parts lose their hair covering, large raised areas of skin resembling papillomas up to 20 mm in diameter are left.

Another similar disease was also described in north America and Australia in the 1940s to the 1960s, termed viral papular dermatitis (McIntyre 1948; Hutchins 1960). Comparison of the clinical, histopathological and virological features of Uasin Gishu and viral papular dermatitis, along with experimental vaccinia infections in horses suggests that these conditions are probably the same disease (Studdert 1989; Taylor 1993).

Pox viruses have also been demonstrated in skin lesions resembling a human disease called molluscum contagiosum. Molluscum contagiosum is a mildly contagious, cutaneous poxvirus infection (caused by molluscipox virus) of man characterised by small, waxy, firm papules occurring principally on the face, trunk and genital region. 'Molluscum bodies', brightly eosinophilic, dyskeratotic keratinocytes containing intracytoplasmic pox virions, are considered pathognomic for this disease (Raheley and Mueller 1983). A similar disease (with similar lesion morphology) has been reported in a small number of horses involving multiple small papules on the cutaneous surface of the prepuce, the penis, neck, thorax, mammary glands and the muzzle (Gribble 1980; Raheley and Mueller 1983; Cooley *et al.* 1987; Lange *et al.* 1991; van Rensburg *et al.* 1991). The papules are typically 2–3 mm in diameter, dome-shaped with a smooth hypopigmented or slightly roughened surface. Affected horses are generally systemically well, but in one reported case, widespread lesions of molluscum contagiosum were identified in association with granulomatous enteritis (Cooley *et al.* 1987); the authors of this report suggested that the widespread lesions in this horse may have been associated with immunosuppression. Mature virions with a typical pox virus morphology have been found in the keratinocytes of the *stratum spinosum* and *stratum granulosum* in this condition. On the basis of very close homology of their viral DNA sequences, the viruses of equine and human molluscum contagiosum are considered to be either identical or very closely related (Thompson *et al.* 1998), and it has been suggested that the disease may have been transmitted from man to the horse.

Diagnosis

The clinical features plus the presence of large, eosinophilic, intracytoplasmic pox inclusions in vacuolated keratinocytes are considered pathognomic for this disease. The virus may be demonstrated by electron microscopy. Definitive identification of the specific poxvirus requires viral isolation and its identification by serological and immunofluorescence techniques (Scott and Miller 2003).

Immunity

Recovery from horsepox leaves considerable immunity (Timoney *et al.* 1988). The bovine and equine diseases reciprocally immunise against each other, and both will infect people who have not been vaccinated against smallpox.

Treatment

Treatment is symptomatic, including supportive care and prevention of secondary bacterial infections (including topical treatment with antibacterial shampoos). Mildly affected horses usually recover in 2–4 weeks.

No reported treatment has been successful for molluscum contagiosum. Horses may remain affected by multiple lesions for many months to years. Some of the lesions may regress with time, but complete resolution is unlikely.

References

Cooley, A.J., Reinhard, M.K., Gross, T.L., Fadok, V.A. and Levy, M. (1987) Molluscum contagiosum in a horse with granulomatous enteritis. *J. comp. Pathol.* **97**, 29-34.

Daubney, R. (1934) Uasin Gishu skin disease of horses. *Kenya Dept. Agric. Annu. Rep.* **3**, 26-27.

DeJong, D.A. (1917) The relationship between contagious pustular stomatitis of the horse, equine variola (horse-pox of Jenner), and vaccinia (cow-pox of Jenner). *J. comp. Path. Therap.* **30**, 242-262.

Gribble, D. (1980) Poxvirus infection in the horse resembling molluscum contagiosum: a case report. *Proc. Am. Coll. vet. Pathol.* **31**, 105.

Hutchins, D.R. (1960) Skin diseases of horses in New South Wales. *N. Z. vet. J.* **8**, 85-95.

Jayo, M.J., Jensen, L.A., Leipold, H.W. and Cook, J.E. (1986) Poxvirus infection in a donkey. *Vet. Pathol.* **23**, 635-637.

Kaminjolo, J.S., Nyaga, P.N. and Gicho, J.N. (1974a) Isolation, cultivation and characterization of a poxvirus from some horses in Kenya. *Zbl. Vet. Med. B.* **21**, 592-601.

Kaminjolo, J.S., Johnson, L.W., Frank, H. and Gicho, J.N. (1974b) Vaccinia-like pox virus identified in a horse with a skin disease. *Zbl. Vet. Med. B.* **21**, 202-206.

Kaminjolo, J.S. and Winquist, G (1975) Histopathology of skin lesions of Uasin Gishu skin disease of horses. *J. comp. Pathol.* **85**, 391-395.

McIntyre, R.W. (1948) Virus papular dermatitis of the horse. *Am. J. vet. Res.* **10**, 229-232.

Lange, L., Marett, S., Maree, C. and Gerdes, T. (1991) Molluscum contagiosum in three horses. *J. S. Afr. vet. Ass.* **62**, 68-71.

Munz, E. and Dumbell, K. (2004) Horsepox. In: *Infectious Diseases of Livestock,* 2nd edn., Eds: J.A.W. Coetzer and R.C. Tustin, Oxford University Press, Cape Town. pp 1298-1299.

Rahaley, R.S. and Mueller, R.E. (1983) Molluscum contagiosum in a horse. *Vet. Pathol.* **20**, 247-250.

Scott, D.W. and Miller, W.H. (2003) Poxvirus infections. In: *Equine Dermatology*, Elsevier, St Louis. pp 376-382.

Studdert, M.J. (1989) Experimental vaccinia virus infection of horses. *Aust. vet. J.* **66**, 157-159.

Taylor, C.E. (1993) Did vaccinia virus come from a horse? *Equine vet. J.* **25**, 8-10.

Thompson, C.H., Yager, J.A. and van Rensburg, I.B. (1998) Close relationship between equine and human molluscum contagiosum viruses demonstrated by *in situ* hybridisation. *Res. vet. Sci.* **64**, 157-161.

Timoney, J.F., Gillespie, J.H., Scott, F.W. and Barlough, J.E. (1988) Horsepox. In: *Hagan and Bruner's Microbiology and Infectious Diseases of Domestic Animals,* 8th edn., Comstock Publishing Associates, Ithaca. p 571.

Van Rensburg, I.B.J., Collett, M.G., Ronen, N. and Gerdes, T. (1991) Molluscum contagiosum in a horse. *J. S. Afr. vet. Ass.* **62**, 72-74.

EQUINE SALMONELLOSIS

H. C. McKenzie III and T. S. Mair*[†]

duPont Scott Equine Medical Center, Virginia/Maryland Regional College of Veterinary Medicine, Virginia Polytechnic and State University, Leesburg, Virginia 20176, USA; and [†]Bell Equine Veterinary Clinic, Mereworth, Maidstone, Kent ME18 5GS, UK.

Keywords: horse; *Salmonella*; salmonellosis; diarrhoea; colitis; zoonosis

Summary

Salmonellosis is a disease caused by an enteric or systemic infection with *Salmonella* spp. Clinically normal horses can transiently shed *Salmonella* organisms, but the prevalence of shedding is higher in horses presented to veterinary hospitals and horses with abdominal diseases. *Salmonella* infections can affect horses of all ages and range in severity from asymptomatic colonisation to severe systemic illness. The clinical signs of salmonellosis are variable and may include fever, mild abdominal pain, anorexia and depression without diarrhoea in some horses, but most horses that are clinically affected have moderate to severe, watery diarrhoea. Foals may develop haemorrhagic diarrhoea, septicaemia, pneumonia, meningitis, and septic arthritis or physitis. Treatments are largely supportive, and include fluid and electrolyte therapy, anti-inflammatory drugs, anti-endotoxin treatments, probiotics, intestinal protectants and nutritional support. Antimicrobial therapy is controversial. Salmonellosis is an important zoonosis.

Introduction

The Gram-negative bacteria of the species *Salmonella enterica* are facultative intracellular anaerobes that are responsible for infections in humans and animals worldwide. *Salmonella enterica* includes 6 subspecies with more than 2000 serovars. Horses are not considered to be carriers of these bacteria, as there are no known strains that are host-adapted to the horse. Clinically normal horses can transiently shed *Salmonella enterica* organisms, however, and the prevalence of shedding in horses presented to veterinary hospitals is reported to range from 6–13% (Palmer *et al.* 1985; Traub-Dargatz *et al.* 1990; Cohen *et al.* 1994, 1995; Mainar-Jaime *et al.* 1998; Kim *et al.* 2001; Ernst *et al.* 2004; Ward *et al.* 2005). These organisms are of particular concern in equine hospitals due to the mixing of large numbers of susceptible individuals and the potential for the development of multidrug resistant strains. Outbreaks typically result in substantial adverse impact on patient wellbeing as well as economic losses to the patient's owner and the facility. *Salmonella* spp. infections affect horses of all ages and can range in severity from asymptomatic colonisation to severe systemic illness. Salmonellosis typically manifests in horses as an acute enterocolitis with severe diarrhoea, but soft tissue infections and bacteraemia can also occur. Salmonellosis presents a substantial biosecurity challenge as the organisms are highly infectious, especially in susceptible individuals, and horses suffering from *Salmonella*-associated diarrhoea shed large numbers of infectious organisms into the environment.

Source of infection

The initial source of infection in individual horses or even in outbreaks of salmonellosis is frequently not identified. Potential sources of infection include consumption of contaminated food or water; contact with contaminated environmental surfaces, equipment or handlers; aerosol exposure; direct contact with shedding animals; and ingestion of contaminated bird/vermin faeces or dead insects (Traub-Dargatz *et al.* 1990; Traub-Dargatz and Besser 2007). The most frequently reported outbreaks of salmonellosis have been in hospitalised horses (Kim *et al.* 2001; Ward *et al.* 2005a; Traub-Dargatz and Besser 2007). Clinically normal horses and other

*Author to whom correspondence should be addressed.

livestock species that shed the organism in their faeces are considered to be an important potential source of contamination of the environment. Horses with abdominal pain have increased shedding (5% identified via culture and up to 40% via polymerase chain reaction [PCR] techniques) suggesting that *Salmonella* spp. are common inhabitants of the gastrointestinal tract, but are generally shed in low numbers in the faeces unless there is an abdominal disorder (Cohen *et al.* 1995; Ernst *et al.* 2004; Ward *et al.* 2005b). Changes in intestinal motility and volatile fatty acid production by normal flora may increase the ability of *Salmonella* spp. to attach to the intestinal mucosa and to proliferate. The increased shedding of *Salmonella* spp. in horses with abdominal pain does not significantly affect mortality, but is undesirable because of the potential for colitis and increased environmental shedding. *Salmonella* organisms can persist in the environment for months to years depending on the serotype, moisture content, and temperature conditions.

Pathophysiology

The development of equine salmonellosis represents the interplay of a number of factors, including the degree of bacterial exposure, the virulence of the *Salmonella* organisms, and the susceptibility of the host. Horses with impaction colic are particularly at risk (**Fig 1**). Outbreaks tend to be more common in large animal hospitals where these factors are common, on brood mare farms with a high-density population of mares and foals, or on farms where horses have been fed feed contaminated with *Salmonella* spp. Hot weather, increasing numbers of horses and foals on a farm, and wet flooring in barns or hospitals all seem to increase infection rates. Disease transmission is faecal-oral in nature and the severity of exposure is directly related to the number of bacteria that an individual horse ingests in contaminated feed or water, with the size of the infective dose being determined by the other factors of virulence and susceptibility. This infective dose may range from hundreds of organisms in particularly susceptible individuals to millions of organisms in a healthy animal (Murray 2002). The number of organisms shed by infected individuals can vary dramatically, with chronically infected cases often passing small numbers of organisms intermittently, while acutely affected individuals may shed very large numbers of organisms. The virulence of any particular *Salmonella* organism is determined by its invasiveness, which depends upon the attachment of the organism to the mucosal epithelium and the production of enzymes and toxins (cytotoxins, endotoxin, and enterotoxins) that damage the epithelium and/or alter epithelial permeability and facilitate bacterial entry into the mucosal cells (Coburn *et al.* 2007) and infection of the *lamina propria*.

In order to reach their sites of colonisation within the lower intestinal tract *Salmonella* spp. must first survive passage through the stomach, where they are exposed to a number of antimicrobial factors including the inherently low pH and the presence of hydrochloric acid. Following gastric passage the organisms must attach to the intestinal epithelium, and this is mediated by *fimbriae* or *pili* on the bacterial surface (Foley and Lynne 2008). Successful infection requires that the *Salmonella* organisms invade the epithelial cells and establish intracellular infection. After the bacteria initially attach to the epithelium they express a type III secretion system (T3SS), which facilitates epithelial invasion by allowing the direct transfer of virulence factors into the host cells. It performs this feat using a needle-like structure that penetrates the epithelial cell membrane and forms a conduit by which these factors are delivered into the epithelial cell (Foley

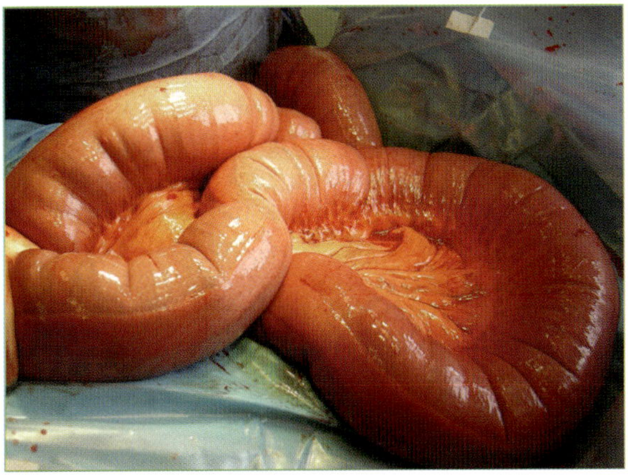

FIGURE 1: Small colon impaction as seen at exploratory celiotomy. The small colon is diffusely inflamed as well as distended; Salmonella enterica *ssp.* enterica *serovar* typhimurium *was cultured from the colonic contents.*

and Lynne 2008). Several different virulence factors can be involved, including *Salmonella* invasion proteins (Sips), endotoxin (LPS) and flagellin (Grassl and Finlay 2008). These factors are all potent inflammatory agents, and it appears that *Salmonella* organisms actually foster and utilise the host inflammatory response to facilitate their invasion of the intestinal epithelium, as their ability to establish infection is correlated with their ability to attract neutrophils to the epithelium (Coburn *et al.* 2007). These virulence factors act to stimulate local proinflammatory cytokine production, particularly of interleukin-1 beta and the neutrophil chemoattractant factor interleukin-8, and also activate cyclooxygenase within the epithelium.

The next step in the establishment of intracellular infection is the movement of the bacterium from the epithelial cell surface into the host cell. This process is also mediated by the T3SS, as several Sips (A, B and C) interact with the actin cytoskeleton of the epithelial cell resulting in the internalisation of the bacterium within a membrane-bound vacuole (Foley and Lynne 2008). This *Salmonella*-containing vacuole (SCV) does not fuse with lysosomes within the cell, and the organism is thus protected from the normal phago-lysosomal fusion process that is necessary for bacterial killing (Foley and Lynne 2008). The SCV moves from the luminal border of the epithelial cell to the basal membrane where the bacteria then interact with and enter macrophages in the submucosa (Foley and Lynne 2008). The gut associated lymphoid tissues, such as the Peyer's patches and mucosa-associated lymphoid tissue, appear to represent a primary target during the initiation of *Salmonella* infection (Grassl and Finlay 2008). The macrophages within these structures play a key role in the initial production of tumour necrosis factor-alpha (TNF-α) and inducible nitric oxide synthase (iNOS), and these mediators play an important role in the up-regulation of the inflammatory response (Grassl and Finlay 2008). This inflammatory response contributes to the development of the diarrhoea that is characteristic of enteric *Salmonella* infections, and increased production of prostaglandin E2 by iNOS appears to be a major contributor to intestinal hypersecretion (Bertelsen *et al.* 2003).

Host susceptibility is increased in the presence of stress, such as that associated with prolonged transport or surgery, or due to the presence of concurrent diseases resulting in impaired immune function. Altered diet, feed withdrawal prior to anaesthesia and treatment with antimicrobial drugs are other potential predisposing factors. Many of these factors will be present in hospitalised horses, and most of the published reports of outbreaks of salmonellosis have originated from veterinary teaching hospitals. In the normal intestine there is a large resident microbial community, termed the 'microbiota', which functions in a symbiotic manner with the host tissues to optimise nutrient utilisation, foster maturation and function of intestinal tissues and enhance the function of the intestinal immune system (Stecher *et al.* 2007). In addition, this microbiota provides an efficient barrier against infection by enteric pathogens. This ability of the enteric population of commensal bacteria to resist the proliferation of pathogenic bacteria, termed colonisation resistance, is impaired in the face of antimicrobial administration or gastrointestinal dysfunction, and loss of this function increases the susceptibility of the host to *Salmonella* infection (Sekirov *et al.* 2008). A history of prior antimicrobial exposure (Baker and Leyland 1973; Smith *et al.* 1978; Hird *et al.* 1986; Ernst *et al.* 2004) and abdominal surgery during hospitalisation (Owen *et al.* 1983; Begg *et al.* 1988; Ernst *et al.* 2004) have been shown to be risk factors associated with shedding of *Salmonella* in equine patients.

Following the establishment of a *Salmonella* infection a local and systemic inflammatory response develops in an effort to eliminate the organism. Mucosal inflammation results in increased mucosal permeability, increased secretion of water and electrolytes, and alterations in motility due to altered enteric nervous system function. The development of this secretory response, in combination with intestinal hypermotility and decreased intestinal transit times, may be beneficial by decreasing mucosal adherence of pathogenic organisms but may also interfere with the normal intestinal microbiota. Impairment of the normal barrier function of the intestinal mucosa, in combination with derangements in the normal flora, increases the pathogenicity of *Salmonella* organisms. This appears to result in part from the negative effects of these changes on the ability of the normal microbiota to effectively compete with the *Salmonella* organisms (Stecher *et al.* 2007).

The loss of fluid, electrolytes and protein that result from the intestinal inflammation and hypersecretion induced by *Salmonella* infection may be severe, requiring aggressive supportive care. Profound intestinal inflammation can occur, leading to permanent dysfunction and overwhelming systemic inflammation, resulting in the death of the affected individual. Bacterial translocation can also occur, resulting in the spread of *Salmonella* organisms to the regional lymph nodes initially, with subsequent entry into the systemic circulation resulting in bacteraemia (Hollis *et al.* 2008).

Clinical signs

The clinical signs of salmonellosis are variable and may include inapparent infections ('silent carriers') (Smith 1981) and a mild infection characterised by fever, mild abdominal pain, anorexia and depression without diarrhoea (Smith 1979). However, most horses that are clinically affected have moderate to severe, watery diarrhoea (Smith 1981) (**Fig 2**). Laminitis may be observed as a sequel to severe *Salmonella*-induced entercolitis. Foals may develop haemorrhagic diarrhoea (rarely seen in adult horses), septicaemia, pneumonia, meningitis and lameness due to either septic arthritis or physitis. Small colon impactions in adult horses frequently have associated salmonellosis (**Fig 1**).

Most clinically affected horses have neutropenia, vacuolated neutrophils (toxic changes), hypochloraemia, hyponatraemia, elevated PCV and azotaemia. Acidosis will be present if the anion gap (lactate) is increased. Hypoproteinaemia generally occurs within a couple of days even in those horses without diarrhoea. A rebound neutrophilia may occur after the initial neutropenia. Coagulation abnormalities such as thrombocytopenia and low antithrombin III may occur in more severe cases resulting in colonic, pulmonary, and limb thrombosis.

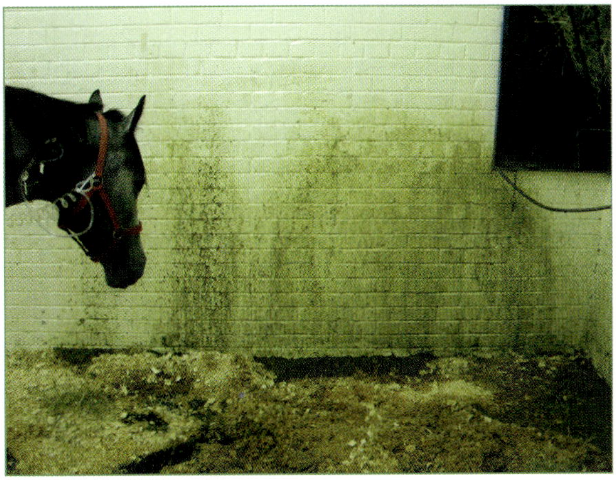

FIGURE 2: Profuse diarrhoea associated with salmonellosis.

In foals complete blood count (CBC), electrolyte, clinical chemistry, and coagulation markers are similar to those in the adult horses, although the number of band cells are often greater, and electrolyte abnormalities are generally more severe. Blood cultures, joint fluid, cerebrospinal fluid, or tracheal aspirates may be *Salmonella* positive in infected foals.

Abortion of mares can arise following infection by *Salmonella* serovar *abortus-equi*. Other clinical syndromes have also been associated with infection by this organism, including fistulous withers, orchitis, septicaemia and septic arthritis. Infection by this agent occurred in an endemic area in Japan (Akiba *et al.* 2003) and has occasionally been recorded in Europe in the past 20 years (Madic *et al.* 1997). Salmonellosis has also been associated with gastric dilation and ileus syndrome in adult horses (Merritt *et al.* 1982). Affected horses may present with fever and ileus with gastric reflux; *Salmonella* spp. may be isolated from the gastric reflux in these cases.

Chronic diarrhoea (i.e. diarrhoea that persists longer than 4 weeks) is not generally associated with salmonellosis (Smith *et al.* 1981). However, horses with chronic diarrhoea of other causes may shed *Salmonella* spp (Merritt 1994), and in some cases treatment with enrofloxacin may be beneficial (assuming that the underlying cause of the diarrhoea is also treated).

Diagnosis

Salmonella is reported to be the most frequently diagnosed aetiological agent in equine infectious diarrhoea (Murray 1996). Thousands of serotypes of *Salmonella* have been identified, although the majority of equine cases of salmonellosis are typically associated with one of a few serotypes, including: *Salmonella enterica* ssp. *enterica* serovars *typhimurium*, *enteritidis*, *krefeld*, *saint-paul*, *serovar anatum*, *newport* and *infantis* (Hird *et al.* 1984; Benson *et al.* 1985; Carter *et al.* 1986; Donahue 1986;

Ikeda *et al.* 1986; Dargatz *et al.* 1990; Traub-Dargatz *et al.* 1990; Walker *et al.* 1991; van Duijkeren *et al.* 1994, 2002; Hartmann *et al.* 1996; Pare *et al.* 1996; Tillotson *et al.* 1997; Weese *et al.* 2001; Schott *et al.* 2001; Ernst *et al.* 2004). The most commonly implicated of these is *Salmonella enterica* ssp. *enterica* serovar typhimurium. Diagnostic testing for *Salmonella* organisms relies primarily on faecal culture, using selective enrichment media (selenite broth, tetrathionate broth, or Rappaport-Vassiliadis enrichment broth) to enhance the detection of *Salmonella* spp. by increasing the number of organisms, and selective isolation media (brilliant green agar, MacConkey agar or xylose lysine desoxycholate [XLD] agar) to decrease the interference of other enteric organisms in the isolation process. Suspected isolates should be cultured on lysine iron agar and triple sugar iron agar to aid in the differentiation of *Salmonella* colonies from other enteric bacteria. Once isolated in culture, *Salmonella* organisms should be further identified by means of standard biochemical techniques or using a biochemical identification kit (API 20E)[1]. All confirmed isolates should then be further characterised by means of antimicrobial sensitivity testing, serotyping and phage typing (Schott *et al.* 2001; van Duijkeren *et al.* 2002).

When performing faecal culture a minimum of 10 g of faecal material should be submitted (Larsen 1997). *Salmonella* organisms are more consistently shed in formed stool than in diarrhoeic stool (Larsen 1997), increasing the likelihood of isolating the organism in the early stages or as the animal recovers from clinical disease. The time required to isolate and identify *Salmonella* organisms from faecal samples using culture represents one of the primary limitations of this approach, as it may require 3–4 days to obtain a definitive result on any single faecal culture. In addition, faecal culture exhibits a low sensitivity for the detection of *Salmonella* shedders in the equine population, although the use of multiple cultures (5), combined with utilisation of selective media, allows for adequate sensitivity levels to be achieved (van Duijkeren *et al.* 1995). Culture of rectal mucosa with faecal material substantially increases the sensitivity of culture techniques (Palmer *et al.* 1985). Faecal culture remains the gold standard for clinical monitoring of equine patients, despite its limitations and the recent development of more sensitive techniques, such as PCR.

Polymerase chain reaction tests are available for the detection of *Salmonella* spp. DNA in faeces, and these offer a more rapid turnaround time and higher sensitivity than culture techniques, but do not allow for further identification of the organisms or for antibacterial susceptibility testing (Cohen *et al.* 1996). The PCR techniques that have been developed for the detection of *Salmonella* DNA in equine faeces have been demonstrated to be both highly sensitive and specific (Amavisit *et al.* 2001; Ewart *et al.* 2001; Gentry-Weeks *et al.* 2002; Kurowski *et al.* 2002; Ward *et al.* 2005). The high sensitivity of these PCR techniques results from the ability of these assays to detect even a single DNA fragment containing the targeted DNA sequence. As a result, PCR testing can result in much higher numbers of positive results than culture techniques, as seen in one study where 40% of clinical faecal samples were positive on PCR testing, as compared to 2% positive results with culture (Amavisit *et al.* 2001). An even more dramatic example of this phenomenon was observed in a study that revealed that 17% of horses presented to the outpatient service of a veterinary teaching hospital were positive for *Salmonella* DNA on faecal PCR testing, yet none of these animals were culture positive, and 65% of hospitalised horses were PCR positive, while only 10% were culture positive (Cohen *et al.* 1996). An even greater disparity was found between PCR and culture techniques when analysing environmental samples, with 0.001% (1/783) of the samples positive on culture and 14% (110/783) of the samples positive on PCR testing (Ewart *et al.* 2001). A recent study reported that 75% of horses hospitalised for problems other than gastrointestinal disease were positive on serial PCR for *Salmonella* DNA, while only 9.5% were positive on serial faecal culture (Ward *et al.* 2005). The wide disparity between the results of culture and PCR techniques likely reflects the ability of the PCR techniques to detect DNA from nonviable (dead or inactivated) organisms in the faeces or the environment. This possibility was supported by the findings of Amavisit *et al.* (2001), who reported that the use of enrichment culture techniques did not increase the detectability of *Salmonella* from clinical faecal samples (Amavisit *et al.* 2001). On the basis of these results it is apparent that PCR techniques are overly sensitive for routine clinical application.

Further characterisation of *Salmonella* organisms cultured from clinical cases is important epidemiologically, both for the equine population and human populations potentially exposed to these organisms, and this can be achieved by means of serotyping and phage typing after the organism has been isolated using culture techniques. Phage typing has recently revealed the emergence of *Salmonella enterica* subspecies *enterica* serovar typhimurium definitive type (DT) 104 as an increasingly common animal pathogen (van Duijkeren *et al.* 2002; Weese *et al.* 2001). Equine salmonellosis due to DT104 represents a serious concern, as the organism exhibits antimicrobial multiresistance and presents an increased risk of zoonosis (van Duijkeren *et al.* 2002; Weese *et al.* 2001). It has been recommended that the phage type distribution of *Salmonella* isolates should be monitored to ascertain if DT104 remains a common equine pathogen (Weese *et al.* 2001; van Duijkeren *et al.* 2002).

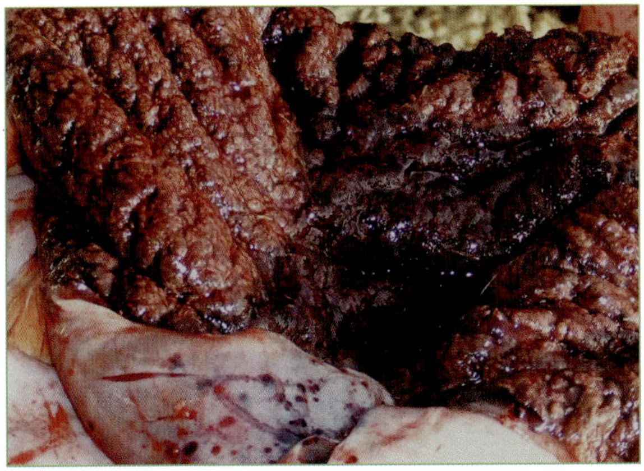

FIGURE 3: Post mortem appearance of salmonellosis. Severe colitis with extensive diphtheritic pseudomembranes over the mucosal surface.

Pathology

The gross pathological findings in horses with salmonellosis are those of enteritis and/or colitis. Typically, diffuse fibrinous or haemorrhagic inflammation of the caecum and large colon will be present. The mucosa may be ulcerated and there may be diphtheritic pseudomembranes adherent to the surface (**Fig 3**). Histologically, the caecum and colon show typhlitis/colitis with haemorrhage and coagulative necrosis (**Fig 4**). Fibrinocellular exudates may be attached to the necrotic epithelium. The capillaries of the *lamina propria* are frequently thrombosed. The mesenteric lymph nodes are typically swollen, haemorrhagic and oedematous (**Fig 5**). Small foci of hepatic necrosis ('paratyphoid nodules') may be observed in the liver.

Treatment

The treatment of salmonellosis is primarily supportive in nature, as the pathogenic bacteria may not respond to specific therapy. Substantial losses of

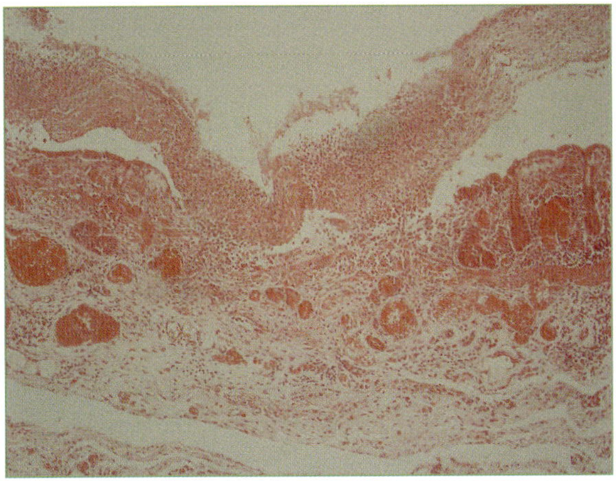

FIGURE 4: Salmonellosis – photomicrograph of the large colon. An ulcer with overlying diphtheritic membrane is present. The mucosa is congested. Haematoxylin and eosin.

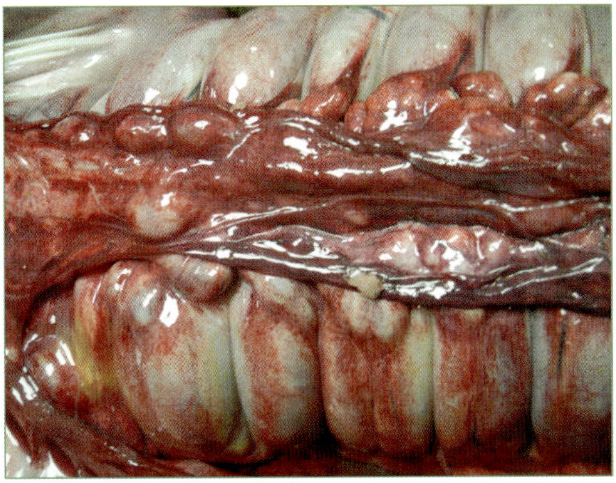

FIGURE 5: Post mortem appearance of salmonellosis. Oedematous and haemorrhagic colonic lymph nodes.

fluid from the circulating volume necessitate supportive fluid therapy in most cases, and accompanying losses of protein may also necessitate colloid therapy. Electrolyte derangements are often present, requiring that supplementation be provided either enterally or parenterally. Anti-inflammatory therapy is indicated in many of these conditions in order to address both the local and systemic components of the inflammatory response. Decreased voluntary feed intake or forced withholding of feed may necessitate nutritional support. Antimicrobial therapy may be indicated in some cases. The management of these cases can be quite intensive and is difficult to perform outside of a hospital environment.

Fluid therapy

Horses with salmonellosis typically present with dehydration secondary to fluid losses in the form of diarrhoea alone or in combination with decreased voluntary fluid intake. The correction of dehydration requires fluid replacement therapy, as these patients are often unable to correct their fluid status by voluntary intake. The fluid therapy plan should address both the correction of existing deficits, and the provision of fluids to replace ongoing losses and provide for basal metabolic requirements. In most cases fluid replacement is best accomplished via the parenteral route, as this allows for the rapid administration of large volumes of fluid in acute cases, and also allows for the ready correction of any electrolyte deficits. Colloid therapy may also be indicated, as hypoproteinaemia can develop due to the loss of protein into the lumen of the intestine. Colloid administration is accomplished by the use of either equine plasma or a synthetic colloid such as hydroxyethyl starch (Hetastarch)[2]. Equine plasma is typically administered at doses ranging from 10–20 ml/kg bwt, with the therapeutic goal of correcting the hypoalbuminaemia. Repeated dosing may be required due to the severity of the presenting hypoalbuminaemia and ongoing losses due to the underlying enteropathy. The use of hydroxyethyl starches can be beneficial in providing additional colloidal support and may have a more prolonged duration of action, but care must be taken to avoid overdosage due to the possibility of haemorrhagic dysfunction. The recommended dosage range for Hetastarch is typically 5–10 ml/kg bwt, but cumulative doses should not exceed a total of 20 ml/kg bwt. The use of hydroxyethyl starches will result in lowering of the measured total protein and albumin concentrations in the patient's serum due to dilution, which renders these values inaccurate as representations of colloid oncotic pressure. This requires that treatment be directed toward resolution of the clinical signs of hypoproteinaemia, rather than correction of the hypoproteinaemia itself.

Enteral fluid therapy has been proposed for cases of colitis, as small intestinal function is typically normal in these cases (Ecke *et al.* 1997; Schott 1998; Lopes *et al.* 2003). The enteral route is intrinsically more physiological, and has the additional advantages of reduced cost and simplicity (Lopes *et al.* 2003). Oral rehydration solutions are widely used in the treatment of human patients with diarrhoea, and the reported outcomes with oral rehydration are equivalent or superior to those reported with i.v. fluid therapy (Atherly-John *et al.* 2002; Nager and Wang 2002). The enteral route of administration can be used successfully in the treatment of horses with mild colitis, but more severely affected patients are usually unable to tolerate the administration of the volumes of fluids required to correct their deficits and replace their ongoing losses, and may exhibit increased discomfort, abdominal distension or even develop enterogastric reflux (Ecke *et al.* 1998; Lopes *et al.* 2003). Administration of enteral fluids in mild cases is easily accomplished using a large bore stomach tube or a smaller indwelling enteral feeding tube[3]. Enteral fluid solutions are easily prepared using tap water, and an isotonic solution can be formulated by combining 5 l of water with 1.5 tablespoons (28 g) of table salt, 0.5 teaspoons (3 g) of Lite salt[4] and 1.5 tablespoons (17 g) of baking soda ($NaHCO_3$) (Lopes *et al.* 2003). Enteral fluids prepared as above are recommended to be administered as repeated bolus doses or as a continuous infusion at rates of up to 6–8 l/h (Ecke *et al.* 1997; Lopes *et al.* 2003). The authors' experience, however, suggests that such aggressive rates of administration can result in substantial worsening of diarrhoea and abdominal discomfort and should be avoided. Preferably the enteral fluids should be administered as smaller bolus doses or as a continuous rate infusion at a rate of 3–6 l/h (Lopes *et al.* 2003).

Anti-inflammatory therapy

Anti-inflammatory therapy is important in the management of salmonellosis, primarily for the control of abdominal discomfort that can be present early in the disease process, but it is also indicated for the control of the systemic inflammatory response that accompanies this disease process. The most commonly utilised anti-inflammatory drug is flunixin meglumine, which is a potent visceral analgesic with a well-demonstrated ability to suppress abdominal pain in equine gastrointestinal diseases when administered at 1.1 mg/kg bwt *per os* or i.v. (Clark and Clark 1999). In addition, flunixin meglumine has been shown to have some 'anti-endotoxaemic' effects, as it suppress the systemic response to endotoxin when given as a pretreatment at doses as low as 0.25 mg/kg bwt, thereby minimising the severity of endotoxaemia-associated hypotension, hypovolaemia, haemoconcentration, pulmonary hypertension, tachypnoea, tachycardia and lactic acidosis (Bottoms *et al.* 1981; Dunkle *et al.* 1985; Ewert *et al.* 1985; Templeton *et al.* 1987). Additionally, flunixin meglumine has been shown to reduce the development of ileus following endotoxin exposure (King and Gerring 1989). It appears that nonsteroidal anti-inflammatory drug therapy may also provide a useful anti-secretory effect in salmonellosis by inhibiting the increased production of prostaglandin E2 that accompanies *Salmonella* infection and which appears to be responsible, in part, for epithelial hypersecretion (Bertelsen *et al.* 2003). There is some evidence that nonsteroidal anti-inflammatory drug administration may impair the recovery of barrier function in equine intestinal mucosa, but this does not appear to be associated with increased absorption of LPS from the intestinal lumen *in vitro* (Tomlinson and Blikslager 2004, 2005).

Anti-endotoxin therapies

As bacterial endotoxin has been shown to play an important role in the development of severe systemic inflammation (endotoxaemia) associated with gastrointestinal disease there has been significant interest in finding ways to inhibit the activity of endotoxin in the systemic circulation. Two basic approaches have been utilised in the attempt to neutralise endotoxin: the administration of anti-endotoxin antibodies and the use of chemical substances that bind to endotoxin (Moore and Barton 2003). The development of antibodies to bacterial endotoxin has been challenging due to the antigenic variation of endotoxin between species of Gram-negative bacteria, and for this reason antibodies have been targeted against the more conserved core and lipid A regions of the endotoxin molecule (Moore and Barton 2003). Studies regarding the efficacy of anti-endotoxin antibodies in experimental equine endotoxaemia, and in horses presenting with colic, have also yielded conflicting results, leading to uncertainty regarding the clinical application of this type of therapy (Morris *et al.* 1986; Garner *et al.* 1988; Spier *et al.* 1989; Durando *et al.* 1994). Furthermore, worsened clinical signs of endotoxaemia and increased systemic inflammation associated with the administration of anti-endotoxin antiserum in a foal model of endotoxaemia has been reported (Durando *et al.* 1994). Serum and plasma products containing anti-endotoxin antibodies are commercially available for use in the horse and are widely used, but the uncertainty from published reports regarding this therapy needs to be resolved before specific recommendations can be made.

The use of the anti-endotoxin agent polymyxin B has been extensively examined in a variety of animal species and in man, and there is good evidence that this substance binds endotoxin and prevents it from initiating or potentiating the systemic inflammatory response. Polymyxin B has been examined in several equine endotoxaemia models. It has been demonstrated to decrease the severity of both the clinical signs of endotoxaemia and the severity of the systemic inflammatory response, even when administered before or after endotoxin exposure, although the best effects were associated with pretreatment (Durando *et al.* 1994; Barton 2000; Parviainen *et al.* 2001; Barton *et al.* 2004). The current recommendation for the clinical use of polymyxin B is to initiate therapy as early as possible using a dosage of 6000 iu/kg bwt (1 mg/kg bwt) diluted in 1 l of 5% dextrose given i.v. over 15 min every 8 h (Morresey and Mackay 2006). Due to the potential for nephrotoxicity it is recommended that horses administered this drug have adequate hydration and that serum creatinine be monitored (Moore and Barton 2003). Prolonged administration should also be avoided to minimise the risk of nephrotoxicity, and a maximum of 3–5 doses should be administered.

Nutritional support

Horses suffering from salmonellosis should ideally have free access to roughage and supplemental feeding *ad libitum* with concentrates to meet at least their maintenance metabolic energy requirements (roughly 67 MJ for a 500 kg horse) (Magdesian 2003). Unfortunately, some horses suffering from salmonellosis may be anorexic due to the illness, impairing the patient's ability to meet their metabolic needs through voluntary intake. Most adult horses can reasonably be maintained without nutritional support for several days, as they will mobilise their endogenous energy reserves (fat, muscle) to meet their metabolic needs. However, some horses and ponies appear predisposed to excessive fat mobilisation and they should not be maintained without nutritional support due to the risks of hypertriglyceridaemia and hyperlipaemia (Dunkel and McKenzie 2003). Nutritional supplementation is most readily accomplished using the parenteral route as these patients are typically already receiving i.v. fluid therapy. Parenteral nutrition can be characterised as partial or complete, based upon whether or not it meets the animal's entire nutritional needs. Total parenteral nutrition requires the use of both carbohydrate and lipid energy sources, in combination with amino acids and strives to supply all of the patient's nutritional requirements. This degree of support is rarely required in adult patients, where partial caloric supplementation is adequate for short term support. Partial parenteral nutrition can be accomplished with carbohydrate or carbohydrate/amino acid solutions. Supplementation of the i.v. fluids with dextrose at a moderate rate of 21–42 kJ/kg bwt/day (1.5–3 l of 50% dextrose per day) appears to be beneficial in clinically ill horses with decreased or absent appetite as it minimises the degree of fat mobilisation secondary to a negative energy balance, and has been shown to correct hypertriglyceridaemia (Dunkel and McKenzie 2003; Magdesian 2003). If the patient requires support beyond a few days then amino acid supplementation should be provided.

Probiotics/prebiotics

Restoration of the microbial flora of the gastrointestinal tract has been shown in many species to aid in the resolution of colitis and this is most readily accomplished by the administration of live beneficial enteric organisms. These organisms are termed probiotics, which have been defined as live microbial feed supplements that are beneficial to health (Fooks and Gibson 2002). A more recent, broader concept is that of 'biotherapeutic agents', which have been defined as living microorganisms used either to prevent or to treat diseases by interacting with the natural microecology of the host (Elmer and McFarland 2001). Much of the research regarding probiotics has been performed in other species, and the types of organism used in equine probiotics are generally the same as have been administered to human patients. As a result it is not clear that the organisms present in many equine probiotics (*Lactobacillus*, *Bifidobacterium*, *Enterococcus*) are necessarily the most relevant to the equine gastrointestinal flora (Weese *et al.* 2004). The fact that probiotics are marketed as feed supplements also means that there is no requirement regarding the demonstration of efficacy of these products, therefore any label claims of efficacy should be viewed with caution. This concern is reinforced by the disappointing results of the few trials that have looked at the effects of probiotics in equine salmonellosis (van Duijkeren *et al.* 1995; Parraga *et al.* 1997; Kim *et al.* 2001) and foal diarrhoea (Weese and Rousseau 2005). The yeast *S. boulardii* has been shown to be beneficial in equine clostridial enterocolitis (Desrochers *et al.* 2005), and could prove useful in the treatment of salmonellosis as it has been reported to have beneficial effects in an experimental salmonellosis model (Czerucka and Rampal 2002). Further work is clearly required in order to better define the types of probiotic organisms most likely to be beneficial in equine colitis.

An alternative means of restoring the normal gastrointestinal flora is the provision of nondigestible oligosaccharides as a 'prebiotic'. The concept behind prebiotics is that of an insoluble fibre that selects for, and stimulates the growth of, beneficial microorganisms in the large intestine that can alter the microbiota to a healthy composition and exert beneficial effects on the host (Bengmark 2001). The substance most studied as a prebiotic is germinated barley feedstuff (GBF), which is generated by the brewing industry as a by-product of the brewing process. GBF has been shown to have anti-inflammatory effects in animal models of colitis, with one study reporting decreased gastrointestinal and systemic inflammation as well as decreased mucosal injury in association with increased levels of the beneficial short-chain fatty acid butyrate (Kanauchi *et al.* 2008). A similar study demonstrated a superior effect of GBF as compared to a probiotic consisting of *Lactobacillus* and *Cl. butyricum* organisms that demonstrated no effect (Fukuda *et al.* 2002). Dried GBF is widely used in dairy cattle feeds and is a component of some commercial horse feeds and appears to be a safe feed supplement, although no specific reports are available regarding GBF administration in the horse. The first author has utilised fresh and frozen GBF in horses with colitis at an empirical dosage rate of 0.2–0.4 kg 3–4 times daily, with some encouraging clinical results. Further work is required, however, to demonstrate efficacy of this treatment in equine enterocolitis and to determine the most appropriate dosage of GBF for feeding to horses with diarrhoea.

Gastrointestinal protectants and adsorbents

An additional means of limiting gastrointestinal inflammation is the administration of products by the enteral route, which may exert anti-inflammatory effects on the mucosa or that impair the activity of the enteric pathogens or their toxins (Tillotson and Traub-Dargatz 2003). Bismuth subsalicylate has been used as an agent to protect the gastrointestinal mucosa and decrease mucosal inflammation, but there is not much evidence that it has a significant effect in secretory diarrhoea in any species (Aranda-Michel and Giannella 1999; Zaman *et al.* 2001). This compound has been reported to stimulate intestinal sodium and water absorption and to have anti-inflammatory and antibacterial effects, including direct binding of bacterial toxins (Aranda-Michel and Giannella 1999). Bismuth subsalicylate is widely regarded as a safe over-the-counter human antidiarrhoeal agent, but there are reports of toxicity associated with overdosage (Vernace *et al.* 1994; Gordon *et al.* 1995). Recommended dosages for bismuth subsalicylate in the horse range from 0.5–4 ml/kg bwt every 4–6 h (Tillotson and Traub-Dargatz 2003).

Recent work has examined the possible application of the adsorptive substance di-tri-octahedral smectite (DTO smectite; Biosponge[5]) in enterocolitis. This product and the related dioctohedral smectite, have been shown to bind *Clostridium difficile* toxins A and B, and *Cl. perfringens* enterotoxins *in vitro* (Martirosian *et al.* 1998; Weese *et al.* 2003). These compounds are thought to act by several mechanisms, including direct binding of bacterial toxins, direct adsorption of bacteria, modification of the gastrointestinal mucus to inhibit toxin absorption and repair of mucosal integrity (Gonzalez *et al.* 2004). A recent study utilising an experimental model of inflammatory colitis in rats has demonstrated that this type of compound may also have direct anti-inflammatory effects within the intestinal mucosa (Gonzalez *et al.* 2004). A small study reported that outcome was substantially improved in horses suffering from clostridial enterocolitis with the use of DTO smectite (Herthel 2000). The recommended dosage is 1.4 kg of powder in water via nasogastric tube, followed by 0.4 kg every 4–6 h. While the indication for using this product in the horse suffering from salmonellosis is less clear than in the case of clostridial colitis, clinical experience suggests that this product may be of some benefit in salmonellosis.

Antimicrobial therapy

The role of antimicrobial therapy in the treatment of salmonellosis is controversial, due to concerns regarding lack of efficacy and the potential development of antimicrobial resistance (Frye and Fedorka-Cray 2007; Vo *et al.* 2007). Often, antimicrobial therapy is used in patients suffering from gastrointestinal disease due to the presence of fever and leucopenia, which may indicate the presence of bacterial infection or may result from the effects of bacterial toxins such as endotoxin. There are additional concerns that severe gastrointestinal disease may be associated with impairment of the barrier function of the gastrointestinal mucosa, resulting in an increased risk of bacterial invasion leading to localised infection or septicaemia and infections distant to the intestine (pneumonia, endocarditis, meningitis etc.). The efficacy of systemic antimicrobial therapy in the prevention of bacterial invasion in gastrointestinal disease is not established (Koratzanis *et al.* 2002).

Antimicrobial resistance is common in the *Salmonella* organisms associated with enterocolitis, especially to the beta-lactams, tetracylines, trimethoprim, and the sulpha drugs (van Duijkeren *et al.* 2002; Randall *et al.* 2004). The intracellular localisation of *Salmonella* organisms limits their susceptibility to antimicrobials that exhibit a limited ability to penetrate the cell wall, such as the aminoglycosides, which decreases the utility of these drugs, even though many isolates are sensitive to amikacin. Increased *in vivo* susceptibility is seen to those antimicrobials that are able to reach therapeutic levels intracellularly, such as the fluoroquinolones, and these drugs are widely used in human salmonellosis patients (van Duijkeren and Houwers 2000). Cephalosporins are also frequently used in human salmonellosis patients, and the third generation cephalosporin ceftiofur has been reported to be effective in the treatment of calves with salmonellosis (Fecteau *et al.* 2003). Many equine and other domestic animal *Salmonella* isolates are reported to be sensitive to ceftiofur and the fluoroquinolones (Seyfarth *et al.* 1997; van Duijkeren *et al.* 2002), although ceftiofur resistance does appear to be increasing (Frye and Fedorka-Cray 2007). Multi-drug resistant strains from several equine nosocomial outbreaks have been reported to be sensitive to ciprofloxacin, which is the active metabolite of enrofloxacin (Dargatz and Traub-Dargatz 2004).

While the treatment of equine patients suffering from salmonellosis with appropriate antimicrobials is controversial it should be considered as it may result in an improved chance of survival. Given the presence of multiresistant strains of *Salmonella* it is important that one determines the antimicrobial sensitivity pattern of any equine isolates and utilise this as a guide to ongoing therapy in the individual patient or concurrently affected individuals. Based upon the available data, empirical treatment with enrofloxacin could represent a reasonable initial approach in the severely affected patient while sensitivity results are pending. Enrofloxacin is the most commonly used fluoroquinolone in the horse and it has a relatively broad spectrum, with excellent activity against Gram-negative organisms. Enrofloxacin is a concentration dependent antimicrobial, and exhibits peak concentration-dependent bactericidal effects with prolonged post antibiotic effects. As a result it can be given at relatively high doses at a decreased frequency. Toxicity is primarily due to adverse effects on cartilage maturation, resulting in a contraindication to its use in growing animals (Beluche *et al.* 1999; Egerbacher *et al.* 2001). Enrofloxacin is administered at 7.5 mg/kg bwt once daily orally or 5 mg/kg bwt once daily i.v. (Giguere *et al.* 1996; Kaartinen *et al.* 1997).

Control

The shedding of *Salmonella* organisms into the environment from horses as well as domestic and wild animals in the vicinity of the facility cannot be entirely prevented; therefore there is always a risk of exposure. As a result, the control of *Salmonella* infections is dependent upon the utilisation of effective biosecurity measures designed to minimise the risk of infection in susceptible individuals and biocontainment procedures to minimise the spread of disease when infection does occur. Segregation of horses likely to shed *Salmonella* organisms, such as those having suffered from intestinal impactions or having undergone colic surgery, can help to reduce the risk of exposure for susceptible individuals in the hospital population. Isolation of animals that develop diarrhoea and/or fever and leucopenia represents a first step in biocontainment, and can be accomplished using barrier procedures within the hospital ward or preferably by moving the individual to a separate housing facility used solely for this purpose. Barrier procedures must be tailored to suit the individual facility but include the wearing of gloves, gowns and boots when working with the affected individual, as well as using foot baths and hand washing and disinfection (Weese 2004). Manure from suspect or confirmed cases should be handled separately from the rest of the facilities waste stream and should never be spread on pastures. Faecal samples for *Salmonella* culture should be collected at the time the animal is isolated, both for surveillance and for the optimisation of patient therapy. Serial cultures should be performed in order to ensure that 3–5 cultures are negative for *Salmonella* prior to removing an animal from isolation and returning them to the hospital or farm population. The stall and any other potentially contaminated surfaces must be thoroughly cleaned and disinfected, and it is recommended that the surfaces be cultured prior to reuse in order to ensure that disinfection has been effective. When used after cleaning to remove organic debris, sodium hypochlorite is an effective disinfectant and is widely used to good effect.

Outcome

Due to the severity of the local and systemic inflammatory responses induced by salmonellosis, the prognosis for survival is somewhat guarded in most cases. It is possible that the prognosis may be improved with aggressive supportive care and specific therapy, but this is difficult to predict given the variability of these organisms with regards to virulence and resistance to antimicrobials. Due to the widespread shedding of *Salmonella* organisms by clinically normal horses and the increased susceptibility to infection in hospitalised horses, surveillance and infection control will remain the mainstays for controlling equine salmonellosis.

Public health risk

Salmonellosis is an important zoonotic disease that is considered to be responsible for more than one million human cases of diarrhoea, 15,000 hospitalisations and 400 deaths annually in the USA (Voetsch *et al.* 2004). Most cases of human infection arise from food-borne exposure, including contamination of horsemeat in parts of the world where horsemeat is used for human consumption (Espie and Weill 2003). Direct contact with infected horses is also an important risk factor for zoonotic transmission (Anon 2001). The emergence of multi-drug resistant strains, such as multidrug resistant *Salmonella* serovar newport, causes particular concern about direct transmission between infected animals and their owners and attending veterinary staff (Traub-Dargatz and Besser 2007).

Manufacturers' addresses

[1]bioMerieux, Hazelwood, Missouri, USA.
[2]Hospira, Lake Forest, Illinois, USA.
[3]MILA international Inc., Erlanger, Kentucky, USA.
[4]Morton Salt, Chicago, Illinois, USA.
[5]Platinum Performance, Los Olivos, California, USA.

References

Akiba, M., Uchida, I., Nishimori, K., Tanaka, K., Anzai, T., Kuwamoto, Y., Wada, R., Ohya, T. and Ito, H. (2003) Comparison of *Salmonella enterica* serovar *Abortus equi* isolates of equine origin by pulsed-field gel electrophoresis and fluorescent amplified-fragment length polymorphism fingerprinting. *Vet. Microbiol.* **92**, 379.

Amavisit, P., Browning, G.F., Lightfoot, D., Church, S., Anderson, G.A., Whithear, K.G. and Markham, P.F. (2001) Rapid PCR detection of *Salmonella* in horse faecal samples. *Vet. Microbiol.* **79**, 63-74.

Anon (2001) Outbreaks of multidrug-resistant *Salmonella typhimurium* associated with veterinary facilities - Idaho, Minnesota, and Washington, 1999. MMWR 50 701. Centers for Disease Control and Prevention.

Aranda-Michel, J. and Giannella, R.A. (1999) Acute diarrhoea: a practical review. *Am. J. Med.* **106**, 670-676.

Atherly-John, Y.C., Cunningham, S.J. and Crain, E.F. (2002) A randomized trial of oral vs intravenous rehydration in a pediatric emergency department. *Arch. Pediatr. Adolesc. Med.* **156**, 1240-1243.

Baker, J.R. and Leyland, A. (1973) Diarrhoea in the horse associated with stress and tetracycline therapy. *Vet. Rec.* **93**, 583-584.

Barton, M.H. (2000) Use of polymyxin B for treatment of endotoxemia in horses. *Comp. cont. Educ. pract. Vet.* **11**, 1056-1059.

Barton, M.H., Parviainen, A. and Norton, N. (2004) Polymyxin B protects horses against induced endotoxaemia *in vivo*. *Equine vet. J.* **36**, 397-401.

Begg, A.P., Johnston, K.G., Hutchins, D.R. and Edwards, D.J. (1988) Some aspects of the epidemiology of equine salmonellosis. *Aust. vet. J.* **65**, 221-223.

Beluche, L.A., Bertone, A.L., Anderson, D.E., Kohn, C.W. and Weisbrode, S.E. (1999) *In vitro* dose-dependent effects of enrofloxacin on equine articular cartilage. *Am. J. vet. Res.* **60**, 577-582.

Bengmark, S. (2001) Pre-, pro- and synbiotics. *Curr. Opin. Clin. Nutr. Metab. Care.* **4**, 571-579.

Benson, C.E., Palmer, J.E. and Bannister, M.F. (1985) Antibiotic susceptibilities of *Salmonella* species isolated at a large animal veterinary medical center: a three year study. *Can. J. Comp. Med.* **49**, 125-128.

Bertelsen, L.S., Paesold, G., Eckmann, L. and Barrett, K.E. (2003) *Salmonella* infection induces a hypersecretory phenotype in human intestinal xenografts by inducing cyclooxygenase 2. *Infect. Immun.* **71**, 2102-2109.

Bottoms, G.D., Fessler, J.F., Roesel, O.F., Moore, A.B. and Frauenfelder, H.C. (1981) Endotoxin-induced hemodynamic changes in ponies: effects of flunixin meglumine. *Am. J. vet. Res.* **42**, 1514-1518.

Carter, J.D., Hird, D.W., Farver, T.B. and Hjerpe, C.A. (1986) Salmonellosis in hospitalized horses: seasonality and case fatality rates. *J. Am. vet. med. Ass.* **188**, 163-167.

Clark, J.O. and Clark, T.P. (1999) Analgesia. *Vet. Clin. N. Am.: Equine Pract.* **15**, 705-723.

Coburn, B., Grassl, G.A. and Finlay, B.B. (2007) *Salmonella*, the host and disease: a brief review. *Immunol. Cell. Biol.* **85**, 112-118.

Cohen, N.D., Wallis, D.E., Neibergs, H.L. and Hargis, B.M. (1995) Detection of *Salmonella enteritidis* in equine feces using the polymerase chain reaction and genus-specific oligonucleotide primers. *J. vet. Diagn. Invest.* **7**, 219-222.

Cohen, N.D., Martin, L.J., Simpson, R.B., Wallis, D.E. and Neibergs, H.L. (1996) Comparison of polymerase chain reaction and microbiological culture for detection of *salmonellae* in equine feces and environmental samples. *Am. J. vet. Res.* **57**, 780-786.

Cohen, N.D., Neibergs, H.L., Wallis, D.E., Simpson, R.B., McGruder, E.D. and Hargis, B.M. (1994) Genus-specific detection of *salmonellae* in equine feces by use of the polymerase chain reaction. *Am. J. vet. Res.* **55**, 1049-1054.

Czerucka, D. and Rampal, P. (2002) Experimental effects of *Saccharomyces boulardii* on diarrhoeal pathogens. *Microbes Infect.* **4**, 733-739.

Dargatz, D.A. and Traub-Dargatz, J.L. (2004) Multidrug-resistant *Salmonella* and nosocomial infections. *Vet. Clin. N. Am.: Equine Pract.* **20**, 587-600.

Desrochers, A.M., Dolente, B.A., Roy, M.F., Boston, R. and Carlisle, S. (2005) Efficacy of *Saccharomyces boulardii* for treatment of horses with acute enterocolitis. *J. Am. vet. med. Ass.* **227**, 954-959.

Donahue, J.M. (1986) Emergence of antibiotic-resistant *Salmonella agona* in horses in Kentucky. *J. Am. vet. med. Ass.* **188**, 592-594.

Dunkel, B. and McKenzie, H.C., 3rd (2003) Severe hypertriglyceridaemia in clinically ill horses: diagnosis, treatment and outcome. *Equine vet. J.* **35**, 590-595.

Dunkle, N.J., Bottoms, G.D., Fessler, J.F., Knox, K. and Roesel, O.F. (1985) Effects of flunixin meglumine on blood pressure and fluid compartment volume changes in ponies given endotoxin. *Am. J. vet. Res.* **46**, 1540-1544.

Durando, M.M., MacKay, R.J., Linda, S. and Skelley, L.A. (1994) Effects of polymyxin B and *Salmonella typhimurium* antiserum on horses given endotoxin intravenously. *Am. J. vet. Res.* **55**, 921-927.

Ecke, P., Hodgson, D.R. and Rose, R.J. (1997) Review of oral rehydration solutions for horses with diarrhoea. *Aust. vet. J.* **75**, 417-420.

Ecke, P., Hodgson, D.R. and Rose, R.J. (1998) Induced diarrhoea in horses. Part 2: Response to administration of an oral rehydration solution. *Vet. J.* **155**, 161-170.

Egerbacher, M., Edinger, J. and Tschulenk, W. (2001) Effects of enrofloxacin and ciprofloxacin hydrochloride on canine and equine chondrocytes in culture. *Am. J. vet. Res.* **62**, 704-708.

Elmer, G.W. and McFarland, L.V. (2001) Biotherapeutic agents in the treatment of infectious diarrhoea. *Gastroenterol. Clin. North. Am.* **30**, 837-854.

Ernst, N.S., Hernandez, J.A., MacKay, R.J., Brown, M.P., Gaskin, J.M., Nguyen, A.D., Giguere, S., Colahan, P.T., Troedsson, M.R., Haines, G.R., Addison, I.R. and Miller, B.J. (2004) Risk factors associated with faecal *Salmonella* shedding among hospitalized horses with signs of gastrointestinal tract disease. *J. Am. vet. med. Ass.* **225**, 275-281.

Espie, E. and Weill, F.X. (2003) Outbreak of multidrug resistant *Salmonella* Newport due to the consumption of horsemeat in France, Eurosurveill Week 7 http://www.eurosurveillance.org/ew/2003/030703.asp

Ewart, S.L., Schott, H.C., 2nd, Robison, R.L., Dwyer, R.M., Eberhart, S.W. and Walker, R.D. (2001) Identification of sources of *Salmonella* organisms in a veterinary teaching hospital and evaluation of the effects of disinfectants on detection of *Salmonella* organisms on surface materials. *J. Am. vet. med. Ass.* **218**, 1145-1151.

Ewert, K.M., Fessler, J.F., Templeton, C.B., Bottoms, G.D., Latshaw, H.S. and Johnson, M.A. (1985) Endotoxin-induced hematologic and blood chemical changes in ponies: effects of flunixin meglumine, dexamethasone, and prednisolone. *Am. J. vet. Res.* **46**, 24-30.

Fecteau, M.E., House, J.K., Kotarski, S.F., Tankersley, N.S., Ontiveros, M.M., Alcantar, C.R. and Smith, B.P. (2003) Efficacy of ceftiofur for treatment of experimental salmonellosis in neonatal calves. *Am. J. vet. Res.* **64**, 918-925.

Foley, S.L. and Lynne, A.M. (2008) Food animal-associated *Salmonella* challenges: pathogenicity and antimicrobial resistance. *J. anim. Sci.* **86**, E173-187.

Fooks, L.J. and Gibson, G.R. (2002) Probiotics as modulators of the gut flora. *Br. J. Nutr.* **88**, *Suppl.* **1**, S39-49.

Frye, J.G. and Fedorka-Cray, P.J. (2007) Prevalence, distribution and characterisation of ceftiofur resistance in *Salmonella enterica* isolated from animals in the USA from 1999 to 2003. *Int. J. Antimicrob. Agents.* **30**, 134-142.

Fukuda, M., Kanauchi, O., Araki, Y., Andoh, A., Mitsuyama, K., Takagi, K., Toyonaga, A., Sata, M., Fujiyama, Y., Fukuoka, M., Matsumoto, Y. and Bamba, T. (2002) Prebiotic treatment of experimental colitis with germinated barley foodstuff: A comparison with probiotic or antibiotic treatment. *Int. J. Mol. Med.* **9**, 65-70.

Garner, H.E., Sprouse, R.F. and Lager, K. (1988) Cross-protection of ponies from sublethal *Escherichia coli* endotoxemia by *Salmonella typhimurium* antiserum. *Equine Pract.* **10**, 10-17.

Gentry-Weeks, C., Hutcheson, H.J., Kim, L.M., Bolte, D., Traub-Dargatz, J., Morley, P., Powers, B. and Jessen, M. (2002) Identification of two phylogenetically related organisms from feces by PCR for detection of *Salmonella* spp. *J. clin. Microbiol.* **40**, 1487-1492.

Giguere, S., Sweeney, R.W. and Belanger, M. (1996) Pharmacokinetics of enrofloxacin in adult horses and concentration of the drug in serum, body fluids, and endometrial tissues after repeated intragastrically administered doses. *Am. J. vet. Res.* **57**, 1025-1030.

Gonzalez, R., de Medina, F.S., Martinez-Augustin, O., Nieto, A., Galvez, J., Risco, S. and Zarzuelo, A. (2004) Anti-inflammatory effect of diosmectite in hapten-induced colitis in the rat. *Br. J. Pharmacol.* **141**, 951-960.

Gordon, M.F., Abrams, R.I., Rubin, D.B., Barr, W.B. and Correa, D.D. (1995) Bismuth subsalicylate toxicity as a cause of prolonged encephalopathy with myoclonus. *Mov. Disord.* **10**, 220-222.

Grassl, G.A. and Finlay, B.B. (2008) Pathogenesis of enteric *Salmonella* infections. *Curr. Opin. Gastroenterol.* **24**, 22-26.

Hartmann, F.A., Callan, R.J., McGuirk, S.M. and West, S.E. (1996) Control of an outbreak of salmonellosis caused by drug-resistant *Salmonella anatum* in horses at a veterinary hospital and measures to prevent future infections. *J. Am. vet. med. Ass.* **209**, 629-631.

Herthel, D. (2000) Preventing and treating colitis with DTO smectite. *J. equine vet. Sci.* **20**, 432.

Hird, D.W., Casebolt, D.B., Carter, J.D., Pappaioanou, M. and Hjerpe, C.A. (1986) Risk factors for salmonellosis in hospitalized horses. *J. Am. vet. med. Ass.* **188**, 173-177.

Hird, D.W., Pappaioanou, M. and Smith, B.P. (1984) Case-control study of risk factors associated with isolation of *Salmonella saintpaul* in hospitalized horses. *Am. J. Epidemiol.* **120**, 852-864.

Hollis, A.R., Wilkins, P.A., Palmer, J.E. and Boston, R.C. (2008) Bacteremia in equine neonatal diarrhoea: A retrospective study (1990-2007). *J. vet. Intern. Med.* **22**, 1203-1209.

Ikeda, J.S., Hirsh, D.C., Jang, S.S. and Biberstein, E.L. (1986)

Characteristics of *Salmonella* isolated from animals at a veterinary medical teaching hospital. *Am. J. vet. Res.* **47**, 232-235.

Kaartinen, L., Panu, S. and Pyorala, S. (1997) Pharmacokinetics of enrofloxacin in horses after single intravenous and intramuscular administration. *Equine vet. J.* **29**, 378-381.

Kanauchi, O., Oshima, T., Andoh, A., Shioya, M. and Mitsuyama, K. (2008) Germinated barley foodstuff ameliorates inflammation in mice with colitis through modulation of mucosal immune system. *Scand. J. Gastroenterol.* **43**, 1-7.

Kim, L.M., Morley, P.S., Traub-Dargatz, J.L., Salman, M.D. and Gentry-Weeks, C. (2001) Factors associated with *Salmonella* shedding among equine colic patients at a veterinary teaching hospital. *J. Am. vet. med. Ass.* **218**, 740-748.

King, J.N. and Gerring, E.L. (1989) Antagonism of endotoxin-induced disruption of equine bowel motility by flunixin and phenylbutazone. *Equine vet. J., Suppl.* **7**, 38-42.

Koratzanis, G., Giamarellos-Bourboulis, E.J., Papalambros, E. and Giamarellou, H. (2002) Bacterial translocation following intrabdominal surgery. Any influence of antimicrobial prophylaxis? *Int. J. Antimicrob. Agents* **20**, 457-460.

Kurowski, P.B., Traub-Dargatz, J.L., Morley, P.S. and Gentry-Weeks, C.R. (2002) Detection of *Salmonella* spp in faecal specimens by use of real-time polymerase chain reaction assay. *Am. J. vet. Res.* **63**, 1265-1268.

Larsen, J. (1997) Acute colitis in adult horses. A review with emphasis on aetiology and pathogenesis. *Vet. Q.* **19**, 72-80.

Lopes, M.A.F., Hepburn, R.J., McKenzie 3rd, H.C. and Sykes, B.W. (2003) Enteral fluid therapy for horses. *Comp. cont. Educ. pract. Vet.* **25**, 390-397.

Madic, J., Hajsig, D., Sostaric, B., Curic, S., Seol, B., Naglic, T. and Cvetnic, Z. (1997) An outbreak of abortion in mares associated with *Salmonella abortusequi* infection. *Equine vet. J.* **29**, 230-233.

Magdesian, G.K. (2003) Nutrition for critical gastrointestinal illness: feeding horses with diarrhoea or colic. *Vet. Clin. N. Am.: Equine Pract.* **19**, 617-644.

Mainar-Jaimc, R.C., House, J.K., Smith, B.P., Hird, D.W., House, A.M. and Kamiya, D.Y. (1998) Influence of faecal shedding of *Salmonella* organisms on mortality in hospitalized horses. *J. Am. vet. med. Ass.* **213**, 1162-1166.

Martirosian, G., Rouyan, G., Zalewski, T. and Meisel-Mikolajczyk, F. (1998) Dioctahedral smectite neutralization activity of *Clostridium difficile* and *Bacteroides fragilis* toxins *in vitro*. *Acta. Microbiol. Pol.* **47**, 177-183.

Merritt, A.M. (1994) Chronic diarrhoea in horses: a summary. *Vet. Med.* **89**, 363.

Merritt, A.M., Bobbins, J. and Brewer, B. (1982) Is *Salmonella* infection a cause of the acute gastric dilatation/ileus syndrome in horses? In: *Proceedings of the Equine Colic Research Symposium*. pp 119-124

Moore, J.N. and Barton, M.H. (2003) Treatment of endotoxemia. *Vet. Clin. N. Am.: Equine Pract.* **19**, 681-695.

Morresey, P.R. and Mackay, R.J. (2006) Endotoxin-neutralizing activity of polymyxin B in blood after IV administration in horses. *Am. J. vet. Res.* **67**, 642-647.

Morris, D.D., Whitlock, R.H. and Corbeil, L.B. (1986) Endotoxemia in horses: protection provided by antiserum to core lipopolysaccharide. *Am. J. vet. Res.* **47**, 544-550.

Murray, M.J. (1996) Salmonellosis in horses. *J. Am. vet. med. Ass.* **209**, 558-560.

Murray, M.J. (2002) Medical disorders of the small intestine In: *Large Animal Internal Medicine*, 3rd edn., Ed: B.P. Smith, Mosby, St Louis. pp 641-649.

Nager, A.L. and Wang, V.J. (2002) Comparison of nasogastric and intravenous methods of rehydration in pediatric patients with acute dehydration. *Pediatrics* **109**, 566-572.

Owen, R.A., Fullerton, J. and Barnum, D.A. (1983) Effects of transportation, surgery, and antibiotic therapy in ponies infected with *Salmonella*. *Am. J. vet. Res.* **44**, 46-50.

Palmer, J.E., Benson, C.E. and Whitlock, R.H. (1985) *Salmonella* shed by horses with colic. *J. Am. vet. med. Ass.* **187**, 256-257.

Pare, J., Carpenter, T.E. and Thurmond, M.C. (1996) Analysis of spatial and temporal clustering of horses with *Salmonella* krefeld in an intensive care unit of a veterinary hospital. *J. Am. vet. med. Ass.* **209**, 626-628.

Parraga, M.E., Spier, S.J., Thurmond, M. and Hirsh, D. (1997) A clinical trial of probiotic administration for prevention of *Salmonella* shedding in the postoperative period in horses with colic. *J. vet. Intern. Med.* **11**, 36-41.

Parviainen, A.K., Barton, M.H. and Norton, N.N. (2001) Evaluation of polymyxin B in an *ex vivo* model of endotoxemia in horses. *Am. J. vet. Res.* **62**, 72-76.

Randall, L.P., Cooles, S.W., Osborn, M.K., Piddock, L.J. and Woodward, M.J. (2004) Antibiotic resistance genes, integrons and multiple antibiotic resistance in thirty-five serotypes of *Salmonella enterica* isolated from humans and animals in the UK. *J. Antimicrob. Chemother.* **53**, 208-216.

Schott, H.C., 2nd (1998) Oral fluids for equine diarrhoea: an underutilized treatment for a costly disease? *Vet. J.* **155**, 119-121.

Schott, H.C., 2nd, Ewart, S.L., Walker, R.D., Dwyer, R.M., Dietrich, S., Eberhart, S.W., Kusey, J., Stick, J.A. and Derksen, F.J. (2001) An outbreak of salmonellosis among horses at a veterinary teaching hospital. *J. Am. vet. med. Ass.* **218**, 1100, 1152-1159.

Sekirov, I., Tam, N.M., Jogova, M., Robertson, M.L., Li, Y., Lupp, C. and Finlay, B.B. (2008) Antibiotic-induced perturbations of the intestinal microbiota alter host susceptibility to enteric infection. *Infect. Immun.* **76**, 4726-4736.

Seyfarth, A.M., Wegener, H.C. and Frimodt-Moller, N. (1997) Antimicrobial resistance in *Salmonella enterica* subsp. *enterica serovar typhimurium* from humans and production animals. *J. Antimicrob. Chemother.* **40**, 67-75.

Smith BP (1979) Atypical salmonellosis in horses: fever and depression without diarrhoea. *J. Am. vet. med. Ass.* **175**, 69.

Smith, B.P. (1981) Equine salmonellosis: a contemporary view. *Equine vet. J.* **13**, 147.

Smith, B.P., Reina-Guerra, M. and Hardy, A.J. (1978) Prevalence and epizootiology of equine salmonellosis. *J. Am. vet. med. Ass.* **172**, 353-356.

Spier, S.J., Lavoie, J.P., Cullor, J.S., Smith, B.P., Snyder, J.R. and Sischo, W.M. (1989) Protection against clinical endotoxemia in horses by using plasma containing antibody to an Rc mutant *E. coli* (J5). *Circ. Shock.* **28**, 235-248.

Stecher, B., Robbiani, R., Walker, A.W., Westendorf, A.M., Barthel, M., Kremer, M., Chaffron, S., Macpherson, A.J., Buer, J., Parkhill, J., Dougan, G., von Mering, C. and Hardt, W.D. (2007) *Salmonella enterica* serovar *typhimurium* exploits inflammation to compete with the intestinal microbiota. *PLoS Biol.* **5**, 2177-2189.

Templeton, C.B., Bottoms, G.D., Fessler, J.F., Ewert, K.M., Roesel, O.F., Johnson, M.A. and Latshaw, H.S. (1987) Endotoxin-induced hemodynamic and prostaglandin changes in ponies: effects of flunixin meglumine, dexamethasone, and prednisolone. *Circ. Shock.* **23**, 231-240.

Tillotson, K., Savage, C.J., Salman, M.D., Gentry-Weeks, C.R., Rice, D., Fedorka-Cray, P.J., Hendrickson, D.A., Jones, R.L., Nelson, W. and Traub-Dargatz, J.L. (1997) Outbreak of *Salmonella infantis* infection in a large animal veterinary teaching hospital. *J. Am. vet. med. Ass.* **211**, 1554-1557.

Tillotson, K. and Traub-Dargatz, J.L. (2003) Gastrointestinal protectants and cathartics. *Vet. Clin. N. Am.: Equine Pract.* **19**, 599-615.

Tomlinson, J.E. and Blikslager, A.T. (2004) Effects of ischemia and the cyclooxygenase inhibitor flunixin on *in vitro* passage of lipopolysaccharide across equine jejunum. *Am. J. vet. Res.* **65**, 1377-1383.

Tomlinson, J.E. and Blikslager, A.T. (2005) Effects of cyclooxygenase inhibitors flunixin and deracoxib on permeability of ischaemic-injured equine jejunum. *Equine vet. J.* **37**, 75-80.

Traub-Dargatz, J.L. and Besser, T.E. (2007) Salomonellosis. In: *Equine Infectious Diseases,* Eds: D. Sellon and M.T. Long, W.B. Saunders, Philadelphia. pp 331-345.

Traub-Dargatz, J.L., Salman, M.D. and Jones, R.L. (1990) Epidemiologic study of salmonellae shedding in the feces of horses and potential risk factors for development of the infection in hospitalized horses. *J. Am. vet. med. Ass.* **196**, 1617-1622.

Van Duijkeren, E. and Houwers, D.J. (2000) A critical assessment of antimicrobial treatment in uncomplicated *Salmonella enteritis*. *Vet. Microbiol.* **73**, 61-73.

Van Duijkeren, E., Sloet van Oldruitenborgh-Oosterbaan, M.M., Houwers, D.J., van Leeuwen, W.J. and Kalsbeek, H.C. (1994) Equine salmonellosis in a Dutch veterinary teaching hospital. *Vet. Rec.* **135**, 248-250.

Van Duijkeren, E., Flemming, C., Sloet van Oldruitenborgh-Oosterbaan, M., Kalsbeek, H.C. and van der Giessen, J.W. (1995) Diagnosing salmonellosis in horses. Culturing of multiple versus single faecal samples. *Vet. Q.* **17**, 63-66.

Van Duijkeren, E., Wannet, W.J., Heck, M.E., van Pelt, W., Sloet van Oldruitenborgh-Oosterbaan, M.M., Smit, J.A. and Houwers, D.J. (2002) Sero types, phage types and antibiotic susceptibilities of *Salmonella* strains isolated from horses in The Netherlands from 1993 to 2000. *Vet. Microbiol.* **86**, 203-212.

Vernace, M.A., Bellucci, A.G. and Wilkes, B.M. (1994) Chronic salicylate toxicity due to consumption of over-the-counter bismuth subsalicylate. *Am. J. Med.* **97**, 308-309.

Vo, A.T., van Duijkeren, E., Fluit, A.C. and Gaastra, W. (2007) A novel *Salmonella* genomic island 1 and rare integron types in *Salmonella Typhimurium* isolates from horses in The Netherlands. *J. Antimicrob. Chemother.* **59**, 594-599.

Voetsch, A.C., Van Gilder, T.J., Angulo, F.J., Farley, M.M., Shallow, S., Marcus, R., Cieslak, P.R., Deneen, V.C., Tauxe, R.V. and Emerging Infections Program, FoodNet Working Group. (2004) FoodNet estimate of the burden of illness caused by nontyphoidal *Salmonella* infections in the United States. *Clin. Infect. Dis.* **38**, S127-S134.

Walker, R.L., Madigan, J.E., Hird, D.W., Case, J.T., Villanueva, M.R. and Bogenrief, D.S. (1991) An outbreak of equine neonatal salmonellosis. *J. vet. Diagn. Invest.* **3**, 223-227.

Ward, M.P., Alinovi, C.A., Couetil, L.L. and Wu, C.C. (2005) Evaluation of a PCR to detect *Salmonella* in faecal samples of horses admitted to a veterinary teaching hospital. *J. Vet. Diagn. Invest.* **17**, 118-123.

Ward, M.P., Brady, T.H., Couetil, L.L., Liljebielke, K., Maurer, J.J. and Wu, C.C. (2005a) Investigation of an outbreak of salmonellosis caused by multidrug-resistant *Salmonella typhimurium* in a population of hospitalised horses. *Vet. Microbiol.* **107**, 233-240

Ward, M.P., Alinovi, C.A., Couetil, L.L. and Wu, C.C. (2005b) Evaluation of a PCR to detect *Salmonella* in faecal samples of horses admitted to a veterinary teaching hospital. *J. vet. Diagn. Invest.* **17**, 118-123.

Weese, J.S. (2004) Barrier precautions, isolation protocols, and personal hygiene in veterinary hospitals. *Vet. Clin. N. Am.: Equine Pract.* **20**, 543-559.

Weese, J.S. and Rousseau, J. (2005) Evaluation of *Lactobacillus pentosus* WE7 for prevention of diarrhoea in neonatal foals. *J. Am. vet. med. Ass.* **226**, 2031-2034.

Weese, J.S., Cote, N.M. and deGannes, R.V. (2003) Evaluation of *in vitro* properties of di-tri-octahedral smectite on clostridial toxins and growth. *Equine vet. J.* **35**, 638-641.

Weese, J.S., Baird, J.D., Poppe, C. and Archambault, M. (2001) Emergence of *Salmonella typhimurium* definitive type 104 (DT104) as an important cause of salmonellosis in horses in Ontario. *Can. vet. J.* 42, 788-792.

Weese, J.S., Anderson, M.E., Lowe, A., Penno, R., da Costa, T.M., Button, L. and Goth, K.C. (2004) Screening of the equine intestinal microflora for potential probiotic organisms. *Equine vet. J.* **36**, 351-355.

Zaman, K., Yunus, M., Rahman, A., Chowdhury, H.R. and Sack, D.A. (2001) Efficacy of a packaged rice oral rehydration solution among children with cholera and cholera-like illness. *Acta. Paediatr.* **90**, 505-510.

CLOSTRIDIAL DISEASES

J. S. Weese

Dept of Pathobiology, Ontario Veterinary College, University of Guelph, Guelph, Ontario N1G 2W1, Canada.

Keywords: horse; colitis; diarrhoea; infectious; gastrointestinal; clostridium

Summary

Clostridia are important equine pathogens that can cause a wide-range of diseases in various body systems. Many clostridial diseases can be rapidly fatal, yet most members of this genus can be found in healthy horses and are widely distributed in the environment. *Clostridium difficile* and *C. perfringens* are considered important causes of colitis in adult horses and foals; however, other clostridia probably also play a role. Toxins produced by *Clostridium tetani* are the cause of tetanus, and those produced by *Clostridium botulinum* cause botulism and have been implicated in equine grass sickness (dysautonomia). Various clostridia, including *C. perfringens*, can cause clostridial myonecrosis. *Clostridium piliforme* is the cause of a rapidly fatal necrotising hepatopathy of foals known as Tyzzer's disease. Equine practitioners probably commonly encounter clostridial diseases, yet diagnosis and management may be challenging. An understanding of the pathophysiology, diagnosis and management of various clostridial diseases is therefore important.

Introduction

The *Clostridium* genus contains a diverse group of bacterial species, many of which are important equine pathogens. All clostridia are Gram-positive spore-forming anaerobic bacteria, with varying degrees of aerotolerance. Many clostridia are normal commensal components of the intestinal microflora in healthy horses and are likely to play an important role in maintenance of digestive tract health. However, some are opportunistic pathogens that can cause a wide range of diseases (**Table 1**). The spore-forming nature of clostridia may also play an important role in disease pathogenesis by allowing for prolonged survival in inhospitable conditions as well as being resistant to disinfectants.

Clostridial enterocolitis

Enterocolitis is a sporadic but potentially devastating disease in the horse. It is likely that numerous clostridia are involved in its aetiopathogenesis, but the most commonly implicated are *C. difficile* and *C. perfringens*.

Clostridium difficile

Clostridium difficile is an important cause of colitis in some regions (Båverud *et al.* 1997, 1998; Gustafsson *et al.* 1997; Weese *et al.* 2001; Magdesian *et al.* 2002), although there appears to be significant geographic variation. Sporadic cases are most common; however, outbreaks can occur, particularly amongst foals on breeding farms and adult horses in veterinary hospitals (Madewell *et al.* 1995). Disease has been reproduced experimentally in foals (Arroyo *et al.* 2004), confirming its role as a significant pathogen in this age of horse.

A small percentage of healthy adult horses and foals carry *C. difficile* in their intestinal tracts (Weese *et al.* 2001; Båverud *et al.* 2003; Gustafsson *et al.* 2004). Whilst the dynamics of colonisation are unknown, it is likely that horses can carry *C. difficile* for long periods without ever developing disease. Carrier status rates are higher among foals and

TABLE 1: Known or suspected syndromes associated with different *Clostridium* spp

Organism	Diseases
Clostridium difficile	Colitis, duodenitis/proximal jejunitis
C. perfringens	Colitis, myonecrosis
C. botulinum	Botulism, equine grass sickness
C. tetani	Tetanus
C. piliforme	Tyzzer's disease
C. sordellii	Colitis, acute pasture myodystrophy
C. bifermentans	Acute pasture myodystrophy

horses treated with antimicrobials (Båverud *et al.* 2003; Gustafsson *et al.* 2004). The pathogenesis of disease is somewhat unclear, but probably involves proliferation of toxigenic strains of *C. difficile* in the intestinal tract, followed by production of bacterial toxins. Three major toxins may be produced by *C. difficile* strains: toxin A (an enterotoxin), toxin B (a cytotoxin) and CDT (a binary toxin) (Arroyo *et al.* 2007). The ability to produce even one of these toxins renders a strain clinically relevant. Reasons for proliferation of *C. difficile* in the intestinal tract are poorly understood, but factors that disrupt the intestinal microflora such as antimicrobial therapy are likely involved. However, despite the strong association between *C. difficile* infection (CDI), previously referred to as *C. difficile* associated diarrhoea (CDAD) and antimicrobials in man, and reports of antimicrobial-associated diarrhoea caused by *C. difficile* in horses (Båverud *et al.* 1997,1998; Gustafsson *et al.* 2004), there is not an absolute association between antimicrobials and CDI (Jones *et al.* 1987; Weese *et al.* 2006). There has been no reported difference in antimicrobial use history in horses with *C. difficile* vs. those with colitis of other aetiologies (Weese *et al.* 2006). Furthermore, a history of preceding antimicrobial therapy in the majority of CDI cases is lacking (Weese *et al.* 2001, 2006). In Sweden, there have been reports of fatal *C. difficile* colitis in mares whose foals were being treated with erythromycin, and experimental induction of disease following the administration of low doses of erythromycin to mares is possible (Båverud *et al.* 1997, 1998; Gustafsson *et al.* 1997). This phenomenon appears to be geographically variable and does not appear to be common in other regions.

Clinical presentation of CDI is highly variable. Signs range from mild diarrhoea with no signs of systemic illness to peracute and rapidly fatal necrotising haemorrhagic enterocolitis (Jones *et al.* 1987; Båverud *et al.* 1997, 1998; Weese *et al.* 2001, 2006). Signs of severe systemic illness may be associated with endotoxaemia and systemic inflammatory response syndrome (SIRS).

There are several suggested options for the diagnosis of CDI, although many of these are of questionable use (**Table 2**). Diagnosis should involve detection of clostridial toxins in faeces, ideally using a test that has been validated in horses (*C. difficile* TOX A/B II)[1] (Medina *et al.* 2008). Tests that detect both toxin A and toxin B are preferred because some equine strains produce only toxin B (Magdesian *et al.* 2006; Arroyo *et al.* 2007). Tests for CDT are not

TABLE 2: Testing options for diagnosis of *C. difficile* infection in horses

Test	Advantages	Disadvantages
Culture	Provides isolates for typing and susceptibility testing.	Nondiagnostic. Healthy horses can shed *C. difficile* and some strains do not produce toxins. Slow. Limited availability.
Culture with PCR testing of isolates	Does not detect nontoxigenic strains.	Healthy horses can shed toxigenic strains. Time consuming. Limited availability.
Common antigen ELISA	Rapid. Low cost. Easy. Good screening test. Excellent negative predictive value.	False positives common. Healthy horses can shed *C. difficile*. Detects nontoxigenic strains.
Toxin A ELISA	Rapid. Low cost. Easy. Detection of toxin that is clinically relevant.	Some strains produce toxin B but not toxin A.
Toxin A/B ELISA	Rapid. Easy. Detects toxin A negative/B positive strains. Good correlation with Gold Standard.	More expensive than antigen ELISA. Not all tests have been validated for use in horses.
Antigen ELISA + toxin detection	Reduces false positives.	More expensive.
Cell cytotoxicity assay	Gold standard. Highly sensitive and specific.	Expensive. Time consuming. Limited availability.
PCR from faeces	Rapid. Potentially highly sensitive and specific. Targets toxin gene so does not detect nontoxigenic strains.	Detects colonised individuals. Not validated for use in horses.
Faecal smear	None	Useless.

currently available. The positive predictive value of toxin detection can be strengthened by concurrent detection of *C. difficile* by culture, antigen ELISA or PCR. Initial screening with a highly sensitive (but less specific) test such as antigen ELISA can be used as a rapid and cost-effective 2-step approach, with positive samples subsequently being tested for toxins by ELISA.

Supportive care is the most important aspect of treatment. Di-tri-octahedral smectite (Bio-Sponge)[2] (1.5 kg loading dose *per os* followed by 450 g *per os* q. 6-8 h) has been shown to bind to clostridial toxins *in vitro* (Weese *et al.* 2003), although clinical efficacy is unclear. Probiotic compounds have been suggested but there is little evidence regarding their efficacy (Pillai and Nelson 2008). In a small trial of horses with acute colitis, administration of the yeast *Saccharomyces boulardii* (10^{10} yeast cells *per os* q. 12 h for 14 days) was reported to shorten the duration of diarrhoea (but it did not affect the overall outcome) (Desrochers *et al.* 2005). However, a specific study of this therapy in CDI has not been reported. If diarrhoea is considered to be associated with antimicrobial therapy, all antimicrobial treatments should be withdrawn, if possible. Metronidazole (15 mg/kg bwt *per os* q. 8 h for 3–5 days) is commonly used and has been associated with increased survival in horses with CDI (Weese *et al.* 2006). A poor response to metronidazole does not necessarily indicate resistance. Metronidazole resistance is very rare but has been reported in isolates from horses in California (Jang *et al.* 1997; Magdesian *et al.* 2002), although this is somewhat controversial. Vancomycin is used in some human cases of CDI, and has anecdotally been used in horses with suspected metronidazole-resistant CDI. However, there are major ethical concerns about the use of vancomycin in horses, and consensus has not been reached as to whether it is appropriate, particularly in the absence of confirmed metronidazole resistance in individual cases.

The prognosis is highly variable and depends on the severity of disease. Variable mortality rates (up to 42%) have been reported (Weese *et al.* 2001, 2006; Magdesian *et al.* 2006), and conflicting data are present regarding whether the CDI carries a worse prognosis than other causes of colitis (Weese *et al.* 2001, 2006). Complications such as laminitis, venous thrombosis and disseminated intravascular coagulation (DIC) can occur, and these will complicate both the treatment and the prognosis. There are no specific preventive measures. Judicious use of antimicrobials and other general practices such as providing a proper diet, minimising diet and management changes and reducing 'stress' may be important. A vaccine is not currently available.

TABLE 3: Toxin production by different *Clostridium perfringens* types

	Toxin					
Type	Alpha	Beta	Epsilon	Iota	Beta2	Enterotoxin
A	+	-	-	-	±	±
B	+	+	+	-	±	±
C	+	+	-	-	±	±
D	+	-	+	-	±	±
E	+	-	-	+	±	±

+ Type produces this toxin; - Type does not produce this toxin; ± Some strains of that type produce this toxin.

Clostridium perfringens

Clostridium perfringens is a ubiquitous species that can be found in the intestinal tract of many animals, and in the environment. It is commonly implicated as a cause of colitis in adult horses and foals (Pearson *et al.* 1986; Dart *et al.* 1988; Browning *et al.* 1991; Netherwood *et al.* 1996; Bueschel *et al.* 1998; East *et al.* 1998; Donaldson and Palmer 1999; Weese *et al.* 2001). *Clostridium perfringens* can be classified into 5 types according to their ability to produce 4 major toxins (**Table 3**). However, other toxins such as enterotoxin and β2 toxins can also be produced. The role of these different toxin types in disease is poorly understood. Enterotoxin producing strains have been evaluated most thoroughly and studies have demonstrated an association between the presence of enterotoxin in feces and diarrhoea (Donaldson and Palmer 1999; Weese *et al.* 2001). β2 toxin-producing strains have received attention recently and this may also be an important virulence factor (Waters *et al.* 2005).

One factor that complicates both our understanding of the role of *C. perfringens* in colitis and diagnosis is the prevalence of *C. perfringens* in the faeces of healthy horses, and particularly in foals. Colonisation rates of up to 90% have been reported in young foals and 35% in apparently healthy adult horses (Weese *et al.* 2001; Tillotson *et al.* 2002). However, certain strains are less commonly present. *Type C* strains are uncommon in healthy foals (Tillotson *et al.* 2002), but have been implicated in severe disease in foals (Howard-Martin *et al.* 1986; Pearson *et al.* 1986; East *et al.* 1998). In contrast, *Type A* strains are commonly isolated from horses with diarrhoea and normal horses, and the relevance of isolation of *Type A C. perfringens* is therefore often unclear.

The pathogenesis is poorly understood but presumably involves proliferation of *C. perfringens* in the intestinal tract with associated toxin production. Whether this occurs following ingestion of *C. perfringens* or from proliferation of endogenous *C. perfringens* remains unclear, as are factors associated with this event. The following were reported as risk factors for *C. perfringens enterocolitis* in foals in one study (East *et al.* 2000): housing in a stall or drylot during the first 3 days of life; the presence of other livestock on the premises; being born on dirt, sand or gravel; low amounts of grass hay or pasture fed to the mare *post partum*; and being of the stock horse type. Feeding broodmares low amounts of grain *prepartum* was associated with decreased risk in the same study.

Clinical presentation is variable and nonspecific as described for *C. difficile*. It has been suggested that *C. perfringens* may cause severe haemorrhagic diarrhoea more often, but this has not been proven.

Definitive diagnosis is challenging. Isolation of *C. perfringens*, quantification of *C. perfringens* and analysis of faecal smears for clostridial spores are all nondiagnostic (Weese *et al.* 2001). Genotyping of isolates, whereby *C. perfringens* isolates are tested to identify what toxigenic genes they possess, can provide some additional information but is rarely, by itself, diagnostic because detection of strains that are able to produce enterotoxin (or another toxin) does not mean that clinically relevant levels of toxins are actually being produced in the intestinal tract. An exception might be detection of *Type C* strains that appear to be more strongly associated with disease (East *et al.* 1998). Detection of enterotoxin is possible by ELISA or reverse passive latex agglutination assay (RPLAA). Neither has been validated for use in horses and there are concerns about poor specificity of the RPLAA (Netherwood *et al.* 1998). Positive ELISA results can be treated as a presumptive diagnosis. Additional confidence in ELISA-positive cases can be achieved by detection of enterotoxin-producing strains by genotyping of *C. perfringens* isolated from faeces or by direct PCR from faeces for the cpe gene. Identification of β2 toxin producing strains may also be suggestive but inadequate information is currently available. The relevance of other strains in the absence of toxin detection testing is questionable.

Supportive therapy is critical. The required intensity of treatment varies greatly depending on the case. Metronidazole (15 mg/kg bwt *per os* q. 8 h for 3–5 days) is commonly used. Zinc bacitracin (5.5 g *per os* q. 12 h for 2 doses, then q. 24 h) has been used with anecdotal success in idiopathic colitis (Staempfli *et al.* 1992) and should be effective against *C. perfringens*. However, objective evidence of efficacy is lacking.

An equine vaccine is not currently available. While ruminant vaccines have been used in horses, particularly during outbreaks on breeding farms, this extra-label use is not recommended because of lack of evidence of efficacy and anecdotal reports of adverse effects.

Duodenitis/proximal jejunitis

This syndrome, also referred to as 'anterior enteritis', is a sporadic disease characterised by inflammation and oedema of the proximal small intestine, with subsequent ileus, small intestinal distention, gastric distension and signs of moderate to severe colic.

Clostridium difficile has been implicated as a cause of this condition based on a high prevalence of isolation of *C. difficile* from gastrointestinal reflux of affected horses, but not controls with gastric reflux from obstructive lesions (Arroyo *et al.* 2006). Despite this association, causation has not yet been demonstrated.

Culture of samples of gastric reflux can be performed but the diagnostic significance is uncertain, and few laboratories are able to isolate *C. difficile*. Other tests such as toxin ELISA or PCR have not been evaluated on reflux and are not currently recommended.

The association between *C. difficile* and duodenitis/proximal jejunitis suggests that empirical treatment for clostridial infection with metronidazole (40–60 mg/kg bwt q. 8–12 h *per rectum* or 10–20 mg/kg bwt i.v q. 6–8 h) or penicillin (sodium or potassium penicillin, 20,000–40,000 iu/kg bwt i.v. q. 6 h) could be considered along with supportive therapy; however, the efficacy is unclear.

Clostridial myonecrosis

Clostridial myonecrosis, often referred to as clostridial myositis, gas gangrene and malignant oedema, is an uncommon but severe disease caused by growth of clostridia in skeletal muscle, with subsequent tissue necrosis and systemic inflammation. *Clostridium perfringens* has been most commonly implicated (Peek *et al.* 2003); however, various clostridia can be involved, including *C. septicum*, *C. sporogenes* and *C. sordellii*.

Clostridial spores can be present in healthy muscle (Vengust *et al.* 2003) but are dormant in the aerobic environment of healthy muscle. Severe tissue necrosis following the injection of irritant substances or trauma can create an anaerobic environment that allows germination of spores. Alternatively, clostridial spores can be introduced into the muscle during injection or with penetrating trauma. If an anaerobic environment results, spore germination can occur. Most reported cases are associated with intramuscular injection. Flunixin meglumine has been implicated as a leading cause of clostridial myonecrosis (Peek *et al.* 2003). Other substances such as ivermectin, antihistamines, phenylbutazone, dipyrone, B vitamins and synthetic prostaglandins have also been implicated (Valberg and McKinnon 1984; Rebhun *et al.* 1985; Peek *et al.* 2003).

Affected animals develop varying degrees of swelling over the infected area. Swelling can progress rapidly and becomes severe within hours of initial onset. Some animals may be found dead without preceeding signs. Subcutaneous emphysema is usually palpable because of gas production in the infected tissues, however, a lack of gas crepitation does not rule out this condition. Signs of systemic inflammation and toxaemia may be present and laminitis is a common secondary problem that can develop quickly.

Clostridial myonecrosis should be considered in all cases of acute muscular inflammation particularly if emphysema is present and if i.m. injection preceded clinical signs. Identification of Gram-positive rods from aspirates is strongly suggestive. Confirmation is based on culture of clostridia from aspirates or tissue samples from the infected site or demonstration of clostridial antigens by fluorescent antibody testing

Prompt, aggressive therapy is required. Antimicrobial treatment should be instigated immediately. High doses of penicillin (40,000 iu/kg bwt i.v. q. 2–6 h) are often used initially, followed by a lower dose (20,000 iu/kg bwt q. 6 h) after a few days. Oxytetracycline, chloramphenicol and metronidazole have also been used as they may have better effects against some clostridia *in vitro*. However oxytetracycline is more commonly reported as a cause of colitis in horses and may pose a higher risk of inducing colitis (Andersson *et al.* 1971; Baker and Leyland 1973). Furthermore, metronidazole is unlikely to achieve effective tissue concentrations. Analgesic therapy with NSAIDs and/or opiods is indicated. Surgical fenestration is also a critical component of treatment (**Figure 1**) and should be performed as soon as there is reasonable suspicion of clostridial myonecrosis. Numerous vertical incisions should be made to remove debris and necrotic tissue, facilitate drainage and to establish an aerobic environment. Ultrasonographic guidance can be useful to identify pockets of fluid or gas.

Even with prompt and aggressive therapy, the prognosis is guarded because of the severity of disease and the incidence of secondary problems such as laminitis (Rebhun *et al.* 1985; Peek *et al.* 2003). Avoiding i.m. injection of irritating drugs is the most effective means of prevention. There is no evidence that any specific pre-injection or injection procedures are protective.

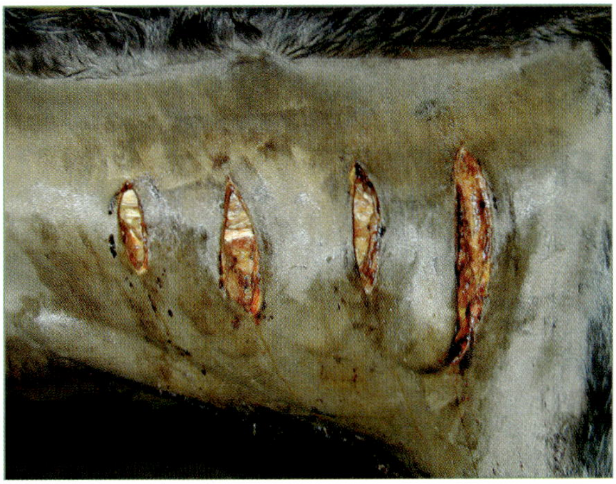

FIGURE 1: Aggressive surgical fenestrations in the neck of a horse with clostridial myonecrosis.

Botulism

Botulism (Barr 2009) is a potentially fatal neuromuscular disease caused by the toxin of *C. botulinum*, the spores of which are universally present in the soil. Strains are classified on the basis of the different neurotoxins produced (A, B, C1, D, E, F and G) with different types predominating in different geographic areas.

Toxicoinfectious botulism (also know as shaker foal syndrome) affects young foals, typically fast growing foals aged 1–2 months, but can cause disease in animals aged as young as 1 week and as old as 6 months (Wilkins and Palmer 2003a). It is caused by the ingestion of *C. botulinum* spores, followed by intestinal spore germination, bacterial growth and toxin production. Toxicoinfectious botulism is rare in adults, possibly because their developed intestinal microflora inhibits *C. botulinum* germination and growth.

The second main form, sometimes referred to as 'forage poisoning,' results from the ingestion of preformed toxin and typically affects adult horses (Galey 2001). Improperly prepared or stored hay, haylage and silage are most commonly implicated (Ricketts *et al.* 1984; Broughton and Parsons 1985; Wichtel and Whitlock 1991; Galey 2001). It has been suggested that the incidence of this disease has increased in Europe because of the growing popularity of feeding haylage (Frey *et al.* 2007). Outbreaks are not uncommon because the contaminated feed source may be fed to several animals.

Botulinum toxin is extremely potent and horses are considered particularly sensitive to its effects (Wilkins 2007). Botulinum toxin interferes with release of acetylcholine at the neuromuscular junction by irreversibly binding to presynaptic membranes (Montecucco and Schiavo 1994). This results in paresis and paralysis, which can progress to death from respiratory failure. The neurotoxins do not affect the central nervous system or sensory nerves.

The typical clinical presentation of toxicoinfectious botulism is flaccid paralysis characterised initially by weakness and muscle tremors, which become more pronounced with exertion (Wilkins and Palmer 2003a). Decreased eyelid, tail and tongue tone and dysphagia are common. Paresis may progress to paralysis and respiratory failure. Aspiration pneumonia may develop as a result of dysphagia.

Similar signs follow ingestion of preformed toxin, and may develop hours to days following ingestion of contaminated feeds. Varying degrees of weakness, muscle tremors, exercise intolerance, recumbency, excessive salivation, dysphagia, and reduced eyelid, tongue and tail tone are common with this form (Wichtel and Whitlock 1991; Schoenbaum *et al.* 2000; Galey 2001). Pupillary light responses may be sluggish. In some situations, sudden death is the only sign.

Diagnosis of botulism can be difficult. Clinical signs are usually sufficiently clear to make a presumptive diagnosis of toxicoinfectious botulism in foals in an endemic area. Faeces can be tested for the presence of *C. botulinum* and *C. botulinum* toxins. Serum, faeces, intestinal contents and liver can be tested for botulinum toxin by the mouse inoculation test; however, a negative result does not rule out botulism because of the relatively low sensitivity of the test and the high susceptibility of horses to the toxins.

Definitive diagnosis of botulism associated with preformed toxin ingestion can be equally problematic. Clinical signs of progressive flaccid paresis or paralysis with normal mental status are supportive, particularly if multiple animals are involved and a high-risk feed source such as silage has been fed. Mouse inoculation testing can be performed but the sensitivity is poor. Isolation of *C. botulinum* from faeces or intestinal contents is not diagnostic as these organisms can be found in some normal individuals.

Prompt treatment of toxicoinfectious botulism is critical. Administration of antitoxin is a critical aspect of treatment (Wilkins 2007). Polyvalent (anti-B and anti-C) and monovalent (anti-B) antitoxins are available commercially, and should be administered as soon as possible. While ineffective against bound toxin, antitoxin may bind to any circulating toxin. There is no cross-reactivity with other toxins so the administered antitoxin must be of the appropriate type to be effective. Supportive therapy is critical. Ventilatory support may be needed in severe cases (Wilkins and Palmer 2003b). Aminoglycosides, tetracyclines and procaine penicillin should be avoided because they may potentiate neuromuscular blockade. With aggressive therapy, survival rates can be high. A survival rate of 96% was reported in one study (Wilkins and Palmer 2003a); however, 30% of those foals required mechanical ventilation, which is not an option for all veterinary clinics and owners. Foals that survive should have a complete recovery unless secondary problems such as severe aspiration pneumonia or septicaemia developed during treatment.

The principles of treatment of botulism associated with ingestion of preformed toxin are similar to those for toxicoinfectious botulism. If available, polyvalent antitoxin (75,000 iu for an adult horse) should be administered as soon as possible. The feed should be evaluated and an alternate source used until the source of the toxin has been identified. While feed can be tested, the possibility of false negative results dictates that all high-risk feeds should be discarded.

The prognosis varies with severity of disease. Mortality rates are much higher in adults than foals with toxicoinfectious botulism (Ricketts *et al.* 1984; Wichtel and Whitlock 1991; Schoenbaum *et al.* 2000). In recumbent animals, the prognosis is grave because of the problems associated with prolonged recumbency and the inability to mechanically ventilate large animals. Complete recovery is typical in surviving animals (Wilkins 2007). Prompt antitoxin administration is probably one of the most important factors; however, the high cost may make this impossible in some cases.

Vaccination of mares with *C. botulinum* toxoid is an effective means of reducing the risk of toxicoinfectious botulism, provided foals ingest an adequate volume of good quality colostrum and the vaccine strain is appropriate since vaccination against one strain does not confer immunity against other strains. Vaccination should be considered in areas where botulism is endemic or when mares and foals may be transported to endemic areas for breeding.

Proper production and handling of feed is important for prevention of feed-associated botulism. Silage and haylage should be considered high-risk feeds and if they are to be fed, it is essential that they be properly prepared with an appropriately acidic pH. Silage with a pH $\geq$4.5 is favourable to *C. botulinum* growth and toxin production. If botulism is present in wild animals in the area, care should be taken to ensure that dead animals are not incorporated into hay, haylage or silage. Vaccination should be considered in endemic areas, particularly if high-risk feeds are fed.

Equine grass sickness (equine dysautonomia)

Equine grass sickness (EGS), also known as equine dysautonomia and mal seco, is a geographically restricted but important disease. It has been most widely reported in the UK but cases have been described in several other European countries and in South America (Doxey *et al.* 1991, 1998; Uzal and Robles 1993; Uzal *et al.* 1994; Böhnel *et al.* 2003), with anecdotal reports from North America. As the name implies, it is strongly associated with access to grass pastures. It is a seasonal disease, with most UK cases occurring in between April and June (Wood *et al.* 1998) and most often affects young adults (Gilmour and Jolly 1974; Wood *et al.* 1998). Virtually all affected animals have access to pasture, and clusters of cases can be identified on specific farms or even on individual pastures. Studies have reported various farm-level risk factors (increased soil nitrogen content, previous cases, pasture or soil disturbance, higher number of horses, presence of younger animals, rearing of domestic birds) and horse-level risk factors (young age, male gender, contact with cases, living on premises with previous cases, field change in preceding 2 weeks) (Wood *et al.* 1998; Newton *et al.* 2004; McCarthy *et al.* 2004). While definitive evidence remains elusive, there is increasing evidence implicating *C. botulinum Type C* as the causative agent (Hunter *et al.* 1999; Nunn *et al.* 2007).

Three different forms are usually described; acute, subacute and chronic. The acute form is severe and invariably fatal (within 48 h). It is characterised by depression, anorexia, sweating, ptyalism and colic, with decreased borborygmi, dehydration and progressive abdominal distention (Doxey *et al.* 1991). Muscle tremors are common and may be severe, particularly over the shoulders, triceps and flank. Nasogastric reflux may be present and stomach rupture, with ensuing peritonitis, may occur if gastric decompression is not performed. Dysphagia can be present but may not be recognised because of anorexia accompanying severe disease.

The subacute form is similar to the acute form, but milder. Tachycardia is usually present, although signs of distress, severe abdominal pain and nasogastric reflux are uncommon. Death usually occurs within 2–5 days.

The chronic form may be of insidious onset, characterised by weight loss, depression, a 'tucked-up' abdomen, weakness and dysphagia. Mastication is typically slow and laboured, and oesophageal spasm may be noted after swallowing. Intermittent diarrhoea, bilateral nasal discharge and chronic rhinitis may also be present.

Clinical signs, signalment, identification of risk factors such as recent change in grazing or previous disease on the premises and exclusion of other differential diagnoses are suggestive for EGS in areas where the disease in endemic. Ileal biopsy with histological identification of changes to enteric nerve plexi provides a definitive diagnosis (Scholes *et al.* 1993). Histological examination of haematoxylin and eosin stained rectal biopsy specimens has been proposed as a rapid and minimally invasive test in live horses (Wales and Whitwell 2006), but further study of this technique in the field is required. *Post mortem* confirmation of the diagnosis is more common, with demonstration of characteristic neural degeneration of autonomic ganglia, intestinal wall nerve plexi, brain and spinal cord. Culture of faeces or intestinal contents is not helpful. Although *Clostridium botulinum Type C* can be more commonly identified in the intestinal contents of horses with EGS, it can also be found in some normal horses.

Treatment of the acute and subacute forms is not indicated because affected horses invariably die. A few horses with chronic EGS can recover with supportive therapy, including i.v. fluid therapy and nutritional support through force-feeding, feeding via nasogastric tube or parenteral feeding (Doxey *et al.* 1995; Doxey *et al.* 1998; Fintl and McGorum 2002). Administration of cisapride (0.8 mg/kg bwt *per os* q. 8 h) has been shown to increase gastrointestinal motility in affected animals (Milne *et al.* 1996) but the effect on outcome was not reported. The majority of survivors can return to a normal level of work (Doxey *et al.* 1995). Recovery to full competitive work may take in excess of 12 months. Long-term difficulty coping with dry fibrous hay may be encountered (Doxey *et al.* 1998). Mild, recurrent colic may persist in some cases, and some animals have persistent or intermittent inappropriate skin sweating.

There is little objective information about methods to prevent, or reduce the risk of grass sickness. Pasture access and management may be important factors; however, inadequate data are currently available to make evidence-based recommendations. Vaccination with *C. botulinum Type C* toxoid is a potential but untested prophylactic option.

Tyzzer's disease

Tyzzer's disease (see Peek 2009) is a rare but usually fatal infection caused by *C. piliforme*. It usually causes sporadic cases of severe and peracute hepatitis in 1–6 week old foals. Outbreaks can occur, but are uncommon.

The pathophysiology is poorly understood, but probably involves ingestion of *C. piliforme* spores from faeces or the environment, followed by germination of spores in the intestinal tract and portal migration to the liver. Risk factors include being born in a specific time of year (13th March–13th April in one study), being born to nonresident mares and foals of mares aged <6 years (Fosgate *et al.* 2002).

Often, affected foals are found moribund or dead. Close observation can identify early cases, which have nonspecific abnormalities such as weakness, lethargy, anorexia, pyrexia, diarrhoea, dehydration and icterus. Terminally, seizures and marked abnormalities in mentation may be observed.

Diagnosis is typically only obtained at necropsy, through identification of bacteria with the characteristic appearance of *C. piliforme* in the liver using Warthin-Starry stain. This organism cannot be grown using standard culture methods. PCR testing of liver biopsy specimens has potential as a rapid *ante mortem* diagnostic test (Borchers *et al.* 2006).

Supportive therapy is indicated but rarely used because of rapid death, with most affected foals being found dead or dying within 24–48 h. Successful treatment of a foal with aggressive supportive therapy along with ampicillin and gentamicin has been reported (Borchers *et al.* 2006). There are no known means of prevention.

Tetanus

Tetanus (see Johnson 2009) is a neuromuscular disease caused by *C. tetani*, an organism that is common in the environment (Wilkins *et al.* 1988). It is now a rare disease in most regions because of widespread and effective vaccination; however, the risk of exposure persists. *Clostridium tetani* spores can persist in the environment for years and horses are considered the most susceptible domestic animal to this disease.

Most cases of tetanus occur secondary to wounds, especially puncture wounds of the foot or lower extremity. In these situations, *C. tetani* spores, which mainly originate from soil, contaminate the wound, proliferate if a local anaerobic environment is created, and produce the exotoxins tetanolysin and tetanospasmin (Goonetilleke and Harris 2004). Tetanolysin causes tissue necrosis and creates a favourable environment for further growth of *C. tetani* whereas tetanospasmin reaches peripheral nerves both locally and through the bloodstream. Once in the nerves, tetanospasmin travels centripetally in axons to the presynaptic inhibitory cells of the spinal cord where it prevents neurotransmitter release, resulting in increased muscle tone and spasm. The interval between infection and the onset of clinical signs is highly variable and influenced by the site of infection and the amount of toxin produced.

Classical signs of tetanus include rigidity of muscles of the head and neck characterised by increased masticatory muscle tone, facial expression rigidity and neck stiffness, and a 'saw-horse' stance with rigid extension of the neck, back and limbs, and an elevated tailhead. It may be impossible to open the mouth (trismus, 'lockjaw'), and dysphagia is common. Prolapse of the nictitans in response to stimulation is common, and often used as a pathognomonic sign. Ambulatory horses have a stiff gait. In more severe cases, animals may become recumbent. Tonic spasms (tetanic convulsions), often initiated by external stimuli such as touch, sound or light, usually develop within a few days of the onset of initial signs. Dysphagia is common. Death can occur from complications of exhaustion, recumbency, respiratory failure from respiratory muscle involvement or from musculoskeletal injuries.

Classical clinical signs in a non- or under-vaccinated horse can provide a presumptive diagnosis, particularly if a history of a recent puncture wound is present. Induction of transient prolapse of the third eyelid by tapping the horse beneath the eye or under the lower jaw has been described as an early and sensitive indicator of tetanus (MacKay 2007). Confirmation can be achieved by isolation of *C. tetani* from an aspirate of an infected site; however, the site of infection can be difficult to locate.

Supportive care is critical. Affected horses should be carefully and quietly moved to a large well-bedded stall with limited visual and auditory stimuli. Lights should be turned down. Earplugs can be used to reduce auditory stimuli, provided placement does not result in excessive stimulation. Feed and water should be raised from the ground to facilitate accessibility. Intravenous fluid therapy may be required in horses that cannot drink. Nutritional support by nasogastric feeding or parenteral nutrition may also be required. A sling may be needed in severe cases. Affected horses should be handled as little as possible and only by experienced personnel because of the potential for injury from involuntary movements or excessive reaction to stimuli.

Sedatives and muscle relaxants may provide some degree of clinical improvement. Chlorpromazine (0.4–1.0 mg/kg bwt i.m. or i.m. q. 6–12 h) and acepromazine (0.02–0.1 mg/kg bwt i.v. or i.m. q. 6–12 h) are most commonly used (MacKay 2007). Diazepam (0.1–0.2 mg/kg bwt i.v. PRN) with or without xylazine (0.25–0.6 mg/kg bwt i.v. or i.m. PRN) may be useful in the short term but long-term diazepam usage can be associated with respiratory and central nervous system depression. Phenobarbital can be administered intravenously (12 mg/kg bwt loading dose i.v. then 6.7–9 mg/kg bwt i.v. over 20 min q. 8–12 h) or orally (11 mg/kg bwt *per os* q. 24 h).

If a wound is present and thought to be the inciting cause, it should be cleaned, debrided and lavaged. Metronidazole (25 mg/kg bwt *per os* q. 6–8) is the drug of choice, but is not available in all countries. If oral treatment is not possible, metronidazole can be administered *per rectum* (40–60 mg/kg bwt q. 8–12 h) or i.v. (10–20 mg/kg bwt q. 6–8 h). Although historically penicillin has been used extensively for the treatment of tetanus, it is believed to have anti-GABA and proconvulsant effects (Tsuda *et al.* 1994) and may be contraindicated.

Tetanus antitoxin has no effect on toxin already bound to nerve tissue and there may be little circulating toxin by the time tetanus is diagnosed. Regardless, antitoxin treatment is indicated because there could be some reduction effect on circulating toxins. Tetanus antitoxin can be administered locally at the site of infection and systemically (10,000–50,000 iu i.m. or subcut. q. 24 h for 3–5 days) (MacKay 2007).

Toxin binding is irreversible and growth of new nerve terminals is required for recovery, a process that may take weeks or months. Mortality rates of 50–75% have been reported (Green *et al.* 1994). One study reported that the prognosis was best for horses that were previously vaccinated, responded clinically to sedation and did not rapidly (within 24–48 h) become recumbent (Green *et al.* 1994).

Tetanus is a highly preventable disease because of the availability of efficacious vaccines. All horses should be vaccinated against tetanus yearly (Anon 2008). Prophylactic tetanus antitoxin should be reserved for unvaccinated horses with contaminated wounds. In these situations, both tetanus antitoxin and tetanus toxoid should be administered at different body sites. Administration of tetanus antitoxin should be reserved for unvaccinated horses and foals from unvaccinated mares because of concerns regarding serum hepatitis (Messer and Johnson 1994).

Conclusion

Clostridial species are responsible for a wide range of diseases, and it is likely that they are associated with many other conditions that are currently considered to be idiopathic. A general understanding of these important pathogens is therefore important for equine practitioners.

Manufacturers' addresses

[1]TechLab, Blacksburg, Virginia, USA.
[2]Platinum Performance, Buellton, California, USA.

References

Anon (2008) *American Association 'of Equine Practitioners Guidelines for the Vaccination of Horses.* http://www.aaep.org/vaccination_guidelines.htm.

Andersson, G., Ekman, L., Mansson, I., Persson, S., Rubarth, S. and Tufvesson, G. (1971) Lethal complications following administration of oxytetracycline in the horse. *Nord. vet. Med.* **23**, 9-22.

Arroyo, L., Staempfli, H. and Weese, J. (2007) Molecular analysis of *Clostridium difficile* isolates recovered from horses with diarrhea. *Vet. Microbiol.* **120**, 179-183.

Arroyo, L., Stämpfli, H. and Weese, J. (2006) Potential role of *Clostridium difficile* as a cause of duodenitis-proximal jejunitis in horses. *J. med. Microbiol.* **55**, 605-608.

Arroyo, L.G., Weese, J.S. and Staempfli, H.R. (2004) Experimental *Clostridium difficile* enterocolitis in foals. *J. vet. intern. Med.* **18**, 734-738.

Baker, J.R. and Leyland, A. (1973) Diarrhoea in the horse associated with stress and tetracycline therapy. *Vet. Rec.* **93**, 583-584.

Barr, B. (2009) Equine botulism. In: *Infectious Diseases of the Horse*, Eds: T.S. Mair and R.E. Hutchinson, Equine Veterinary Journal Ltd., Newmarket. pp 305-311.

Båverud, V., Gustafsson, A., Franklin, A., Lindholm, A. and Gunnarsson, A. (1997) *Clostridium difficile* associated with acute colitis in mature horses treated with antibiotics. *Equine vet. J.* **29**, 279-284.

Båverud, V., Franklin, A., Gunnarsson, A., Gustafsson, A. and Hellander-Edman, A. (1998) *Clostridium difficile* associated with acute colitis in mares when their foals are treated with erythromycin and rifampicin for *Rhodococcus equi* pneumonia. *Equine vet. J.* **30**, 482-488.

Båverud, V., Gustafsson, A., Franklin, A., Aspán, A. and Gunnarsson, A. (2003) *Clostridium difficile*: prevalence in horses and environment, and antimicrobial susceptibility. *Equine vet. J.* **35**, 465-471.

Böhnel, H., Wernery, U. and Gessler, F. (2003) Two cases of equine grass sickness with evidence for soil-borne origin involving botulinum neurotoxin. *J. vet. Med. B. Infect. Dis. vet. Public Health* **50**, 178-182.

Borchers, A., Magdesian, K.G., Halland, S., Pusterla, N. and Wilson, W.D. (2006) Successful treatment and polymerase chain reaction (PCR) confirmation of Tyzzer's disease in a foal and clinical and pathologic characteristics of 6 additional foals (1986-2005). *J. vet. intern. Med.* **20**, 1212-1218.

Broughton, J. and Parsons, L. (1985) Botulism in horses fed big bale silage. *Vet. Rec.* **117**, 674.

Browning, G.F., Chalmers, R.M., Snodgrass, D.R., Batt, R.M., Hart, C.A., Ormarod, S.E., Leadon, D., Stoneham, S.J. and Rossdale, P.D. (1991) The prevalence of enteric pathogens in diarrhoeic Thoroughbred foals in Britain and Ireland. *Equine vet. J.* **23**, 405-409.

Bueschel, D., Walker, R., Woods, L., Kokai-Kun, J., McClane, B. and Songer, J.G. (1998) Enterotoxigenic *Clostridium perfringens* type A necrotic enteritis in a foal. *J. Am. vet. med. Ass.* **213**, 1305-1307, 1280.

Dart, A.J., Pascoe, R.R., Gibson, J.A. and Harrower, B.J. (1988) Enterotoxaemia in a foal due to *Clostridium perfringens* type A. *Aust. vet. J.* **65**, 330-331.

Desrochers, A., Dolente, B., Roy, M., Boston, R. and Carlisle, S. (2005) Efficacy of *Saccharomyces boulardii* for treatment of horses with acute enterocolitis. *J. Am. vet. med. Ass.* **227**, 954-959.

Donaldson, M.T. and Palmer, J.E. (1999) Prevalence of *Clostridium perfringens* enterotoxin and *Clostridium difficile* toxin A in feces of horses with diarrhea and colic. *J. Am. vet. med. Ass.* **215**, 358-361.

Doxey, D.L., Milne, E.M. and Harter, A. (1995) Recovery of horses from dysautonomia (grass sickness). *Vet. Rec.* **137**, 585-588.

Doxey, D.L., Milne, E.M., Gilmour, J.S. and Pogson, D.M. (1991) Clinical and biochemical features of grass sickness (equine dysautonomia). *Equine vet. J.* **23**, 360-364.

Doxey, D.L., Milne, E.M., Ellison, J. and Curry, P.J. (1998) Long-term prospects for horses with grass sickness (dysautonomia). *Vet. Rec.* **142**, 207-209.

East, L.M., Dargatz, D.A., Traub-Dargatz, J.L. and Savage, C.J. (2000) Foaling-management practices associated with the occurrence of enterocolitis attributed to *Clostridium perfringens* infection in the equine neonate. *Prev. vet. Med.* **46**, 61-74.

East, L.M., Savage, C.J., Traub-Dargatz, J.L., Dickinson, C.E. and Ellis, R.P. (1998) Enterocolitis associated with *Clostridium perfringens* infection in neonatal foals: 54 cases (1988-1997). *J. Am. vet. med. Ass.* **212**, 1751-1756.

Fintl, C. and McGorum, B.C. (2002) Evaluation of three ancillary treatments in the management of equine grass sickness. *Vet. Rec.* **151**, 381-383.

Fosgate, G.T., Hird, D.W., Read, D.H. and Walker, R.L. (2002) Risk factors for *Clostridium piliforme* infection in foals. *J. Am. vet. med. Ass.* **220**, 785-790.

Frey, J., Eberle, S., Stahl, C., Mazuet, C., Popoff, M., Schatzmann, E., Gerber, V., Dungu, B. and Straub, R. (2007) Alternative vaccination against equine botulism (BoNT/C). *Equine vet. J.* **39**, 516-520.

Galey, F.D. (2001) Botulism in the horse. *Vet. Clin. N. Am.: Equine Pract.* **17**, 579-588.

Gilmour, J.S. and Jolly, G.M. (1974) Some aspects of the epidemiology of equine grass sickness. *Vet. Rec.* **95**, 77-81.

Goonetilleke, A. and Harris, J.B. (2004) Clostridial neurotoxins. *J. Neurol. Neurosurg. Psychiatr.* **75**, *Suppl.* **3**, iii35-39.

Green, S.L., Little, C.B., Baird, J.D., Tremblay, R.R. and Smith-Maxie, L.L. (1994) Tetanus in the horse: a review of 20 cases (1970 to 1990). *J. vet. intern. Med.* **8**, 128-132.

Gustafsson, A., Båverud, V., Gunnarsson, A., Pringle, J. and Franklin, A. (2004) Study of faecal shedding of *Clostridium difficile* in horses treated with penicillin. *Equine vet. J.* **36**, 180-182.

Gustafsson, A., Båverud, V., Gunnarsson, A., Rantzien, M.H., Lindholm, A. and Franklin, A. (1997) The association of erythromycin ethylsuccinate with acute colitis in horses in Sweden. *Equine vet. J.* **29**, 314-318.

Howard-Martin, M., Morton, R.J., Qualls, C.W. and MacAllister, C.G. (1986) *Clostridium perfringens type C* enterotoxemia in a newborn foal. *J. Am. vet. med. Ass.* **189**, 564-565.

Hunter, L.C., Miller, J.K. and Poxton, I.R. (1999) The association of *Clostridium botulinum type C* with equine grass sickness: a toxicoinfection? *Equine vet. J.* **31**, 492-499.

Jang, S., Hansen, L., Breher, J., Riley, D., Magdesian, K., Madigan, J., Tang, Y., Silva, J. and Hirsh, D. (1997) Antimicrobial susceptibilities of equine isolates of *Clostridium difficile* and molecular characterization of metronidazole-resistant strains. *Clin. Infect. Dis.* **25**, *Suppl.* 2, S266-267.

Johnson, A.L. (2009) Tetanus. In: *Infectious Diseases of the Horse*, Eds: T.S. Mair and R.E. Hutchinson, Equine Veterinary Journal Ltd., Newmarket. pp 298-304.

Jones, R.L., Adney, W.S. and Shideler, R.K. (1987) Isolation of *Clostridium difficile* and detection of cytotoxin in the feces of diarrheic foals in the absence of antimicrobial treatment. *J. clin. Microbiol.* **25**, 1225-1227.

MacKay, R.J. (2007) Tetanus. In: *Equine Infectious Diseases*, 1st edn., Eds: D.C. Sellon and M.T. Long, Saunders Elsevier, St Louis. pp 376-380.

Madewell, B.R., Tang, Y.J., Jang, S., Madigan, J.E., Hirsh, D.C., Gumerlock, P.H. and Silva, J.J. (1995) Apparent outbreak of *Clostridium difficile*-associated diarrhea in horses in a veterinary teaching hospital. *J. vet. diagn. Invest.* **7**, 343-346.

Magdesian, K.G., Hirsh, D.C., Jang, S.S., Hansen, L.M. and Madigan, J.E. (2002) Characterization of *Clostridium difficile* isolates from foals with diarrhea: 28 cases (1993-1997). *J. Am. vet. med. Ass.* **220**, 67-73.

Magdesian, K., Dujowich, M., Madigan, J., Hansen, L., Hirsh, D. and Jang, S. (2006) Molecular characterization of *Clostridium difficile* isolates from horses in an intensive care unit and association of disease severity with strain type. *J. Am. vet. med. Ass.* **228**, 751-755.

McCarthy, H.E., French, N.P., Edwards, G.B., Miller, K. and Proudman, C.J. (2004) Why are certain premises at increased risk of equine grass sickness? A matched case-control study. *Equine vet. J.* **36**, 130-134.

Medina, C., Weese, J.S. and Staempfli, H. (2008) Validation of a commercial enzyme immunoassay for detection of *Clostridium difficile* toxins in feces of horses with acute diarrhea. In: *26th Annual Conference of the American Association of Veterinary Internal Medicine*, San Antonio.

Messer, N.T. and Johnson, P.J. (1994) Idiopathic acute hepatic disease in horses: 12 cases (1982-1992). *J. Am. vet. med. Ass.* **204**, 1934-1937.

Milne, E.M., Doxey, D.L., Woodman, M.P., Cuddeford, D. and Pearson, R.A. (1996) An evaluation of the use of cisapride in horses with chronic grass sickness (equine dysautonomia). *Br. vet. J.* **152**, 537-549.

Montecucco, C. and Schiavo, G. (1994) Mechanism of action of tetanus and botulinum neurotoxins. *Mol. Microbiol.* **13**, 1-8.

Netherwood, T., Wood, J., Townsend, H., Mumford, J. and Chanter, N. (1996) Foal diarrhoea between 1991 and 1994 in the United Kingdom associated with *Clostridium perfringens*, rotavirus, *Strongyloides westeri* and *Cryptosporidium* spp. *Epidemiol. Infect.* **117**, 375-383.

Netherwood, T., Binns, M., Townsend, H., Wood, J.L., Mumford, J.A. and Chanter, N. (1998) The *Clostridium perfringens* enterotoxin from equine isolates; its characterization, sequence and role in foal diarrhoea. *Epidemiol. Infect.* **120**, 193-200.

Newton, J.R., Hedderson, E.J., Adams, V.J., McGorum, B.C., Proudman, C.J. and Wood, J.L. (2004) An epidemiological study of risk factors associated with the recurrence of equine grass sickness (dysautonomia) on previously affected premises. *Equine vet. J.* **36**, 105-112.

Nunn, F.G., Pirie, R.S., McGorum, B., Wernery, U. and Poxton, I.R. (2007) Comparison of IgG antibody levels to *Clostridium botulinum* antigens between euthanased and surviving cases of chronic grass sickness. *Res. vet. Sci.* **83**, 82-84.

Pearson, E.G., Hedstrom, O.R., Sonn, R. and Wedam, J. (1986) Hemorrhagic enteritis caused by *Clostridium perfringens type C* in a foal. *J. Am. vet. med. Ass.* **188**, 1309-1310.

Peek, S.F. (2009) Tyzzer's disease. In: *Infectious Diseases of the Horse*, Eds: T.S. Mair and R.E. Hutchinson, Equine Veterinary Journal Ltd., Newmarket. pp 293-297.

Peek, S., Semrad, S. and Perkins, G. (2003) Clostridial myonecrosis in horses (37 cases 1985-2000). *Equine vet. J.* **35**, 86-92.

Pillai, A. and Nelson, R. (2008) Probiotics for treatment of *Clostridium difficile*-associated colitis in adults. *Cochrane Database of Systematic Reviews* (Online), CD004611.

Rebhun, W.C., Shin, S.J., King, J.M., Baum, K.H. and Patten, V. (1985) Malignant edema in horses. *J. Am. vet. med. Ass.* **187**, 732-736.

Ricketts, S.W., Greet, T.R., Glyn, P.J., Ginnett, C.D., McAllister, E.P., McCaig, J., Skinner, P.H., Webbon, P.M., Frape, D.L. and Smith, G.R. (1984) Thirteen cases of botulism in horses fed big bale silage. *Equine vet. J.* **16**, 515-518.

Schoenbaum, M.A., Hall, S.M., Glock, R.D., Grant, K., Jenny, A.L., Schiefer, T.J., Sciglibaglio, P. and Whitlock, R.H. (2000) An outbreak of type C botulism in 12 horses and a mule. *J. Am. vet. med. Ass.* **217**, 365-368, 340.

Scholes, S.F., Vaillant, C., Peacock, P., Edwards, G.B. and Kelly, D.F. (1993) Diagnosis of grass sickness by ileal biopsy. *Vet. Rec.* **133**, 7-10.

Staempfli, H.R., Prescott, J.F., Carman, R.J. and McCutcheon, L.J. (1992) Use of bacitracin in the prevention and treatment of experimentally-induced idiopathic colitis in horses. *Can. J. vet. Res.* **56**, 233-236.

Tillotson, K., Traub-Dargatz, J., Dickinson, C., Ellis, R., Morley, P., Hyatt, D., Magnuson, R., Riddle, W., Bolte, D. and Salman, M. (2002) Population-based study of fecal shedding of *Clostridium perfringens* in broodmares and foals. *J. Am. vet. med. Ass.* **220**, 342-348.

Tsuda, A., Ito, M., Kishi, K., Shiraishi, H., Tsuda, H. and Mori, C. (1994) Effect of penicillin on GABA-gated chloride ion influx. *Neurochem. Res.* **19**, 1-4.

Uzal, F.A. and Robles, C.A. (1993) Mal seco, a grass sickness-like syndrome of horses in Argentina. *Vet. Res. Comm.* **17**, 449-457.

Uzal, F.A., Doxey, D.L., Robles, C.A., Woodman, M.P. and Milne, E.M. (1994) Histopathology of the brain-stem nuclei of horses with "Mal seco", an equine dysautonomia. *J. comp. Pathol.* **111**, 297-301.

Valberg, S.J. and McKinnon, A.O. (1984) Clostridial cellulitis in the horse: A report of five cases. *Can. vet. J.* **25**, 67-71.

Vengust, M., Arroyo, L., Weese, J. and Baird, J. (2003) Preliminary evidence for dormant clostridial spores in equine skeletal muscle. *Equine vet. J.* **35**, 514-516.

Wales, A.D. and Whitwell, K.E. (2006) Potential role of multiple rectal biopsies in the diagnosis of equine grass sickness. *Vet. Rec.* **158**, 372-377.

Waters, M., Raju, D., Garmory, H., Popoff, M. and Sarker, M. (2005) Regulated expression of the beta2-toxin gene (cpb2) in *Clostridium perfringens* type a isolates from horses with gastrointestinal diseases. *J. clin. Microbiol.* **43**, 4002-4009.

Weese, J.S., Cote, N.M. and deGannes, R.V. (2003) Evaluation of *in vitro* properties of di-tri-octahedral smectite on clostridial toxins and growth. *Equine vet. J.* **35**, 638-641.

Weese, J.S., Staempfli, H.R. and Prescott, J.F. (2001) A prospective study of the roles of *clostridium difficile* and enterotoxigenic *Clostridium perfringens* in equine diarrhoea. *Equine vet. J.* **33**, 403-409.

Weese, J.S., Toxopeus, L. and Arroyo, L. (2006) *Clostridium difficile* associated diarrhoea in horses within the community: predictors, clinical presentation and outcome. *Equine vet. J.* **38**, 185-188.

Wichtel, J.J. and Whitlock, R.H. (1991) Botulism associated with feeding alfalfa hay to horses. *J. Am. vet. med. Ass.* **199**, 471-472.

Wilkins, C.A., Richter, M.B., Hobbs, W.B., Whitcomb, M., Bergh, N. and Carstens, J. (1988) Occurrence of *Clostridium tetani* in soil and horses. *S. Afr. Med. J.* **73**, 718-720.

Wilkins, P.A. (2007) Botulism. In: *Equine Infectious Diseases*, 1st edn., Eds: D.C. Sellon and M.T. Long, Saunders Elsevier, St Louis. pp 372-376.

Wilkins, P.A. and Palmer, J.E. (2003a) Botulism in foals less than 6 months of age: 30 cases (1989-2002). *J. vet. intern. Med.* **17**, 702-707.

Wilkins, P.A. and Palmer, J.E. (2003b) Mechanical ventilation in foals with botulism: 9 cases (1989-2002). *J. vet. intern. Med.* **17**, 708-712.

Wood, J.L., Milne, E.M. and Doxey, D.L. (1998) A case-control study of grass sickness (equine dysautonomia) in the United Kingdom. *Vet. J.* **156**, 7-14.

EQUINE PROLIFERATIVE ENTEROPATHY: *LAWSONIA INTRACELLULARIS*

H. C. McKenzie III

Marion duPont Scott Equine Medical Center, Virginia/Maryland Regional College of Veterinary Medicine, Virginia Polytechnic and State University, Leesburg, Virginia 20176, USA.

Keywords: horse; proliferative; enteropathy; oedema; hypoalbuminaemia; foal

Summary

Proliferative enteropathy is an infectious disease that affects young horses and is caused by the bacterium *Lawsonia intracellularis*. This disease causes dramatic structural changes in the mucosal epithelium of the small intestine due to proliferation of the crypt epithelial cells. These alterations lead to a protein-losing enteropathy that can result in variable degrees of hypoalbuminaemia, hypoproteinaemia, ventral oedema, lethargy, diarrhoea, fever, weight loss and colic. Diagnosis of proliferative enteropathy is by a combination of clinical signs (ventral oedema), clinicopathological abnormalities (hypoalbuminaemia), abdominal ultrasonographic examination, immunoperoxidase monolayer assay serology and faecal PCR testing for *Lawsonia* DNA. Treatment is best accomplished using lipophilic antimicrobials such as the tetracyclines (oxytetracycline, doxycycline), the macrolides (erythromycin, azithromycin, clarithromycin) or chloramphenicol. The prognosis for survival with appropriate treatment is good, but affected animals often exhibit a decrease in growth rate and as a result may be at a slight disadvantage relative to their peers for several months.

Introduction

Proliferative enteropathy is an increasingly recognised condition in young horses caused by the obligate intracellular bacterium *Lawsonia intracellularis*. This organism has been identified as an enteropathogen in numerous species, including swine, hamsters, horses, rats, rabbits, emu, ostrich, monkeys, sheep, white-tailed deer, dogs, foxes, ferrets and guinea pigs (Cooper and Gebhart 1998; Klein *et al.* 1999; Lawson and Gebhart 2000). Although the disease now recognised as proliferative enteropathy was first described as intestinal adenomatosis in swine in 1931 (Biester and Schwartze 1931) the aetiological agent remained a mystery 1973 when the presence of bacteria in the enteric lesions was first described (Rowland *et al.* 1973). With the development of improved diagnostic tools, including novel serological and PCR methods, it has become clear that *Lawsonia* infections are widespread in the swine population, with prevalence rates as high as 90% reported in Europe (McOrist 2005). The first equine case of proliferative enteropathy was described in a foal in 1982 (Duhamel and Wheeldon 1982), but it was not until 1996 that a case of equine proliferative enteropathy was associated with *Lawsonia intracellularis* infection (Williams *et al.* 1996). Since that time the condition has been reported in young horses from North America, Europe and Australia, which suggests that the distribution is worldwide (Cooper *et al.* 1997a; Frank *et al.* 1998; Brees *et al.* 1999; Lavoie *et al.* 2000; Schumacher *et al.* 2000; Bihr 2003; McClintock and Collins 2004; Deprez *et al.* 2005; Dauvillier *et al.* 2006; Wuersch *et al.* 2006; Feary *et al.* 2007; McGurrin *et al.* 2007; Frazer 2008).

Lawsonia intracellularis infections are associated with profound intestinal hyperplasia due to proliferation of infected crypt epithelial cells of the small intestine. This proliferation results in loss of the normal villous structure, leading to impaired intestinal absorption and subsequent protein losing enteropathy. *Lawsonia* infections show a strong predisposition for young horses, typically from age 2–8 months, probably due to impaired immune function, although the exact nature of this dysfunction is not yet well characterised. The frequency with which proliferative enteropathy is being diagnosed in horses has increased dramatically over the last decade, probably due to increased clinician awareness and the development of effective *ante mortem* diagnostic tests. This disease can have devastating effects, with progressive weight loss, intermittent colic, profound hypoproteinaemia and peripheral oedema frequently reported. Fatal outcomes are reported, especially in cases that are severely debilitated or in which timely appropriate treatment is not initiated (Williams *et al.* 1996; Frank *et al.* 1998; Brees *et al.* 1999). Successful treatment is possible with early diagnosis and aggressive intervention, although affected animals may show decreased growth rates for several months.

Description and classification

The microaerophilic obligate intracellular nature of this bacterium has made it difficult to isolate, identify and investigate. As a result little was known about this organism for nearly 20 years following the first histological association of the organism with porcine adenomatosis (Rowland *et al.* 1973). The organism can be most readily identified in the enterocytes of infected animals using the Warthin-Starry silver stain and the microscopic characteristics consist of nonspore forming curved rods with a Gram-negative staining pattern (McOrist *et al.* 1995a). The bacteria characteristically replicate within the apical cytoplasm of enterocytes, and are not enclosed by any membranous vacuoles. Following the development of appropriate cell culture techniques the organism was cultivated *in vitro* and McOrist *et al.* (1995a) were able to establish the taxonomic classification of the organism. Based upon phenotypic and genetic analysis they determined that *L. intracellularis* represents a unique organism that is most closely related to but distinct from *Desulfovibrio* spp. organisms. They proposed the novel genus name of *Lawsonia* in honour of G. H. K. Lawson, who first discovered the bacterium, and the species name of *intracellularis* as indicative of the fastidious intracellular nature of the organism. Subsequent investigators have determined that *L. intracellularis* is also closely related to the human pathogen *Bilophila wadsworthia* (Lawson and Gebhart 2000).

Ample evidence exists to support the role of *L. intracellularis* in the development of proliferative intestinal lesions in a number of species and no other organisms have been shown to induce similar lesions. It appears that the organism is not host-specific, as porcine strains are capable of inducing disease in other species, including hamsters, rats and mice (Smith and Lawson 2001). In addition, there is 98–100% genetic similarity of 16s rRNA between isolates obtained from multiple species, including pigs, hamsters, horses, ferret, deer and ostrich, which further supports the suggestion that these organisms are very closely related and probably represent a single species (Cooper *et al.* 1997a,b; Lawson and Gebhart 2000).

Pathophysiology

Transmission of *L. intracellularis* is thought to be faecal-oral in nature, as the organism is shed in the faeces and the disease has been experimentally induced by feeding infected intestinal cells to naïve animals (Cooper and Gebhart 1998). Interestingly, exposure to *L. intracellularis* alone is not adequate to achieve infection in swine, as commensal intestinal bacteria must be present for infection to occur (McOrist *et al.* 1994). The role of these commensal organisms is unclear, but it appears that the normal flora supports the ability of *L. intracellularis* to invade the enterocytes and colonise the intestinal tract (Smith and Lawson 2001). The development of clinical disease also appears to require some degree of immune dysfunction, as weanling age animals appear to be most susceptible in all species (Cooper and Gebhart 1998). It has been proposed that the decline of maternal antibodies that occurs at several months of age in foals may predispose them to *Lawsonia* infection (Frazer 2008). Cell-mediated immune responses rather than humoural responses appear to be central to preventing clinical disease in other species, however, as interferon-gamma has been shown to be critical in mounting an appropriate immune response in murine models of *L. intracellularis* infection. Two studies have demonstrated that normal mice develop mild self-limiting *Lawsonia* infections whereas mice lacking the interferon-gamma receptor develop severe, persistent infections resulting in a high fatality rate (Smith *et al.* 2000; Go *et al.* 2005). There is evidence that foals do suffer from an age-related relative immunodeficiency characterised by decreased interferon-gamma production in young foals (Breathnach *et al.* 2006), and this may contribute to their predisposition to *Lawsonia* infection. However, this immunodeficiency is generally resolving by the time that most foals develop clinical signs of proliferative enteropathy as weanlings. Another possible immunosuppressive influence that may predispose foals to proliferative enteropathy is stress induced by management changes, such as weaning, conditioning and transport (Frazer 2008). This seems likely to be a contributing factor in the susceptibility of weanling age foals, as clinical signs are generally observed in swine within 2 weeks after substantial management stress, particularly weaning (Cooper and Gebhart 1998). A study investigating the role of genetic variation on the susceptibility of foals to *R. equi* and *Lawsonia infections* reported an association between certain equine immune response gene polymorphisms and PCR detection of faecal shedding of *Lawsonia* in a group of foals, which may suggest that there could be breed-related or familial predispositions as well (Horrin *et al.* 2004).

The mechanisms by which *L. intracellularis* organisms invade the host cells following ingestion are not completely understood. Entry into the enterocytes requires that the organism initially attaches to the enterocyte cell membrane, which has been shown to be an active process dependent upon enterocyte cell viability, but not bacterial viability (Lawson *et al.* 1995). The organism is then phagocytosed in a short-lived vacuole that breaks down and releases the bacteria into the cytoplasm, allowing the organism to avoid the damaging effects of phagolysosomal fusion (Smith and Lawson 2001). Viable organisms replicate free within the apical cytoplasm, frequently in association with mitochondria (McOrist *et al.* 2006). The organism exhibits tropism for crypt cells, rather than mature epithelial cells, and this appears to be related to the mechanism by which the bacteria colonise the epithelium (Smith and Lawson 2001). The crypt cells represent a rapidly dividing cell population that supports normal epithelial restitution, and the division of infected cells results in the production of infected daughter cells leading to population of the epithelium with infected cells (Lawson and Gebhart 2000).

Characteristic findings on histopathological evaluation of tissue specimens from infected animals are the presence of numerous curved bacteria within the apical cytoplasm of the infected enterocytes, profound mucosal hyperplasia and the relative absence of an active inflammatory response (Cooper and Gebhart 1998; Smith and Lawson 2001). The presence of the organism within the enterocytes results in an increased rate of cellular replication as early as 2 days after infection, and the rate of replication can increase to as much as 4 times normal (Smith and Lawson 2001). The mechanism by which *Lawsonia* induces this proliferation is unknown, but may be due to impaired apoptosis or the stimulation of a host response resulting in proliferation (McOrist *et al.* 1996a). The rapid proliferation and accumulation of infected crypt epithelial cells within the intestinal wall results in the development of the epithelial hyperplasia that is characteristic of this disease. Dramatic thickening and corrugation of the small intestinal mucosa represent the characteristic gross lesions. The small intestine is affected in foals, with gross lesions detected most often in the distal portion of the small intestine (terminal jejunum to ileum), but in severe cases the entirety of the small intestine can be involved (Lavoie *et al.* 2000; Schumacher *et al.* 2000; Deprez *et al.* 2005; Wuersch *et al.* 2006; McGurrin *et al.* 2007). The combined effects of the loss of villous architecture, which is primarily absorptive, and the proliferation of the crypt epithelium, which is secretory in nature (Cunningham 1997), are probably responsible for the loss of fluid and protein into the intestinal lumen that occurs with this disease, as little or no inflammation is present within the affected intestinal segment.

The presenting signs of proliferative enteropathy can include anorexia, depression, lethargy, weight loss, fever, diarrhoea, colic and ventral oedema. While there is some variation amongst reports, ventral oedema appears to be the most common presenting complaint in foals (Frazer 2008). Colic, diarrhoea and fever are also very common, however, and it is typical for foals to present with more than one problem (Lavoie *et al.* 2000; Atherton and McKenzie 2006; Sampieri *et al.* 2006; McGurrin *et al.* 2007; Frazer 2008). Clinicopathological abnormalities at presentation can include panhypoproteinaemia, hypoalbuminaemia, leukocytosis, hyperfibrinogenaemia and increased haemoglobin concentration and packed cell volume (PCV). Of these abnormalities, hypoalbuminaemia is the most common, as it is a consistent feature of the reported equine cases in which it was measured (Lavoie *et al.* 2000; McClintock and Collins 2004; Atherton and McKenzie 2006; Dauvillier *et al.* 2006; Sampieri *et al.* 2006; Wuersch *et al.* 2006; Feary *et al.*

2007; McGurrin *et al.* 2007; Frazer 2008). All of the other reported cases demonstrated hypoproteinaemia (Schumacher *et al.* 2000; Bihr 2003; Deprez *et al.* 2005). This finding is to be expected given the characteristics of the lesion in the small intestine, which causes a protein losing enteropathy (Rowan and Lawrence 1982).

Epidemiology

Equine proliferative enteropathy is a disease of young animals, with foals from 2–8 months most commonly affected, (Lavoie *et al.* 2000; Frazer 2008) although one case was reported in a yearling (Deprez *et al.* 2005). Equine proliferative enteropathy is typically sporadic in nature, but herd outbreaks have been reported. Given that the organism is shed in the faeces it is likely that environmental contamination with infected manure represents the route of transmission of this disease. Survival of *L. intracellularis* for up to 2 weeks outside of host cells has been demonstrated, along with some resistance to disinfectants, so environmental persistence may occur (Cooper and Gebhart 1998; Collins *et al.* 2000). The actual source of *L. intracellularis* organisms in equine infections remains unknown at this time. Documented exposure to swine is rare in published case reports of equine proliferative enteropathy, which suggests that pigs are an unlikely source of *L. intracellularis* in equine infections. It seems likely that other domestic species or wildlife play a role as carriers of this organism, given the variety of species that can be infected with this organism and the variety of species present in most farm environments. Alternatively it is possible that adult horses with subclinical infections may represent a reservoir. Pregnant animals have been shown to be susceptible in other species (Starek and Bilkei 2004). While epidemiological data regarding *Lawsonia* is limited in the horse, some studies have examined the serological status of horses on farms with documented cases of proliferative enteropathy (Lavoie *et al.* 2000; Schumacher *et al.* 2000; Dauvillier *et al.* 2006; Feary *et al.* 2007; Pusterla *et al.* 2008). Several of these studies demonstrated serological evidence of exposure to *Lawsonia* in foals housed with affected foals (Lavoie *et al.* 2000; Feary *et al.* 2007; Frazer 2008; Pusterla *et al.* 2008). One recent study showed that not only were clinically normal herdmates sometimes seropositive, but it also demonstrated that these individuals could be positive on fecal PCR testing, although this was less common than serological evidence of exposure (Frazer 2008). Two studies have also demonstrated *L. intracellularis*-specific antibodies in adult horses housed with affected foal(s) (Schumacher *et al.* 2000; Feary *et al.* 2007). Interestingly, Feary *et al.* (2007) also examined numerous other species of animals on the farm of interest, using both serology and PCR, and found that one dog was transiently positive for *L. intracellularis* on faecal PCR testing.

Diagnosis

Definitive diagnosis of equine proliferative enteropathy requires histological examination of affected tissues from the small intestine; however, this is not practical in most cases as surgical biopsy is not appropriate and most affected animals can survive with appropriate treatment. Histological examination using haematoxylin and eosin staining reveals the characteristic epithelial hyperplasia and loss of normal villous structure, and silver staining techniques reveal the curved bacilli within the apical cytoplasm of the affected crypt cells (Guedes *et al.* 2002a). Additional evaluation of fixed tissues can be performed using immunohistochemical staining with *L. intracellularis*-specific antibodies or PCR-based detection of *L. intracellularis* DNA (Kim *et al.* 2000; Guedes *et al.* 2002a). *Ante mortem* testing consists of serological testing, using either the indirect fluorescent antibody test (IFAT), ELISA or immunoperoxidase monolayer assays (IPMA), or faecal testing using PCR techniques. Serology is of questionable utility in the diagnosis of proliferative enteropathy in the clinical setting, as some clinically normal foals may test positive yet never develop clinical disease (Lavoie *et al.* 2000; Feary *et al.* 2007; Frazer 2008; Pusterla *et al.* 2008). In addition, it is possible for serological testing to yield false negative results early in the course of infection (Dauvillier *et al.* 2006; Sampieri *et al.* 2006; Feary *et al.* 2007; Pusterla *et al.* 2008). For these reasons serology is most useful in assessing the epidemiological status of the herd (Guedes *et al.* 2002a). Despite these limitations, serology is considered useful by some clinicians as one component of the clinical evaluation of foals showing clinical signs that are suspicious of proliferative enteropathy. When evaluating the individual patient, serological testing should be repeated if possible in order to detect delayed seroconversion, or paired with other testing modalities, primarily faecal PCR and clinical evaluation.

There are currently 2 primary serological tests available, namely an IFAT and an IPMA (Guedes *et al.* 2002b), although a recent study has reported the development of an enzyme-linked immunosorbent assay (Wattanaphansak *et al.* 2008). Most of the recent equine studies have utilised the IPMA methodology, which has technical advantages over the IFAT assay (Atherton and McKenzie 2006; Feary *et al.* 2007; Frazer 2008; Pusterla *et al.* 2008). While there has been some debate regarding the appropriate cutoff value for the IPMA test in equine cases, most reports use a value of 1:30 as the cutoff (Atherton and McKenzie 2006; Feary *et al.* 2007; Frazer 2008; Pusterla *et al.* 2008), which is consistent with the usage of the test in the swine population (Guedes *et al.* 2002b).

Due to the limitations of histology and serology in the diagnosis of proliferative enteropathy, there has been a great deal of interest in developing DNA-based testing using polymerase chain reaction (PCR) techniques. These techniques have the substantial benefits of being both highly specific, due to the identification of species specific DNA, and highly sensitive, due to their ability to amplify and detect the target DNA even at very low concentrations. The primary limitation of PCR techniques is that they can detect the DNA of nonviable organisms, meaning that infection is not always present even when the DNA of the organism is detected. Another limitation of PCR techniques for the detection of *L. intracellularis* is that despite their high sensitivity these tests can yield false negative results if the animal is not shedding the organism at the time of testing. Several studies in pigs have demonstrated very low sensitivities for PCR testing following experimental infection (Knittel *et al.* 1998; Guedes *et al.* 2002a). One recent equine study reported a false negative rate of 19% using faecal PCR in foals (Frazer 2008). In addition to these concerns regarding low sensitivity, it appears that the likelihood of obtaining a positive test result on faecal PCR decreases dramatically following the initiation of antimicrobial treatment (Kyriakis *et al.* 2002; Dauvillier *et al.* 2006). Often faecal PCR testing is combined with serological testing in evaluating foals suspected of suffering from proliferative enteropathy, and by using both tests the likelihood of detection is substantially increased (Frazer 2008).

Due to the limitations of both serology and faecal PCR it is clear that the equine clinician must use clinical parameters to identify foals suspected of suffering from this disease, and the initial identification of suspected cases is always based upon clinical evaluation. The most common clinical abnormalities observed at presentation are progressive weight loss, intermittent colic, lethargy,

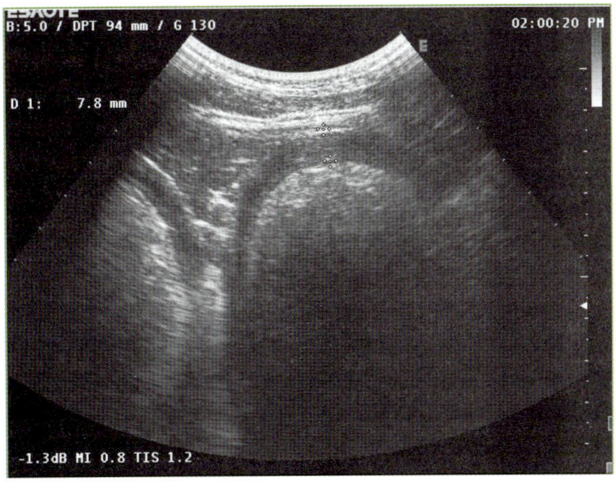

FIGURE 1: Thickened small intestinal wall (7.8 mm) on transabdominal ultrasonographic using 5 MHz frequency.

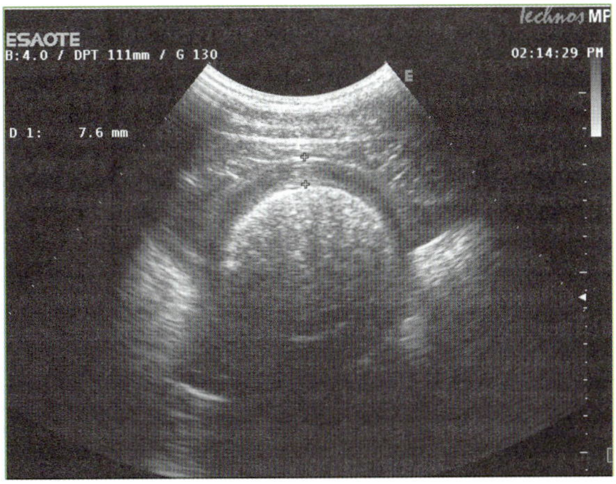

FIGURE 2: Thickened small intestinal wall (7.6 mm) on transabdominal ultrasonographic using 4 MHz frequency.

diarrhoea, fever and peripheral oedema. A recent retrospective study of 57 equine cases confirmed that ventral oedema is the most common clinical sign (Frazer 2008). Additional clinical diagnostics may be used to aid in confirming a diagnosis of proliferative enteropathy. One that is frequently mentioned is the use of ultrasonography to evaluate the thickness of the small intestinal wall. A small intestinal wall thickness exceeding the normal value of ≤3 mm (Reef 1998) is considered strongly suggestive of proliferative enteropathy (see **Figs 1** and **2**). This test is not always definitive, however, as while positive results are common and strongly reinforce the suspected diagnosis (Atherton and McKenzie 2006), false negatives can occur (Frazer 2008).

Clinicopathological evaluation is also helpful in supporting a diagnosis of proliferative enteropathy. Hypoalbuminaemia is the most common clinicopathological finding, as supported by multiple studies (Frank *et al.* 1998; Lavoie *et al.* 2000; McClintock and Collins 2004; Atherton and McKenzie 2006; Dauvillier *et al.* 2006; Wuersch *et al.* 2006; Feary *et al.* 2007; McGurrin *et al.* 2007; Frazer 2008). Panhypoproteinaemia is also common, but this can be masked by dehydration and hyperglobulinaemia. Other common clinicopathological abnormalities are leucocytosis, hyperfibrinogenaemia and increased PCV and haemoglobin concentration. Of these leucocytosis and hyperfibrinogenaemia are the most commonly mentioned in the literature (Atherton and McKenzie 2006; Dauvillier *et al.* 2006; Sampieri *et al.* 2006; Wuersch *et al.* 2006; Feary *et al.* 2007; McGurrin *et al.* 2007; Frazer 2008). Additional nonspecific abnormalities reported on serum biochemical testing have included: hyponatraemia, hypochloraemia, hypokalaemia, hypocalcaemia, elevated blood urea nitrogen (BUN), elevated serum creatinine, elevated creatine kinase (CK), elevated lactate dehydrogenase (LDH) and elevated aspartate aminotransferase (AST) (Lavoie *et al.* 2000; Sampieri *et al.* 2006; Frazer 2008).

Clinical diagnosis of proliferative enteropathy is ultimately based upon a combination of clinical, clinicopathological and diagnostic findings. A foal presenting with ventral oedema, hypoalbuminaemia and thickened small intestine on abdominal ultrasound is likely to be affected by proliferative enteropathy. Definitive diagnosis is elusive, but positive test results on either serum IPMA or faecal PCR would reinforce this diagnosis. Unfortunately not all foals will present with such definitive signs, but, by integrating the clinical presentation, clinicopathological data, ultrasonographic findings, serology and faecal PCR results, the clinician can maximise the likelihood of appropriately identifying the foal with proliferative enteropathy.

Treatment

Treatment of proliferative enteropathy consists of supportive therapy in combination with specific therapies directed towards *Lawsonia intracellularis*. Supportive therapy is primarily directed towards correction of the hypoalbuminaemia, although fluid therapy, nutritional support and analgesic therapy are often indicated as well. Colloid administration is the cornerstone of the treatment of hypoalbuminaemia, and this is accomplished by the use of either equine plasma or a synthetic colloid such as hydroxyethyl starch (Hetastarch)[1]. Equine plasma is typically administered at dose rates ranging from 10–20 ml/kg bwt, with the therapeutic goal of correcting the hypoalbuminaemia. Repeated dosing may be required due to the severity of the presenting hypoalbuminaemia and ongoing losses due to the underlying enteropathy.

The use of hydroxyethyl starches can be beneficial in providing additional colloidal support of the severely hypoalbuminaemic foal, but care must be taken to avoid overdosage, due to the possibility of haemorrhagic dysfunction. The recommended dosage range for Hetastarch is typically 5–10 ml/kg bwt, but cumulative doses should not exceed a total dose of 20 ml/kg bwt. The use of hydroxyethyl starches will result in lowering of the measured total protein and albumin concentrations in the patient's blood, which renders these values inaccurate as representations of colloid oncotic pressure, requiring that treatment be directed toward resolution of the clinical signs of hypoproteinaemia, rather than correction of the hypoproteinaemia itself. The use of crystalloid fluids is indicated in the dehydrated patient, but care must be taken to ensure that worsening of the hypoalbuminaemia does not result due to haemodilution. It is wise to provide colloids in conjunction with crystalloids and to administer the crystalloid solutions at the slowest rate possible while supporting the patient appropriately.

Specific therapy for *L. intracellularis* requires the use of antimicrobials that are able to reach therapeutic concentrations within the cytoplasm of the infected enterocyte, due to the fastidious intracellular nature of this organism. This limits the selection of appropriate antimicrobials to those drugs with high lipid solubility, which includes the macrolides, rifampin, tetracyclines and chloramphenicol.

In the horse, proliferative enteropathy was first treated with erythromycin (25 mg/kg bwt orally every 6–8 h), with or without rifampin (5 mg/kg bwt orally every 12 h) (Frank *et al.* 1998; Lavoie *et al.* 2000; Schumacher *et al.* 2000; Bihr 2003; McClintock and Collins 2004). The rationale for this choice of antibiotic was that erythromycin was found to have the lowest minimum inhibitory concentration against 2 strains of *L. intracellularis in vitro* (McOrist *et al.* 1995b). Erythromycin has often been combined with rifampin in the treatment of equine proliferative enteropathy due to the potential synergy associated with this combination, and probably due to the familiarity of equine clinicians with this combination from its use in the treatment of rhodococcal pneumonia. However, the use of erythromycin is associated with an increased risk of diarrhoea. In addition, erythromycin has been associated with the development of hyperthermia in foals treated for rhodococcal pneumonia. Erythromycin is a motilin-receptor agonist (Scarpignato and Pelosini 1999) and this effect may contribute to the development of diarrhoea. Erythromycin may also reduce the normal thermoregulatory response to hyperthermia, resulting in fever (Stratton-Phelps *et al.* 2000). The macrolides azithromycin and clarithromycin are associated with a lower incidence of hyperthermia in foals when used for the treatment of rhodococcal pneumonia (Giguere *et al.* 2004), and therefore may represent safer therapeutic options for the treatment of equine proliferative enteropathy. The successful use of azithromycin (10 mg/kg bwt orally once daily for 5–7 days then every other day) as a treatment for equine proliferative enteropathy has been reported in a few studies (Atherton and McKenzie 2006; Feary *et al.* 2007), as has the use of clarithromycin (7.5 mg/kg bwt orally every 12 h) (Atherton and McKenzie 2006; Frazer 2008).

As a result of the limitations of erythromycin therapy there has been interest in exploring the use of other antimicrobial agents. Several studies in swine have yielded data that support the use of a wider range of antimicrobials for the treatment of *Lawsonia* infections, including the tetracyclines (McOrist *et al.* 1995b, 1996b, 1997; Kyriakis *et al.* 2002). The tetracyclines are good choices in the treatment of intracellular pathogens, due to their ability to penetrate into and accumulate within the cytoplasm (Tulkens 1991; Womble *et al.* 2007). Both oral doxycycline (10 mg/kg bwt orally every 12 h) and i.v. oxytetracycline (6.6 mg/kg bwt i.v. every 12 h) have been reported to be effective in the treatment of equine proliferative enteropathy (Atherton and McKenzie 2006; Sampieri *et al.* 2006; Frazer 2008). Given the safety of these treatments and their reasonable cost to the client, doxycycline and oxytetracycline appear to be gaining favour as the primary therapies for this disease in foals.

Chloramphenicol has also been of some interest in the treatment of proliferative enteropathy, primarily due to the excellent intracellular penetration of this agent (Buonpane *et al.* 1988). There are concerns regarding possible human exposure to chloramphenicol, primarily due to the risk of aplastic anaemia, and while there is some debate regarding the actual magnitude of this risk (Laporte *et al.* 1998), chloramphenicol cannot be administered to food animals in the USA and is not available for veterinary use in Europe. In countries where chloramphenicol can be administered to horses it may represent a reasonable therapeutic option, as it has been reported to be effective in several studies when administered at 50 mg/kg bwt orally every 6–8 h (Lavoie *et al.* 2000; Atherton and McKenzie 2006; McGurrin *et al.* 2007; Frazer 2008).

While there is some *in vitro* evidence that suggest that the penicillins, cephalosporins and aminoglycosides may have efficacy against *L. intracellularis*, these drugs are very unlikely to be clinically effective due to their limited ability to achieve significant intracytoplasmic concentrations (Atherton and McKenzie 2006). The fluoroquinolones can achieve significant intracellular concentrations and may have activity against *Lawsonia* (McOrist *et al.* 1995b), but the use of these drugs in growing animals is contraindicated due to the potential for cartilage injury (Vivrette *et al.* 2001). In addition, the one reported case where enrofloxacin was administered in the treatment of a yearling suffering from proliferative enteropathy resulted in therapeutic failure (Deprez *et al.* 2005).

Expected outcomes

While the reported survival rates for foals suffering from proliferative enteropathy vary substantially, some of the most recent reports document survival rates ranging from 81% (9/11) to 93% (53/57) and 100% (7/7) (Atherton and McKenzie 2006; Sampieri *et al.* 2006; Frazer 2008). These results reinforce the fact that with early detection and appropriate therapy most foals should survive. The gastrointestinal pathology that is characteristic of this disease is not permanent in nature, but the impaired growth that results from the protein losing enteropathy does appear to slow the growth of affected foals. Most foals appear to regain normal growth rates after several months, and eventually may 'catch up' with their peers, but Frazer (2008) determined that as yearlings the affected Thoroughbred foals in one study achieved only 68% of the sales price of their peers.

Manufacturer's address

[1]Hospira, Lake Forest, Illinois, USA.

References

Atherton, R.P. and McKenzie, H.C. (2006) Alternative antimicrobial agents in the treatment of proliferative enteropathy in horses. *J. equine vet. Sci.* **26**, 535-541.

Biester, H.E. and Schwartze, L.H. (1931) Intestinal adenoma in swine. *Am. J. Pathol.* **7**, 175-185.

Bihr, T.P. (2003) Protein-losing enteropathy caused by *Lawsonia intracellularis* in a weanling foal. *Can. vet. J.* **44**, 65-66.

Breathnach, C.C., Sturgill-Wright, T., Stiltner, J.L., Adams, A.A., Lunn, D.P. and Horohov, D.W. (2006) Foals are interferon gamma-deficient at birth. *Vet. Immunol. Immunopathol.* **112**, 199-209.

Brees, D.J., Sondhoff, A.H., Kluge, J.P., Andreasen, C.B. and Brown, C.M. (1999) *Lawsonia intracellularis*-like organism infection in a miniature foal. *J. Am. vet. med. Ass.* **215**, 511-514, 483.

Buonpane, N.A., Brown, M.P., Gronwall, R., Stone, H.W. and Miles, N. (1988) Serum concentrations and pharmacokinetics of chloramphenicol in foals after a single oral dose. *Equine vet. J.* **20**, 59-61.

Collins, A.M., Love, R.J., Pozo, J., Smith, S.H. and McOrist, A.L. (2000) Studies on the *ex-vivo* survival of *Lawsonia intracellularis*. *Swine Health Prod.* **8**, 211-215.

Cooper, D.M. and Gebhart, C.J. (1998) Comparative aspects of proliferative enteritis. *J. Am. vet. med. Ass.* **212**, 1446-1451.

Cooper, D.M., Swanson, D.L. and Gebhart, C.J. (1997a) Diagnosis of proliferative enteritis in frozen and formalin-fixed, paraffin-embedded tissues from a hamster, horse, deer and ostrich using a *Lawsonia intracellularis*-specific multiplex PCR assay. *Vet. Microbiol.* **54**, 47-62.

Cooper, D.M., Swanson, D.L., Barns, S.M. and Gebhart, C.J. (1997b) Comparison of the 16S ribosomal DNA sequences from the intracellular agents of proliferative enteritis in a hamster, deer, and ostrich with the sequence of a porcine isolate of *Lawsonia intracellularis*. *Int. J. Syst. Bacteriol.* **47**, 635-639.

Cunningham, J.G. (1997) Digestion and absorption: The nonfermentative processes. In: *Textbook of Veterinary Physiology*, Ed: J.G. Cunningham, W.B. Saunders, Philadelphia. pp 301-330.

Dauvillier, J., Picandet, V., Harel, J., Gottschalk, M., Desrosiers, R., Jean, D. and Lavoie, J.P. (2006) Diagnostic and epidemiological features of *Lawsonia intracellularis* enteropathy in 2 foals. *Can. vet. J.* **47**, 689-691.

Deprez, P., Chiers, K., Gebhart, C.J., Ducatelle, R., Lefere, L., Vanschandevijl, K. and van Loon, G. (2005) *Lawsonia intracellularis* infection in a 12-month-old colt in Belgium. *Vet. Rec.* **157**, 774-776.

Duhamel, G.E. and Wheeldon, E.B. (1982) Intestinal adenomatosis in a foal. *Vet. Pathol.* **19**, 447-450.

Feary, D.J., Gebhart, C.J. and Pusterla, N. (2007) *Lawsonia intracellularis* proliferative enteropathy in a foal. *Schweiz. Arch. Tierheilkd.* **149**, 129-133.

Frank, N., Fishman, C.E., Gebhart, C.J. and Levy, M. (1998) *Lawsonia intracellularis* proliferative enteropathy in a weanling foal. *Equine vet. J.* **30**, 549-552.

Frazer, M.L. (2008) *Lawsonia intracellularis* infection in horses: 2005-2007. *J. vet. Intern. Med.* **22**, 1243-1248.

Giguere, S., Jacks, S., Roberts, G.D., Hernandez, J., Long, M.T. and Ellis, C. (2004) Retrospective comparison of azithromycin, clarithromycin, and erythromycin for the treatment of foals with *Rhodococcus equi* pneumonia. *J. vet. intern. Med.* **18**, 568-573.

Go, Y.Y., Lee, J.K., Ye, J.Y., Lee, J.B., Park, S.Y., Song, C.S., Kim, S.K. and Choi, I.S. (2005) Experimental reproduction of proliferative enteropathy and the role of IFN-gamma in protective immunity against *Lawsonia intracellularis* in mice. *J. vet. Sci.* **6**, 357-359.

Guedes, R.M., Gebhart, C.J., Winkelman, N.L., Mackie-Nuss, R.A., Marsteller, T.A. and Deen, J. (2002a) Comparison of different methods for diagnosis of porcine proliferative enteropathy. *Can. J. vet. Res.* **66**, 99-107.

Guedes, R.M., Gebhart, C.J., Winkelman, N.L. and Mackie-Nuss, R.A. (2002b) A comparative study of an indirect fluorescent antibody test and an immunoperoxidase monolayer assay for the diagnosis of porcine proliferative enteropathy. *J. vet. diagn. Invest.* **14**, 420-423.

Horrin, P., Smola, J., Matiasovic, J., Vyskocil, M., Lukeszova, L., Tomanova, K., Kralik, P., Glasnak, V., Schroffelova, D., Knoll, A., Sedlinska, M., Krenkova, L. and Jahn, P. (2004) Polymorphisms in equine immune response genes and their associations with infections. *Mamm. Genome* **15**, 843-850.

Kim, J., Choi, C., Cho, W.S. and Chae, C. (2000) Immunohistochemistry and polymerase chain reaction for the detection of *Lawsonia intracellularis* in porcine intestinal tissues with proliferative enteropathy. *J. vet. med. Sci.* **62**, 771-773.

Klein, E.C., Gebhart, C.J. and Duhamel, G.E. (1999) Fatal outbreaks of proliferative enteritis caused by *Lawsonia intracellularis* in young colony-raised rhesus macaques. *J. Med. Primatol.* **28**, 11-18.

Knittel, J.P., Jordan, D.M., Schwartz, K.J., Janke, B.H., Roof, M.B., McOrist, S. and Harris, D.L. (1998) Evaluation of *antemortem* polymerase chain reaction and serologic methods for detection of *Lawsonia intracellularis*-exposed pigs. *Am. J. vet. Res.* **59**, 722-726.

Kyriakis, S.C., Bourtzi-Hatzopoulou, E., Alexopoulos, C., Kritas, S.K., Polyzopoulou, Z., Lekkas, S. and Gardey, L. (2002) Field evaluation of the effect of in-feed doxycycline for the control of ileitis in weaned piglets. *J. vet. Med. B. Infect. Dis. Vet. Public. Health* **49**, 317-321.

Laporte, J.R., Vidal, X., Ballarin, E. and Ibanez, L. (1998) Possible association between ocular chloramphenicol and aplastic anaemia--the absolute risk is very low. *Br. J. Clin. Pharmacol.* **46**, 181-184.

Lavoie, J.P., Drolet, R., Parsons, D., Leguillette, R., Sauvageau, R., Shapiro, J., Houle, L., Halle, G. and Gebhart, C.J. (2000) Equine proliferative enteropathy: a cause of weight loss, colic, diarrhoea and hypoproteinaemia in foals on three breeding farms in Canada. *Equine vet. J.* **32**, 418-425.

Lawson, G.H. and Gebhart, C.J. (2000) Proliferative enteropathy. *J. comp. Pathol.* **122**, 77-100.

Lawson, G.H., Mackie, R.A., Smith, D.G. and McOrist, S. (1995) Infection of cultured rat enterocytes by ileal symbiont *intracellularis* depends on host cell function and actin polymerisation. *Vet. Microbiol.* **45**, 339-350.

McClintock, S.A. and Collins, A.M. (2004) *Lawsonia intracellularis* proliferative enteropathy in a weanling foal in Australia. *Aust. vet. J.* **82**, 750-752.

McGurrin, M.K., Vengust, M., Arroyo, L.G. and Baird, J.D. (2007) An outbreak of *Lawsonia intracellularis* infection in a Standardbred herd in Ontario. *Can. vet. J.* **48**, 927-930.

McOrist, S. (2005) Defining the full costs of endemic porcine proliferative enteropathy. *Vet. J.* **170**, 8-9.

McOrist, S., Gebhart, C.J. and Bosworth, B.T. (2006) Evaluation of porcine ileum models of enterocyte infection by *Lawsonia intracellularis*. *Can. J. vet. Res.* **70**, 155-159.

McOrist, S., Gebhart, C.J., Boid, R. and Barns, S.M. (1995a) Characterization of *Lawsonia intracellularis* gen. nov., sp. nov., the obligately intracellular bacterium of porcine proliferative enteropathy. *Int. J. Syst. Bacteriol.* **45**, 820-825.

McOrist, S., Mackie, R.A. and Lawson, G.H. (1995b) Antimicrobial susceptibility of ileal symbiont *intracellularis* isolated from pigs with proliferative enteropathy. *J. clin. Microbiol.* **33**, 1314-1317.

McOrist, S., Mackie, R.A., Neef, N., Aitken, I. and Lawson, G.H. (1994) Synergism of ileal symbiont *intracellularis* and gut bacteria in the reproduction of porcine proliferative enteropathy. *Vet. Rec.* **134**, 331-332.

McOrist, S., Morgan, J., Veenhuizen, M.F., Lawrence, K. and Kroger, H.W. (1997) Oral administration of tylosin phosphate for treatment and prevention of proliferative enteropathy in pigs. *Am. J. vet. Res.* **58**, 136-139.

McOrist, S., Roberts, L., Jasni, S., Rowland, A.C., Lawson, G.H., Gebhart, C.J. and Bosworth, B. (1996a) Developed and resolving lesions in porcine proliferative enteropathy: possible pathogenetic mechanisms. *J. comp. Pathol.* **115**, 35-45.

McOrist, S., Smith, S.H., Shearn, M.F., Carr, M.M. and Miller, D.J. (1996b) Treatment and prevention of porcine proliferative enteropathy with oral tiamulin. *Vet. Rec.* **139**, 615-618.

Pusterla, N., Higgins, J.C., Smith, P., Mapes, S. and Gebhart, C. (2008) Epidemiological survey on farms with documented occurrence of equine proliferative enteropathy due to *Lawsonia intracellularis*. *Vet. Rec.* **163**, 156-158.

Reef, V.B. (1998) Pediatric abdominal ultrasonography. In: *Equine Diagnostic Ultrasound*, 1st edn., Ed: V.B. Reef, W.B. Saunders, Philadelphia. pp 364-403.

Rowan, T.G. and Lawrence, T.L. (1982) Amino acid digestibility in pigs with signs of porcine intestinal adenomatosis. *Vet. Rec.* **110**, 306-307.

Rowland, A.C., Lawson, G.H. and Maxwell, A. (1973) Intestinal adenomatosis in the pig: occurrence of a bacterium in affected cells. *Nature* **243**, 417.

Sampieri, F., Hinchcliff, K.W. and Toribio, R.E. (2006) Tetracycline therapy of *Lawsonia intracellularis* enteropathy in foals. *Equine vet. J.* **38**, 89-92.

Scarpignato, C. and Pelosini, I. (1999) Management of irritable bowel syndrome: novel approaches to the pharmacology of gut motility. *Can. J. Gastroenterol.* **13**, *Suppl.* A, 50A-65A.

Schumacher, J., Rolsma, M., Brock, K.V. and Gebhart, C.J. (2000) Surgical and medical treatment of an Arabian filly with proliferative enteropathy caused by *Lawsonia intracellularis*. *J. vet. int. Med.* **14**, 630-632.

Smith, D.G. and Lawson, G.H. (2001) *Lawsonia intracellularis*: getting inside the pathogenesis of proliferative enteropathy. *Vet. Microbiol.* **82**, 331-345.

Smith, D.G., Mitchell, S.C., Nash, T. and Rhind, S. (2000) Gamma interferon influences intestinal epithelial hyperplasia caused by *Lawsonia intracellularis* infection in mice. *Infect. Immun.* **68**, 6737-6743.

Starek, M. and Bilkei, G. (2004) Sows seropositive to *Lawsonia intracellularis* (LI) influence performance and LI seropositivity of their offspring. *Acta. Vet. Brno.* **73**, 341-345.

Stratton-Phelps, M., Wilson, W.D. and Gardner, I.A. (2000) Risk of adverse effects in pneumonic foals treated with erythromycin versus other antibiotics: 143 cases (1986-1996). *J. Am. vet. med. Ass.* **217**, 68-73.

Tulkens, P.M. (1991) Intracellular distribution and activity of antibiotics. *Eur. J. Clin. Microbiol. Infect. Dis.* **10**, 100-106.

Vivrette, S.L., Bostian, A., Bermingham, E. and Papich, M.G. (2001) Quinolone-induced arthropathy in neonatal foals. *Proc. Am. Ass. equine Practnrs.* **47**, 376-377.

Wattanaphansak, S., Asawakarn, T., Gebhart, C.J. and Deen, J. (2008) Development and validation of an enzyme-linked immunosorbent assay for the diagnosis of porcine proliferative enteropathy. *J. vet. Diagn. Invest.* **20**, 170-177.

Williams, N.M., Harrison, L.R. and Gebhart, C.J. (1996) Proliferative enteropathy in a foal caused by *Lawsonia intracellularis*-like bacterium. *J. vet. Diagn. Invest.* **8**, 254-256.

Womble, A., Giguere, S. and Lee, E.A. (2007) Pharmacokinetics of oral doxycycline and concentrations in body fluids and bronchoalveolar cells of foals. *J. vet. Pharmacol. Therap.* **30**, 187-193.

Wuersch, K., Huessy, D., Koch, C. and Oevermann, A. (2006) *Lawsonia intracellularis* proliferative enteropathy in a filly. *J. vet. Med. A. Physiol. Pathol. Clin. Med.* **53**, 17-21.

A REVIEW OF *STREPTOCOCCUS EQUI* INFECTION IN THE HORSE

A. M. House*, L. H. Javsicas and D. N. Zimmel

University of Florida College of Veterinary Medicine, Large Animal Clinical Sciences, PO Box 100136, Gainesville, Florida 32610-0136, USA.

Keywords: horse; strangles; vaccination; infection control

Summary

Strangles is a result of bacterial infection with *Streptococcus equi* ssp. *equi* (*S. equi*). The disease has been in the equine population for centuries and was first reported in 1251 (Sweeney *et al.* 2005). The infection is highly contagious in horse populations and can become endemic on farms with previous outbreaks of the disease. Diagnosis of the disease has often been made based on clinical examination, however, confirmation via culture and/or PCR is recommended. Routine abscessation of lymph nodes localised to the submandibular region and the head generally requires supportive care with anti-inflammatory drugs and drainage when possible. Treatment of *S. equi* infection with antimicrobials is generally reserved for complicated cases. Complications from *S. equi* infection include metastatic infection, purpura haemorrhagica, myositis, and rarely glomerulonephritis, myocarditis, or agalactia (Sweeney *et al.* 1987; Divers *et al.* 1992). Control of outbreaks can be attainable through strict management and identification of exposed and infected horses in conjunction with implementation of barrier control, isolation, and disinfection procedures. Vaccination is generally not recommended during outbreaks, but remains a valuable tool for possible disease prevention and mitigation of clinical signs. Serology with the SeM-specific ELISA is useful to detect recent infections and determine the need for vaccination.

Aetiology and pathogenesis

Streptococcus equi ssp. *equi* (*S. equi*) is a Gram-positive beta-haemolytic bacterium of the Lancefield Group C that results in the purulent lymphadenitis and pharyngitis recognised as equine strangles. Studies indicate that *S. equi* is a clone derived from the more genetically diverse *S. zooepidemicus* (Timoney *et al.* 1997). However, *S. equi* is not a normal inhabitant of the equine upper respiratory tract. The bacterium enters the horse through inhalation into the nose or ingestion into the mouth. *S. equi* attaches to cells in the crypt of the lingual and palatine tonsils and to the follicular-associated epithelium of the pharyngeal and tubal tonsils. The bacterium gains access to the local lymphatics and lymph nodes where extracellular replication occurs within hours of attachment (Timoney 1993). Multiple virulence factors contribute to the pathogenicity of *S. equi*, including the antiphagocytic SeM protein, the hyaluronic acid capsule, Mac protein, and other undetermined factors and/or cytotoxins (Muhktar and Timoney 1988; Sweeney *et al.* 2005). The SeM protein, also known as fibrinogen-binding protein, is a 58-kD cell wall antigen that prevents activation of the alternative complement pathway by limiting deposition of C3b on the bacterium's surface. SeM also disrupts neutrophil killing of the bacterium and binds fibrinogen (Timoney *et al.* 1997). The hyaluronic acid capsule aids in repelling phagocytes due to its negative charge. These factors favour conditions for abscess formation due to the accumulation of large numbers of extracellular bacteria surrounded by degenerating neutrophils.

Infection with *S. equi* occurs primarily but not exclusively in young horses aged 1–5 years. Transmission of the bacterium occurs via direct contact with nasal or lymph node discharge from infected horses or from exposure to contaminated fomites such as halters, brushes or clothing. New

*Author to whom correspondence should be addressed.

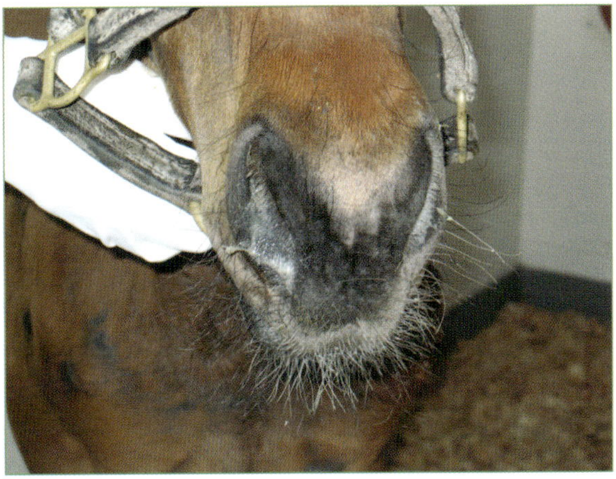

FIGURE 1: Nasal discharge due to strangles.

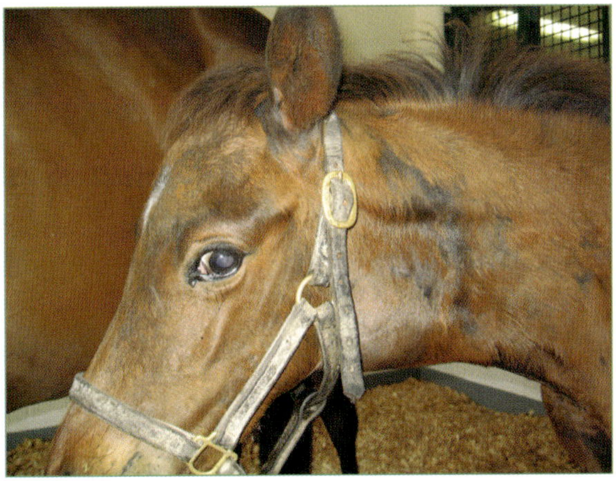

FIGURE 2: Severely enlarged throat latch region associated with strangles.

additions to a farm are a potential source of exposure to naïve herds. The incubation period ranges from 2–6 days prior to the onset of clinical signs. Nasal shedding occurs from infected horses 2–3 days after the onset of fever and typically continues for 2–3 weeks in most cases. Shedding may persist for months to years in rare cases, especially when guttural pouch infection is present (Newton *et al.* 1997). A recovered horse may be a potential source of infection for at least 6 weeks after clinical signs have resolved (Sweeney *et al.* 2005). Periodic subclinical carrier horses present a challenge for identification and prevention of further herd outbreaks. The carrier state develops in up to 10% of infected horses, and may result in chronic empyema of the guttural pouch.

Clinical signs

Strangles acquired its name because affected horses were sometimes suffocated by large, infected lymph nodes that obstructed their upper airway or trachea. The hallmark clinical signs of infection are fever, mucopurulent nasal discharge, and lymphadenopathy of the submandibular and/or retropharyngeal lymph nodes with subsequent abscessation. Lymph nodes usually rupture and drain 7–10 days after the initial onset of clinical signs. Purulent nasal discharge is typically present (**Fig 1**), although it may initially be serous. Mucopurulent ocular discharge may also occur, and the nasal and ocular mucosal membranes are often hyperaemic. Depression, pharyngitis and rhinitis are frequently seen. Anorexia and dysphagia may occur secondary to pharyngitis and/or lymph node compression of the throat. Swelling may become so severe that respiratory distress ensues and tracheostomy may be required (**Fig 2**). Peripheral lymph node abscessation is occasionally disseminated (**Figs 3** and **4**). Coughing is not a significant clinical sign in many cases, although some horses will develop a soft moist cough that worsens with disease progression. The average clinical course of the disease is about 3 weeks. Disease severity appears dependent on challenge load and duration. Inocula of $<10^6$ CFU are not consistently effective in causing disease because such low numbers are efficiently removed via mucociliary clearance (Sweeney *et al.* 2005).

Guttural pouch empyema can result from retropharyngeal lymph nodes that abscess and

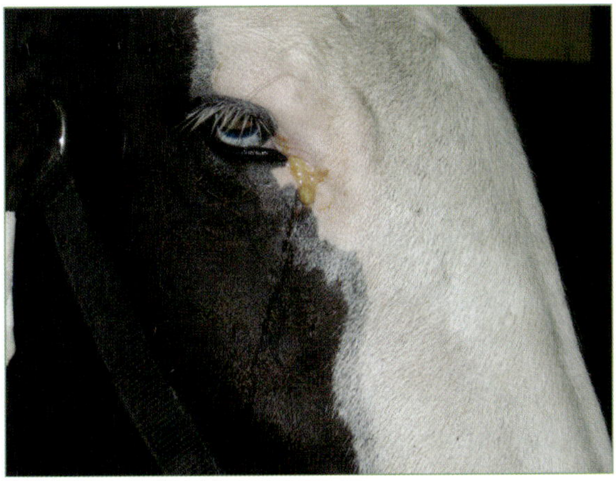

FIGURE 3: Strangles abscess near the eye.

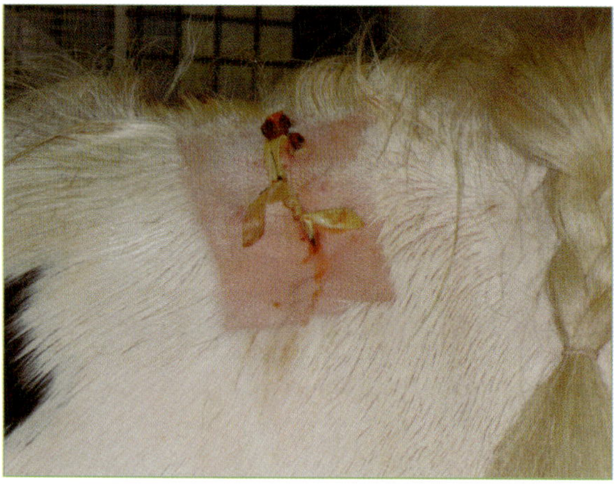

FIGURE 4: Abscess along the withers

rupture into the guttural pouches (**Fig 5**, endoscopy) or from bacterial entrance through the pharynx. Purulent secretions that persist in the guttural pouch may form hard, inspissated chondroids. Chondroid formation can present a treatment challenge, and removal is typically performed endoscopically with a basket or via a surgical approach to the guttural pouch (**Fig 6**). Undiagnosed guttural pouch empyema or chrondroids can result in persistent shedding of *S. equi* into the environment.

Complications of infection

Fortunately, although strangles' morbidity is high, the mortality rate for uncomplicated infections remains relatively low. Complications are reported to occur in approximately 20% of strangles cases (Sweeney *et al.* 1987; Sweeney *et al.* 2005). The occurrence of complications will increase the likelihood of death from 8% to 40% of cases (Sweeney *et al.* 1987). Metastatic spread of infection (also known as bastard strangles) with internal abscessation, purpura haemorrhagica, myositis from muscle infarction, rhabdomyolysis, glomerulonephritis, myocarditis, agalactia in periparturient mares and septicaemia with spread to the lungs, joints or central nervous system are all possible complications associated with *S. equi* infection (Sweeney *et al.* 1987, 2005; Yelle 1987; Divers *et al.* 1992; Pusterla *et al.* 2003; Spoormakers *et al.* 2003; Sponseller *et al.* 2005; Finno *et al.* 2006; Pusterla *et al.* 2007). Horses that develop complicated infection typically require antimicrobial and additional supportive therapies.

Metastatic spread of *S. equi* can infect the thorax, brain, mesentery, liver, spleen, or kidneys. Although metastatic infection is classically associated with a poor prognosis, one study that evaluated horses with abdominal abscesses reported a long-term survival rate of 40% (Pusterla *et al.* 2007). Diagnostic evaluation to determine the presence of metastatic infection may include rectal examination, abdominocentesis, abdominal and/or thoracic ultrasound, radiographs, and/or transtracheal aspiration. The horse's clinical signs will typically dictate the appropriate modalities for disease investigation. Long-term administration of antimicrobials is necessary for treatment of internal abscesses; the mean duration in the study by Pusterla *et al.* (2007) was 72 days. There is not strong evidence

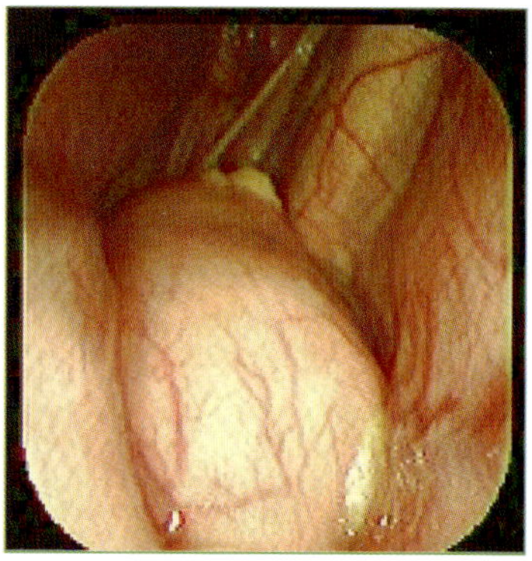

FIGURE 5: Endoscopy: guttural pouch with ruptured lymph node protruding from the floor of the pouch.

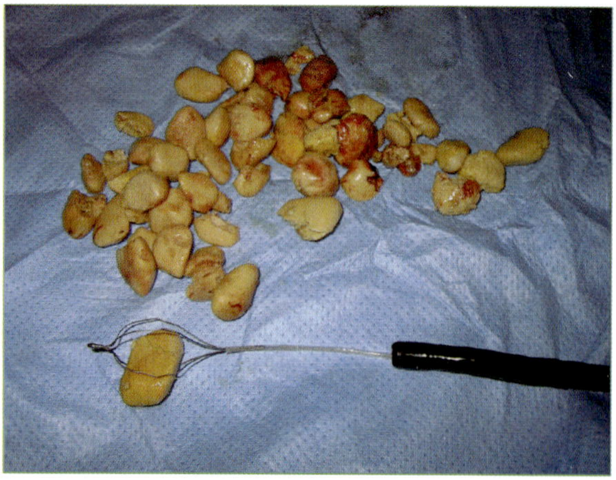

FIGURE 6: Chondroids removed from the guttural pouch using endoscopic basket forceps.

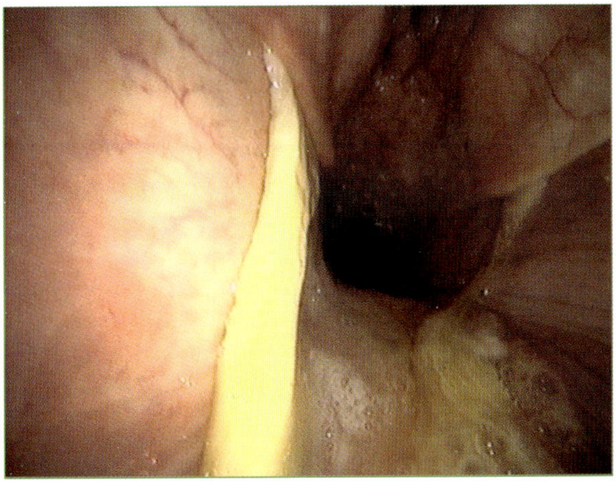

FIGURE 7: Mucopurulent discharge from guttural pouch ostia into the nasopharynx.

to support the belief that antimicrobial use early in the course of disease contributes to metastatic infection with *S. equi* (Ramey 2007).

Purpura haemorrhagica is an aseptic vasculitis characterised primarily by oedema of the limbs and petechial or ecchymotic haemorrhages. The clinical signs of purpura haemorrhagica can vary from a mild, transient reaction to a severe or even fatal disease (Pusterla *et al.* 2003). The oedema may become severe enough to cause serum seepage and/or sloughing of the skin. In addition to the limbs, the oedema may affect the head or trunk. In some cases, the vasculitis may result in colic, respiratory difficulty, and muscle pain from its effect on the gastrointestinal tract, muscle and respiratory system. Colic and muscle stiffness may be the primary clinical signs in horses with muscle infarctions due to purpura haemorrhagica (Kaese *et al.* 2005). Early recognition of muscle swelling, abdominal pain, neutrophilia, hypoalbuminaemia and high creatine kinase levels may improve the outcome for horses with infarctive purpura; however, 4 of the 5 horses in the study by Kaese *et al.* (2005) were subjected to euthanasia. In addition to muscle infarctions, rhabdomyolysis and immune-mediated myositis have also been described in horses following exposure to *S. equi* (Sponseller *et al.* 2005; Lewis *et al.* 2007).

The pathogenesis of purpura haemorrhagica is not completely understood but it appears to be secondary to immune complex deposition within blood vessel walls. It can occur following vaccination for *S. equi* or from re-exposure to the organism in natural infection, but may also be due to other organisms. In a study of 53 horses with purpura, 17 were exposed to or infected with *S. equi* and 5 had been vaccinated with the *S. equi* M protein; the remaining 31 cases were associated with other organisms or had no known aetiology (Pusterla *et al.* 2003). A pre-existing high serum antibody titre to *S. equi* antigens may predispose horses to the development of purpura (Sweeney *et al.* 2005). Therefore, vaccination is contraindicated for horses with antibody levels of >1:1600. Diagnosis of purpura can be confirmed by the identification of a leucocytoclastic vasculitis on skin biopsy, isolation of the organism or increased antibody levels (>1:12,800). Treatment typically consists of corticosteroids, supportive care and frequently antimicrobials such as penicillin. Dexamethasone at 0.1–0.2 mg/kg bwt is typically used for initial therapy and then tapered. Hydrotherapy and bandaging can be beneficial adjunctive therapies for oedema and serum exudation from the skin. In the study of 53 horses with purpura haemorrhagica, the majority required treatment for more than 7 days (Pusterla *et al.* 2003).

Diagnosis

Clinical signs of strangles are highly suggestive of the diagnosis. However, definitive diagnosis is made by culture of the bacteria from a nasal swab, aspirate of an abscessed lymph node, or a nasal-pharyngeal wash. Culture remains the gold standard diagnostic modality for *S. equi*. When compared to culture for the diagnosis of strangles, polymerase chair reaction (PCR) is considered to be 2–3 times more sensitive (Timoney and Artiushin 1997; Newton *et al.* 2000; Gronbaek *et al.* 2006). The PCR detects the DNA sequence of SeM, the antiphagocytic protein of the bacteria (Sweeney *et al.* 2005). Although an allele of this gene is found on some strains of *S. zooepidemicus*, the sequence is of low homology and PCR of *S. zooepidemicus* is unlikely to yield a false positive result. Additionally, there is no evidence that an SeM-like protein is expressed by *S. zooepidemicus* (Sweeney *et al.* 2005). PCR cannot differentiate between live and dead bacteria, so is ideally used in conjunction with culture for confirmation of strangles. However, if consecutive PCRs are negative when screening for infection or subclinical carrier status, the horse is unlikely to have strangles. Nasal washes are also considered superior to swabs for diagnosis because a larger surface area within the nares is sampled (Timoney and Artiushin 1997). The real challenge is diagnosing horses that are asymptomatic carriers. Anywhere from 4–50% of the horses on farms with recurring strangles are carriers of the infection, although it is estimated that the carrier state develops in up to 10% of affected horses and results in chronic empyema of the guttural pouch (Sweeney *et al.* 2005). Endoscopy is an excellent adjunctive tool for diagnosis of asymptomatic carriers, and can facilitate obtaining samples via guttural pouch lavage (**Fig 7**). Most horses will begin shedding the bacteria from their nasal passages a couple of days after the onset of fever. Bacterial shedding occurs intermittently for several weeks. Some horses may continue to shed the bacteria for months or even years, serving as a continual source of new infections on the farm.

A recent study that used a nested PCR assay suggests that *S. equi* DNA can be detected longer in convalescent horses, and that horses in the group without disease may also be infected (Gronbaek *et al.* 2006). Further work is required to confirm how long such animals can be detected by PCR analysis and, most importantly, what proportion is actually harbouring viable *S. equi* (Prescott and Timoney 2007).

Serology can be a useful diagnostic test to determine recent (but not necessarily current) *S. equi* infection, determine the need for vaccination, and to aid in the diagnosis of metastatic infection and purpura haemorrhagica. An SeM-specific antibody ELISA is commercially available[1], but cannot distinguish between the response to vaccination and natural infection (**Table 1**). Serum titres peak about 5 weeks after exposure and remain high for at least 6 months, while the response to commercial vaccines peaks at about 2 weeks and also remains high for 6 months (Sheoran *et al.* 1997). Interpretation of results should consider that there may be considerable variation in the response of individual horses. Horses with a titre >1:1600 should never be vaccinated (Sweeney *et al.* 2005).

Treatment

Antimicrobial therapy remains controversial for the treatment of strangles. Uncomplicated cases of submandibular lymph node abscessation do not require antimicrobial therapy in the authors' opinion. Complicated cases and those requiring tracheostomy for management of respiratory distress generally do require antimicrobial and other supportive therapies. There is some evidence that treatment with antimicrobials at the first sign of fever and in horses with no lymph node enlargement may prevent infection. However, early antimicrobial treatment will also prevent these cases from developing immunity to the infection, and subsequently makes them susceptible to reinfection sooner.

In horses with uncomplicated lymphadenopathy, treatment should be aimed at encouraging maturation and rupture of effected lymph nodes. Antimicrobial therapy is not necessary and may prolong the course of the disease. To encourage maturation of abscesses, topical poultice application and hot packing is recommended by some authors (Sweeney *et al.* 2005). Once abscesses mature and an area of thinning forms

TABLE 1: Interpretation of SeM-specific ELISA (adapted from Sweeney *et al.* 2005)

	Antibody titre	Interpretation
Negative	No antibodies detected	Horse has no previous exposure or was exposed in last 7 days.
Weak positive	1:200–1:400	Equivocal result could indicate very recent exposure or residual vaccination response. Repeat testing recommended in 7–14 days.
Moderate positive	1:800–1:1600	Intermediate positive response, which could indicate exposure 2–3 weeks ago or infection 6 months to 2 years ago.
High positive	1:3200–1:6400	Antibodies detected at a high level. Could indicate infection 4–12 weeks ago or be post vaccination (1–2 weeks post injectable vaccine or 2–4 weeks post intranasal vaccine). Vaccination is contraindicated in horses with titres >1:1600.
Very high positive	>1:12,800	SeM specific antibodies very high. Can be seen in horses with metastatic infection or purpura haemorrhagica.

on the ventral skin surface, they can be lanced to promote drainage. Care should be taken in transcutaneous drainage of retropharyngeal abscesses due to the proximity of large vessels. Ultrasonographic examination is recommended to determine the exact depth of the abscess. After lancing, abscesses can be flushed frequently with a dilute povidone-iodine solution to aid in healing (Sweeney *et al.* 2005). Guttural pouch empyema following rupture of the retropharyngeal lymph nodes should be treated with copious lavage, as accumulation of purulent material in the guttural pouches promotes chondroid formation (**Fig 6**), making resolution of disease and carrier status more difficult. Depending on the amount and character of guttural pouch empyema, lavage can be performed transendoscopically using a pressure bag or fluid pump, indwelling catheter, or with a small bore stomach tube (Adkins *et al.* 1997; Judy *et al.* 1999; Sweeney *et al.* 2005). Although sterile saline is ideal, the authors have also used nonsterile saline made with tap water and salt (100 g of salt in 16 l of water). During lavage, it is essential that the horse be adequately sedated to keep the head lowered and decrease the risk of aspiration. Frequent re-evaluation of the guttural pouches endoscopically allows determination of ongoing drainage from the retropharyngeal lymph nodes and the need for further lavage.

Retropharyngeal abscessation causing respiratory distress may require placement of a temporary tracheostomy. Though antimicrobial therapy has been recommended in these cases to prevent lower airway infection, the author has successfully treated horses with *S. equi* with a tracheostomy without antimicrobials with no complications. Antimicrobial therapy has been recommended by some authors (Sweeney *et al.* 2005) once drainage from abscesses has been established, as it may promote a more rapid recovery. However, it is important to bear in mind that it is often difficult to determine when all affected lymph nodes have matured and are draining.

Horses that develop chondroids become significantly more challenging to treat. Complete removal of all chondroids is essential to eliminate carrier status (Verheyen *et al.* 2000). Nonsurgical approaches to chondroid removal include copious lavage, suction and use of an endoscopically guided memory-helical polyp retrieval basket (**Fig 6**) (Seahorn and Schumacher 1991; Adkins *et al.* 1997; Judy *et al.* 1999; Sweeney *et al.* 2005). In cases with significant chondroid accumulation, surgical approaches to the guttural pouch may be required (Schaaf *et al.* 2006). Techniques have been described for surgical approaches to the guttural pouch under general anaesthesia (Schaaf *et al.* 2006) and standing (Gehlen and Ohnesorge 2005; Perkins *et al.* 2006). Complete removal of chondroids may not be accomplished intraoperatively and it is vital to examine the guttural pouches endoscopically after surgery as continued lavage may be necessary.

Antimicrobial therapy is warranted in horses that are severely anorexic, depressed, persistently febrile despite NSAID therapy, dysphagic, or have metastatic abscessation to the abdominal or thoracic lymph nodes. Penicillin is the antimicrobial of choice for *S. equi* as it is consistently sensitive to this agent (Sweeney *et al.* 2005). Although many isolates may be sensitive *in vitro* to TMP-SMZ, there are concerns as to the *in vivo* activity based on work done with *S. equi* ssp. *zooepidemicus*, casting doubt on the effectiveness of this drug to treat all strangles infections (Ensink *et al.* 2003). The length of antimicrobial therapy depends on the clinical signs of the horse, but for horses with unresolved lymphadenopathy, a 3 week course is often required. Long-term antimicrobial treatment is indicated for treatment of metastatic abscesses (Pusterla *et al.* 2007). Topical application of a penicillin gelatin solution into the guttural pouches can achieve high concentrations within the guttural pouch and may be indicated for treating guttural pouch empyema and chronic carriers (Verheyen *et al.* 2000; Sweeney *et al.* 2005). The recipe for 50 ml of penicillin/gelatin solution as reported in Sweeney *et al.* (2005) is:

- Weigh out 2 g of gelatin (Sigma G-6650 or household grade) and add 40 ml sterile water.
- Heat or microwave to dissolve the gelatin.
- Cool gelatin to 45–50°C.
- Meanwhile add 10 ml sterile water to 10,000,000 units (10 Mega) sodium benzylpenicillin G.
- Mix penicillin solution with the cooled gelatin to make a total volume of 50 ml.
- Dispense into syringes and leave overnight at 48°C to set.

The gelatin solution can be instilled through an endoscope and is retained in the guttural pouch better than an aqueous solution (Sweeney *et al.* 2005).

Adjunctive treatment appropriate in most cases includes NSAIDs (flunixin or phenylbutazone) to control fever and pain associated with lymphadenitis and pharyngitis, adequate nutrition, and maintenance of hydration. Nutrition and hydration are of particular importance in horses with dysphagia.

Outbreak management and prevention

In an outbreak of strangles, movement of all horses on or off the farm should be stopped, and new horses should not be introduced. The temperature of all horses on the farm should be taken twice daily to identify new cases as early as possible. Monitoring the rectal temperature and isolating horses at the first sign of fever is one of the most effective ways to stop the spread of infection, since infected horses can transmit the bacteria to healthy horses 2–3 days after onset of fever once shedding has commenced (Sweeney *et al.* 2005). Strangles is also a reportable disease in some states of the USA, and the state veterinarian may need to be notified. To determine if strangles is reportable in your state, contact the state veterinarian's office. Most states have a list of reportable diseases posted on the web. Strangles is not considered a reportable disease in the UK. Strategies to eradicate and prevent strangles (STEPS) in the UK can be found on line at http://www.equine-strangles.co.uk/.

An isolated area should be set up for horses with fever and/or other clinical signs. Extreme care should be taken not to mix either horses with infection or horses exposed to horses with strangles with unexposed horses. Ideally, 3 groups of horses should be created: 1) infected horses; 2) horses that have been exposed to or contacted infected horses; and 3) clean horses with no exposure. No nose to nose contact or shared water buckets should occur among the groups. Unexposed horses should be kept in a 'clean' area, and ideally should have separate caretakers, cleaning equipment, grooming equipment, water troughs and pasture. People and equipment can act as fomites for disease transmission. Extreme care, handwashing and disinfection of supplies must be observed by everyone involved. If different individuals cannot care for infected and healthy horses, then healthy horses should always be dealt with first. Dedicated protective clothing such as boots, gowns or coveralls, and gloves should be utilised when dealing with infected horses.

Thorough cleaning and disinfection is critical when dealing with any infectious disease. All water troughs should be thoroughly cleaned and disinfected daily during an outbreak. The label instructions on disinfectants should be read to be sure they are used at the correct dilution and are active against *S. equi*. All surfaces and stalls should be disinfected following removal of manure and organic material. Manure will inactivate bleach and iodine type solutions. Manure and waste feed from infected horses should be composted in an isolated location, and not spread on the pastures. Pastures that were utilised for sick horses should be rested for a minimum of 4 weeks. There is a lack of field-based proof for prolonged environmental persistence of *S. equi*, which is sensitive to bacteriocins from environmental bacteria and does not readily survive in the presence of other soil-borne flora (Sweeney *et al.* 2005).

A significant challenge when dealing with an outbreak of strangles is identifying the horses that are subclinical shedders. These horses can shed the bacteria for weeks, months or even years, and serve as a continual source of reinfection for a farm (Newton *et al.* 1997; Chanter *et al.* 1998; Sweeney *et al.* 2005). Ideally, all horses on an infected farm should be tested for strangles. Use of bacterial culture and PCR combined identifies carriers with an improved success rate. Nasal pharyngeal swabs or washes can be done to sample the horses for infection. The washes improve the chance of identifying carrier horses. Additionally, all infected horses should be tested 3 consecutive times and be negative all 3 times before being put back with healthy horses (Sweeney *et al.* 2005). Since previously infected horses can shed the bacteria for weeks to months, or even years in rare cases, 3 negative test samples are recommended prior to reintroduction to the healthy herd. For the most accurate diagnosis of carriers and horses without obvious clinical signs, upper airway and guttural pouch endoscopy can be performed. This procedure allows for identification of infections that can develop in the guttural pouch, and subsequent culture of that area.

Vaccination

Vaccination is one method for prevention and control of infection by *S. equi*. Vaccination is recommended on farms where *S. equi* has been an endemic problem or for horses expected to be at a high risk of exposure. With strangles, vaccination will probably reduce the severity of disease in the majority of horses that are infected, but will not result in complete disease prevention. Available vaccines in the USA can be administered by i.m. (Strepguard[2], Strepvax II[3]) and intranasal routes (Pinnacle I.N.)[4]. To the authors' knowledge, Equilis StrepE[2] from Intervet is the only vaccine licensed for use in the EU, and is labelled for subcutaneous administration inside the upper lip. Improper administration of the vaccine can result in poor protection against infection and/or complications at the site of injection. The inactivated vaccines have reduced the severity of clinical signs and reduced the incidence of disease by as much as 50% during outbreaks (Hoffman *et al.* 1991). The injectable vaccines are associated with increased injection site reactions when compared to other equine immunisations. The intranasal vaccination has stimulated high levels of immunity against experimental infection, and will result in excellent local immunity if properly administered. Slowly developing submandibular abscesses have occurred in a very small percent of cases due to residual vaccinal organism in the modified live product (Kemp-Symonds *et al.* 2007). Cervical abscesses may also result from i.m. administration of the modified live product or inadvertent needle contamination when administering other vaccinations, hence the recommendation that other vaccinations be administered prior to or on a different date from the live strangles vaccination (Sweeney *et al.* 2005).

Vaccination is generally not recommended during an outbreak of strangles. If there are horses on the farm with no clinical signs of infection and no known contact with sick horses, vaccination may be considered. Horses that have had the disease within the previous year also do not need to be vaccinated. Once recovered from an active infection, approximately 75% of horses have immunity for 5 years or longer (Hamlen *et al.* 1994). It is generally recommended that recovered horses have titres checked prior to additional vaccination. Vaccination of horses recently exposed to strangles may result in purpura haemorrhagica. Vaccination is generally only recommended in healthy horses with no fever or nasal discharge. Manufacturer recommendations may vary slightly; however, vaccination with inactivated products may have improved efficacy if a primary series of 3 doses of vaccine is followed by booster doses at 6 month intervals. Vaccination with the modified live intranasal product requires a 2 dose series and annual or semi-annual booster for adults. Pregnant mares should be vaccinated 30 days prior to foaling with the inactivated i.m. vaccine to induce colostral antibody production. Foals should begin their vaccination series aged 4–6 months when using the inactivated i.m. vaccine. They will require 3 doses 4–6 weeks apart. Foals vaccinated with the modified attenuated live vaccine should start the series at age 6–9 months and require 2 doses 3 weeks apart.

Manufacturers' addresses

[1]IDEXX, Westbrook, Maine, USA.
[2]Intervet, Boxmeer, The Netherlands.
[3]Boehringer Ingelheim, Ingelheim, Germany.
[4]Fort Dodge, Fort Dodge, Iowa, USA.

References

Adkins, A.R., Yovich, J.V. and Colbourne, C.M. (1997) Nonsurgical treatment of chondroids of the guttural pouch in a horse. *Aust. vet. J.* **75**, 332-333.

Chanter, N., Newton, J.R., Wood, J.L., Verheyen, K. and Hannant, D. (1998) Detection of strangles carriers. *Vet. Rec.* **142**, 496.

Divers, T.J., Timoney, J.F., Lewis, R.M. and Smith, C.A. (1992) Equine glomerulonephritis and renal-failure associated with complexes of Group-C streptococcal antigen and Igg antibody. *Vet. Immunol. Immunopathol.* **32**, 93-102.

Ensink, J.M., Smit, J.A. and Van, D.E. (2003) Clinical efficacy of trimethoprim/sulfadiazine and procaine penicillin G in a *Streptococcus equi* subsp. *zooepidemicus* infection model in ponies. *J. vet. Pharmacol. Ther.* **26**, 247-252.

Finno, C., Pusterla, N., Aleman, M., Mohr, F.C., Price, T., George, J., and Holmberg, T. (2006) *Streptococcus equi* meningoencephalomyelitis in a foal. *J. Am. vet. med. Ass.* **229**, 721-724.

Gehlen, H. and Ohnesorge, B. (2005) Laser fenestration of the mesial septum for treatment of guttural pouch chondroids in a pony. *Vet. Surg.* **34**, 383-386.

Gronbaek, L.M., Angen, O., Vigre, H. and Olsen, S.N. (2006) Evaluation of a nested PCR test and bacterial culture of swabs from the nasal passages and from abscesses in relation to diagnosis of *Streptococcus equi* infection (strangles). *Equine vet. J.* **38**, 59-63.

Hamlen, H.J., Timoney, J.F. and Bell, R.J. (1994) Epidemiologic and immunologic characteristics of *Streptococcus equi* infection in foals. *J. Am. vet. med. Ass.* **204**, 768-775.

Hoffman, A.M., Staempfli, H.R., Prescott, J.F. and Viel, L. (1991) Field evaluation of a commercial M-protein vaccine against *Streptococcus equi* infection in foals. *Am. J. vet. Res.* **52**, 589-592.

Judy, C.E., Chaffin, M.K. and Cohen, N.D. (1999) Empyema of the guttural pouch (auditory tube diverticulum) in horses: 91 cases (1977-1997). *J. Am. vet. med. Ass.* **215**, 1666-1670.

Kaese, H.J., Valberg, S.J., Hayden, D.W., Wilson, J.H., Charlton, P., Ames, T.R. and Al-Ghamdi, G.M. (2005) Infarctive purpura haemorrhagica in five horses. *J. Am. vet. med. Ass.* **226**, 1893-1898, 1845.

Kemp-Symonds, J., Kemble, T. and Waller, A. (2007) Modified live *Streptococcus equi* ('strangles') vaccination followed by clinically adverse reactions associated with bacterial replication. *Equine vet. J.* **39**, 284-286.

Lewis, S.S., Valberg, S.J. and Nielsen, I.L. (2007) Suspected immune-mediated myositis in horses. *J. vet. Intern. Med.* **21**, 495-503.

Muhktar, M.M. and Timoney, J.F. (1988) Chemotactic response of equine polymorphonuclear leucocytes to *Streptococcus equi*. *Res. vet. Sci.* **45**, 225-229.

Newton, J.R., Verheyen, K., Talbot, N.C., Timoney, J.F., Wood, J.L., Lakhani, K.H. and Chanter, N. (2000) Control of strangles outbreaks by isolation of guttural pouch carriers identified using PCR and culture of *Streptococcus equi*. *Equine vet. J.* **32**, 515-526.

Newton, J.R., Wood, J.L., Dunn, K.A., DeBrauwere, M.N. and Chanter, N. (1997) Naturally occurring persistent and asymptomatic infection of the guttural pouches of horses with *Streptococcus equi*. *Vet. Rec.* **140**, 84-90.

Perkins, J.D., Schumacher, J., Kelly, G., Gomez, J.H. and Schumacher, J. (2006) Standing surgical removal of inspissated guttural pouch exudate (chondroids) in ten horses. *Vet. Surg.* **35**, 658-662.

Prescott, J.F. and Timoney, J.F. (2007) Could we eradicate strangles in equids? *J. Am. vet. med. Ass.* **231**, 377-378.

Pusterla, N., Watson, J.L., Affolter, V.K., Magdesian, K.G., Wilson, W.D. and Carlson, G.P. (2003) Purpura haemorrhagica in 53 horses. *Vet. Rec.* **153**, 118-121.

Pusterla, N., Whitcomb, M.B. and Wilson, W.D. (2007) Internal abdominal abscesses caused by *Streptococcus equi* subspecies *equi* in 10 horses in California between 1989 and 2004. *Vet. Rec.* **160**, 589-592.

Ramey, D. (2007) Does early antibiotic use in horses with 'strangles' cause metastatic *Streptococcus equi* bacterial infections? *Equine vet. Educ.* **19**, 14-15.

Schaaf, K.L., Kannegieter, N.J. and Lovell, D.K. (2006) Surgical treatment of extensive chondroid formation in the guttural pouch of a Warmblood horse. *Aust. vet. J.* **84**, 297-300.

Seahorn, T.L. and Schumacher, J. (1991) Nonsurgical removal of chondroid masses from the guttural pouches of 2 horses. *J. Am. vet. med. Ass.* **199**, 368-369.

Sheoran, A.S., Sponseller, B.T., Holmes, M.A. and Timoney, J.F. (1997) Serum and mucosal antibody isotype responses to M-like protein (SeM) of *Streptococcus equi* in convalescent and vaccinated horses. *Vet. Immunol. Immunopathol.* **59**, 239-251.

Sponseller, B.T., Valberg, S.J., Tennent-Brown, B.S., Foreman, J.H., Kumar, P. and Timoney, J.F. (2005) Severe acute rhabdomyolysis associated with *Streptococcus equi* infection in four horses. *J. Am. vet. med. Ass.* **227**, 1800-1804.

Spoormakers, T.J., Ensink, J.M., Goehring, L.S., Koeman, J.P., Ter, B.F., van der Vlugt-Meijer, R.H. and van den Belt, A.J. (2003) Brain abscesses as a metastatic manifestation of strangles: symptomatology and the use of magnetic resonance imaging as a diagnostic aid. *Equine vet. J.* **35**, 146-151.

Sweeney, C.R., Timoney, J.F., Newton, J.R. and Hines, M.T. (2005) *Streptococcus equi* infections in horses: guidelines for treatment, control, and prevention of strangles. *J. vet. intern. Med.* **19**, 123-134.

Sweeney, C.R., Whitlock, R.H., Meirs, D.A., Whitehead, S.C. and Barningham, S.O. (1987) Complications associated with *Streptococcus equi* infection on a horse farm. *J. Am. vet. med. Ass.* **191**, 1446-1448.

Timoney, J.F. (1993) Strangles. *Vet. Clin. N. Am.: Equine Pract.* **9**, 365-374.

Timoney, J.F. and Artiushin, S.C. (1997) Detection of *Streptococcus equi* in equine nasal swabs and washes by DNA amplification. *Vet. Rec.* **141**, 446-447.

Timoney, J.F., Artiushin, S.C. and Boschwitz, J.S. (1997) Comparison of the sequences and functions of *Streptococcus equi* M-like proteins SeM and SzPSe. *Infect. Immun.* **65**, 3600-3605.

Verheyen, K., Newton, J.R., Talbot, N.C., de Brauwere, M.N. and Chanter, N. (2000) Elimination of guttural pouch infection and inflammation in asymptomatic carriers of *Streptococcus equi*. *Equine vet. J.* **32**, 527-532.

Yelle, M.T. (1987) Clinical aspects of *Streptococcus equi* infection. *Equine vet. J.* **19**, 158-162.

CONTAGIOUS EQUINE METRITIS AND OTHER EQUINE VENEREAL INFECTIONS

S. W. Ricketts

Rossdale and Partners, Beaufort Cottage Equine Hospital, Cotton End Road, Exning, Newmarket, Suffolk CB8 7NN, UK.

Keywords: horse; venereal infection; *Taylorella equigenitalis*; contagious equine metritis; *Klebsiella pneumoniae*; *Pseudomonas aeruginosa*; equine herpesvirus 3; equine viral arteritis

Summary

Currently, 2 viral infections (equine herpesvirus 3, EHV-3, and equine arteritis virus, EAV), 3 bacterial infections (*Taylorella equigenitalis*, *Klebsiella pneumoniae* and *Pseudomonas aeruginosa*) and one protozoan infection (*Trypanosoma equiperdum*, which causes dourine) are recognised as venereal diseases in the horse. In addition, equine infectious anaemia virus may be spread by this route. Equine coital exanthema is a predominantly sexually transmitted infection, caused by EHV-3. Typical 'pox-like' skin lesions appear on the penis of stallions and the vulva of mares. The virus is endemic in the UK and most horse breeding populations internationally. EAV is a togavirus that causes pyrexia, depression, conjunctivitis, increased respiratory rate, skin lesions, and oedema of the limbs, head and trunk. Mares may be infected at natural mating or during artificial insemination with semen (raw, extended or frozen/thawed) from virus-shedding stallions. EAV is also spread by the respiratory aerosol route by actively infected horses. Mares who are infected during pregnancy may abort, following placental arteritis. Contagious equine metritis, caused by *Taylorella equigenitalis*, originally caused a copious greyish/ opalescent vaginal discharge and conception failure in a high proportion of infected mares, but recently the disease appears to have become endemic in much of the mainland European non-Thoroughbred horse populations, and can cause sub-clinical infections. Capsule types 1, 2 and 5 of *Klebsiella pneumoniae* can cause epidemics of acute endometritis, with a variable cream-coloured vaginal discharge that may be first seen as early as 3–4 days after mating. Some strains of *Pseudomonas aeruginosa* can cause venereal disease, with a variable cream-coloured vaginal discharge which may be first seen as early as 3–4 days after mating.

Introduction

Venereal diseases are specific infectious conditions that may be specifically transmitted by mares and stallions at mating. Currently, 2 viral infections (equine herpesvirus 3, EHV-3, and equine arteritis virus, EAV) and 3 bacterial infections (*Taylorella equigenitalis*, *Klebsiella pneumoniae* and *Pseudomonas aeruginosa*) are recognised as such. It is probable that equine infectious anaemia may be transmitted at mating by viraemic mares and stallions, but this has not been specifically documented. The protozoan *Trypanosoma equiperdum* (which causes dourine) is transmitted at mating and artificial insemination (AI) in horse populations in Africa, Asia, South America and isolated areas of southern Europe and southern USA.

In France, Germany, Ireland, Italy and the UK, the Horserace Betting Levy Board's (HBLB) voluntary Code of Practice, which was first developed in 1977 (**Fig 1**) and which has since been updated annually (**Fig 2**), provides a useful framework for the control of equine venereal diseases in horse populations. This document is widely circulated in its updated form annually and has become an indispensable reference manual of 'standard operating procedures' for owners, managers and veterinary surgeons involved with horse breeding. The UK and Irish Thoroughbred industries first adopted the Code of Practice but many other breed societies have since adapted similar codes and it is in the interests of all horse populations that these guidelines (or other appropriate codes or guidelines in other countries) are followed by everyone. Clinicians in countries other than France, Germany, Ireland, Italy and the UK are recommended to seek the guidance of their own appropriate industry and veterinary organisations.

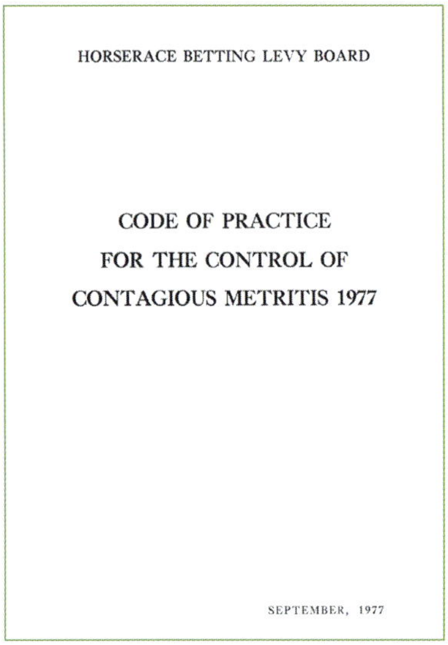

FIGURE 1: Cover of the first Horserace Betting Levy Board Code of Practice for Contagious Metritis 1977, published in 1977.

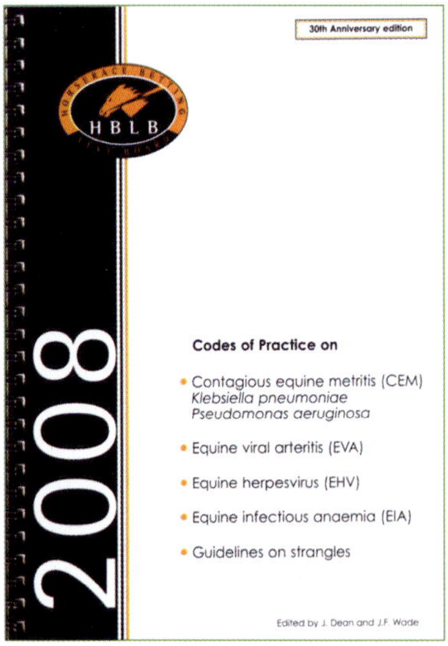

FIGURE 2: Cover of the 30th Horserace Betting Levy Board Codes of Practice, published in 2008.

Pathophysiology of equine uterine infections

To understand the difference between sporadic and venereal infections in mares it is important to consider the mare's unusual cervicouterine physiology. During oestrus, her cervix relaxes to allow intrauterine ejaculation by the stallion. This contrasts with the 'norm' for most other species, i.e. intravaginal ejaculation with a closed and mucus-plugged cervix. The endometria of all mares are therefore challenged at natural mating by the variety of micro-organisms that normally contaminate and inhabit the skin of the external genitalia of both mare and stallion. Normal, genitally healthy mares are able to resolve this transient acute (characterised by polymorphonuclear leucocytic infiltration) endometritis (**Fig 3**), associated with opportunist infection, within 72 h, returning the endometrium to a healthy state (free from acute endometritis) (**Fig 4**) for conception and developing pregnancy by the time that the fertilised ovum enters the uterus from the fallopian tube at approximately Day 5 after ovulation. The uteri of all mares are therefore transiently inflamed, if not infected, at natural mating.

Some aged mares and those who have sustained or developed perineal, vaginal, cervical or uterine

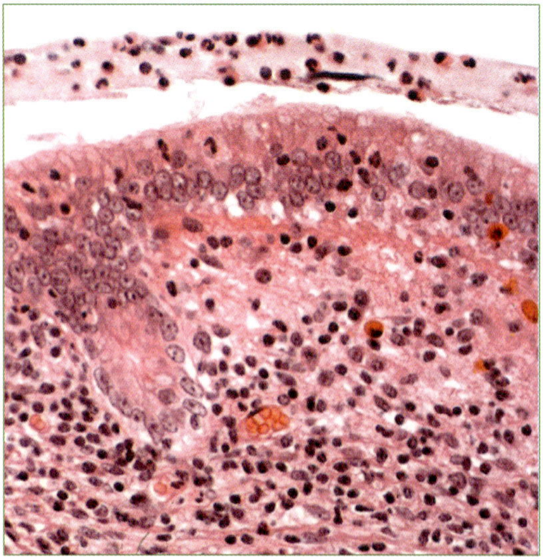

FIGURE 3: Endometrial biopsy section (H&E) taken from a mare showing acute endometritis (polymorphonuclear cell infiltration of superficial stroma overlying the luminal epithelium) in the uterine lumen.

structural or functional injuries or abnormalities, particularly those who are unable to clear fluid from their uteri, become unable to resolve this acute endometritis. In these individuals, this results in persistent acute endometritis, which usually causes conception or gestational failure. These compromised mares may also succumb to persistent acute endometritis spontaneously or following foaling or veterinary examination. Recurrent and/or persistent acute endometritis and uterine fluid pooling are thought to be significant accelerating causes of chronic endometrial degenerative disease (involving endometrial gland degeneration and malfunction and endometrial stromal fibrosis), which may contribute to the linear decline in fertility potential that is recognised to occur in the Thoroughbred broodmare population.

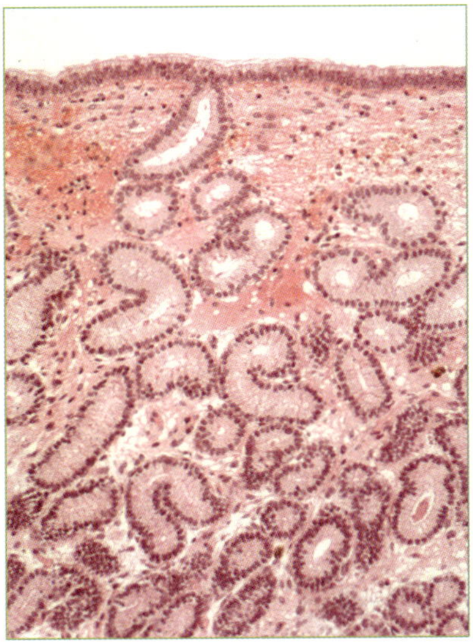

FIGURE 4: Endometrial biopsy section (H&E) taken from a mare showing a normal oestral endometrium.

Transient and persistent acute endometritis is caused by a variety of equine environmental and genital skin contaminant bacteria (most commonly *Streptococcus zooepidemicus*, *Escherichia coli* and *Staphylococcus aureus*). Although infections may occur after and as a consequence of mating, they relate to the mare's compromised genital state, do not produce epidemic disease and are therefore sporadic and not considered true venereal diseases. However, experience suggests that *T. equigenitalis*, some capsule types of *K. pneumoniae* and some strains of *P. aeruginosa* are capable of infecting not only genitally compromised mares but young healthy maiden mares and multiparous mares with no evidence of genital injury or underlying abnormality. They may result in epidemics of post mating infection and may be transmitted between mares and stallions in both directions. Therefore, these are considered true potential equine venereal disease bacteria.

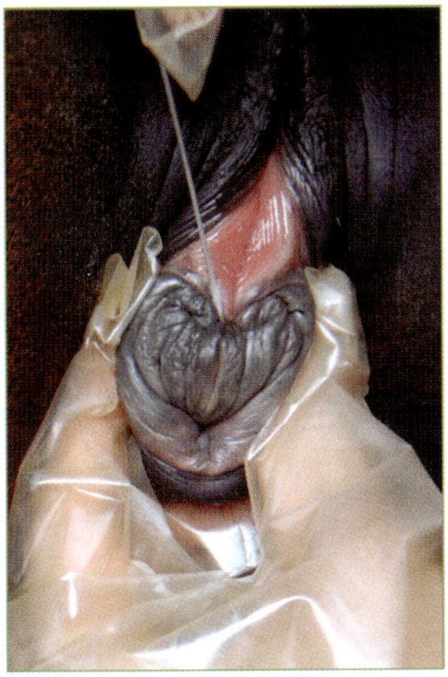

FIGURE 5: Swab sample (narrow tipped) being taken from the clitoral sinus of a mare.

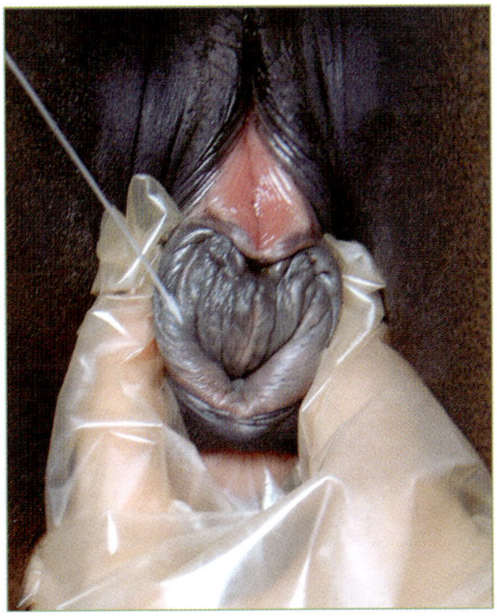

FIGURE 6: Swab sample being taken from the clitoral fossa of a mare.

It has been established that *T. equigenitalis*, *K. pneumoniae* and *P. aeruginosa* may live in the smegma associated with the clitoral fossa and sinuses of mares and the urethral fossa and diverticulum and the prepuce of stallions, producing a symptomless carrier state. To diagnose or rule out active infection or to diagnose or confirm freedom from the carrier state, swab samples are collected from the clitoral fossa and sinus (with narrow tipped paediatric-type swabs) (**Figs 5** and **6**) and the endometrium (with extended normal tipped swabs, via the open oestrous cervix) (**Fig 7**) of mares and from the urethra (**Fig 8**), urethral fossa and diverticulum (**Fig 9**), penile shaft and preputial smegma (**Fig 10**) and pre-ejaculatory fluid of stallions. Swabs are placed immediately into Amies charcoal transport medium and transported, without exposure to extreme temperatures, within 24–48 h, to an HBLB quality assured and designated laboratory for aerobic (48 h on blood and McConkey's agar) and microaerophilic culture (at least 7 days on special haemolysed blood agar). In the UK, designated laboratories are quality assurance (QA) tested twice yearly and they work to a recommended common laboratory protocol.

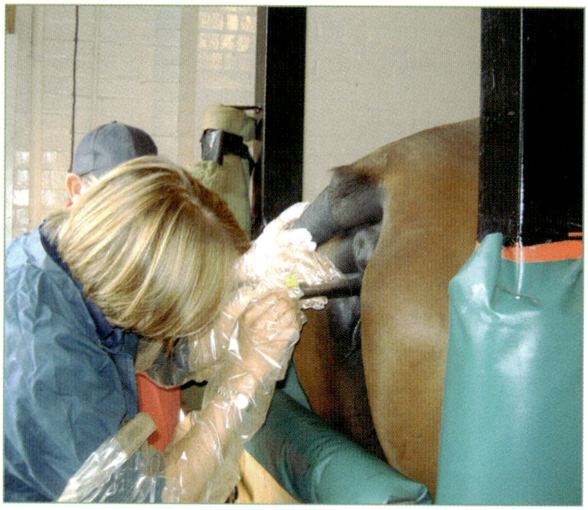

FIGURE 7: Swab sample (extended) being taken from the endometrium of a mare via a sterile disposable speculum through the open oestral cervix.

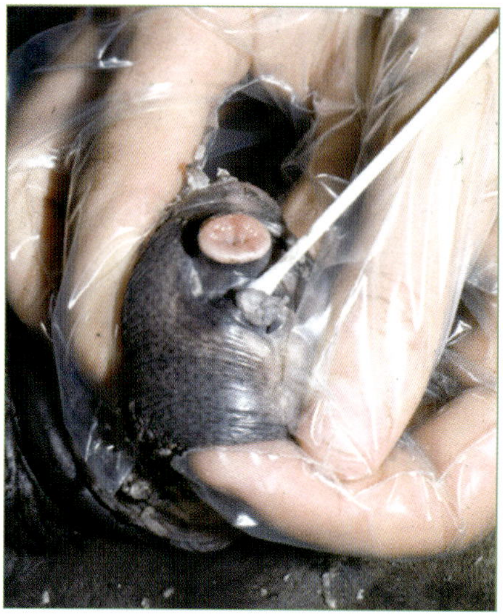

FIGURE 9: Swab sample being taken from the urethral fossa and diverticulum of a stallion (demonstrating a 'pea' of smegma in the fossa).

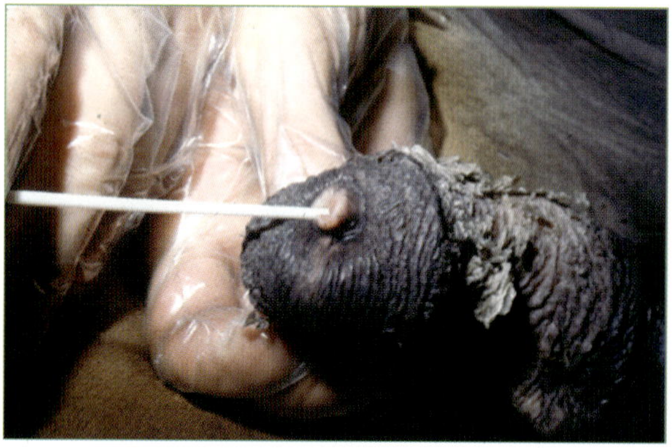

FIGURE 8: Swab sample being taken from the urethra of a stallion.

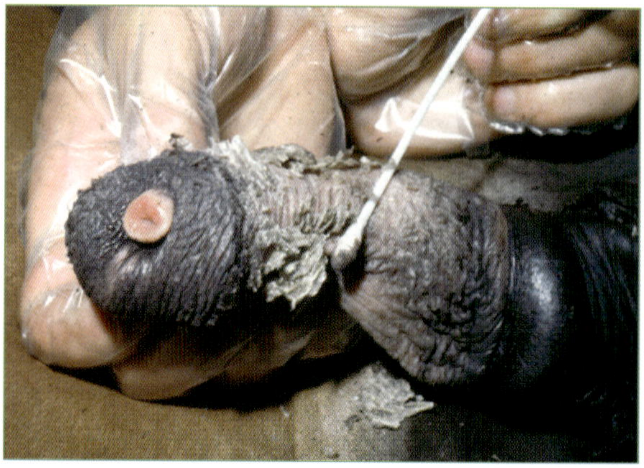

FIGURE 10: Swab sample being taken from the preputial smegma of a stallion.

Taylorella equigenitalis

This small, slow-growing (3–4 days on specialised haemolysed blood agar) (**Fig 11**) Gram-negative, microaerophilic, catalase-positive, oxidase-positive, but otherwise biochemically unreactive coccobacillus is the cause of contagious equine metritis (CEM), a 'new' equine epidemic venereal disease, which was first reported in Newmarket in 1977. Two main strains (streptomycin resistant and sensitive) have been isolated, both in association with epidemic acute endometritis. The streptomycin resistant strain was the original isolate in Newmarket in 1977. The streptomycin sensitive strain has since been intermittently isolated in the UK from imported mares and male horses. Whereas the disease that was originally recognised in Thoroughbred horses was quite virulent, causing copious greyish/opalescent vaginal discharge (**Fig 12**) and conception failure in a high proportion of mares mated, the disease that now appears to be endemic in much of the mainland European non-Thoroughbred horse populations, is reported to be more insidious, less virulent and mostly symptomless in infected mares. This has resulted in a large 'pool' of carrier mares. Owners of horses in disease-free horse populations must be very careful to avoid contact with these carrier mares and, of course, carrier stallions.

Taylorella equigenitalis may cause epidemic acute endometritis in mares, with clinical signs varying from a copious mucoid/grey vaginal discharge that may be first seen as early as 2 days after mating, to no gross signs of abnormality. The acute endometritis usually causes conception failure, with premature luteolysis, but some mares may not succumb or may resolve the acute infection soon enough to allow conception and normal pregnancy to proceed. Nonpregnant and pregnant mares may become symptomless carriers, the clitoral fossa and sinuses being the important sites of persistence. These sites contain many surface folds, in which smegma forms, producing ideal conditions for the persistent carrier state. The diagnosis is confirmed by the growth of the organism or detection of its specific DNA by PCR test from endometrial (acute infection) and/or clitoral (carrier state) fossa and/or sinus swab samples.

Acute endometritis can be successfully treated by repeated intrauterine irrigation with penicillin, ceftiofur sodium or many other antibiotics or antiseptics, relatively easily. At the same time the clitoral fossa and sinuses must be thoroughly and repeatedly treated by washing with chlorhexidine solution. Nitrofurazone ointment, which was used to pack the clitoral fossa and sinuses of carrier mares after chlorhexidine washing, is no longer available in the European Union (EU) for veterinary use, but is usually unnecessary. Following this external genital

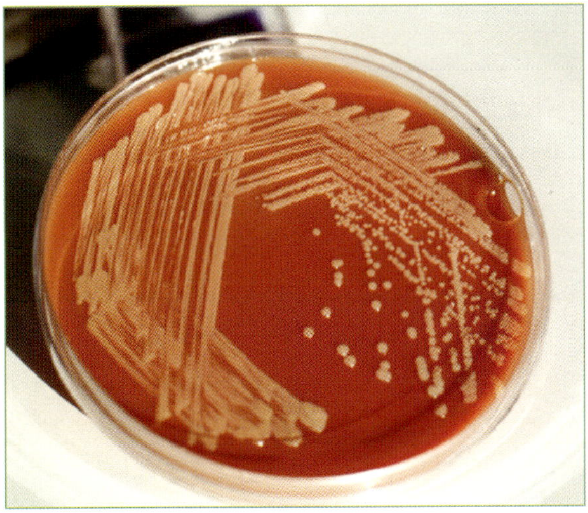

FIGURE 11: Taylorella equigenitalis growing on haemolysed CEMO agar after 4 days microaerophilic incubation.

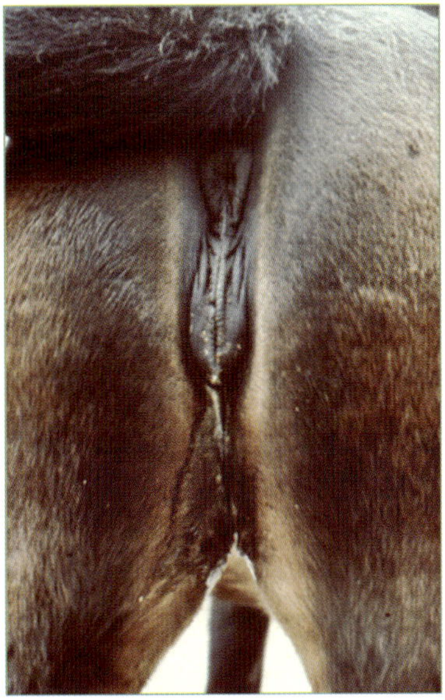

FIGURE 12: Mare with a vaginal discharge with Taylorella equigenitalis infection.

'sterilisation' it is prudent to treat the clitoral fossa and sinuses with an actively growing bacterial broth, purpose-made from normal equine external genital commensal microflora, to establish normal skin microflora quickly and to discourage opportunist overgrowth with environmental *Pseudomonas* spp. or *Klebsiella* spp.

In intractable carrier cases, clitoral sinusectomy or clitorectomy, performed under local infiltration anaesthesia with the mare sedated and restrained in the standing position, may be required to remove all remaining organisms.

In stallions, *T. equigenitalis* infection causes no local or systemic disease but causes a symptomless mechanical carrier state in the smegma of the urethral fossa and diverticulum and of the preputial skin folds and clefts. It is treated by daily washing of the erect penis with clean water and nonantiseptic soap to remove all smegma from the urethral fossa and diverticulum, penile shaft and prepuce, drying these areas with disposable paper towels and then thoroughly treating/massaging them with 2% chlorhexidine scrub. As with mares, this should be followed by treating with equine external genital commensal microflora.

Successful treatment is confirmed in mares and stallions by the collection of 3 sets of swab samples (clitoral fossa and, if clitorectomy has not been performed, sinus swabs in mares and urethral, urethral fossa and diverticulum, preputial smegma and pre-ejaculatory fluid in stallions) with negative results. For some cases, specific *T. equigenitalis* DNA (polymerase chain reaction, i.e. PCR) and/or test mating and follow-up swabbing of the mares may be helpful to give added reassurance before recommencing mating.

Contagious equine metritis is a notifiable disease in the UK, France and Ireland. In the UK, the isolation of *T. equigenitalis* must be reported by the isolating laboratory to a Divisional Veterinary Manager (DVM) of the Department for Environment, Food and Rural Affairs (Defra).

Taylorella equigenitalis was eradicated from the Thoroughbred horse population of the UK by the vigorous application of the HBLB's Code of Practice. It remains endemic in many non-Thoroughbred horse populations in mainland Europe and therefore the potential for reintroduction remains. It has been occasionally isolated in the UK, since eradication, from non-Thoroughbred horses imported for competitive sports and in non-Thoroughbred horses imported into UK quarantine facilities prior to re-export to southern hemisphere countries.

A distinct but related organism, *Taylorella asinigenitalis*, has been isolated from donkeys and horses without recognisable clinical signs of infection. The 2 organisms must be differentiated by specific PCR testing.

Klebsiella pneumoniae

Some strains (capsule types) of this Gram-negative, lactose-fermenting, aerobic bacillus, which produces luxuriant mucoid pink colonies on McConkey's agar after overnight aerobic incubation (**Fig 13**), can cause equine venereal disease. Capsule types 1, 2 and 5 have been known to cause epidemics of acute endometritis, with a variable cream-coloured vaginal discharge (**Fig 14**) that may be first seen as early as 3–4 days after mating. Capsule type 7 (sometimes isolated from horse faeces) and many other capsule types have not yet been reliably associated with true epidemic venereal disease, but may, as other bacteria may, cause opportunist acute endometritis in genitally-compromised mares. Acute endometritis usually causes conception failure, with premature luteolysis, but some mares resolve the acute infection soon enough to allow conception and pregnancy to proceed, sometimes followed by placentitis,

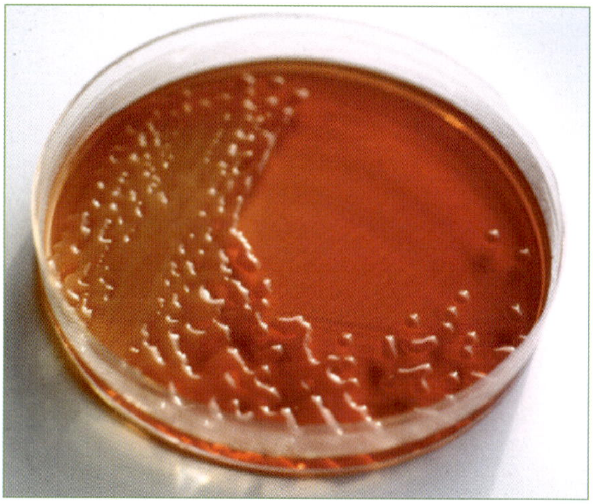

FIGURE 13: Klebsiella pneumoniae growing on McConkey's agar after 24 h aerobic incubation, showing pink, mucoid, coalescing colonies.

gestational failure or the eventual birth of a septicaemic foal, suggesting that the organism can persist. Mares may become symptomless carriers, the clitoral fossa and urethra being the most important sites of persistence. Diagnosis is confirmed by the growth of the organism from endometrial (acute infection) and/or clitoral fossa and sinus and urethral (carrier state) swab samples.

Acute endometritis can be successfully treated by repeated (5–7 days) daily intrauterine irrigation with gentamicin. At the same time the clitoral fossa, sinuses and urethral opening must be thoroughly and repeatedly treated with gentamicin. Some mares may be sensitive to gentamicin and may develop dermatitis of the ventral vulva, clitoris and fossa. Following this external genital 'sterilisation' in both mares and stallions, the clitoral fossa and sinuses or penis and prepuce should be treated with an actively growing bacterial broth, purpose-made from normal equine external genital commensals, to encourage the rapid re-establishment of a normal external genital microflora. In intractable cases, clitorectomy, performed under local infiltration anaesthesia with the mare sedated and restrained in the standing position, followed by appropriate antibiotic treatment of the empty clitoral fossa, followed by normal commensal broth culture treatment, may be required to resolve the problem.

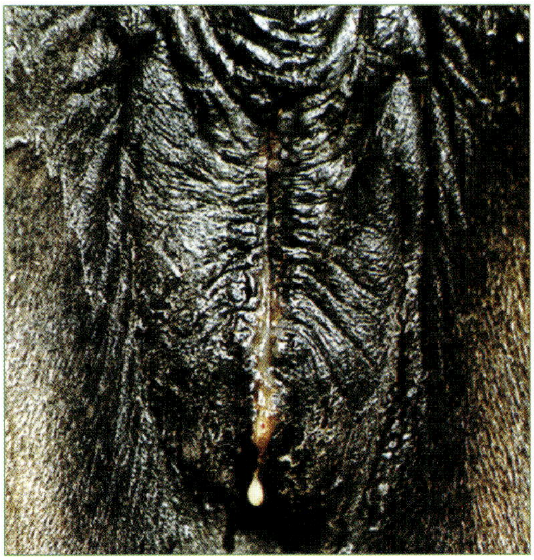

FIGURE 14: Mare with a vaginal discharge with Klebsiella pneumoniae *infection.*

In stallions, *K. pneumoniae* (capsule types 1, 2 or 5) infection causes a symptomless mechanical carrier state in the smegma of the urethral fossa and diverticulum and of the preputial skin folds. It is treated by daily washing of the erect penis with clean water and nonantiseptic soap to remove all smegma from the urethral fossa and diverticulum, penile shaft and prepuce, drying with disposable paper towels and then thoroughly treating/massaging with 1% hypochlorite solution and then 50 mg/ml gentamicin solution. Gentamicin cream or ointment, which were used to treat stallions for *K. pneumoniae* infections, is no longer available in the EU. A 7–10 day treatment programme is usually required and some stallions become sensitive to gentamicin and develop penile dermatitis.

In some intractable *K. pneumoniae* infections, clearance of the organism has followed the packing of the clitoral fossa in mares and the urethral fossa and diverticulum in stallions with gentamicin surgical sponge. This causes local soreness and sometimes ulceration, which resolves following the removal of the sponge after 7–10 days.

In one reported stallion, intractable *K. pneumoniae* genital infection resulted in ascending infection to the bladder and kidneys. Necropsy investigations revealed positive cultures from multiple organs. Urine cultures should be considered in intractable cases. Some stallions have been treated systemically with gentamicin (4.4 mg/kg bwt b.i.d., i.v., for up to 34 days) with apparently useful results. Great care should be taken with such systemic treatments to avoid local injection reactions and intestinal microflora damage, which may result in potentially fatal colitis.

Some stallions with *K. pneumoniae* genital infections have been successfully treated with a 50% aqueous solution of 10% enrofloxacin, repeatedly applied locally. *In vitro* antibiotic sensitivity testing should be confirmed before starting treatment, or the problem may become worse following the sterilisation of the normal penile skin flora and superinfection with the more resistant *K. pneumoniae.*

Successful treatment is confirmed in mares and stallions by the collection of 3 sets of swab samples (clitoral fossa and, if clitorectomy has not been performed, sinus swabs in mares and urethral, urethral fossa and diverticulum, preputial smegma and pre-ejaculatory fluid in stallions) with negative results. Test mating and follow-up swabbing of the mares may then be helpful to give added reassurance before recommencing mating, in some cases.

The incidence of isolation of *K. pneumoniae* (capsule types 1, 2 and 5) from Thoroughbred mares in the UK has been significantly reduced by the application of the HBLB's Code of Practice.

Pseudomonas aeruginosa

Some strains of this Gram-negative, lactose-fermenting, aerobic bacillus, which produces luxuriant greenish, foul-smelling colonies on blood (**Fig 15**) or specialised *Pseudomonas* agar overnight, can cause venereal disease, with a variable cream-coloured vaginal discharge, which may be first seen as early as 3–4 days after mating. Occasionally, isolates require 48 h aerobic culture to become recognisable. Strain typing may be performed but, unfortunately, no reliable association between strain type and the potential to produce true epidemic venereal disease has yet been identified. 'Nonvenereal' strains, as with any other bacteria, may cause acute endometritis in so-called 'susceptible' mares. The acute endometritis usually causes conception failure, with premature luteolysis, but some mares resolve the acute infection soon enough to allow conception and pregnancy to proceed, sometimes followed by placentitis, gestational failure or the eventual birth of a septicaemic foal, suggesting persistence. Mares may become symptomless carriers, the clitoral fossa being the most important site of persistence. Diagnosis is confirmed by the growth of the organism from endometrial (acute infection) and/or clitoral (carrier state) swab samples.

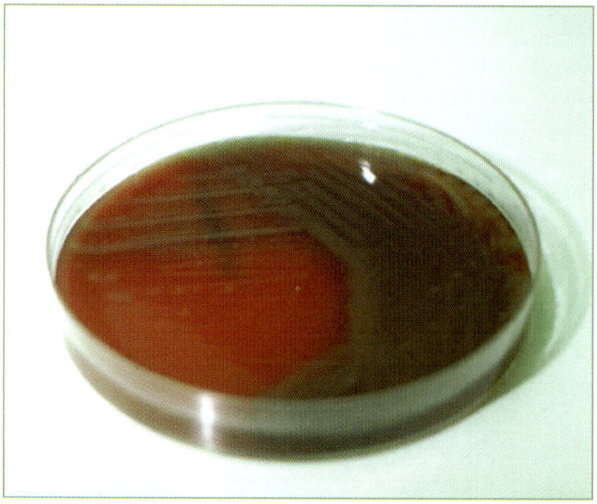

FIGURE 15: Pseudomonas aeruginosa growing on blood agar after 24 h aerobic incubation, showing greenish pigmentation.

Acute endometritis can be successfully treated by repeated intrauterine irrigation with gentamicin, or ticarcillin and clavulanic acid. At the same time the clitoral fossa and sinuses must be thoroughly and repeatedly treated with gentamicin or ticarcillin/clavulanate or repeatedly treated with 1% silver nitrate solution (for its desiccant effect). Following this external genital 'sterilisation' it is prudent to treat the clitoral fossa and sinuses with an actively growing bacterial broth purpose-made from normal equine external genital commensals, to encourage the rapid re-establishment of a normal external genital microflora. In intractable cases, clitorectomy, performed under local infiltration anaesthesia with the mare sedated and restrained in the standing position, followed by appropriate antibiotic treatment of the empty clitoral fossa, followed by normal commensal broth culture treatment, may be required to resolve the problem.

In stallions, *P. aeruginosa* infection causes a symptomless mechanical carrier state in the smegma of the urethral fossa and diverticulum and of the preputial skin folds. It is treated by daily washing of the erect penis with clean water and nonantiseptic soap to remove all smegma from the urethral fossa and diverticulum, penile shaft and prepuce, drying with disposable paper towels and then thoroughly treating/massaging with 50 mg/ml gentamicin solution. Gentamicin cream or ointment, which was used to treat stallions for *P. aeruginosa* infections, is no longer available in the EU. A 7–10 day treatment programme is usually required and some stallions become sensitive to gentamicin and develop penile skin inflammation and soreness.

Pseudomonas aeruginosa usually fluoresces (**Fig 16**) and it is sometimes helpful to examine the erect penis and prepuce of an infected stallion with a Woods lamp to identify areas of bright fluorescence in order to locate areas on which to concentrate treatment and monitor clearance. In some stallions with focal or very sparse colonisation, 1% silver nitrate solution has been applied, as a desiccant, via a household plant sprayer to the identified focal areas, daily for up to 30 days, with helpful results.

The penis should be periodically treated with sterile petroleum jelly or lanolin to replace skin oils in order to prevent the penile skin from cracking. One percent silver sulphadiazine cream has been used to treat stallions with *P. aeruginosa* infections with disappointing results.

In some intractable *P. aeruginosa* infections clearance of the organism has followed the packing of the clitoral fossa in mares and the urethral fossa and diverticulum in stallions with gentamicin surgical sponge. This causes local soreness and sometimes ulceration, which resolves following the removal of the sponge after 7–10 days.

Some stallions with *P. aeruginosa* genital infections have been successfully treated with a 50% aqueous solution of 10% enrofloxacin. *In vitro* antibiotic sensitivity testing should be confirmed before starting treatment.

Successful treatment is confirmed in mares and stallions by the collection of 3 sets of swab samples (clitoral fossa and, if clitorectomy has not been performed, sinus swabs in mares and urethral, urethral fossa and diverticulum, preputial smegma and pre-ejaculatory fluid in stallions) with negative results. Test mating and follow-up swabbing of the mares may then be helpful to give added reassurance before recommencing mating, in some cases.

The incidence of isolation of *P. aeruginosa* from Thoroughbred mares in the UK has been significantly reduced by the application of the HBLB's Code of Practice.

Whilst transmission of *T. equigenitalis*, *K. pneumoniae* and *P. aeruginosa* infections should be avoidable by the careful use of AI (where allowed by registration authorities) with effective barrier management, the potential for bacterial spread during AI remains if careful management procedures are not adopted. *T. equigenitalis* transmission between stallions in an AI unit has been reported, presumably associated with lateral infections via unprotected phantoms and/or commonly used semen collection utensils. Antibiotic containing seminal extenders cannot be relied upon to eliminate *K. pneumoniae* and *P. aeruginosa* infection in contaminated ejaculates.

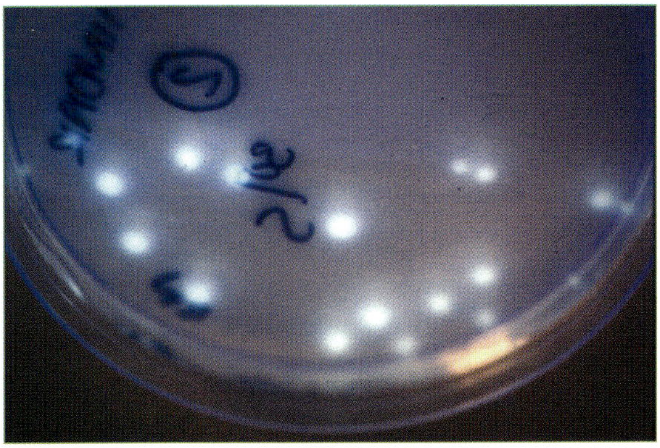

FIGURE 16: Pseudomonas aeruginosa fluorescing (Woods lamp) on Pseudomonas agar after 24 h incubation.

Nasogenital transmission of *T. equigenitalis*, *K. pneumoniae* and *P. aeruginosa* between mares at pasture and at teasing has been suspected. The role of stable flies for potential vulval to vulval transmission is unproven.

Whereas *T. equigenitalis* is quickly destroyed in the environment by lipid solvents, detergents, heat, drying and commonly used disinfectants, *K. pneumoniae* and *P. aeruginosa* are notoriously resistant to disinfectants and their use where these organisms occur may encourage their selective overgrowth. *K. pneumoniae* and *P. aeruginosa* can remain viable in 2% chlorhexidine and perhaps other disinfectant solutions and can be transmitted between mares when contaminated disinfectant is used to wash vulvas prior to veterinary examinations or before mating. The repeated disinfection of horse genitalia should be avoided where *K. pneumoniae* and *P. aeruginosa* are commonly found in the environment. The washing of mares is better done with clean warm water spraying and the use of disposable paper towels. Hygienic management of mare examination stocks and handling areas, particularly at covering barns, is important to prevent the lateral spread of all sexually transmitted diseases.

Equine coital exanthema

Equine coital exanthema (ECE) is a predominantly sexually transmitted infection, caused by EHV-3, a highly contagious but otherwise noninvasive and relatively benign virus. EHV-3 is distinct from the other equine herpesviruses. Typical 'pox-like' skin lesions appear on the penis of stallions (**Fig 17**) and the vulva of mares (**Fig 18**). The virus is endemic in UK and most horse breeding populations internationally.

Signs of systemic illness and genital discomfort are unusual but some stallions become uncomfortable enough to be unwilling to mate mares until lesions have healed. Some infected stallions take longer to recover and may develop secondary complications. Mares seldom show signs of systemic illness and lesions usually heal within 10–14 days, often leaving white (depigmented) skin scars.

Latent carrier infection occurs in both mares and stallions. These individuals may or may not have shown previously recognisable signs of disease at primary infection or reinfection and usually do not do so at recrudescence. The anatomical site of virus latency is unproven.

A nonvenereal form of EHV-3 infection occurs uncommonly in maiden colts and fillies, causing pyrexia (raised temperature) and very painful coalescing skin lesions around the anus and vulva (in fillies), over the perineum and between the hindlegs and on the scrotum (in colts).

In breeding horses, the infection causes no immediate or longer-term direct effect on the fertility of stallions or mares who are infected but temporarily disrupts mating schedules while the stallion recovers and becomes no longer infectious. Where infection occurs towards the end of the breeding season, missed mating opportunities may result in reduced pregnancy rates. The virus has not been reported to cause abortion in mares.

Equine herpesvirus-3 infection may currently be more common, or is being reported more frequently, in the horse population of the UK than it has been previously. Also, where this infection has previously been considered 'nuisance value', more infected stallions now appear to be showing signs of systemic illness and/or debilitating genital discomfort and are more commonly developing secondary complications and therefore taking longer to recover and return to mating. This is having important effects on busy mating schedules. It is unclear whether this is associated with increased viral virulence or other factors, e.g. the much busier mating schedules for popular stallions covering large numbers of mares.

There are no legal notification requirements for ECE in the UK although it may be helpful to inform the relevant breeders' association if infection occurs. The owners/managers of mares and stallions who have or will be in sexual contact should be informed.

After an incubation period of 5–9 days, small (1–3 mm) raised papules, which are often not noticed, appear on the skin of the penis of stallions and the vulva of mares. Over the next 24–48 h these progress to fluid-filled vesicles, which burst to form pustules that mature and rupture leaving purulent 'pox-like' craterous lesions, which may remain as individual lesions or may coalesce into a raw or encrusted skin erosion or ulcer, before healing usually by 10–14 days. Secondary infection with bacteria will delay healing and may require local antiseptic or antibiotic treatment.

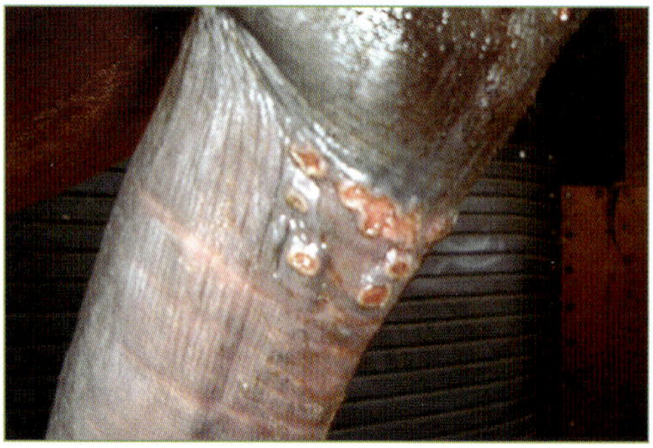

FIGURE 17: Punctate, coalescing ulcers on the penile shaft of a stallion with equine herpesvirus-3 infection (equine coital exanthema) at the acute stage.

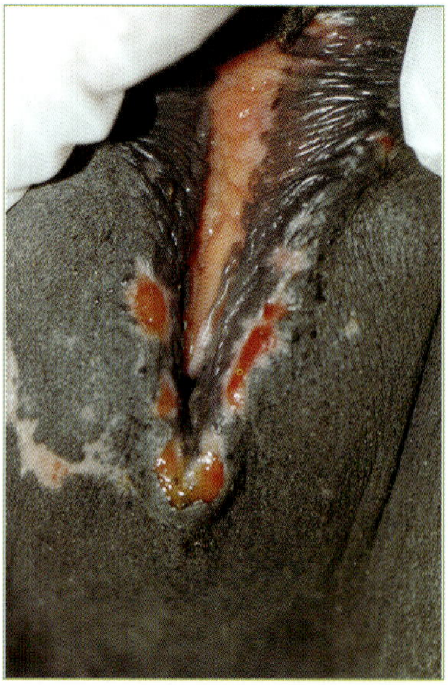

FIGURE 18: Punctate, coalescing ulcers on the ventral aspects of the vulval lips of a mare with equine herpesvirus-3 infection (equine coital exanthema) at the early healing stage.

Infection usually produces minimal signs of systemic illness and genital discomfort but some stallions develop pyrexia and associated lethargy and may become uncomfortable enough to be unwilling to mate mares until lesions have healed. Lesions specifically on the urethral process of the stallion sometimes result in pain at or inability/unwillingness to ejaculate. Some infected stallions have taken up to a month to heal and recover from infection and others have become quite ill with hindlimb swelling associated with inguinal lymph node enlargement. Mares seldom show signs of systemic illness and lesions, which often look purulent and secondarily infected, usually heal within 10–14 days, often leaving white (depigmented) skin scars, which may persist permanently.

Equine herpesvirus-3 is highly infectious between susceptible horses and may be transmitted by direct or indirect genital contact. The virus may be transmitted from subclinical carriers that have no recognisable signs of skin lesions. Horses that have recovered from infection and those that have shown no recognisable signs of typical skin lesions may become latent carriers of EHV-3. It is believed that the most common source of infection for ECE is the periodically recrudescing (viral shedding) symptomless latent carrier mare or stallion. These individuals are currently nondetectable.

Nevertheless, all stallions and mares should be routinely and carefully inspected for signs of papules, vesicles, pustules or 'pox-like' craterous lesions on the skin of their penis/prepuce and vulva/perineum before mating proceeds. If there is any suspicion of infection, veterinary advice should be sought before mating is allowed to proceed. The presence of such lesions , with a connected history of natural mating, is usually sufficient to allow diagnosis of ECE. If confirmation is necessary, paired serum (clotted blood) samples (collected at the time of first diagnosis and 14–21 days later) may be submitted for EHV-3 neutralising (SN) antibody testing. A significant rise in antibody titre (concentration) between the first (acute) and second (convalescent) sample confirms seroconversion, indicating challenge by EHV-3. It is reported that SN antibody production may be low in magnitude in some cases and so ECE cannot be conclusively ruled out on the basis of a <4-fold rise in antibody titre. It is reported that detection of serum EHV-3 complement fixing (CF) antibody is indicative of infection within the previous 60 days.

It is seldom, if ever, necessary or appropriate to biopsy fresh vesicular lesions to demonstrate typical herpesviral microscopic pathology (eosinophilic intranuclear inclusion bodies in degenerate epithelial cells) or to attempt viral isolation or demonstrate the presence of viral DNA by polymerase chain reaction (PCR) testing.

If signs of illness occur (pyrexia, lethargy, local inflammation and soreness), systemic treatment with nonsteroidal anti-inflammatory medication and local treatment with antiseptics may be indicated. Where secondary bacterial infection of the lesions occurs, specific local antibiotic treatment may be indicated. Where stallions become systemically ill, they may require systemic treatment with antibiotics and nonsteroidal anti-inflammatory medication.

Anti-herpesviral medication (acyclovir), licensed for human use, has been used for the treatment of EHV-3 skin lesions in stallions and mares but there is insufficient data to assess its efficacy or usefulness.

Treatment of skin lesions is palliative rather than curative and is directed at aiding speedy natural resolution of the infection and healing of the skin lesions. The infected penis and prepuce of stallions and the vulva of mares should be washed daily with clean saline solution, to discourage secondary bacterial invasion and infection of the ruptured vesicles.

Veterinary surgeons or assistants who are handling the genitalia of horses, irrespective of their infection status, should wear disposable gloves that are changed between horses and veterinary surgeons should use disposable vaginascopes. Utensils, such as jugs/buckets and washing water or saline solution should not be shared between horses and disposable paper towels should be used rather than shared sponges.

There is no commercially available vaccine for EHV-3 infection. Although it is unusual for stallions or mares to show signs of infection again after natural infection, natural immunity is believed to be short-lived and individuals have shown recurrent ECE in sequential breeding seasons.

In horse populations with endemic EHV-3, where occasional reactivations of latent virus with shedding by symptomless carriers is undetectable and therefore unavoidable, early diagnosis and containment of spread of infection is most important. Staff involved with stallion mating management should be trained in the recognition of genital skin lesions characteristic of ECE and what to do should signs be suspected.

When infection is suspected or diagnosed in a stallion, mating should cease until the stallion is confirmed free of disease. This usually takes 10–14 days but may take longer in individual stallions. Although for stallions with no systemic signs of illness, it is tempting for managers of busy commercial stallions, with the encouragement of some mare owners, to continue to mate mares, this is inadvisable because:

1. The stallion may become sore and unwilling to mate/ejaculate and the potential for development of systemic signs of illness and secondary complications will be increased.
2. The stallion's healing and recovery process may be prolonged.
3. The numbers of mares infected may be increased.
4. The numbers of symptomless latent carriers in the horse population may be increased.
5. The incidence of disease in the horse population may be increased, resulting in increased disruption of mating schedules.

When infection is diagnosed in a stallion, all mare owners mated by and booked to that stallion should be informed so that they may ask their attending veterinary surgeon to examine their mares for signs of infection so that treatment may be applied, if indicated, and so that they may be warned of the timing that is anticipated for the stallion to be temporarily unavailable for mating.

When infection is diagnosed in a mare that has been mated within 3 weeks, the mating stallion owner/manager should be informed so that he/she may cease mating with the stallion and ask the attending veterinary surgeon to examine the stallion for signs of infection. The stallion owner/manager should then notify owners/managers of other mares mated by that stallion within the previous 3–4 weeks so that their veterinary surgeons may examine for signs of infection. Mating should only recommence when the stallion is free from signs of infection and/or when reports reveal no signs of infection in other mares that he has mated and veterinary opinion is that he is not in the stage of incubating the infection.

Whilst ECE should be avoidable by the careful use of AI (where allowed by registration authorities) with effective barrier management, the potential for virus spread during AI has not been explored.

Nasogenital transmission of EHV-3 between mares at pasture and at teasing, with demonstrable nasal, lip and nostril lesions, has been reported. The role of stable flies for potential vulval to vulval transmission is unproven.

The virus is quickly destroyed in the environment by lipid solvents, detergents, heat, drying and commonly used disinfectants. Hygienic management of mare examination stocks and handling areas, particularly at covering barns, is important for the prevention of ECE and other sexually transmitted diseases.

Resumption of mating should be based upon freedom from clinical signs of infective lesions rather than set time periods, as the latter will vary with individual circumstances. However, stallions that are immediately rested and palliatively treated are usually ready for resumption of mating by 10–14 days. Stallions may be considered recovered when any systemic signs of illness have resolved and the penis and prepuce have been thoroughly examined, with the penis erect, and no vesicular or pox-like skin lesions are visible or previously diagnosed lesions have healed over, leaving noninflamed, smooth scars. The vulvas of mares should be examined thoroughly after washing and no vesicular or pox-like skin lesions should be visible or previously diagnosed lesions should have healed over, leaving noninflamed, smooth scars.

Equine viral arteritis

Equine arteritis virus (EAV) (see Timoney 2009) is a togavirus, which causes pyrexia, depression, conjunctivitis (**Fig 19**), increased respiratory rate, skin lesions, and oedema of the limbs, head and trunk. Mares may be infected at natural mating or during AI with semen (raw, extended or frozen/thawed) from virus-shedding stallions. EAV is also spread by the respiratory aerosol route by actively infected horses. Mares that are infected during pregnancy may abort, following placental arteritis.

In the UK, equine viral arteritis (EVA) is

notifiable by law under the Equine Viral Arteritis Order 1995, where:

1. EVA is suspected in a stallion, either on the basis of clinical signs or following blood or semen testing.
2. EVA is suspected, either on the basis of clinical signs or following blood testing, in a mare that has been mated or artificially inseminated within the past 14 days.

The incubation period for EVA ranges from 3–14 days with an average of 7 days and the infective period is considered to be 28 days. Diagnosis is confirmed by virus isolation from respiratory secretions or urine, or by a >4-fold increase in serum neutralising (SN) EAV antibody titre (seroconversion). Enzyme-linked immunosorbent assay (ELISA) provides a rapid and cost-effective screening test for horses that are not being examined for official export purposes. Immunity following infection or vaccination may be life-long and therefore viral serological tests may indicate past challenge rather than active infection. The carrier state has not been identified in mares and so a seropositive mare with no signs of active infection and a static or falling SN EAV titre is considered immune and of no risk for transmission of infection to other horses.

Equine viral arteritis is endemic in some populations of horses, notably Standardbreds and Warmbloods, throughout the world, as judged by levels of seropositivity. In the UK the incidence of seropositivity in indigenous horses is extremely low and it must be assumed that the UK mare population is very susceptible to the clinical disease. A case of EVA was diagnosed in a foal from a Thoroughbred mare imported from Italy to Newmarket in 1975. The first small and limited outbreak of EVA occurred in the UK in 1993. This outbreak followed the importation of an infected non-Thoroughbred stallion from Poland and was spread by AI with transported chilled semen. Cases were isolated and the outbreak was successfully controlled. The occasional imported seropositive non-Thoroughbred male horse has been identified in the UK since then, most commonly in temporary quarantine pending re-export to southern hemisphere countries. Outbreaks of EVA, involving stallions, have since occurred in France, Ireland and other mainland EU countries. Measures designed to prevent the occurrence of EVA in France, Germany, Ireland, Italy and the UK are recommended in the voluntary Code of Practice reviewed and re-published annually by HBLB.

All stallions, teasers and mares to be used for breeding should be blood tested (ELISA) before the start of the breeding season and any horses with positive titres that cannot be explained by vaccination should be isolated, examined for clinical signs, tested by SN test and retested 14 days later (SN tests should be performed at the same laboratory with both samples tested in the same assay) to test for seroconversion. Mares can be released from isolation if their titres are static or declining, as the carrier status has not been recognised in mares. This is in contrast to stallions where semen samples must be collected from unvaccinated seropositive stallions, under direction by Defra, and examined for EAV to look for seminal virus shedding.

Owners/managers of non-Thoroughbred mares who are planning to use AI should make sure that the stallion, whose semen they intend to use is not an EAV semen shedder and that the ejaculate from which their mare's dose was processed did not contain EAV. Any mares that show clinical signs of EVA (pyrexia, depression, conjunctivitis, increased respiratory rate, skin lesions, and oedema of the limbs, head and trunk) within 14 days of insemination should be isolated and blood tested, under direction by Defra.

EVA should be considered when mares abort and *post mortem* examinations fail to reveal evidence of

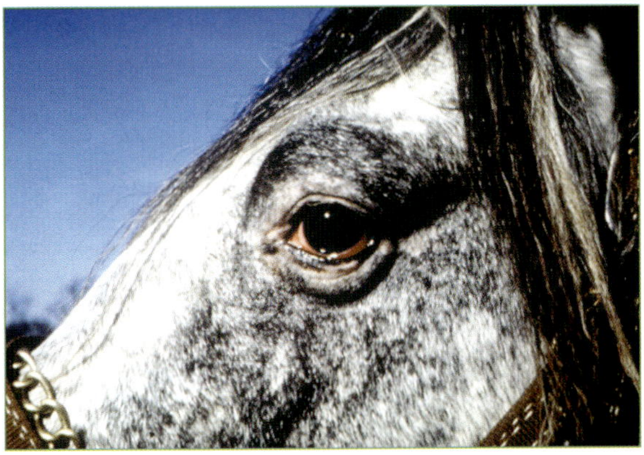

FIGURE 19: Horse with conjunctivitis associated with acute equine viral arteritis (EVA) infection (image courtesy of Professor Peter Timoney).

equine herpesvirus infection or other plausible explanations. Foetal and placental tissue samples may be examined by PCR and viral isolation tests.

Treatment of EVA, where clinical signs occur, is palliative. Clinical signs should not last more than 14–28 days. Isolation to prevent spread to susceptible horses is most important. To prevent respiratory spread it is most important that infected horses are not housed with susceptible horses, in barn-type stabling.

A formalin-inactivated EVA vaccine is licensed for use in horses in the UK and some other EU countries. It is widely used for stallions and teasers, to reduce their chances of becoming seminal shedders if infected. With the very low incidence of seropositivity in UK, mares are not vaccinated so that they may remain 'sentinels' of infection, when routinely blood tested before the start of each breeding season.

The symptomless semen shedding EAV carrier stallion is the most important risk for transmission of infection, both at natural mating and at AI, for susceptible mares and the horse breeding industries of all nations should work towards the diagnosis and elimination of these carriers from their equine populations.

Equine infectious anaemia

Equine infectious anaemia (EIA, swamp fever) (see Cook *et al.* 2009) is caused by a lentivirus that occurs worldwide, including in parts of mainland Europe, in all horse populations. It is not proven that it is sexually transmitted but there would appear to be no reason why it should not be, during natural mating with a viraemic mare or stallion or AI with EIA contaminated semen.

In the UK, EIA is notifiable by law under the Infectious Diseases of Horses Order 1987. Under the Order, anyone who owns, manages, inspects or examines a horse that is affected or is suspected of being affected by EIA must notify the appropriate Divisional Veterinary Manager (DVM) of Defra, who are based in the Animal Health Divisional Offices of Defra.

Under the Order, Defra may declare the premises where EIA is suspected as an infected place and impose restrictions on horses at those premises. A veterinary enquiry will be carried out under the direction of the DVM to determine if EIA is present. The Order also provides Defra with powers to enforce measures for vector control and disinfection.

As there is currently no cure for EIA, any horse testing positive will be subject to compulsory slaughter and disposal under the control of the DVM, without significant compensation. The Equine Infectious Anaemia (Compensation) (England) Order 2006, which came into force in 2006, stipulates compensation to the value of £1 per animal for horses subject to compulsory slaughter for EIA.

Measures designed to prevent the occurrence of EIA in France, Germany, Ireland, Italy and the UK are recommended in the voluntary Code of Practice reviewed and re-published annually by HBLB.

Equine infectious anaemia may take an acute, chronic or sub-clinical form and clinical signs are extremely variable. Outward signs of the acute form include fever, depression, anaemia, increased heart and respiratory rate, haemorrhaging, bloody diarrhoea, loss of coordination, poor performance, ataxia, rapid weight loss, skin swelling and jaundice (**Fig 20**). Acutely infected horses are potently viraemic and are potentially infectious to other horses and donkeys. The chronic form may be characterised by recurring bouts of fever, depression, anaemia, weakness or weight loss, interspersed with periods of normality.

Any horse with severe, unexplained anaemia should be isolated and tested for EIA. Sub-clinically

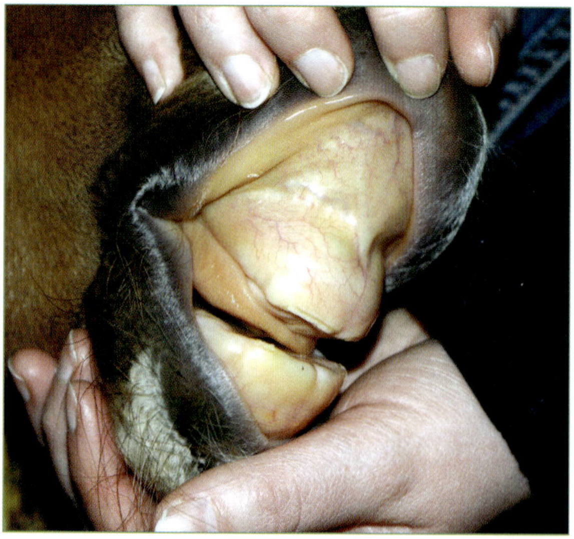

FIGURE 20: Foal with anaemic, jaundiced mucous membranes.

infected horses may not show any clinical signs of disease.

EIA is transmitted between horses by transfer of infected blood or blood products. This can occur in the following ways:

1. By insect vectors such as biting flies (including horse, deer and stable flies) and (rarely) mosquitoes.
2. By administration of infected blood products (including plasma) and unauthorised blood-based veterinary medicinal products.
3. By contaminated veterinary or dental equipment.
4. By other equipment that may become contaminated by blood and act as a vector between animals, e.g. twitches and curry combs.
5. From mare to foal via the placenta, or, rarely, via virus-contaminated colostrum or milk in newborn foals.

Transmission through semen is considered to be a potential, although unproven, risk.

Both clinically and sub-clinically affected horses can be a source of infection for life for other horses, although animals suffering acute disease or recurring bouts of chronic disease are likely to be the most highly infectious.

There is no vaccine available for EIA. Prevention of EIA is therefore based on the establishment of freedom from infection by blood testing and the avoidance of contact with infected horses.

All mares, stallions and teasers (who are not suspected of showing clinical signs and who are not being examined for official export purposes) should be routinely blood tested (ELISA) before the start of each breeding season. This includes all resident horses and horses due to visit the premises, prior to arrival. All horses with positive titres should be isolated in a vector-proof stable, examined for clinical signs and retested immediately by agar gel immunodiffusion (Coggins) test at the Veterinary Laboratories Agency (VLA) laboratory. The Coggins test is currently the only test recognised officially for the purpose of international movement of horses.

Owners temporarily exporting horses for competition or breeding purposes should attempt to ensure, as far as possible, that their horse will not come into direct contact with horses at risk of EIA infection while in a country where EIA is endemic or has occurred recently. On return home these horses should be segregated and monitored for signs of infection. Due to the variability and possible absence of outward signs of EIA, clinical diagnosis is not always possible and laboratory diagnosis, through blood testing, is essential.

Detectable antibodies are usually present in the blood 7–14 days after infection and remain present for the rest of the horse's life.

Control of EIA is primarily by preventing transmission of infection to other horses through insect vector control, avoiding high-risk procedures and detection of infected animals and their prompt destruction.

It is recommended that if infection is suspected, or a horse is suspected of having been in contact with an infected horse:

1. Isolate the horse (ideally in a vector-proof stable) and notify the DVM of Defra immediately. Isolate any other horses with which the horse has had contact.
2. Any directions given by the DVM must be followed, including implementation of vector control.
3. Treat the horse(s) as advised by the DVM and as required to satisfy the immediate welfare needs of the horse.
4. Stop all movement of horses on and off the premises.
5. Group all other horses on the premises away from in contact horses until freedom from infection is confirmed.
6. Any nonurgent actions that could pose a risk of transmission of infection between horses on the premises (such as nonessential veterinary treatment or nonessential contact with staff) should be halted. For essential treatment, the principle of one syringe and one needle for each horse should be strictly followed, as should always be the case for all veterinary treatments.
7. Veterinary procedures represent a particular risk. Veterinary equipment must therefore be either destroyed after use or appropriately sterilised.
8. In addition to the DVM of Defra, inform:
    a. Owners (or persons authorised to act on their behalf) of horses at, or due to arrive at, the premises.
    b. Owners (or persons authorised to act on their

behalf) of horses that have recently left the premises.
   c. The relevant breeders' association.
9. Stables, equipment and vehicles used for horse transport must be cleaned and disinfected.
10. Good hygiene must be exercised, including the use of different staff and equipment for each group of horses, where possible. If this is not possible, staff who have handled infected or in contact horses must disinfect their hands and change clothes before handling other horses. If separate equipment cannot be used for different groups of horses, it must be sterilised or appropriately disinfected before each use.
11. EIA virus can survive in blood, faeces and tissue so all such material must be removed and destroyed promptly and surfaces disinfected.

Horses that have come into contact with an infected horse or a horse that is suspected of being infected must be quarantined for a minimum of 90 days post exposure. Blood testing must be repeated as directed by the DVM until freedom from disease is confirmed.

Any horse tested positive for EIA will be subject to compulsory slaughter and disposal under the Infectious Diseases of Horses Order 1987.

There is currently no effective treatment for EIA. Treatment to alleviate the signs of the disease and otherwise support the horse should be applied, as appropriate for the horse's welfare, until such time as a positive diagnosis is confirmed by Coggins testing and compulsory slaughter is carried out.

Restrictions on the affected premises and/or the horses in it may only be lifted, and any breeding activities resumed, after authorisation by the DVM and approval by the attending veterinary surgeon, who must be satisfied that all in-contact horses have been investigated and found to be negative for EIA virus. If statutory restrictions have been imposed, the requirements of the supervising Defra officials must be met in order that the restrictions can be lifted.

Trypanosoma equiperdum

Trypanosoma equiperdum (see van den Bossche 2009) is a protozoan organism. The disease dourine was prevalent in western Europe during the earlier part of the 20th century but has not been reported to occur there for many years. In the UK it is notifiable by law to Defra. Dourine is still seen in horses in Asia, Africa, South America, southern and eastern Europe, and Mexico. It is sexually transmitted during natural mating or during AI with contaminated semen.

Clinical signs appear from 5–6 days to several weeks after infection and include pyrexia, anorexia, oedema of the genitalia, discharge from the urethra and characteristic raised urticarial skin plaques (2–10 cm in diameter), which appear on the lower parts of the body and then disappear within hours. If these plaques persist they leave depigmented areas. Small pustules develop in waves on the penis and prepuce. They ulcerate and heal slowly leaving slightly elevated nonpigmented scars reminiscent of those seen following EHV-3 infection. Penile and generalised muscular paralysis can develop, leading eventually to emaciation, lameness and death. Differential diagnosis includes EHV-3 and the paralytic form of equine herpesvirus 1. Diagnosis is confirmed serologically with complement fixation test or demonstration of the organism in smears of exudative fluid. Treatment is attempted with quinapyramine sulphate (3 mg/kg subcut.) but it is not known whether recovered stallions are safe for breeding purposes and so eradication is the best policy.

Further reading

Allen, G.P. and Umphenour, N.W. (2004) Equine coital exanthema, In: *Infectious Diseases of Livestock*, Eds: J.A.W. Coetzer and R.C. Tustin, Oxford Press, Cape Town. pp 860-867.

Atherton, J.G. (1975) The identification of equine genital strains of *Klebsiella* and *Enterobacter species*. *Equine vet. J.* **7**, 207-209.

Bryans, J.D. and Hendrick, J.B. (1979) Epidemiological observations on contagious equine metritis in Kentucky 1978. *J. Reprod. Fert., Suppl.* **27**, 343-349.

Conboy, H.S. (2007) Significance of bacteria affecting the stallion's reproductive system. In: *Current Therapy in Equine Reproduction,* Eds: J.C. Samper, J.F. Pycock and A.O. McKinnon, W.B. Saunders, Philadelphia. pp 231-236.

Cook, R.F., Cook, S.J. and Issel, C.J. (2009) Equine infectious anaemia. In: *Infectious Diseases of the Horse*, Eds: T.S. Mair and R.E. Hutchinson, Equine Veterinary Journal Ltd., Newmarket. pp 56-71.

Crouch, J.R.F., Atherton, J.G. and Platt, H. (1972) Venereal transmission of *Klebsiella aerogenes* in a Thoroughbred stud from a persistently infected stallion. *Vet. Rec.* **90**, 21-24.

Crowhurst, R.C. (1977) Genital infection in mares. *Vet. Rec.* **100**, 476.

Crowhurst, R.C., Simpson, D.J., Greenwood, R.E.S. and Ellis, D.J. (1979) Contagious equine metritis. *Vet. Rec.* **104**, 465.

David, J.S.E., Frank, C.J. and Powell, D.G. (1977) Contagious metritis 1977. *Vet. Rec.* **101**, 189-190.

Day, F.T., Crowhurst, R.C., Simpson, D.J., Greenwood, R.E.S., Ellis, D.R. and Eaton-Evans, W. (1979) An outbreak of contagious equine metritis in 1977 and its effect the following season. *J. Reprod. Fert., Suppl.* **27**, 351-354.

Dimmock, W.W. (1939) Equine breeding hygiene. *J. Am. vet. med. Ass.* **94**, 469.

Dimmock, W.W. and Edwards, P.R. (1928) Pathology and bacteriology of the reproductive organs of mares in relation to sterility. *Res. Bull. Ky. Agric. Exp. Stn.* 286.

Gibbs, E.P.J., Roberts, M.C. and Morris, J.M. (1972) Equine coital exanthema in the United Kingdom. *Equine vet. J.* **4**, 74-80.

Greenwood, R.E.S. and Ellis, D.R. (1976) *Klebsiella aerogenes* in mares. *Vet. Rec.* **99**, 439.

Hamm, D.H. (1978) Gentamicin therapy of genital tract infections in stallions. *J. Equine Med. Surg.* **2**, 243-245.

Hazard, G.H., Hughes, K.L. and Penson, P.J. (1979) Contagious equine metritis in Australia. *J. Reprod. Fert., Suppl.* **27**, 337-342.

Heath, P. and Roest, H.-J. (2007) *Proceedings of the First International Conference on Contagious Equine Metritis.* VLA/CIDC-Lelystad, Holland.

Horserace Betting Levy Board (2009) Codes of Practice on Contagious Equine Metritis (CEM), *Klebsiella pneumoniae, Pseudomonas aeruginosa*; Equine Viral Arteritis (EVA); Equine Herpesvirus (EHV); Equine Infectious Anaemia (EIA) and guidelines on strangles. Horserace Betting Levy Board, London. www.hblb.org.uk/document.php?id=43

Hunt, M.D.N. and Rossdale, P.D. (1963) A specific venereal disease of Thoroughbred mares. *Vet. Rec.* **75**, 1092.

Jackson, P.S., Allen, W.R., Ricketts, S.W. and Hall, R. (1979) The irritancy of chlorhexidine gluconate in the genital tract of the mare. *Vet. Rec.* **105**, 122-124.

Jang, S.S., Donahue, J.M., Arata, A.B., Goris, J., Hansen, L.M., Earley, D.L., Vandamme, P.A., Timoney, P.J. and Hirsh, D.C. (2001) *Taylorella asinigenitalis sp. nov.*, a bacterium isolated from the genital tract of male donkeys (*Equus asinus*). *Int. J. Syst. Evol. Microbiol.* **51**, 971-976.

Parlevliet, J.M. and Samper, J.C. (2000) Disease transmission through semen. In: *Equine Breeding Management and Artificial Insemination,* Ed: J.C. Samper, W.B. Saunders, Philadelphia. pp 133-140.

Platt, H., Atherton, J.G. and Ørskov, I. (1976) *Klebsiella* and *Enterobacter* organisms isolated from horses. *J. Hyg. Camb.* **77**, 401-408.

Platt, H., Atherton, J.G., Simpson, D.J., Taylor, C.E.D., Rosenthal, R.O., Brown, D.F.J. and Wreghitt, T.G. (1977) Genital infections in mares. *Vet. Rec.* **101**, 20.

Powell, D.G., David, J.S.E. and Frank, C.J. (1978) Contagious equine metritis. The present situation reviewed and a revised code of practice for control. *Vet. Rec.* **101**, 399-402.

Powell, D.G. and Whitwell, K.E. (1979) The epidemiology of contagious equine metritis (CEM) in England, 1977-1978. *J. Reprod. Fert., Suppl.*, **27**, 331-335.

Ricketts, S.W. (1976) *Klebsiella aerogenes* in mares. *Vet. Rec.* **99**, 489.

Ricketts, S.W. (1981) Bacteriological examinations of the mare's cervix: techniques and interpretation of results. *Vet. Rec.* **108**, 46-51.

Ricketts, S.W. (1985) Dealing with the 'problem mare'. *Equine vet. J.* **17**, 3-4.

Ricketts, S.W. (1987) Uterine abnormalities. In: *Current Therapy in Equine Medicine*, 2nd edn., Ed: N.E. Robinson, W.B. Saunders, Philadelphia. p 503.

Ricketts, S.W. (1987) Vaginal discharge in the mare. *In Pract.* **9**, 117-123.

Ricketts, S.W. (1995) The non-pregnant mare. In: *The Equine Manual*, Eds: A.J. Higgins and I.M. Wright, W.B. Saunders, Philadelphia. pp 606-617.

Ricketts, S.W. (1996) Contagious equine metritis. *Equine vet. Educ.* **8**, 166-170.

Ricketts, S.W. (1997) Treatment of equine endometritis with intrauterine irrigations of ceftiofur sodium: a comparison with mares treated in a similar manner with a mixture of sodium benzylpenicillin, neomycin sulphate, polymixin B sulphate and furaltadone hydrochloride. *Pferdeheilkunde* **5**, 486-489.

Ricketts, S.W. (1999) The treatment of equine endometritis in studfarm practice. *Pferdeheilkunde* **6**, 588-593.

Ricketts, S.W. and Alonso, S. (1991) The effect of age and parity on the development of equine chronic endometrial disease. *Equine vet. J.* **23**, 189-192.

Ricketts, S.W. and Mackintosh, M.E. (1987) The role of anaerobic bacteria in equine endometritis. *J. Reprod. Fertil., Suppl.* **35**, 343-351.

Ricketts, S.W. and Troedsson, M. (2007) Female reproductive problems: Diagnosis and management – Chapter 8: Fertility expectations and management for optimal fertility. In: *Current Therapy in Equine Reproduction,* Eds: J.C. Samper, J.F. Pycock and A.O. McKinnon, W.B. Saunders, Philadelphia. pp 53-69.

Ricketts, S.W., Barrelet, A. and Whitwell, K.E. (2003) Equine abortion. In: *Reproduction. Foaling: Part 2: Fetal and Neonatal Aspects*, Eds: P.D. Rossdale, T.S. Mair and R.E. Green. Equine Veterinary Journal Ltd., Newmarket. pp 18-21.

Ricketts, S.W., Young, A. and Medici, E.B. (1993) Uterine and clitoral cultures. In: *Equine Reproduction,* Eds: A.O. McKinnon and J.L. Voss. Lea & Febiger, Philadelphia. pp 234-245.

Ricketts, S.W., Rossdale, P.D., Wingfield Digby, N.J., Falk, M.M., Hopes, R., Hunt, M.D.N. and Peace, C.K. (1977) Genital infection in mares. *Vet. Rec.* **101**, 65.

Rossdale, P.D., Hunt, M.D.N., Peace, C.K., Hopes, R. and Ricketts, S.W. (1975) A case of equine infectious anaemia in Newmarket. *Vet. Rec.* **97**, 207-208.

Rossdale, P.D. and Ricketts, S.W. (1980) *Equine Studfarm Medicine,* 2nd edn., Baillière Tindall, London.

Simpson, D.J. and Eaton-Evans, W.E. (1978) Developments in contagious equine metritis. *Vet. Rec.* **102**, 19-20.

Simpson, D.J. and Eaton-Evans, W.E. (1978) Sites of CEM infection. *Vet. Rec.* **102**, 488.

Taylor, C.E.D., Rosenthal, R.G. and Brown, D.F.J. (1978) The causative organisms of contagious equine metritis 1977; Proposal for a new species to be known as *Haemophilus equigenitalis. Equine vet. J.* **10**, 136-144.

Timoney, P.J. (2009) Equine viral arteritis. In: *Infectious Diseases of the Horse*, Eds: T.S. Mair and R.E. Hutchinson, Equine Veterinary Journal Ltd., Newmarket. pp 29-40.

Timoney, P.J., Ward, J. and Kelly, P. (1977) A contagious genital infection of mares. *Vet. Rec.* **101**, 103.

Van den Bossche, P., Geerts, S. and Claes, F. (2009) Equine trypanosomiasis. In: *Infectious Diseases of the Horse*, Eds: T.S. Mair and R.E. Hutchinson, Equine Veterinary Journal Ltd., Newmarket. pp 354-365.

Wakeley, P.R., Errington, J., Hannon, S, Roest, H.I., Carson, T., Hunt, B., Sawyer, J. and Heath, P. (2006) Development of a real time PCR for the detection of *Taylorella equigenitalis* directly from genital swabs and discrimination from *Taylorella asinigenitalis*. *Vet. Microbiol.* **118**, 247-254.

Wingfield Digby, N.J. and Ricketts, S.W. (1982) A method for clitoral sinusectomy in mares. *In Pract.* **4**, 145-147.

Wingfield Digby, N.J. and Ricketts, S.W. (1982) Results of concurrent bacteriological and cytological examinations ofthe endometrium of mares in routine studfarm practice 1978-81. *J. Reprod. Fert., Suppl.* **32**, 181-185.

Wood, J.L.N., Cardwell, J.M., Castillo-Olivares, J. and Irwin, V. (2007) Transmission of diseases through semen. In: *Current Therapy in Equine Reproduction,* Eds: J.C. Samper, J.F. Pycock and A.O. McKinnon, W.B. Saunders, Philadelphia. pp 266-274.

RHODOCOCCUS EQUI FOAL PNEUMONIA

N. Cohen* and S. Giguère[†]

Department of Large Animal Clinical Sciences, College of Veterinary, Medicine and Biomedical Sciences, Texas A&M University College Station, Texas 77843-4475; and [†]Department of Large Animal Medicine, College of Veterinary Medicine, University of Georgia, Athens, Georgia 30602, USA.

Keywords: horse; *Rhodococcus equi*; foal pneumonia; extrapulmonary manifestations; treatment; epidemiology; prevention

Summary

Pneumonia caused by the bacterium *Rhodococcus equi* is an important cause of disease and death in foals worldwide. The purpose of this report is to review information about the epidemiology, clinical signs, treatment, and control and prevention of *R. equi* pneumonia, with emphasis on newer findings.

Epidemiology

Pneumonia in foals caused by *R. equi* has been described as occurring recurrently at some farms (so-called *R. equi* endemic farms), sporadically at others, while some farms appear to be unaffected (Prescott 1991). This distribution complicates efforts to generate descriptive statistics describing the cumulative incidence of the disease in foals. Generally, the cumulative incidence of clinical signs of pneumonia attributed to *R. equi* at endemic farms is approximately 10–20% from birth to weaning; however, some farms may experience markedly greater incidences, even reaching 100% on rare occasions (Chaffin *et al.* 2003a; Cohen *et al.* 2005a). A further complication in describing the epidemiology of *R. equi* pneumonia is that the disease appears to be changing with the advent of the use of ultrasonography (and other screening techniques) for detecting pre- or sub-clinical disease. At *R. equi* endemic farms, foals with sonographic evidence of focal or multifocal pulmonary consolidation and/or abscessation are often presumptively diagnosed with *R. equi* pneumonia, particularly when the farm has a history of the disease or results of microbiological culture and cytological examination of fluid obtained by tracheobronchial aspiration are used in one or more foals from the farm to confirm the diagnosis. In the authors' experience, the cumulative incidence of foals at *R. equi* endemic farms with sonographic evidence of pulmonary abscessation or consolidation is generally 30–60%. To the authors' knowledge, the probability of developing clinical signs of pneumonia in foals with pre-/sub-clinical sonographic lesions has not been described. The finding that reported cumulative incidences of clinical disease are considerably lower than those for sonographically detectable lesions suggests that many if not most pre-/sub-clinically affected foals may spontaneously resolve without intervention. However, because it is unknown what proportion or which specific foals might recover spontaneously, and because the disease can be severe, many breeding farms elect to treat all foals with sonographic lesions (sometimes, a threshold for the size or number of sonographic lesions is used as an indicator for the need for therapy) (Slovis 2005). Thus, the widespread application of screening with ultrasonography or other methods appears to have increased the cumulative incidence of disease. Moreover, the practice of early identification of (often presumptive) cases appears to be reducing the severity of pulmonary disease: foals with large, multifocal pyogranulomatous lesions (such as those represented in the radiograph in **Fig 1a**) and moderate to marked clinical signs of pneumonia are observed less frequently, and the disease is more often characterised by foals with smaller, multifocal areas of abscessation or consolidation (similar to the sonographic lesion represented in **Fig 1b**).

*Author to whom correspondence should be addressed.

In considering the epidemiology of an infectious disease, it is common to consider the triad of agent-, environment- and host-related factors. It appears that a given farm can be expected to be affected by multiple strains, indicating that any isolate bearing the virulence-associated plasmid has the capacity to cause disease in foals. A number of recent studies indicate that virulent isolates of *R. equi* are widespread in the environment (including air, soil and faeces of mares) to which foals are exposed from birth (Martens *et al.* 2000; Morton *et al.* 2001; Muscatello *et al.* 2006a,b, 2007; Grimm *et al.* 2007; Cohen *et al.* 2008). Farm-level risk factors include density of horses and the use of management practices deemed desirable, such as checking for evidence of passive transfer of immunity to foals, attending foalings, etc. (Chaffin *et al.* 2003b; Cohen *et al.* 2005a). The latter association is not likely to be causal but is an indication that practices which help reduce the incidence of other infectious diseases do not appear to be effective for preventing *R. equi* pneumonia. Evidence also exists that foaling in pasture and maintaining foals in pastures/paddocks may reduce the cumulative incidence of *R. equi* pneumonia (Cohen *et al.* 2005a, Malschitzky *et al.* 2005); controlled trials of such management practices, however, are lacking. Absence of important agent factors other than possession of the virulence plasmid and widespread environmental exposure suggest that host factors (presumably host immunity) play a critical role in determining which foals develop disease. Many important questions regarding the epidemiology of *R. equi* pneumonia remain unresolved.

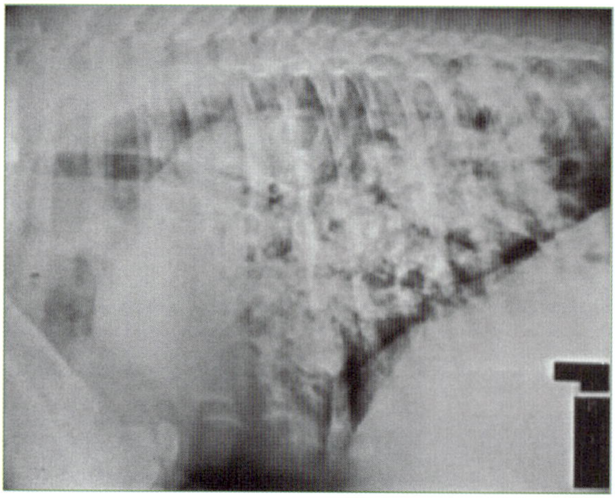

FIGURE 1a: Thoracic radiograph of a foal with large, multifocal opacities in the thorax associated with severe Rhodococcus equi pneumonia.

Clinical signs

The classical clinical signs of *R. equi* pneumonia are described elsewhere (Giguère and Prescott 1997). The disease often is insidiously progressive and foals may have extensive pulmonary pathology before clinical signs of increased effort or rate of respirations, coughing or nasal discharge are detected. As noted above, the clinical signs and pathological severity of lesions appear to be diminishing because of greater use of screening tests by farm veterinarians or farm staff.

Extrapulmonary manifestations of infection with *R. equi* can occur. To the author's knowledge, the frequency of extrapulmonary disorders (EPDs) among

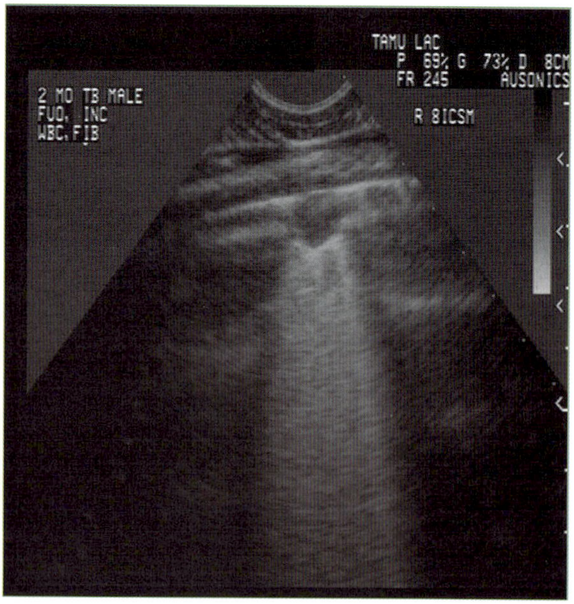

FIGURE 1b: Ultrasonographic image of the right 8th intercostal space obtained shortly after admission to the hospital from a foal from a farm with history of R. equi foal pneumonia. The foal was noted at admission to be bright and alert, but with fever and history of occasional coughing. The observed round, subpleural lesion is approximately 1 cm in diameter. A few other similar lesions were observed in other right intercostal spaces, and fluid obtained by tracheobronchial aspiration yielded cytological evidence of sepsis and a virulent isolate of R. equi.

foals with *R. equi* infections has not been reported from farm-based populations. Among 150 foals with *R. equi* infection admitted to Texas A&M University's Veterinary Teaching Hospital, 115 (77%) were documented as having EPDs (Reuss *et al.* 2008). A plethora (n = 39) of EPDs were identified, of which diarrhoea, presumed immune-mediated synovitis (**Fig 2**), ulcerative enterotyphlocolitis (**Fig 3**), intra-abdominal abscessation (**Fig 4**), and intra-abdominal lymphadenitis occurred most commonly. Many foals developed diarrhoea subsequent to antimicrobial therapy with a macrolide as treatment for *R. equi* pneumonia, and less than half the foals determined to have ulcerative enteritis or typhlocolitis developed diarrhoea. EPDs may be the first clinical signs noted by owners (such as effusion of multiple joints), and EPDs may result in the foal's demise despite resolution of pneumonia attributed to the same bacterium. Enhanced recognition of the frequency with which EPDs occur may lead to earlier recognition of the EPDs or to *R. equi* disease. Although many foals with EPDs had normal blood concentrations of WBCs or neutrophils, most foals without EPDs had concentrations of these blood cells that were within the reference range (Reuss *et al.* 2008); if these findings are true in other settings, the index of suspicion for an EPD should be higher in a foal with *R. equi* pneumonia that has an increased blood concentration of WBCs or neutrophils.

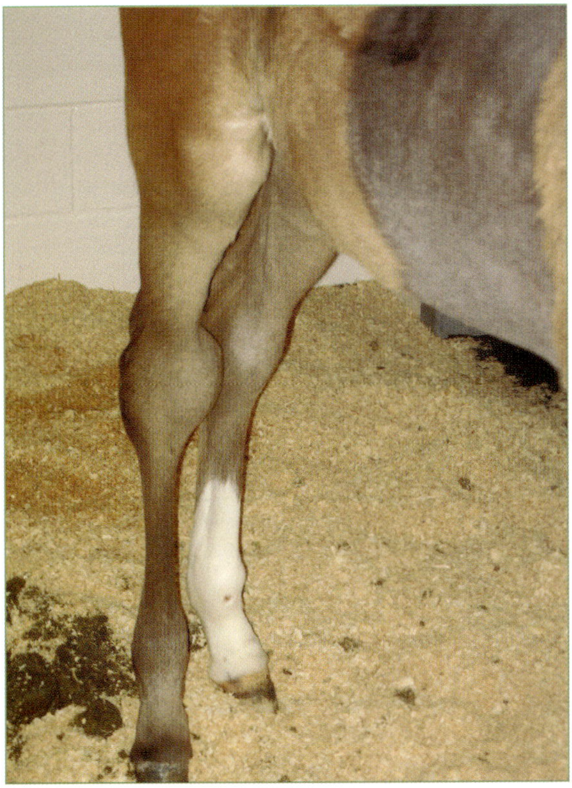

FIGURE 2: Bilateral tarsocrural joint effusion in a foal with presumed immune-mediated polysynovitis associated with R. equi pneumonia.

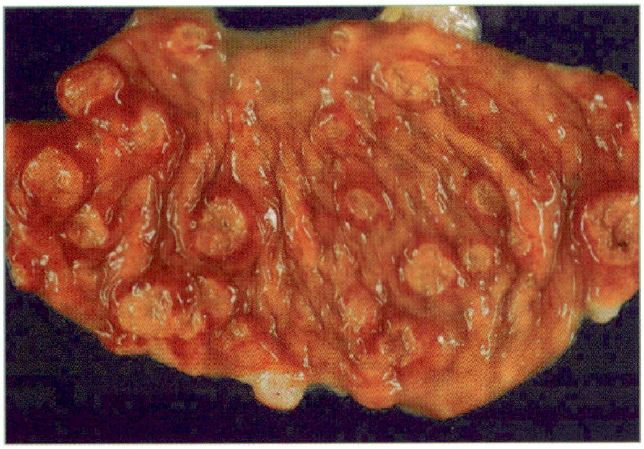

FIGURE 3: Mucosal surface of the colon of a foal with ulcerative enterocolitis caused by infection with R. equi. Note the diffuse, multifocal round areas of ulceration.

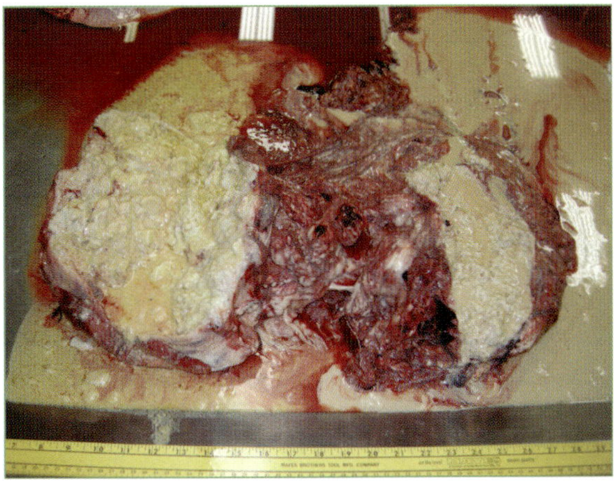

FIGURE 4: A large intra-abdominal abscess caused by R. equi in a foal; the abscess was sectioned during necropsy (photograph courtesy of Ms Jackie Smith and Dr Craig Carter, University of Kentucky Livestock Disease Diagnostic Laboratory).

Treatment

For decades, the standard treatment in North America for *R. equi* has been the combination of erythromycin (a macrolide antimicrobial) and rifampin (Hillidge 1987; Sweeney *et al.* 1987). The rationale for combining the 2 drugs is evidence for *in vitro* synergism against *R. equi*, the ability of both drugs to achieve high intracellular concentrations, the likelihood that the use of 2 synergistic drugs with differing mechanisms of action is likely to reduce the opportunity for resistance (Prescott and Nicholson 1984; Prescott and Sweeney 1985; Nordmann and Ronco 1992), and evidence in nude mice that erythromycin in combination with rifampin was significantly more effective than erythromycin alone (Nordmann *et al.* 1994). Most clinical reports describing outcome of foals with *R. equi* pneumonia have described the use of a combination of a macrolide in combination with rifampin (Hillidge 1987; Sweeney *et al.* 1988; Ainsworth *et al.* 1998; Giguère *et al.* 2004; Reuss *et al.* 2008). For these reasons, despite the absence of clinical trials comparing combination therapy with macrolide monotherapy, the authors recommend that treatment of *R. equi* pneumonia be the combination of a macrolide with rifampin. Rifampin is generally administered to foals at a dosage of 5–10 mg/kg bwt by mouth every 12–24 h. Interestingly, there is evidence from human and laboratory animal studies that the combination of rifampin and the macrolide clarithromycin results in decreased serum concentrations of the latter via stimulation of the hepatic cytochrome P450 enzyme system (Wallace *et al.* 1995; Peloquin and Berning 1996; Yamomoto *et al.* 2004; Grau *et al.* 2006). Although serum concentrations of macrolides are a poor reflection of their clinical activity (because they attain high intracellular concentrations), evidence exists that the principal metabolite of clarithromycin is less able to penetrate leucocytes and lung tissue. Whether this interaction occurs in foals and whether it has clinical relevance remains to be determined from valid patient-based and experimental studies of foals.

Dosing regimens for erythromycin range from 25 mg/kg bwt orally every 6–8 h, to 37.5 mg/kg bwt orally every 12 h (Ewing *et al.* 1994; Lakritz and Wilson 2002). The drug is generally better absorbed when hay is withheld (Lakritz *et al.* 2000). Several formulations are available, including base, estolate, ethylsuccinate, phosphate and stearate. Of these, the ethylsuccinate ester is most poorly absorbed from the gastrointestinal tract; thus, its use should be avoided (Lakritz and Wilson 2002). A number of side-effects have been reported following oral administration of erythromycin to foals, including diarrhoea in the foal, diarrhoea in dams of affected foals and an environmentally-mediated hyperthermia (Baverud *et al.* 1998; Phelps *et al.* 2000). A respiratory distress syndrome resulting from anti-inflammatory effects of a metabolite of erythromycin also has been proposed (Lakritz *et al.* 1997).

In recent years, there has been increasing use in North America of 2 other macrolides to treat *R. equi* foal pneumonia, *viz.*, azithromycin and clarithromycin. These macrolides each enjoy certain advantages relative to erythromycin. Compared to erythromycin, azithromycin generally has higher oral bioavailability, increased distribution into pulmonary tissues and phagocytic cells and fluid recovered by brocho-alveolar lavage (BAL), a longer elimination half-life, and a longer duration of pulmonary epithelial lining fluid and bronchoalveolar cells concentrations above the MIC_{90} for isolates of *R. equi* when administered at an equivalent dose (Jacks *et al.* 2001, 2003). The recommended treatment regimen for azithromycin is 10 mg/kg bwt orally every 24 h for 5 days, then every 48 h as needed. Relative to erythromycin and clarithromycin, azithromycin has a longer terminal half-life in BAL cells and pulmonary epithelial lining fluid (Suarez-Mier *et al.* 2007). The drug is slowly released from cells and sustains high tissue concentrations (Fietta *et al.* 1997; Bosnar *et al.* 2005). Consequently, it has been suggested that daily treatment may be unnecessary, and that administration of higher doses with a longer dose interval and shorter course of treatment may be feasible (Suarez-Mier *et al.* 2007). Side-effects noted with azithromycin include environmentally-mediated hyperthermia and diarrhoea.

Clarithromycin also has pharmacological advantages relative to erythromycin for treatment of *R. equi* pneumonia, including higher oral bioavailability, larger volume of distribution, increased distribution into pulmonary epithelial lining fluid and BAL cells, a longer elimination half-life, and a longer duration of concentrations above the MIC_{90} for *R. equi* when administered at an equivalent dose (Jacks *et al.*

2002; Womble *et al.* 2006a; Suarez-Mier *et al.* 2007). Moreover, concentrations in BAL fluid are significantly higher than those attained with azithromycin, and the MIC_{90} for isolates of *R. equi* is lower for clarithromycin than for either azithromycin or erythromycin (Suarez-Mier *et al.* 2007). The combination of clarithromycin with rifampin appeared to be more effective than rifampin in combination with either erythromycin or azithromycin for treatment of foals with severe *R. equi* pneumonia (Giguère *et al.* 2004). Clarithromycin appears to be more likely than azithromycin or erythromycin to contribute to development of diarrhoea in foals (Giguère *et al.* 2004). The recommended treatment regimen for clarithromycin is 7.5 mg/kg bwt by mouth every 12 h (Jacks *et al.* 2002); however, based on the fact that clarithromycin concentrations in pulmonary fluid and BAL cells are above the MIC_{90} of *R. equi* for at least 24 h after a single dose, it is possible (clinical data are lacking) that once daily administration of a higher dose of clarithromycin would be sufficient (Suarez-Mier *et al.* 2007). The latter dosing regimen might be expected to improve compliance, reduce cost of treatment, and perhaps reduce the incidence of diarrhoea.

Tulathromycin is an injectable macrolide that is approved in the USA for treating respiratory tract disease in cattle and swine. It has a long elimination half-life and attains high pulmonary tissue concentrations in cattle and swine, such that the dosage interval is prolonged (i.e. every 7 days). Although the drug has been used with apparent success to treat abscessing pneumonia in foals, the duration of therapy in foals receiving tulathromycin was significantly longer than that of foals treated with a combination of azithromycin and rifampin (Venner *et al.* 2007). Evidence exists that tulathromycin is rapidly absorbed, widely distributed, and slowly eliminated following i.m. administration to foals (Scheuch *et al.* 2007). Moreover, concentrations in cells recovered by BAL were higher than corresponding plasma concentrations. The use of tulathromycin is not recommended at present for the following reasons. First, MIC data for *R. equi* are lacking for tulathromycin. Because this drug was developed to treat Gram-negative pulmonary infections, it is conceivable that its efficacy against Gram-positive agents such as *R. equi* may be diminished relative to other macrolides. Second, the incidence of side-effects (principally diarrhoea and local reactions at injection sites) was relatively high (Venner *et al.* 2007).

Resistance to macrolide antibiotics is generally class-specific, such that resistance to one macrolide infers resistance to others (Leclercq and Courvalin 2002). After >25 years of macrolides being the standard of treatment for *R. equi*, it is not surprising that isolates of *R. equi* resistant to macrolides have been identified (Giguère *et al.* 2008). This recent report of macrolide-resistant isolates of *R. equi* highlighted several important points. First, some isolates of *R. equi* susceptible to macrolides are misclassified as resistant; therefore, it is reasonable to request re-testing/ validation of resistance by the testing laboratory. Second, infection with macrolide-resistant isolates was associated with significantly poorer prognosis for survival than was infection with macrolide-susceptible isolates, representing an ominous correlation. Finally, the MICs of clarithromycin for resistant isolates were generally below the intracellular concentrations obtained for this antimicrobial, suggesting that clarithromycin might be effective in treatment of foals whose isolates were identified as resistant to macrolides.

Tilmicosin is a macrolide derived from tylosin. In the USA, the drug is approved for treating respiratory tract disease in cattle, sheep, and pigs. The pulmonary disposition of a proprietary fatty acid-salt formulation of tilmicosin was examined in foals, along with the *in vitro* susceptibility of isolates of *R. equi* to this antimicrobial. Although the drug obtained high concentrations (relative to serum) in BAL cells, pulmonary epithelial lining fluid and lung tissue, these concentrations were below the MIC_{90} of *R. equi* observed *in vitro* (Womble *et al.* 2006b). Five of 6 foals exhibited local reactions to the product at the site of injection, and one foal experienced tachypnoea and profuse sweating. Evidence exists that the faecal flora of foals is altered by the drug (Clark 2008), indicating the potential for antimicrobial-associated diarrhoea.

The occurrence of side-effects and resistance to macrolides has created the interest in and need for seeking alternative antimicrobials for treating *R. equi* pneumonia. Unfortunately, options that are currently available are of limited value. Recently, the pharmacokinetics of doxycycline in foals was reported (Womble *et al.* 2007). The drug was well absorbed when administered to foals at a dosage of 10 mg/kg bwt orally (the recommended interval is every 12 h), and concentrations in serum, pulmonary epithelial lining fluid, and cells obtained by BAL exceeded the MIC_{90} of *R. equi* isolates observed in vitro. Many veterinarians combine doxycycline with rifampin to treat foals with *R. equi*. In the authors' limited experience, foals with severe *R. equi* pneumonia may fail to respond to doxycycline despite the aforementioned pharmacokinetic and *in vitro* susceptibility data. Chloramphenicol is probably not a good alternative to macrolides for treating *R. equi* pneumonia because the maximal serum concentration reported in foals for this drug is well below the reported MICs for most *R. equi* isolates (Prescott 1981; Jacks *et al.* 2003).

The duration of antimicrobial treatment of foals with *R. equi* pneumonia is generally prolonged; however, screening to detect sub- or pre-clinical disease is probably associated with shorter duration of treatment. A variety of different strategies for monitoring the response to treatment have been proposed as valuable for determining duration of treatment, but almost none have been systematically evaluated. Concentrations of fibrinogen and WBCs, when values exceed the reference range, have been proposed as tools for monitoring duration of treatment (e.g. treatment for 7–10 days after the WBC concentration is within the reference range). Serum amyloid A (SAA) concentration has been suggested as being more sensitive than concentrations of leucocytes, neutrophils or fibrinogen (Hultén and Demmers 2002) for monitoring foals with *R. equi*, but SAA may fall quite rapidly and values often are not increased among foals with *R. equi* (Cohen *et al.* 2005b). Thoracic imaging may be used to monitor progression of disease, but some foals will maintain radiographic abnormalities despite resolution of clinical signs and infection with *R. equi*. With the caveat that lesions of the central portion of the lung may be missed, sonographic evaluation of areas of pulmonary abscessation or consolidation – in conjunction with clinical signs – is a convenient and effective way for monitoring progress and deciding the duration of treatment: treatment in a clinically healthy foal may be discontinued within days of resolution of sonographic evidence of pulmonary abscessation or consolidation.

Some other aspects of treatment merit mention. When using macrolides, avoidance of heat and humidity is desirable. This may entail the use of misting fans, providing shade and cooling, or moving foals to another geographical region. Foals with respiratory distress probably benefit from intranasal oxygen treatment. Some foals may benefit from the administration of a bronchodilator (such as clenbuterol), and administration of a nonsteroidal anti-inflammatory drug (such as flunixin meglumine) may reduce inflammation and fever in affected foals. The authors often administer a pro-biotic/pre-biotic (such as *Saccharomyces boulardii*) to foals receiving macrolides for *R. equi* in an effort to reduce the incidence of diarrhoea (clinical evidence of the value of this practice is lacking). The value of administration of hyperimmune plasma as an adjunct to treatment has not been examined. Foals that fail to thrive, including those in which pneumonia appears to be improving, should be examined for an intra-abdominal abscess or other EPD.

Treatment of EPDs will vary according to the type of lesion. Intra-abdominal abscesses generally carry a poor prognosis (Reuss *et al.* 2008), although successful treatment has been reported (Valdes and Johnson 2005). Treatment of these cases is generally prolonged, and surgical approaches such as marsupialisation or extirpation yield poor results. Immune-mediated EPDs, such as polysynovitis, generally resolve with successful treatment of the accompanying pneumonia. Exercise should be limited but not eliminated in foals with polysynovitis. Although the authors have occasionally used systemic or intra-articular corticosteroids to manage cases of polysynovitis, this practice is generally discouraged because septic arthritis can occur with *R. equi* infection (Reuss *et al.* 2008) and corticosteroid use might worsen the severity of this potentially life-threatening EPD. Other septic EPDs may require drainage of abscesses/pyogranulomas, curettage of bone or intravenous or intraosseous regional limb perfusion with antimicrobial agents for osteomyelitis etc. Many EPDs are not detected until necropsy, while some (such as intra-abdominal abscessation) are associated with poor prognosis.

Control and prevention

As for any infectious disease, it is better to control or prevent the occurrence of disease rather than to attempt to treat affected cases. The authors advocate a 3-tined approach to control and prevention of *R.*

equi foal pneumonia for affected farms: 1) treating affected foals; 2) screening foals to detect pre-clinical disease; and, 3) preventing foals from developing the disease.

Treatment of foals was discussed in the preceding section. One aspect of treatment that was not covered but that is germane to control and prevention is whether affected foals should be isolated. The fact that virulent isolates are widespread in the environment of foals, that the disease course is insidious (such that exposure of other foals has probably been long-standing by the time a diagnosis is made), and that clinical or epidemiological evidence of foal-to-foal transmission is lacking argue against the need for isolation. On the other hand, the fact that foals amplify the organism in their intestinal tract (Takai *et al.* 1986) indicates that they may contribute to the environmental burden of virulent *R. equi*. Because the airborne burden of virulent *R. equi* has been associated with farm incidence of disease (Muscatello *et al.* 2006a, 2007), it is conceivable that isolating foals might help to confine the extent to which they contribute to environmental contamination. Whether isolation of affected foals might impact incidence of disease is unknown, and to the authors' knowledge most farms and hospitals do not isolate affected foals.

The rationale for screening is that detecting the disease early in its course will shorten the duration and improve the clinical outcome of treatment. A variety of screening methods exist, including visual inspection, physical examination, haematological or serumal assays, and thoracic imaging. These methods can be applied individually, in sequence/series, or in parallel.

Visual inspection by farm personnel to detect changes in attitude, increased respiratory effort, coughing, nasal discharge, or detectable EPDs such as polyarthritis can be useful to detect foals that may have *R. equi* pneumonia. Performing a physical examination, including measuring rectal temperature and auscultation of lung sounds may be useful for screening. The latter, however, is often of limited sensitivity early in the course of disease.

Evidence exists that concentration of WBCs may be useful for screening purposes: a WBC concentration >15 x 10^9 cells/l was observed to have a sensitivity of 79% and specificity of 91% among foals at an endemic farm (Giguère *et al.* 2003a). Although sensitivity of fibrinogen concentration >4 g/l was 91%, the corresponding specificity was only 51% in that same study.

Various serological tests for detecting antibodies against *R. equi* in serum have been developed, including tests using enzyme-linked immunosorbent assay (ELISA), agar-gel immunodiffusion (AGID), and serum haemolysis inhibition (SHI) methodologies. Independently, our laboratories have demonstrated that these tests lack adequate accuracy for diagnostic purposes (Martens *et al.* 2002; Giguère *et al.* 2003b). Moreover, these tests appear to lack accuracy as screening tests (Martens *et al.* 2002). The accuracy of SAA also appears to be too limited to be of value for screening (Cohen *et al.* 2005b). Recently, clinically reasonable sensitivities (i.e. >75%) have been reported using either polymerase chain reaction (PCR) or microbiological culture for detection of *R. equi* in the faeces of foals with *R. equi* pneumonia (Pusterla *et al.* 2007; Lämmer and Venner 2008). The value of testing faeces for virulent *R. equi* using culture or PCR as a screening test for *R. equi* pneumonia remains to be determined.

Thoracic imaging can be useful to screen foals for evidence of *R. equi* pneumonia. Radiography has the advantages of being able to detect either axial or peripheral pulmonary lesions in foals that may be showing few or no clinical signs of disease, and of being more specific for screening than visual inspection, physical examination and haematological findings. Disadvantages include the time, effort, and expense required to apply radiography to multiple foals on a repetitive basis, the requirement for multiple individuals to participate in the process, the time required to process images, radiation exposure of personnel involved, and the fact that early lesions may be subtle and easily missed.

Ultrasonography is increasingly being used in North America to screen foals to detect pre- or sub-clinical pneumonia attributed to *R. equi* (Slovis *et al.* 2005). Advantages of screening with *R. equi* include the fact that it should be more specific than results of visual inspection, physical examination and haematological findings, and results are available in real time. Disadvantages include the fact that the presence of ultrasonographically apparent pulmonary abscessation or consolidation does not equate to a microbiological diagnosis of *R. equi* (i.e. other agents might cause such lesions), that only peripheral pulmonary lesions can be visualised, the costs associated with repetitive thoracic ultrasonography, and the dilemmas that result from detecting an increased prevalence of apparent disease. Ultrasonographic detection appears to be increasing the apparent prevalence of disease because of the identification of foals that have sub-clinical disease, which might regress spontaneously without development of apparent clinical signs. The ratio of foals that are pre-clinical to those that will remain sub-clinical is not known, but it is assumed to be large. Although detecting and managing preclinical infection probably improves clinical outcomes, it appears that foals with pulmonary lesions that would have remained sub-clinical are being identified and treated. Thus, the number of foals being treated for presumed *R. equi* pneumonia at breeding farms is increasing, thereby increasing both the risk of adverse events (such as antimicrobial-associated diarrhoea) and the pressure for development of resistance. To the authors' knowledge, systematic evaluation of the cost-benefit of sonographic screening has not been examined.

Screening tests for *R. equi* pneumonia generally must be applied iteratively. Screening should be initiated when foals are aged 2–3 weeks. The testing strategy and the frequency with which tests should be applied will vary according to the test (e.g. visual inspection vs. thoracic radiography) used, and the preferences of the individual veterinarians and farm staff responsible for farm health management. The approach to screening must be tailored to the needs and resources of the farm and veterinarian(s) providing care. Nevertheless, examinations performed monthly are probably too far apart to be valuable for screening.

It is important to recall that a positive result of a screening test (a screening diagnosis) is not the same as the result of a definitive diagnostic test (a definitive diagnosis). As for diagnostic tests, not all positive results of screening tests will be truly positive, and a test with high sensitivity and specificity may perform disappointingly depending on the prevalence of disease at the farm where screening is to be applied. The goal is to maximise the positive- and negative-predictive values of the screening test(s) being used. It is important to consider both the risks and benefits of treating false-positive screening test results. This requires a good understanding of the principles of screening test performance (a topic beyond the scope of this report), and discussing the principles and goals of screening, in practical terms, with all interested parties.

It is the authors' opinion that screening is undervalued as an approach for controlling pneumonia caused by *R. equi*. Although screening for *R. equi* is generally labourious, diligent attention to existing methods (such as careful visual inspection, efficient but expert physical examination, CBCs and thoracic imaging) will probably have the greatest impact on mortality from this disease at farms with affected foals. Moreover, morbidity might also eventually decline with dedicated efforts to screening, along with updating screening approaches to account for reduced positive-predictive value of positive results with falling prevalence of the disease.

Methods for preventing *R. equi* pneumonia are exiguous. An effective vaccine is not currently available, although many skilled and innovative experts continue to pursue this aim. To date, only transfusion of hyperimmune plasma and chemoprophylaxis with azithromycin have been documented to be effective for preventing *R. equi* pneumonia. As described below, evidence of failure also exists for both of these approaches.

Transfusion of hyperimmune plasma was the first documented approach for reducing disease incidence and death attributable to both experimental and naturally occurring infection in foals (Martens *et al.* 1989; Madigan *et al.* 1991; Muller and Madigan 1992). Subsequent to those pioneering studies, a number of reports have yielded information regarding the effectiveness of *R. equi* hyperimmune plasma (**Table 1**). Although the data are conflicting, all studies apart from Hurley and Begg (1995) identified positive values of the relative risk reduction, indicating that transfusion of hyperimmune plasma has some ameliorating effects but that the process is not completely (i.e. 100%) effective. The optimal amount of plasma that needs to be transfused and the optimal age at which transfusion should occur remain to be determined. Although the initial report of experimental protection (Martens *et al.* 1989) described transfusion of 40 ml/kg bwt of plasma to pony foals (equivalent to the administration of 2 l to a 50 kg/foal), most veterinarians administer 1 l at a given time to each foal. Because of evidence that most foals become infected early in life, we recommend that

TABLE 1: Effectiveness of transfusion of hyperimmune plasma to prevent *R. equi* foal pneumonia: published reports of studies with contemporaneous controls

Incidence* with plasma	Incidence* without plasma	Relative risk reduction#	P<0.05[!]	Source
3%	43%	93%	Yes	Madigan *et al.* (1991)
8%	50%	84%	Yes	Muller and Madigan (1992)
17%	30%	43%	Yes	Malschitzky *et al.* (2005)
4%	30%	87%	Yes	Malschitzky *et al.* (2005)
6%	26%	77%	No	Higuchi *et al.* (1999)
19%	30%	37%	No	Giguère *et al.* (2002)
6%	15%	60%	No	Chaffin *et al.* (2003a)
27%	21%	-30%	No	Hurley and Begg (1995)

*Incidence = cumulative incidence of *R. equi* pneumonia among foals transfused with hyperimmune plasma (first column) or foals from the same farm that did not receive plasma. #Relative risk reduction = ([incidence without plasma – incidence with plasma]/incidence without plasma] X 100%. [!]P value for statistical comparison of incidence of *R. equi* pneumonia among foals that received plasma and those that did not receive plasma.

foals receive transfusion of 1 or 2 l of hyperimmune plasma no later than the second day *post partum*. Many veterinarians also administer a second transfusion at 3–4 weeks of age. Because endemicity of *R. equi* at farms does not appear to be explained by farm-specific isolates (Cohen *et al.* 2003), there is no need to administer plasma that is produced from immunising horses with isolates of *R. equi* obtained from a given farm; transfusion of plasma from horses that have been immunised against a virulent strain of *R. equi* should suffice. Transfusion of hyperimmune plasma is not completely effective and therefore does not eliminate the need for screening. In addition to being incompletely effective, transfusion of hyperimmune plasma carries some risk to foals, both in terms of trauma that may occur during handling and adverse reactions to transfusions. The process is also time- and labour-intensive, and plasma is expensive (although administration is generally cost-effective when transfusion leads to reduced morbidity and mortality).

Because of the aforementioned limitations of transfusion of hyperimmune plasma, our laboratories (and others) have explored approaches for chemoprophylaxis or immunoprophylaxis. Recently, it was demonstrated that chemoprophylaxis with azithromycin (10 mg/kg bwt *per os* every 48 h for 7 total doses beginning on the first day *post partum*) resulted in a statistically significant relative risk reduction of approximately 80% among 338 foals at 10 farms in the United States (Chaffin *et al.* 2008). Overall, the cumulative incidence was reduced from 21% in controls to 5% in treated foals. Interestingly, at a farm with cumulative incidence of abscessing pneumonia in foals attributed primarily to *R. equi* of approximately 75%/year, use of azithromycin (10 mg/kg bwt by mouth every 48 h for 14 doses beginning on the first day *post partum*) was not effective (Venner *et al.* 2009). The reason for this discrepancy is unclear, and merits further investigation.

Because of concerns of development of resistance to an antimicrobial widely used to treat people and other animals, the authors DO NOT advocate widespread use of azithromycin for chemoprophylaxis against *R. equi* pneumonia. Nevertheless, the study by Chaffin *et al.* (2008) provides important data for proof-of-concept for chemoprophylaxis against *R. equi* pneumonia with alternative anti-infective strategies. One such strategy is administration of the trivalent semi-metal gallium maltolate. Gallium accumulates in areas of inflammation, infection, macrophages, neutrophils, and many bacteria (Bernstein 1998; Bernstein *et al.* 2000). Trivalent gallium competes with trivalent iron for binding sites on iron-binding proteins, but unlike trivalent iron it cannot be reduced to the divalent state under physiological conditions. Thus, it does not enter ferrous-bearing molecules such as haem and does not interfere with oxygen transport or other vital bodily functions. Protein-bound trivalent gallium is acquired by bacteria instead of protein-bound trivalent iron. Because the trivalent gallium cannot be reduced, DNA polymerases of bacteria that require reduced (divalent) iron as a co-factor fail, and bacterial replication is inhibited. It has been demonstrated that gallium nitrate: kills virulent *R. equi* and that this effect is mediated by interfering with iron metabolism; can reduce tissue concentrations of virulent *R. equi* in experimentally infected mice; can kill virulent *R. equi* within macrophages; is well absorbed from the intestinal tract of foals; and is safe when administered orally or by gavage in foals (Harrington *et al.* 2006; Martens *et al.* 2006, 2007a,b). A randomised, blinded, placebo-controlled clinical trial to evaluate the effectiveness of gallium maltolate for preventing *R. equi* pneumonia is ongoing, and results are expected by the spring of 2009 (M.K. Chaffin, unpublished data).

Immunity plays an important role in protecting against *R. equi* infection (Hines *et al.* 1997). Deficiencies in expression of cytokines such as interferon-gamma (IFN-γ) have been documented in neonatal foals (Boyd *et al.* 2003; Breathnach *et al.* 2006). Investigators have therefore examined the effects of various immunomodulators on cellular responses of foals (Sturgill and Horohov 2006; Liu *et al.* 2008; Ryan and Giguère 2008). None of these immunomodulators, however, has been examined in the field using a randomised, controlled clinical trial. Thus, the effectiveness of such an approach remains to be determined.

References

Ainsworth, D.M,, Eicker, S.W., Yeager, A.E., Sweeney, C.R., Viel, L., Tesarowski, D., Lavoie, J.P., Hoffman, A., Paradis, M.R, Reed, S.M. and Erb, H.N. (1998) Associations between physical examination, laboratory, and radiographic findings and outcome and subsequent racing performance of foals with *Rhodococcus equi* infection: 115 cases (1984-1992). *J. Am. vet. med. Ass.* **213**, 510-515.

Baverud, V., Franklin, A., Gunnarsson, A., Gustafsson, A. and Hellander-Edman, A. (1998) *Clostridium difficile* associated with acute colitis in mares when their foals are treated with erythromycin and rifampicin for *Rhodococcus equi* pneumonia. *Equine vet. J.* **30**, 482-488.

Bernstein, L.R. (1998) Mechanisms of therapeutic activity for gallium. *Pharmacol. Rev.* **50**, 665-682.

Bernstein, L.R., Tanner, T., Godfrey, C. and Noll, B. (2000) Chemistry and pharmacokinetics of gallium maltolate, a compound with high oral gallium bioavailability. *Met. Based Drugs* **7**, 33-47.

Bosnar, M., Keleneric, Z., Munic, V., Erakovic, V. and Parnham, M.J. (2005) Cellular uptake and efflux of azithromycin, erythromycin, clarithromycin, telithromycin, and cethromycin. *Antimicrob. Agents Chemother.* **49**, 2372-2377.

Boyd, N.K., Cohen, N.D., Lim, W.S., Martens, R.J., Chaffin, M.K., and Ball, J.M. (2003) Temporal changes in cytokine expression of foals during the first month of life. *Vet. Immunol. Immunopathol.* **92**, 75-85.

Breathnach, C.C., Sturgill-Wright, T., Stiltner, J.L., Adams, A.A., Lunn, D.P. and Horohov, D.W. (2006) Foals are interferon gamma-deficient at birth. *Vet. Immunol. Immunopathol.* **112**, 199-209.

Chaffin, M.K., Cohen, N.D. and Martens, R.J. (2003a) Foal-related risk factors associated with development of *Rhodococcus equi* pneumonia on farms with endemic infection. *J. Am. vet. med. Ass.* **222**,476-485.

Chaffin, M.K., Cohen, N.D. and Martens, R.J. (2003b) Evaluation of equine breeding farm management and preventative health practices as risk factors for development of *Rhodococcus equi* pneumonia in foals. *J. Am. vet. med. Ass.* **222**, 467-75.

Chaffin, M.K., Cohen, N.D. and Martens, R.J. (2008) Chemoprophylactic effects of azithromycin against *Rhodococcus equi*-induced pneumonia among foals at equine breeding farms with endemic infections. *J. Am. vet. med. Ass.* **232**, 1035-1047.

Clark, C.R. (2008) *Investigation of the Potential use, Pharmacokinetics, and Safety of Tilmicosin in Horses.* Doctoral Thesis, Department of Veterinary Biomedical Sciences, University of Saskatchewan, Saskatoon, Canada. Accessed on 30th October 2008 at http://sundog.usask.ca/search~S5/?searchtype=a&searcharg=Clark%2CChristopher+Robert&searchscope=5&SORT=D&extended=0&SUBMIT=Search&searchlimits=&searchorigarg=aChristopher+Clark

Cohen, N.D., O'Conor, M.S., Chaffin, M.K. and Martens, R.J. (2005a) Farm characteristics and management practices associated with development of *Rhodococcus equi* pneumonia in foals. *J. Am. vet. med. Ass.* **226**, 404-413.

Cohen, N.D., Chaffin, M.K., Vandenplas, M.L., Edwards, R.F., Nevill, M., Moore, J.N. and Martens, R.J. (2005b) Study of serum amyloid A concentrations as a means of achieving early diagnosis of *Rhodococcus equi* pneumonia. *Equine vet. J.* **37**, 212-216.

Cohen, N.D., Carter, C.N., Scott, H.M., Chaffin, M.K., Smith, J.L., Grimm, M.B., Kuskie, K.R., Takai, S. and Martens, R.J. (2008) Association of soil concentrations of *Rhodococcus equi* and incidence of pneumonia attributable to *Rhodococcus equi* in foals on farms in central Kentucky. *Am. J. vet. Res.* **69**, 385-95.

Cohen, N.D., Smith, K.E., Ficht, T.A., Takai, S., Libal, M.C., West, B.R., DelRosario, L.S., Becu, T., Leadon, D.P., Buckley, T., Chaffin, M.K. and Martens, R.J. (2003) Epidemiologic study of pulsed-field gel electrophoresis of isolates of *Rhodococcus equi* obtained from horses and horse farms. *Am. J. vet. Res.* **64**,153-161.

Ewing, P.J., Burrrows, G., MacAllister, C. and Clarke, C. (1994) Comparison of oral erythromycin formulations in the horse using pharmacokinetic profiles. *J. vet. Pharmacol. Ther.* **17**, 17-23.

Fietta, A., Merlini, C. and Gialdroni Grassi, G. (1997) Requirements for intracellular accumulation and release of clarithromycin and azithromycin by human phagocytes. *J. Chemother.* **9**, 23-31.

Giguère, S. and Prescott, J.F. (1997) Clinical manifestations, diagnosis, treatment, and prevention of *Rhodococcus equi* infection in foals. *Vet. Microbiol.* **56**, 313-334.

Giguère, S., Gaskin, J.M., Miller, C. and Bowman, J.L. (2002) Evaluation of a commercially available hyperimmune plasma product for prevention of naturally acquired pneumonia caused by *Rhodococcus equi* in foals. *J. Am. vet. med. Ass.* **220**, 59-63.

Giguère, S., Hernandez, J., Gaskin, J. and Miller, C. (2003a) Evaluation of white blood cell concentration, plasma fibrinogen concentration, and an agar gel immunodiffusion test for early identification of foals with *Rhodococcus equi* pneumonia. *J. Am. vet. med. Ass.* **222**, 775-781.

Giguère, S., Hernandez, J., Gaskin, J., Prescott, J.F., Takai, S. and Miller, C. (2003b) Performance of five serological assays for diagnosis of *Rhodococcus equi* pneumonia in foals. *Clin. Diagn. Lab. Immunol.* **10**, 241-245.

Giguère, S., Jacks, S., Roberts, G.D., Hernandez, J., Long, M.T. and, Ellis, C. (2004) Retrospective comparison of azithromycin, clarithromycin, and erythromycin for the treatment of foals with *Rhodococcus equi* pneumonia. *J. vet. Intern. Med.* **18**, 568-573.

Giguère, S., Lee, E., Cohen, N.D., Chaffin, M.K., Halbert, N., Martens, R.J., Franklin, R.P. and Clark, C.C. (2008) Prevalence of *Rhodococcus equi* isolates resistant to macrolides or rifampin and outcome of infected foals. *J. vet. intern. Med.* **22**, 737 (abstract).

Grau, S., Mateu-de Antonio, J., Ribes, E., Salvado, M., Garces, J.M., and Garau, J. (2006) Impact of rifampicin addition to clarithromycin in *Legionella pneumophila* pneumonia. *Int. J. Antimicrob. Agents* **28**, 249-252.

Grimm, M.B., Cohen, N.D., Slovis, N.M., Mundy, G.D., Harrington, J.R., Libal, M.C., Takai, S. and Martens, R.J. (2007) Evaluation of fecal samples from mares as a source of *Rhodococcus equi* for their foals by use of quantitative bacteriologic culture and colony immunoblot analysis. *Am. J. vet. Res.* **68**, 63-71.

Harrington, J.R., Martens, R.J., Cohen, N.D. and Bernstein, L.R. (2006) Antimicrobial activity of gallium against virulent *Rhodococcus equi in vitro* and *in vivo*. *J. vet. Pharmacol. Therap.* **29**, 121-127.

Higuchi, T., Arakawa, T., Hashikura, S., Inui, T., Senba, S. and Takai, S. (1999) Effect of prophylactic administration of hyperimmune plasma to prevent *Rhodococcus equi* infection on foals from endemically affected farms. *Zentralbl. veterinaermed. B.* **46**, 641-648.

Hillidge, C.J. (1987) Use of erythromycin-rifampin combination in treatment of *Rhodococcus equi* pneumonia. *Vet. Microbiol.* **14**, 337-342.

Hines, S.A., Kanaly, S.T., Byrne, B.A., and Palmer, G.H. (1997) Immunity to *Rhodococcus equi*. *Vet. Microbiol.* **56**,177-185.

Hultén, C. and Demmers, S. (2002) Serum amyloid A (SAA) as an aid in the management of infectious disease in the foal: comparison with total leucocyte count, neutrophil count and fibrinogen. *Equine vet. J.* **34**, 693-698.

Hurley, J.R. and Begg, A.P. (1995) Failure of hyperimmune plasma to prevent pneumonia caused by *Rhodococcus equi* in foals. *Aust. vet. J.* **72**, 418-420.

Jacks, S., Giguère, S. and Nguyen, A. (2003) *In vitro* susceptibilities of *Rhodococcus equi* and other common equine pathogens to azithromycin, clarithromycin, and 20 other antimicrobials. *Antimicrob. Agents Chemoth.* **47**,1742-1745.

Jacks, S., Giguère, S., Gronwall, P.R., Brown, M.P. and Merritt, K.A.. (2001) Pharmacokinetics of azithromycin and concentration in body fluids and bronchoalveolar cells in foals. *Am. J. vet. Res.* **62**,1870-1875.

Jacks, S., Giguère, S., Gronwall, R.R., Brown, M.P. and Merritt K.A. (2002) Disposition of oral clarithromycin in foals. *J. vet. Pharmacol. Therap.* **25**, 359-62.

Lakritz, J. and Wilson, W.D. (2002) Erythromycin and other macrolide antibiotics for treating *Rhodococcus equi* pneumonia in foals. *Comp. cont. Educ. pract. Vet.* **24**, 256-261.

Lakritz, J., Wilson, W.D., Marsh, A.E. and Mihalyi, J.E. (2000) Effects of prior feeding on pharmacokinetics and estimated bioavailability after oral administration of a single dose of microencapsulated erythromycin base in healthy foals. *Am. J. vet. Res.* **61**,1011-5.

Lakritz, J., Wilson, W.D., Watson, J.L., Hyde, D.M., Mihalyi, J. and Plopper, C.G. (1997) Effect of treatment with erythromycin on bronchoalveolar lavage fluid cell populations in foals. *Am. J. vet. Res.* **58**, 56-61.

Lämmer, M. and Venner, M. (2008) Shedding of *Rhodococcus equi* in faecal and tracheal secretions of foals with pulmonary abscesses. In: *Proceedings of the 4th Havemeyer Workshop on* Rhodococcus equi **4**, 76 (abstract).

Leclercq, R. and Courvalin, P. (2002) Resistance to macrolides and related antibiotics in *Streptococcus pneumoniae*. *Antimicrob. Agents Chemother.* **46**, 2727-2734.

Liu, T., Nerrren, J., Murrell, J., Juillard, V., El Garch, H., Martens, R.J. and Cohen, N.D. (2008) CpG-induced stimulation of cytokine expression by peripheral blood mononuclear cells of foals and their dams. *J. equine vet. Sci.* **28**, 419-426.

Madigan, J.E., Hietala, S. and Muller, N. (1991) Protection against naturally acquired *Rhodococcus equi* pneumonia in foals by administration of hyperimmune plasma. *J. Reprod. Fertil.*, Suppl. **44**, 571-578.

Malschitzky, E., Neves, A.P., Gregory, R.M. and Mattos, R.C. (2005) Reduzir o uso da cocheira a incidencia de infeccoes por *Rhodococcus equi* em potros. *A Hora vet.* **24**, 27-30.

Martens, R.J., Martens, J.G., Fiske, R.A. and Hietala, S.K. (1989) *Rhodococcus equi* foal pneumonia: protective effects of immune plasma in experimentally infected foals. *Equine vet. J.* **21**, 249-255.

Martens, R.J., Takai, S., Cohen, N.D., Chaffin, M.K., Liu, H., Sakurai, K., Sugimoto, H. and Lingsweiler, S.W. (2000) Association of disease with isolation and virulence of *Rhodococcus equi* from farm soil and foals with pneumonia. *J. Am. vet. med. Ass.* **217**, 220-225.

Martens, R.J., Harrington, J.R., Cohen, N.D., Chaffin, M.K., Mealey, K., Tayor, R.J. and Bernstein, L.R. (2006) Gallium therapy: a novel metal-based antimicrobial strategy for potential control of *Rhodococcus equi* foal pneumonia. *Proc. Am. Ass. equine Practnrs.* **52**, 219-221.

Martens, R.J., Mealey, K., Cohen, N.D., Harrington, J.R., Chaffin, M.K., Taylor, R.J. and Bernstein, L.R. (2007a) Pharmacokinetics of gallium maltolate after intragastric administration in neonatal foals. *Am. J. vet. Res.* **68**, 1041-1044.

Martens, R.J., Miller, N.A., Cohen, N.D., Harrington, J.R. and Bernstein, L.R. (2007b) Chemoprophylactic antimicrobial activity of gallium maltolate against intracellular *Rhodococcus equi*. *J. equine vet. Sci.* **27**, 341-345.

Martens, R.J., Cohen, N.D., Chaffin, M.K., Takai, S., Doherty, C.L., Angulo, A.B. and Edwards, R.E. (2002) Evaluation of 5 serologic assays to detect *Rhodococcus equi* pneumonia in foals. *J. Am. vet. med. Ass.* **221**, 825-33.

Moron, A.C., Begg, A.P., Anderson, G.A., Takai, S. Lämmler, C. and Browning, G.F. (2001) Epidemiology of *Rhodococcus equi* strains on Thoroughbred horse farms. *Appl. Environ. Microbiol.* **67**, 2167-2175.

Muller, N. and Madigan, J.E. (1992) Methods of implementation of an immunoprophylaxisis program for the prevention of *Rhodococcus equi* pneumonia: results of 5 years study. *Proc. Am. Ass. equine Practnrs.* **38**, 274-278.

Muscatello, G., Anderson, G.A., Gilkerson, J.R. and Browning, G.F. (2006) Associations between the ecology of virulent *Rhodococcus equi* and the epidemiology of *R. equi* pneumonia on Australian Thoroughbred farms. *Appl. Environ. Microbiol.* **72**, 6152–6160.

Muscatello, G.,Lowe, J.M., Flash, M.L., McBride, K.L., Browning, G.F. and Gilkerson, J.F. (2007) Review of the epidemiology and ecology of *Rhodococcus equi. Proc. Am. Ass. equine Practnrs.* **53**, 214-217.

Muscatello, G., Gerbaud, S., Kennedy, C., Gilkerson, J.R., Buckley, T., Klay, M., Leadon, D.P. and Browning, G.F. (2006) Comparison of concentrations of *Rhodococcus equi* and virulent *R. equi* in air of stables and paddocks on horse breeding farms in a temperate climate. *Equine vet. J.* **38**, 263-265.

Nordmann, P. and Ronco, E. (1992) *In-vitro* antimicrobial susceptibility of *Rhodococcus equi. J. Antimicrob. Chemother.* **29**, 383-393.

Nordmann, P., Kerestedjian, J.J. and Ronco, E. (1994) Therapy of *Rhodococcus equi* disseminated infections in nude mice. *J. Antimicrob. Chemother.* **36**,1244-1248.

Peloquin, C.A. and Berning, S.E. (1996) Evaluation of the drug interaction between clarithromycin and rifampin. *J. Infect. Dis. Pharmacother.* **38**, 830-835.

Phelps, M.S., Wilson, W.D. and Gardner, I.A. (2000) Risk of adverse effects in pneumonic foals treated with erythromycin versus other antibiotics: 143 cases (1986-1996). *J. Am. vet. Med. Ass.* **217**, 68-73.

Prescott, J.F. (1981) The susceptibility of *Corynebacterium equi* to antimicrobial drugs. *J. vet. Pharmacol. Therap.* **4**, 27-31.

Prescott, J.F. (1991) *Rhodococcus equi*: an animal and human pathogen. *Clinical Microbiol. Rev.* **4**, 20-34.

Prescott, J.F., and Nicholson, V.M. (1984) The effects of combinations of selected antibiotics on the growth of Corynebacterium equi. *J. vet. Pharmacol. Therap.* **7**, 61-64.

Prescott, J.F. and Sweeney, C.R. (1985) Treatment of *Corynebacterium equi* pneumonia of foals. *J. Am. vet. med. Ass.* **187**, 725-728.

Pusterla, N., Wilson, W.D., Mapes, S. and Leutenegger, C.M. (2007) Diagnostic evaluation of real-time PCR in the detection of *Rhodococcus equi* in faeces and nasopharyngeal swabs from foals with pneumonia. *Vet. Rec.* **161**, 272-275.

Reuss, S.M., Chaffin, M.K. and Cohen, N.D. (2008) Extrapulmonary disorders associated with *Rhodococcus equi* infection in foals: a retrospective study of 150 cases (1987-2007). *Proc. Am. Ass. equine Practnrs.* **54**, 528.

Ryan, C. and Giguère, S. (2008) Treatment of neonatal foals with immunostimulants enhances phagocytic cell activity against *ex vivo* infection with *Rhodococcus equi. J. vet. intern. Med.* **22**, 712 (abstract).

Scheuch, E., Spieker, J., Venner, M. and Siegmund, W. (2007) Quantitative determination of the macrolide antibiotic tulathromycin in plasma and broncho-alveolar cells of foals using tandem mass spectroscopy. *J. Chromatograph. B* **850**, 464-470.

Slovis, N.M., McCracken, J.L. and Mundy, G.D. (2005). How to use thoracic ultrasound to screen foals for *Rhodococcus equi* at affected farms. *Proc. Am. Ass. equine Practnrs.* **51**, 274-278.

Sturgill, T.L. and Horohov, D.W. (2006) Interferon-gamma expression in young foals when treated with an immunostimulant or plasma. *Proc. Am. Ass. equine Practnrs.* **52**, 237-241.

Suarez-Mier, G., Giguère, S. and Lee, E.A. (2007) Pulmonary disposition of erythromycin, azithromycin, and clarithromycin in foals. *J. vet. Pharmacol. Therap.* **30**, 109-115.

Sweeney, C.R., Sweeney, R.W. and Divers, T.J. (1987) *Rhodococcus equi* pneumonia in 48 foals:response to antimicrobial therapy. *Vet. Microbiol.* **14**, 326-329.

Takai, S., Ohkura, H., Watanabe, Y. and Tsubaki, S. (1986) Quantitative aspects of fecal *Rhodococcus (Corynebacterium) equi* in foals. *J. Clin. Microbiol.* **23**, 794-796.

Valdes, A. and Johnson, J.R. (2005) Septic pleuritis and abdominal abscess formation caused by *Rhodococcus equi* in a foal. *J. Am. vet. med. Ass.* **227**, 960-963.

Venner, M., Kerth, R. and Klug, E. (2007) Evaluation of tulathromycin in the treatment of pulmonary abscesses in foals. *Vet. J.* **174**, 418-421.

Venner, M., Reinhold, B., Beyerbach, M. and Feige, K. (2009) Efficacy of azithromycin in preventing pulmonary abscesses in foals. *Vet. J.* **179**, 301-303.

Wallace Jr., R.J., Brown, B.A., Griffith, D.E., Girard, W. and Tanaka, K. (1995) Reduced serum levels of clarithromycin in patients treated with multi-drug regimens including rifampin or rifabutin for *Mycobacterium avium-M. intracellulare* infection. *J. Infect. Dis.* **171**, 747-750.

Womble, A.Y., Giguère, S. and Lee, E.A. (2007) Pharmacokinetics of oral doxycycline and concentrations in body fluids and bronchoalveolar cells of foals. *J. vet. Pharmacol. Therap.* **30**, 187-193.

Womble, A.Y., Giguère, S., Lee, E.A. and Vickroy, T.W. (2006a) Pharmacokinetics of clarithromycin and concentrations in body fluids and bronchoalveolar cells of foals. *Am. J. vet. Res.* **67**, 181-186.

Womble, A.Y., Giguère, S., Murthy, Y.V., Cox, C. and Obare, E. (2006b) Pulmonary disposition of tilmicosin in foals and in vitro activity against *Rhodococcus equi* and other common equine bacterial pathogens. *J. vet. Pharmacol. Therap.* **29**, 561-568.

Yamomoto, F., Harada, S., Misuyama, T., Harada, Y. and Kitahara, Y. (2004) Concentration of clarithromycin and 14-R-hydroxy clarithromycin in plasma of patients with Mycobacterium avium complex infection, before and after the addition of rifampicin. *Jap. J. Antbiot.* **57**, 124-133.

CORYNEBACTERIUM PSEUDOTUBERCULOSIS INFECTIONS IN HORSES

S. J. Spier

Dept. of Medicine and Epidemiology, School of Veterinary Medicine, University of California, Davis, California 95616, USA.

Keywords: horse; *Corynebacterium pseudotuberculosis*; pectoral abscess, internal abscess; ulcerative lymphangitis; fly vector

Summary

Corynebacterium pseudotuberculosis is a Gram-positive pleomorphic rod-shaped, intracellular, facultative anaerobe with worldwide distribution. Infection of horses with the organism is most commonly seen in the western USA, particularly California. Infections tend to occur both as sporadic cases on a farm or as outbreaks involving hundreds to thousands of horses in a region. Evidence exists that infection is increasing in incidence, possibly associated with climate change. Three forms have been described in horses: ulcerative lymphangitis or limb infection, external abscesses and internal infection. Treatment of external abscesses requires establishment of drainage. Antimicrobial therapy is indicated for horses with ulcerative lymphangitis and for horses with internal abscesses.

Introduction

Infection caused by *Corynebacterium pseudotuberculosis* in horses assumes many forms. Deep intramuscular abscesses in horses caused by *Corynebacterium pseudotuberculosis* were first reported in San Mateo County, California, USA in 1915 (Hall and Fisher 1915). Since that time, disease caused by these bacteria can be considered one of the most frequent infectious diseases in the western USA, particularly California. Infections tend to occur both as sporadic cases on a farm or as outbreaks involving hundreds to thousands of horses in a region. Evidence exists that infection is increasing in incidence, possibly associated with climate change. Unprecedented epidemics in the past decade have affected thousands of horses in Colorado, New Mexico, Utah, Wyoming, Kentucky, Oregon and Idaho; all states historically low in prevalence (Foley *et al.* 2004; Anon 2007). In 2005, hundreds of horses were affected in southern California, leading to speculation that a new bacterial strain had emerged (Conaughton 2005). High environmental temperatures and drought conditions preceded all reported outbreaks of this soil-dwelling organism. The most common clinical form of the disease, characterised by external abscesses in the pectoral or ventral abdomen, is often called 'pigeon fever', due to the swelling of the horse's pectoral region resembling a pigeon's breast (**Fig 1**), or 'dryland distemper', reflecting the prevalence in arid regions of the western USA. Two other clinical forms of the disease include internal organ involvement such as hepatic, renal or splenic abscesses and infection of the limbs, termed 'ulcerative lymphangitis'.

Aetiology

Corynebacterium pseudotuberculosis is a Gram-positive pleomorphic rod-shaped, intracellular, facultative anaerobe with worldwide distribution. Cases have been reported throughout the USA. Infection has been reported in sheep, goats, cattle, buffalo, camelids, equids and man. *Corynebacterium pseudotuberculosis* grows well at 36°C on blood agar in 24–48 h, and it forms small, pinpoint in diameter, whitish, opaque colonies that are surrounded by a weak zone of haemolysis (Aleman and Spier 2002).

The high content of lipids may facilitate survival of the organism in macrophages (Hard 1975). Two species-specific biotypes of *C. pseudotuberculosis* have been identified based on differences in nitrate reduction (Biberstein *et al.* 1971), and DNA fingerprinting techniques have revealed multiple strains (Sutherland *et al.* 1996; Costa *et al.* 1998; Foley *et al.* 2004). Biotypes isolated from small ruminants are nitrate negative, while those from horses are nitrate positive. Natural cross-species transmission does not seem to occur between sheep and horses; however, cattle can have infection from either biotype (Biberstein *et al.* 1971). *Corynebacterium. pseudotuberculosis* produces various extracellular exotoxins, which play a role in virulence; the most studied is phospholipase D (PLD). Phospholipases are a group of enzymes that share the ability to hydrolyse one or more ester linkage in glycerophospholipids. Phospholipase D is important in the pathogenesis of the disease by its action on cell membranes causing hydrolysis and degradation of sphingomyelin in endothelial cells and increasing vascular permeability, facilitating the spread of the bacteria and persistence in the host. The bacterial phospholipase D is similar to the PLD of the brown recluse spider, which explains the presence of pain and oedema at the site of infection. (Coyle and Lipsky 1990; McNamara 1994). The synergistic activity of *C. pseudotuberculosis* exotoxins with the exotoxins of *Rhodococcus equi* in lysing red blood cells in agar forms the basis for the synergistic haemolysis inhibition (SHI) test (Knight 1978). The SHI test is presently the most useful serological test available to detect IgG antibody to *C. pseudotuberculosis* in horses with internal infections.

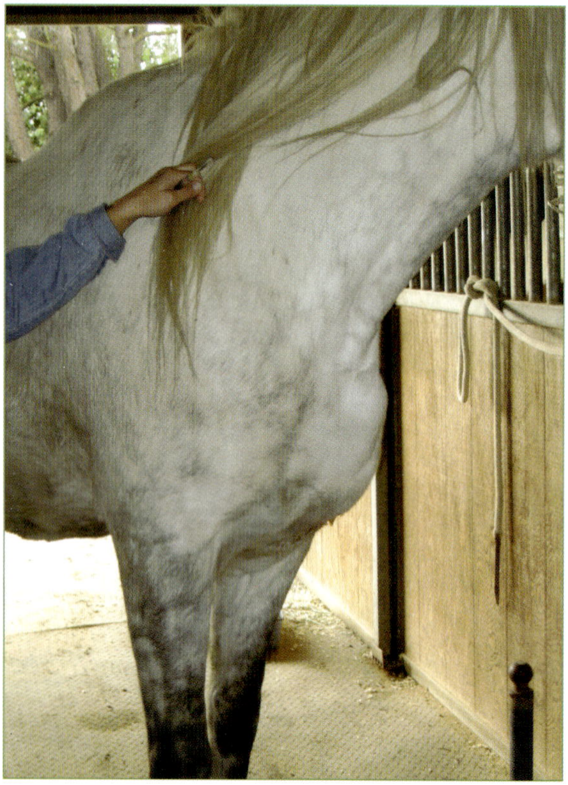

FIGURE 1: Typical pectoral abscess caused by *Corynebacterium pseudotuberculosis.*

Epidemiology

Three forms have been described in horses: ulcerative lymphangitis or limb infection, external abscesses and internal infection. Ulcerative lymphangitis appears as a severe cellulitis, where the lymphatics are affected in one or more limbs with multiple draining ulcerative lesions. In a retrospective study of *C. pseudotuberculosis* infection in horses from California, horses with ulcerative lymphangitis comprised only 1% of the cases, whereas external abscesses occurred in 91%, and internal abscesses in 8% of the cases (Aleman *et al.* 1996). There appears to be no breed or sex predilection for the development of the infection or for any of the 3 forms of disease.

The portal of entry of this soil-dwelling organism is thought to be through abrasions or wounds in the skin or mucous membranes. Many insects have been incriminated as vectors for the transmission of the disease to horses, and studies have shown that *Haematobia irritans*, *Musca domestica* and *Stomoxys calcitrans* can act as mechanical vectors of this

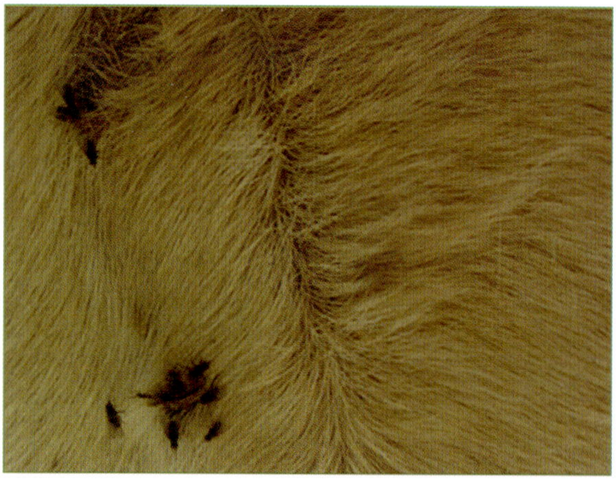

FIGURE 2: Horn flies (*Haematobia irritans*) on the ventral midline of a horse.

disease (Spier *et al.* 2004). The regional location of abscesses suggests that ventral midline dermatitis is a predisposing cause of infection (**Fig 2**). Due to the variable incubation period, ventral midline dermatitis may not be present at the time of maturation of the abscesses.

Temporal and special analysis indicated an incubation period of 3–4 weeks. Within a geographic area, the disease appeared to be transmitted between 7 and 56 days throughout a 4.3–6.5 km distance, strongly suggesting that the disease could be transmitted through horse-to-horse contact or from infected to susceptible horses via insects, other vectors, or contaminated soil (Doherr *et al.* 1999). The organism has been shown to survive for up to 2 months in hay and shavings, and >8 months in soil samples at environmental temperatures (Augustine and Renshaw 1982, 1986). The incidence of disease fluctuates considerably from year to year presumably due to herd immunity and environmental factors such rainfall and temperature. To date, the definitive environmental factors supporting the spread of infection have not been proven (Doherr 1997). Disease incidence is seasonal, with highest number of cases occurring during the dry months of the year, which is late summer and autumn in the southwestern USA, although cases may be seen all year. Horses with internal infection are more frequently seen 1–2 months following the peak number of cases with external abscesses (Vaughan *et al.* 2004).

Horses of all ages may be affected, although the low incidence of disease in foals aged <6 months suggests that passive transfer of immunoglobulins offer protection in foals born in endemic areas. A case-control study in an endemic area revealed that young adults (<5 years), and horses in contact with other horses on summer pasture had increased risk of infection. Horses housed outside or with access to an outside paddock appeared to be at higher risk than stabled horses (Doherr *et al.* 1998).

Clinical findings

External abscesses may occur anywhere on the body, but most frequently develop in the pectoral region and along the ventral midline of the abdomen. Abscesses contain tan, odour-free purulent exudate and are usually well encapsulated. Additional sites for abscess formation are the prepuce, mammary gland, axilla, limbs and head. Other less common areas are the thorax, neck, parotid gland, guttural pouches, larynx, flanks, umbilicus, tail and rectum. Septic joints and osteomyelitis have been reported (Aleman *et al.* 1996). Horses may have an abscess involving a single site, or involving multiple regions of the body. Generally, horses with external abscesses do not usually develop signs of systemic illness, although 25% will develop fever (Aleman *et al.* 1996). If signs of systemic illness are present, further diagnostics to rule out internal infection are warranted. The case fatality for horses with external abscesses is very low (0.8%) (Aleman *et al.* 1996). Clinical pathological abnormalities that may be observed include anaemia of chronic disease, leucocytosis with neutrophilia, hyperfibrinogenaemia and hyperproteinaemia. These haematological parameters can occur with either internal or external abscesses but are more consistently observed with internal abscesses.

Internal infection occurs in approximately 8% of affected horses, which is associated with a case fatality rate of 30–40% (Aleman *et al.* 1996). Diagnosis can be challenging, and long-term antimicrobial therapy is imperative for successful outcome. In a retrospective study, the organs most commonly involved were liver and lungs, with kidney and spleen being affected less often. Abdominal ultrasound was a useful diagnostic technique to specifically identify affected abdominal organs (Vaughan *et al.* 2004; Pratt *et al.* 2005) (**Fig 3**).

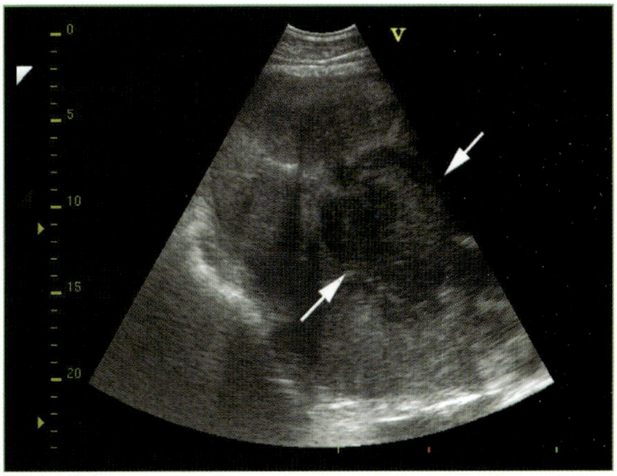

FIGURE 3: Renal abscess (arrows); Courtesy of MaryBeth Whitcomb.

A diagnosis of internal infection is based on clinical signs, clinicopathological data, serology, diagnostic imaging and bacterial culture. The most common clinical signs are concurrent external abscesses, decreased appetite, fever, lethargy, weight loss, and signs of respiratory disease or abdominal pain. Other signs observed in horses with internal abscesses include ventral oedema, ventral dermatitis, ataxia, haematuria (due to renal abscesses) and, uncommonly, abortion.

Serological testing using the synergistic haemolysis inhibition (SHI) test can be useful in aiding the diagnosis of internal abscesses (Knight 1978; Pratt *et al.* 2005). The SHI test measures IgG to the exotoxin of *C. pseudotuberculosis* and is available through the California Animal Health and Food Safety Laboratory System in Davis, California, and the Colorado State University Veterinary Diagnostic Laboratories in Fort Collins, Colorado. Serology is generally not helpful for diagnosis of external abscesses and may be negative early in the course of disease and even the time of abscess drainage. Positive SHI titres must be interpreted carefully and combined with clinical signs to distinguish active infection from exposure or convalescence. Both published and unpublished data from the University of California suggest that a reciprocal titre of ≥256 is indicative of active infection. Horses with internal abscesses generally have SHI titres ≥512. Titres ≤16 are considered negative, while titres between 16 and 128 are considered suspicious or indicative of exposure (S.K. Hietala, personal communication). These are rough guidelines, however, as there is considerable overlap in results from horses with active disease, exposure and recovery from infection.

Ulcerative lymphangitis is the least common form seen in North America, although this form of disease has been reported worldwide. Limb swelling (more commonly hindlimbs are affected), cellulitis and draining tracts following the lymphatics are seen. Horses often develop a severe lameness, fever, lethargy and anorexia. Aggressive medical therapy (antimicrobial and anti-inflammatory) is necessary or the disease often becomes chronic, resulting in limb oedema, prolonged or recurrent infection, lameness, weakness, and weight loss (**Fig 4**).

Therapy

The treatment regimen for external abscesses must be individualised for each horse depending on the severity of disease, including the presence of systemic illness such as fever or anorexia, the extent of soft tissue inflammation, the maturity of the abscess and the ability to successfully establish drainage of purulent exudate. Establishing drainage is the most important treatment and ultimately leads to faster resolution and return to athletic performance. The proximity of the fibrous abscess capsule to the skin varies, often being <1 cm deep for ventral midline abscesses, to >10 cm deep underlying muscle for some pectoral, axillary, triceps or inguinal abscesses. Aspiration and drainage of superficial abscesses is easily performed; however, the use of diagnostic ultrasound is helpful for localisation of deeper abscesses and to judge maturity of the abscess and proximity to the skin. The abscess contents and

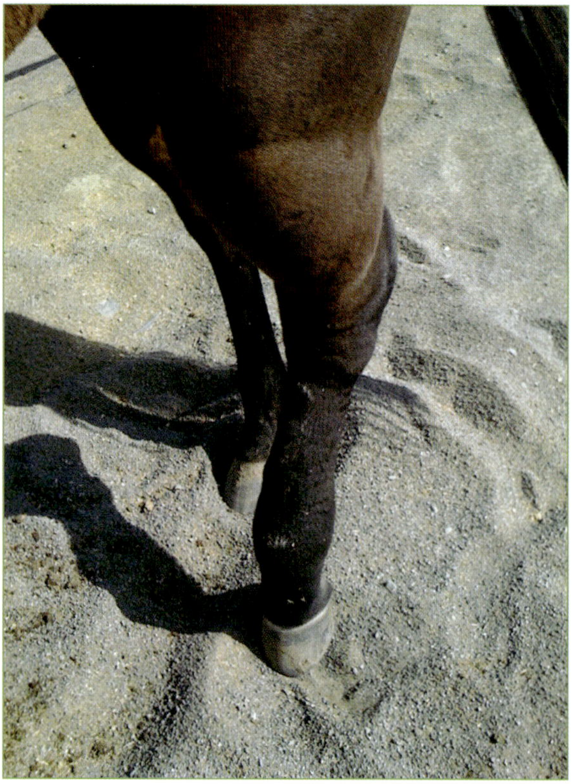

FIGURE 4: Ulcerative lymphangitis is the term used for infection involving the limbs. Aggressive antimicrobial and anti-inflammatory medication is indicated for resolution.

lavage solutions, such as saline with or without antiseptic, should be retrieved and disposed of to prevent further contamination of the immediate environment.

Antimicrobial therapy

Antimicrobials are indicated for horses with ulcerative lymphangitis and for horses with internal abscesses. The use of antimicrobials for external abscesses is not necessary in most horses and may prolong the time to resolution (Aleman *et al.* 1996). Antimicrobial therapy may be justified when signs of systemic illness are present, such as fever, depression and anorexia, or when extensive cellulitis is present. Horses with deep intramuscular abscesses that are lanced and draining through healthy tissue may also benefit from antimicrobial therapy.

Corynebacterium pseudotuberculosis is susceptible *in vitro* to many antimicrobials commonly used in horses, including penicillin G, macrolides, tetracyclines, cephalosporins, chloramphenicol fluoroquinolones and rifampicin, but some isolates may be resistant to aminoglycosides (Adamson *et al.* 1985; Judson and Songer 1991; Foley *et al.* 2004). Several factors should be considered when choosing an antimicrobial. The intracellular location of the organism, the presence of exudates and a thick abscess capsule, and the duration of therapy are important as are the cost of the drug and the convenience of administration. Despite *in vitro* susceptibility, the nature of the bacterium and the copious exudate render certain antimicrobials ineffective for some cases. Trimethoprim-sulpha (5 mg/kg bwt based on the trimethoprim fraction, twice daily orally) or procaine penicillin (20,000 iu/kg bwt twice daily i.m.) are effective for external abscesses especially on the ventral midline. Rifampicin (2.5–5 mg/kg bwt twice daily orally) in combination with ceftiofur (2.5–5 mg/kg bwt twice daily i.v. or i.m.) appears highly effective for treatment of internal abscesses. Internal abscesses have reportedly responded to procaine penicillin (dose as above), trimethoprim-sulpha (dose as above), and potassium penicillin (20,000–40,000 iu/kg bwt 4 times daily i.v.) (Pratt *et al.* 2005).

Horses with ulcerative lymphangitis or cellulitis should be treated early and aggressively with antimicrobials or residual lameness or limb swelling may occur. Typically i.v. antimicrobials (ceftiofur or penicillin G) alone or in combination with rifampicin (orally) are used until lameness and swelling improves, and then therapy with orally administered antimicrobials such as trimethoprim sulphamethoxazole or rifampicin are continued to prevent relapse. The time to resolution reported in one study was approximately 35 days (Aleman *et al.* 1996). Physical therapy, including hydrotherapy, hand walking and leg wraps, as well as NSAIDs are recommended.

Prevention

Until a protective bacterin or toxoid is developed for horses, we can only suggest that horse owners in endemic areas practice good sanitation and fly control and avoid unnecessary environmental contamination from diseased horses. Oil based fly repellents provide longer lasting protection than aqueous products. Presently there is no evidence that diseased horses within a stable should be quarantined, other than paying strict attention to insect control. The feed through products containing cyromazine (Solitude)[1] (a chitin inhibitor) are safer than organophosphate products, and may reduce the incidence of disease by controlling vector populations. Proper sanitation, disposal of contaminated bedding, and disinfection may reduce the incidence of new cases. Proper wound care is also important to prevent infection from a contaminated environment.

Research is being performed to develop a protective vaccine for horses. Commercial bacterin-toxoids (Caseous D-T; Glanvac)[2,3] have been used in small ruminants with success and is approved in some countries (Piontkowski and Shivyers 1998). The safety and effectiveness of these sheep and goat products has not been tested in horses and their use is not advised. Use of autogenous bacterin-toxoids designed for horses demonstrated increased SHI titres following 2 injections; however, the level of protection remains to be established. The lack of experimental challenge models to reproduce the disease, and the sporadic incidence of disease complicate research efforts.

Manufacturers' addresses

[1]Pfizer Animal Health, New York, New York, USA.
[2]Colorado Serum Co., Denver, Colorado, USA.
[3]Pfizer Animal Health, West Ryde, New South Wales, Australia.

References

Adamson, P.J.W., Wilson, W.D., Hirsh, D.C., Baggot, J.D. and Martin, L.D. (1985) Susceptibility of equine bacterial isolates to antimicrobial agents. *Am. J. vet. Res.* **46**, 447-450.

Aleman, M.R. and Spier, S.J. (2002) *Corynebacterium pseudotuberculosis* infection. In: *Large Animal Internal Medicine*, 3rd edn., Ed: BP Smith, C.V. Mosby, St Louis. pp 1078-1084.

Aleman, M., Spier, S.J., Wilson, W.D. and Doherr, M. (1996) Retrospective study of *Corynebacterium pseudotuberculosis* infection in horses: 538 cases. *J. Am. vet. med. Ass.* **209**, 804-809.

Anon (2007) The Seattle Times, Oregon horses coming down with pigeon fever. The Associated Press 18th October 2007 http://seattletimes.nwsource.com/html/localnews/2003958953_web pigeionfever18.html

Augustine, J.L. and Renshaw, H.W. (1982) *Corynebacterium pseudotuberculosis* survival in soil samples amended with water. In: *Proceedings of the Third International Conference on Goat Productivity and Diseases.* p 526.

Augustine, J.L. and Renshaw, H.W. (1986) Survival of *Corynebacterium pseudotuberculosis* in axenic purulent exudate on common barnyard fomites. *Am. J. vet. Res.* **47**, 713-715.

Biberstein, E.L., Knight, H.D. and Jang, S. (1971) Two biotypes of *Corynebacterium pseudotuberculosis. Vet. Rec.* **89**, 691-692.

Conaughton, G. (2005) Outbreaks of horse, goat disease stirs area concern. *North County Times*, **121**, No. 261: A1, A6.

Costa, L.R.R., Spier, S.J. and Hirsh, C.H. (1998) Comparative molecular characterization of *Corynebacterium pseudotuberculosis* of different origin. *Vet. Microbiol.* **62**, 135-143.

Coyle, M.B. and Lipsky, B.A. (1990) Coryneform bacteria in infectious diseases: clinical and laboratory aspects. *Clin. Microbiol. Rev.* **3**, 227-246.

Doherr, M.G. (1997) *Epidemiology of Equine* Corynebacterium pseudotuberculosis *Infection in California*, PhD Dissertation, University of California, Davis.

Doherr, M.G., Carpenter, T.E., Wilson W.D. and Gardner, I.A. (1999) Evaluation of temporal and spatial clustering of horses with *Corynebacterium pseudotuberculosis* infection. *Am. J. vet. Res.* **60**, 284-291.

Doherr, M.G., Carpenter, T.E., Hanson, K.M., Wilson, W.D. and Gardner, I.A. (1998) Risk factors associated with *Corynebacterium pseudotuberculosis* infection in California horses. *Prev. vet. Med.* **35**, 229-239.

Foley, J.E., Spier, S.J., Mihalyi, J., Drazenovich, N. and Leutenegger, C.M. (2004) Molecular epidemiologic features of *Corynebacterium pseudotuberculosis* isolated from horses. *Am. J. vet. Res.* **65**, 1734-1737.

Hall, I.C. and Fisher, C.W. (1915) Suppurative lesions in horses and a calf of California due to the diptheroid bacillus of Preisz-Nocard. *J. Am. vet. med. Ass.* **1**, 18-30.

Hard, G.C. (1975) Comparative toxic effect of the surface lipid of *Corynebacterium ovis* on peritoneal macrophages. *Infect. Immun.* **12**, 1439-1449.

Judson, R. and Songer, J.G. (1991) *Corynebacterium pseudotuberculosis: in vitro* susceptibility to 39 antimicrobial agents. *Vet. Microbiol.* **27**, 145-150.

Knight, H.D. (1978) A serologic method for the detection of *Corynebacterium pseudotuberculosis* in horses. *Cornell Vet.* **68**, 220-237.

McNamara, P.J., Bradley, G.A. and Songer, J.G. (1994) Targeted mutagenesis of the phospholipase D gene results in decreased virulence of *Corynebacterium pseudotuberculosis. Mol. Microbiol.* **12**, 921-930.

Piontkowski, M.D. and Shivvers, D.W. (1998) Evaluation of a commercially available vaccine against *Corynebacterium pseudotuberculosis* for use in sheep. *J. Am. vet. med. Ass.* **212**, 1765-1768.

Pratt, S.M., Spier, S.J., Vaughan, B., Whitcomb, M.B. and Wilson, W.D. (2005) Clinical characteristics and diagnostic test results in horses with internal infection caused by *Corynebacterium pseudotuberculosis*: 30 cases (1995-2003). *J. Am. vet. med. Ass.* **227**, 441-448.

Spier, S.J., Leutenegger, C.M., Carroll, S.P., Loye, J.E., Pusterla, J.B., Carpenter, T.E., Mihalyi, J.E. and Madigan, J.E. (2004) Use of real-time polymerase chain reaction-based fluorogenic 5' nuclease assay to evaluate insect vectors of *Corynebacterium pseudotuberculosis* infections in horses. *Am. J. vet. Res.* **65**, 829-834.

Sutherland, S.S., Hart, R.A. and Buller, N.B. (1996) Genetic differences between nitrate-negative and nitrate-positive *C. pseudotuberculosis* strains using restriction fragment length polymorphisms. *Vet. Microbiol.* **49**, 1-9.

Vaughan, B., Whitcomb, M.B., Pratt, S.M. and Spier, S.J. (2004) Ultrasonographic appearance of abdominal organs in 14 horses with systemic *Corynebacterium pseudotuberculosis* infection. *Proc. Am. Ass. equine Practnrs.* **50**, 63-69.

GLANDERS

U. Wernery

Central Veterinary Research Laboratory, PO Box 597, Dubai, United Arab Emirates.

Keywords: horse; donkey; glanders; *Burkholderia mallei*

Summary

Glanders is a highly contagious disease of equids caused by the Gram-negative bacterium *Burkholderia mallei*. The organism is obligatory aerobic, nonspore forming and nonmotile. The disease is currently confined to some areas of Asia, the Middle East, Africa and South America. The disease is characterised by nodules and ulcers in the skin, and by choanal and lung granulomas. Both acute (especially in donkeys) and chronic (especially in horses) forms of the disease occur. No vaccines are currently available against this disease. Glanders is a potential zoonosis.

Introduction

Glanders is a highly contagious disease mainly affecting equids that can occur in both an acute and chronic form. Aristotle (384–322 BC) was the first to describe the disease in donkeys in his book 'History of Animals', and the causal agent was eventually identified in 1882 by Löffler and Schütz in Germany, and by Bouchard and Charrin in France.

The disease is caused by the Gram-negative bacterium *Burkholderia mallei*, and is characterised by nodules or ulcers in the skin, and by choanal and lung granulomas. Glanders is considered to be a major zoonosis and a biological agent by important national and international organisations such as CDC (USA) or WHO (Switzerland). Recently there has been an increasing number of glanders outbreaks in horses in Asia and South America with severe economic impact on the international trade of horses.

Geographic distribution

In previous centuries, when horses were used extensively for traveling, transportation and in wars, glanders was almost ubiquitous and a much-feared disease around the world. However, glanders has almost disappeared now. Nevertheless, sporadic cases are reported in some countries of Asia (India, Pakistan, Afghanistan, Indonesia, Myanmar) (Verma 1981), the Middle East (Iraq, Lebanon, Turkey, UAE) (Arun *et al.* 1999; Wittig *et al.* 2006), Africa (Mauritania, Senegal, Sudan) and South America (Brazil). In many countries the exact prevalence of glanders is unknown, and cases may not be correctly diagnosed or officially reported due to fear of restrictions. The presence of glanders may only be identified when equids are tested for import/export purposes.

Susceptibility

Susceptible animals are primarily equids. Morbidity, pathogenicity and mortality vary between and within species. Donkeys are particularly susceptible and frequently develop the acute form of glanders, whereas horses are more likely to suffer from the chronic form of the disease. Mules are usually affected with an intermediate, subacute form. Occasionally, domestic and wild carnivores, mainly in zoos (Alibasoglu *et al.* 1986), may become infected, as may camelids.

Cattle, sheep and pigs are resistant to glanders. Among laboratory animals, guinea pigs are the most susceptible and therefore the most suitable for isolation of the pathogen (Straus reaction). Human subjects can also contract the disease sometimes with fatal consequences (Srinivasan *et al.* 2001).

The pathogen

Glanders is caused by *Burkholderia (B.) mallei*, previously called *Pseudomonas mallei*, which is a 2–4 μm long and 0.5 μm wide Gram-negative bacterium. It is obligatory aerobic, nonspore forming and nonmotile. The new genus *Burkholderia*, which was created in 1992, encompasses *B. mallei* and *B. pseudomallei*, a very closely related bacillus that is the causative agent of melioidosis. The bacterium is often poorly stained and has a bipolar appearance. Lesions typically contain only a few bacteria (**Fig 1**).

Evidence suggests that *B. mallei* is a mutant of *B. pseudomallei* that lost its flagellae, as well as some enzymes, and the ability to infect several hosts. In previous years glanders was classified in various bacterial genera, which are found in literature before 1992, namely: *Actinobacillus*, *Loefflerella*, *Malleomyces*, *Pfeifferella*, *Pseudomonas*.

B. mallei is best isolated from choanal pus lesions and farcy pipes, but can be impossible to isolate from skin ulcers. Although *B. mallei* grows on a ordinary culture media, optimal growth is obtained on agars containing glycerol, such as brain heart infusion (BHI) agar with 3% glycerol. When culture attempts are carried out, blood agar, MacConkey agar, potato dextrose agar and BHI agar should be included. Growth is slow and agar plates must, therefore, be incubated for at least 72 h at 37°C. *B. mallei* is extremely difficult to isolate due to competitive growth of other bacterial species such as *B. cepacia*, *Pseudomonas* (*Ps.*) *pickettii*, *Ps. fluorescens*, *Ps. alcaligenes*, *Ps. aeruginosa* and *Pasteurella* spp. It grows well on blood agar after 48 h as small round, smooth edged, concave, cream-coloured colonies. On MacConkey agar a moderate growth of small pale-coloured colonies is observed. Good growth is observed on BHI with glycerol after 48 h of incubation showing 3 mm in diameter round, smooth-edged cream-coloured colonies (**Fig 2**).

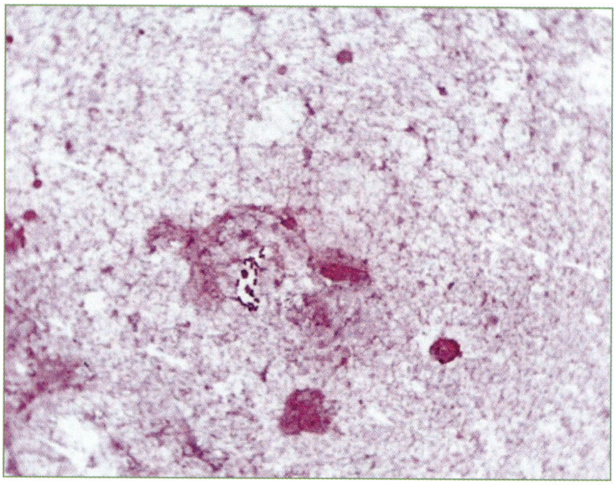

FIGURE 1: Gram stain of choanal lesion showing few Gram-negative rods. B. mallei was isolated from these lesions.

None of the currently available biochemical test kits can clearly differentiate between *B. mallei* and *B. pseudomallei*. *B. mallei* shows positive reaction to arginine dehydrolase (ADA), reduction of nitrites to nitrates, m-acetyl glucosamine assimilation, gluconate assimilation, sodium pyruvate (VP) reaction, glucose, oxidase and catalase (weak) reactions on API 20 NE and E test systems. Differentiation between *B. mallei* and *B. pseudomallei* is performed by polymerase chain reaction (PCR) and genetic typing (Gravelat 1997; Neubauer *et al.* 2006; Scholz *et al.* 2006; Wattiau *et al.* 2007). PCR can even identify the pathogen from formalin-fixed samples.

Resistance

Burkholderia mallei is not very resistant, and is destroyed in 1 min by exposure to a temperature of 61°C, and in 24 h by exposure to direct light. It can survive for 3–5 weeks in damp substrates, one month in tap water and 20–30 days in decomposing material such as pus, nasal discharge or carcasses. In contaminated stables, it can remain viable for at least 6 weeks. It is easily destroyed by common disinfectants such as sodium chloride, 3% cresol, potassium permanganate, copper sulphate and formalin. Burning sulphur (60 g/m^2) on contaminated premises can also be useful for decontamination.

Pathogenesis

The incubation period ranges from 3–14 days, but latent infections can also occur, during which clinical signs may not be evident for several years. Entry of *B.*

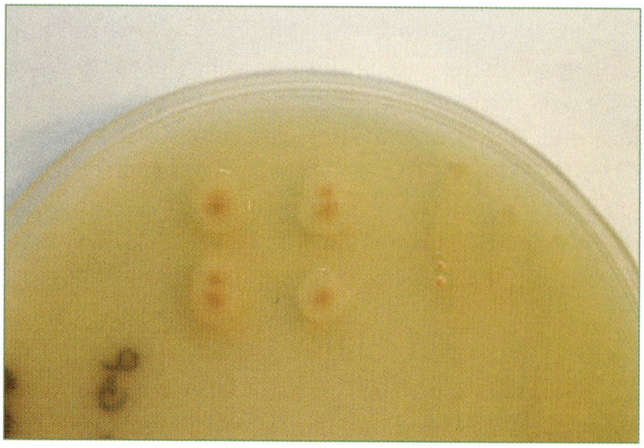

FIGURE 2: B. mallei colonies grown on glycerol potato agar at 37°C for 7 days.

mallei into the body usually takes place through the digestive tract or the skin. In most cases, contaminated feed, water or fomites are the source of infection. Close contact with infected equids or sharing the same feed or water troughs with infected animals are the most common modes of infection. Aerosol infection does not appear to play a role. Carnivores may contract the disease by eating the meat of infected animals. Human subjects contract the disease by direct contact through the skin, nasal or ocular mucosae.

In acute forms of the disease, the organism is distributed throughout the body and also in exudates or secretions, namely pus and other discharges, as well as tears, saliva, urine and faeces. However, the blood of glanderous equids is poorly virulent, unlike the blood of infected human patients and carnivores. In chronic forms of the disease, the organisms are confined to the affected organs and exudates. The danger of chronically infected, asymptomatic carriers must be emphasised. Some animals suffering from latent lung infection may not excrete *B. mallei* until lesions are reactivated when the animals are stressed or kept in poor conditions.

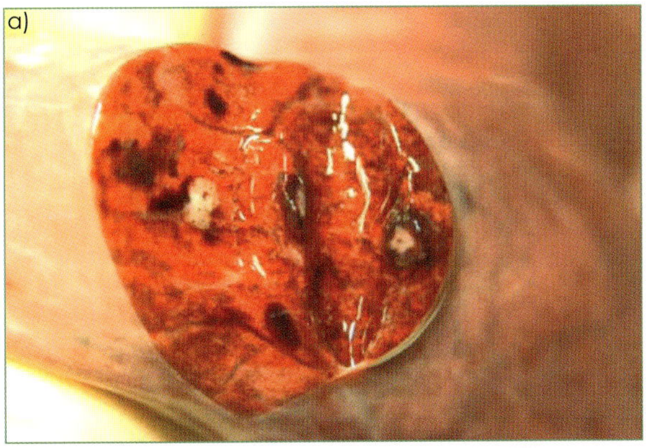

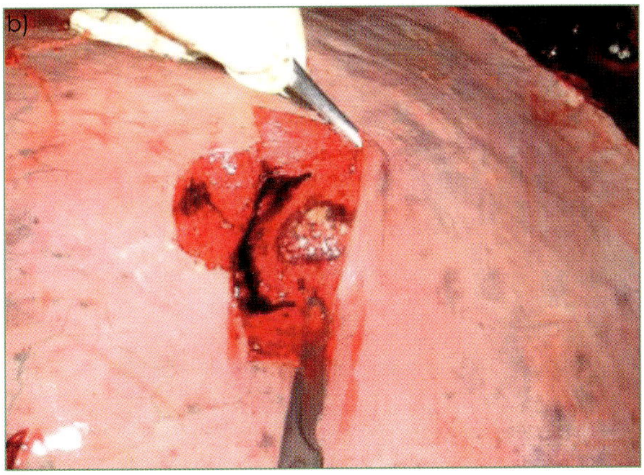

FIGURE 3: a) Typical small reddish pulmonary nodule with central grey necrosis. b) Small lung abscess with 'gun-shot nodules'.

Pathological lesions

After entering the body, usually *per os* or through a wound, *B. mallei* first multiplies at its site of entry and produces a 'primary nodule' from where it is transported via lymphatic vessels or blood into various tissues. In the infected organs, the bacterium multiplies again with the following consequences. In the lungs, reddish nodules resembling small tubercles with a central grey necrotic zone develop; later, some caseous nodules and peripheral fibrous reaction may occur (**Fig 3**). In the choanae and nasal septae, small 3–4 mm vesicular pustules develop which become ulcers and nodules. Nodules are crater-shaped with raised and irregular borders. The base is covered by yellowish-brown granulation tissue and yellowish pus (**Figs 4** and **5**). Nasal discharge, which is usually unilateral, becomes mucous, purulent, yellowish-green. Pus-filled lacrimation may also occur (**Fig 6**). Glanderous lesions may also exist in other organs causing orchitis, arthritis, synovitis and sinusitis. Lesions are sometimes observed in liver or spleen (**Fig 7**). Cutaneous lesions occur as a result of a direct contamination, for example through a wound or by metastases from infected lungs (**Figs 8**, **9** and **10**).

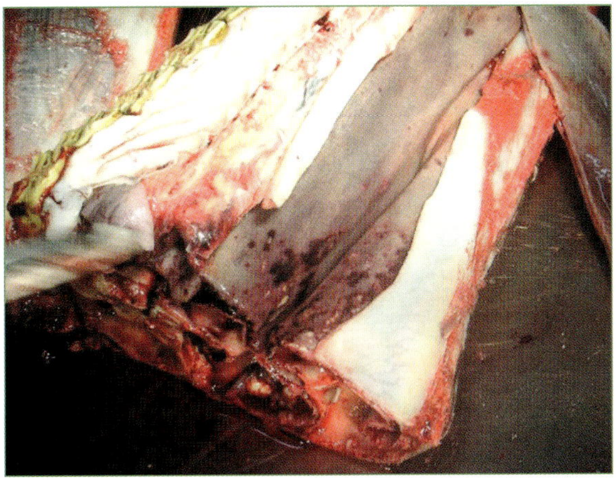

FIGURE 4: Nasal septum with ulcers showing 'punched out' appearance covered with blood or yellow pus.

Classical descriptions of glanders distinguish between respiratory and cutaneous forms of disease, and acute and chronic forms. However, it is very important to remember that in most outbreaks these forms are not clearly distinct and may occur simultaneously in one animal. In horses, slow progression of the disease is more common, but in donkeys and mules the acute form with death within a week may occur. The disease is always fatal. After losing a considerable amount of weight (up to 50 kg/day), the glanderous animals finally die within 1–4 weeks. Donkey and mules die more rapidly than horses.

Microscopic lesions

Glanders lesions are disseminated throughout the lung parenchyma as very small hard granulomas which are easily palpable. As they undergo the same evolution as tubercle lesions, they are named 'pseudo-tubercles'. Microscopically, they are also characterised by central necrosis and liquefaction, and later by the formation of caseous nodules and mineralisation of their centre surrounded by a mixture of inflammatory cells. These comprise many neutrophils, some lymphocytes, macrophages, epithelial and a few giant cells. In the earlier stages, the entire lesions are surrounded by a collection of red blood cells (see also **Fig 3**) and at a later stage enclosed by a fibrous capsule (**Figs 11** and **12**) (Anon 2004).

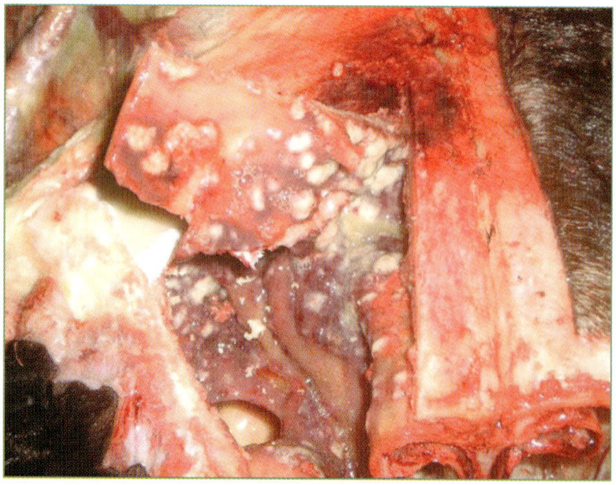

FIGURE 5: Right choanae of a glanderous horse with stellate scars, ulcers, honey-comb necrotic patches and yellow pus production.

Diagnosis

In enzootic areas, all equids exhibiting respiratory symptoms, nasal discharge and/or ulcers should be considered infected with glanders. If infection is confirmed, a thorough epidemiological investigation, including a comprehensive trace-back of the infected

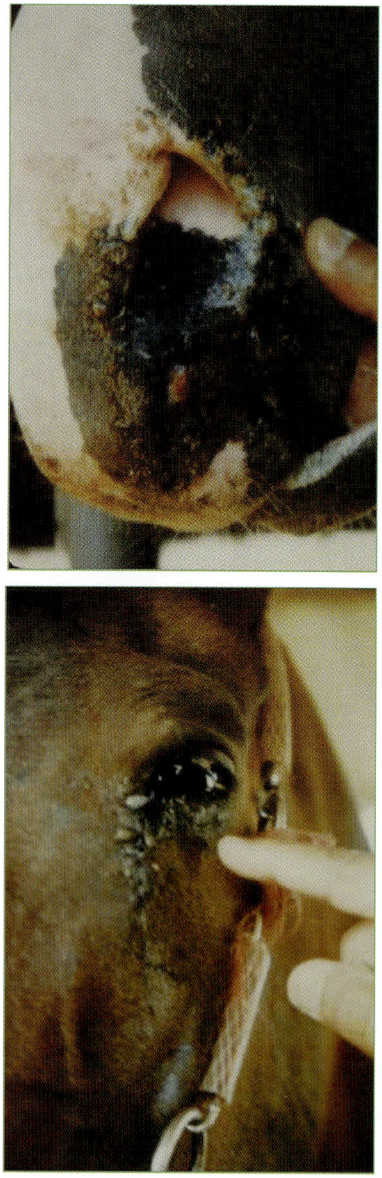

FIGURE 6: Unilateral nasal discharge with ulcers on the inside of the nostril and lacrimation.

animals and all contacts, is essential. The respiratory form of glanders may be confused with melioidosis (*B. pseudomallei*), equine viral arteritis, strangles (*Streptococcus equi equi*) and fungal pneumonia. The cutaneous form of the disease (farcy) may be confused with epizootic lymphangitis caused by *Histoplasma farciminosum* and with *Yersinia pseudotuberculosis*. In all of these cases, laboratory examinations are essential for a proper diagnosis.

The optimal sample for isolating the organism is pus recovered from swabs of lung, choanal and organ abscesses. As mentioned before these abscesses do not contain many bacteria, and therefore several samples must be collected. These samples are also often contaminated with other bacterial species especially *Pseudomonas* spp. and *Pasteurella* spp. which makes isolation very difficult (Anon 2004). Glanderous subcutaneous abscesses contain good numbers of pathogens whereas ulcers are usually free of *B. mallei*.

As glanders is a zoonosis, all samples must be handled with great care in a laboratory that meets the requirements for 'containment group 3' pathogens (Anon 2004). Suspected material should also be inoculated intraperitoneally into a male adult guinea pig. Positive material will cause severe localised peritonitis and orchitis (Straus reaction), but this is not pathognomic and *B. mallei* must be re-isolated from the lesions (**Fig 13**). *B. mallei* cannot be differentiated

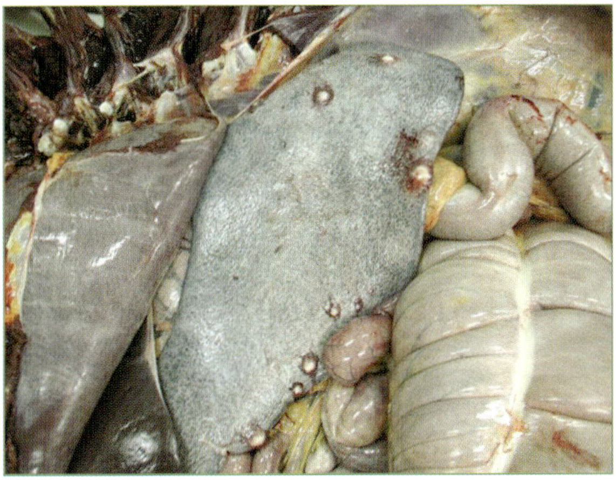

FIGURE 7: Multiple abscess formation in the spleen of a horse with glanders from which B. mallei was isolated.

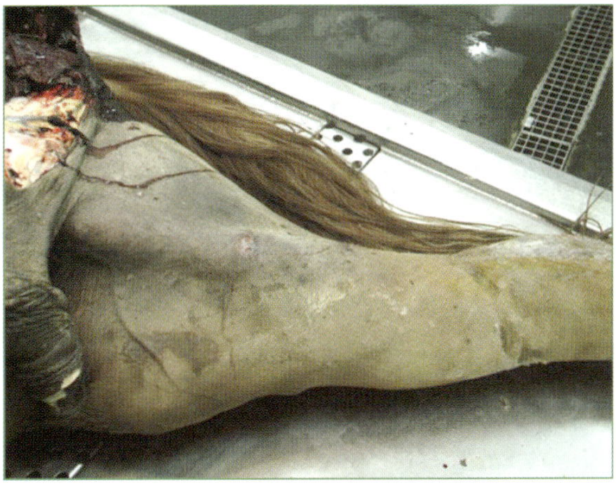

FIGURE 9: A severely swollen lymph vessel (farcy pipe) on the medial side of a hind leg of a horse affected by farcy.

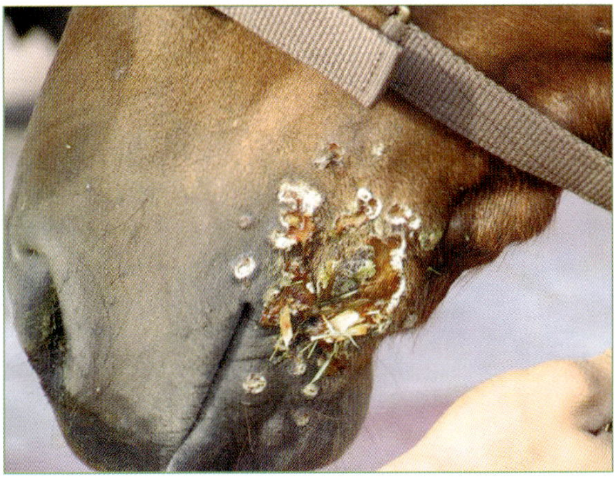

FIGURE 8: Farcy on the head of a glanders horse.

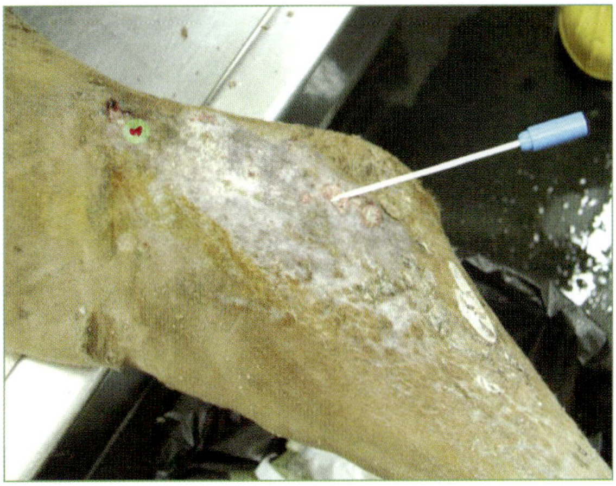

FIGURE 10: Abscess formation along lymph vessel of the same horse as in Figure 9.

from *B. pseudomallei* on metabolic properties and must therefore be tested in PCR. The PCR technique has recently been fully validated, and hopefully will in future gain acceptance as a safe and rapid method of confirming infection (Neubauer *et al.* 2005).

The complement fixation test (CFT) is an accurate serological test that has been used for glanders diagnosis for many years (Neubauer *et al.* 2005). It is reported to have a sensitivity of 90–95%, serum being positive within one week of infection and remaining positive (sometimes) in chronic cases. It is presently the only test described by the OIE for international trade of equids. However, it has been shown that around 1% of the tested equine sera show false positive reaction (cross reactions), which causes uncertainty in times of ever increasing horse transport (Wernery *et al.* 2005). Therefore other serological tests have been developed. None of these tests can differentiate between *B. mallei* and *B. pseudomallei* infection although a cELISA with a specificity of 100% for serodiagnosis of human melioidosis has recently been developed using a monoclonal antibody to a specific epitope on the lipopolysaccharide (LPS) of *B. pseudomallei* (Thepthai *et al.* 2005). A competitive ELISA for *B. mallei* that also uses an anti-LPS monoclonal antibody (mab 3D11) is currently being validated. It has the advantage that, so far, no cross reactivities have been observed. Other techniques such as western blot, avidin-biotin dot ELISA, counter-immunoelectrophoresis as well as Rose Bengal plate agglutination are all in use in different countries. None of these tests have been validated by the OIE. Malleinisation detects the delayed hypersensitivity of infected animals to *B. mallei*. The technique is

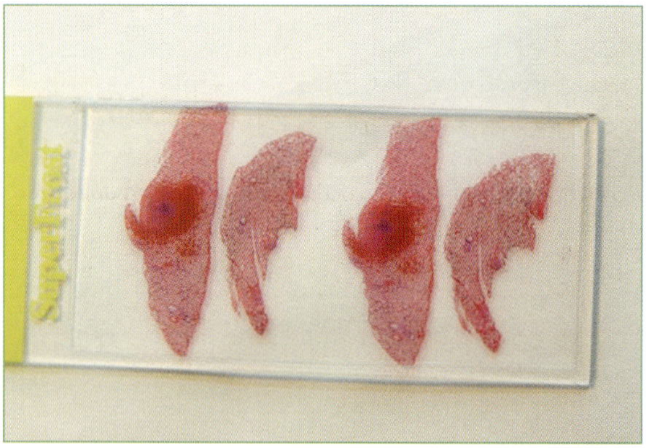

FIGURE 11: Histological sections of lung tissue stained with HE showing miliary necrosis with dark centers surrounded by a cuff of red blood cells typical of a glanders tubercle.

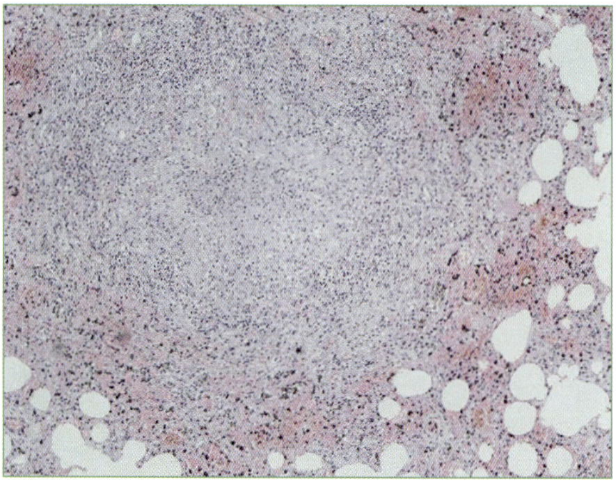

FIGURE 12: Histological section of lung tissue stained with HE showing a glanderous pyogranuloma.

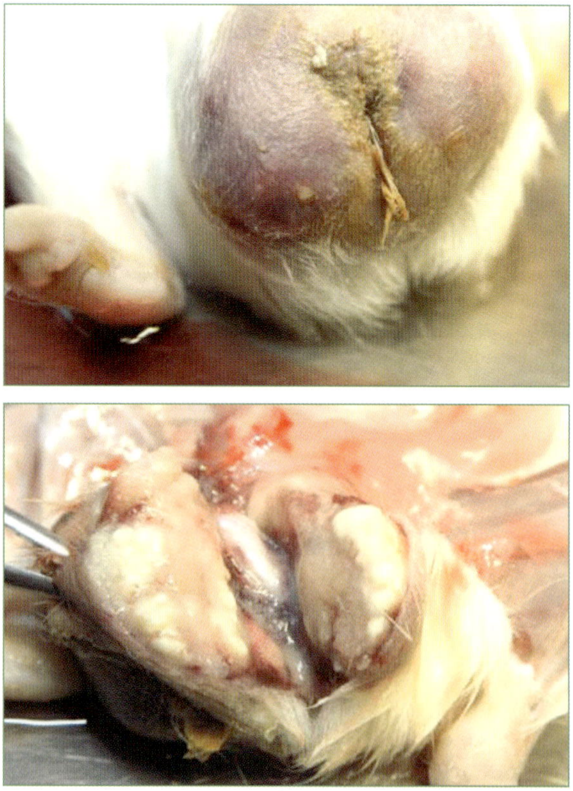

FIGURE 13: Typical Straus reaction in a guinea pig: purulent orchitis 12 days after intraperitoneal infection with material from choanal malleous lesions.

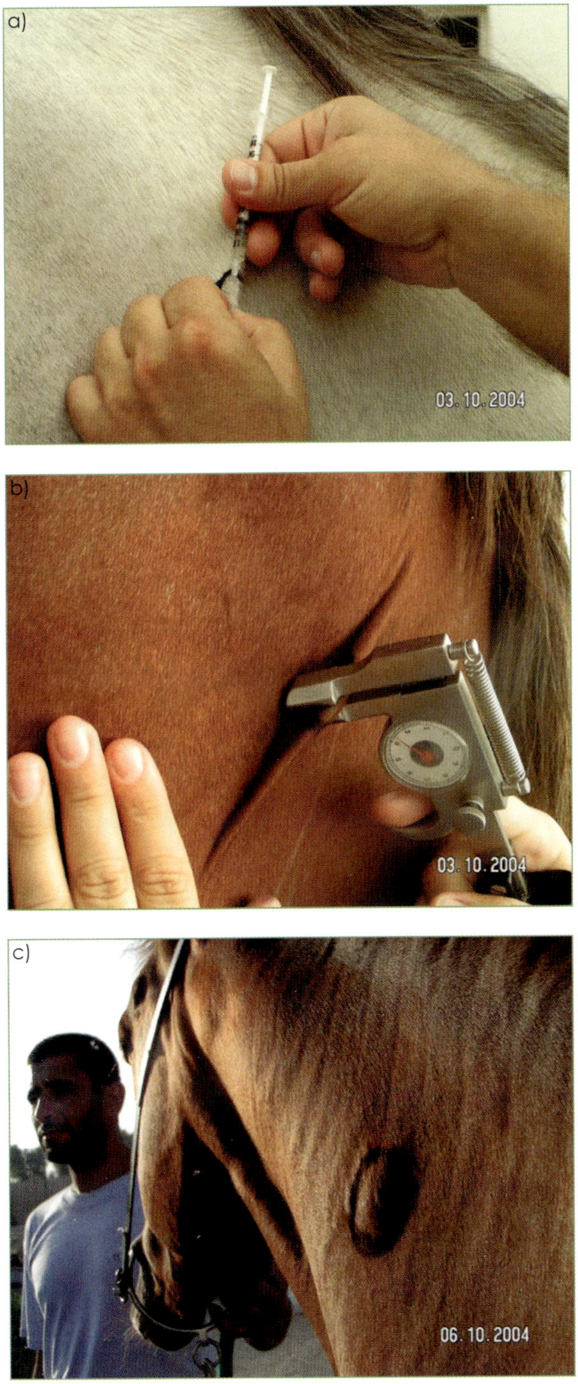

FIGURE 14: a) Intradermal injection of 0.2 ml of PPD into the middle of the neck. b) Measuring of skin thickness. c) Positive skin reaction (above 5 mm) of a glanderous horse 72 h after injection.

recommended by the OIE, and the mallein-purified protein derivate (PPD) is currently available in the Netherlands, Turkey and Romania. The technique recommended is the intradermo-palpebral method which is not easy to perform if large numbers of equids have to be malleinised. In these cases, the intradermal malleinisation with 0.2 ml of PPD in the middle of the neck is recommended by the Turkish manufacturers. The results are read 72 h after injection. A skin thickness of 3–5 mm is suspicious, whereas a thickness of equal or above 5 mm is positive (**Fig 14**). Horses often rub the neck against different objects because the allergic skin reaction is sometimes itchy. The technique has largely replaced the ophthalmic and subcutaneous tests. With the intradermo-palpebral method 0.1 ml of PPD is injected intradermally into the lower eyelid, and the test is read after 24 and 48 h. A positive reaction is characterised by marked oedematous swelling of the eyelid, and there may be a purulent discharge from the inner canthus. This is usually accompanied by a rise in temperature. It must be borne in mind that seroconversion is often observed after subcutaneous injection, which should be avoided, but in many cases specific glanders antibodies are also detected after intradermal malleinisation, which may last for several months. Sensitivity and specificity of this test is comparable to the CFT.

Control

No vaccines are available against glanders. The disease can only be prevented by sanitary measures, although *B. mallei* is sensitive to antibiotics and sulphadiazine, but treatment is prohibited. Positive animals must be subjected to euthanasia and carcasses properly disposed of. Disinfection of the premises must be carried out, and complete quarantine of affected stables must take place. Equine movement should be closely monitored. Glanders is an OIE B list equine disease and is notifiable.

References

Alibasoglu, M., Yesildere, T., Calislar, T., Inal, T. and Calsikan, U. (1986) Outbreak of glanders in lions in Istanbul zoological garden. *Berl. Münch. Tierärztl Wschrift.* **99**, 57-63.

Anon (2004) *Manual for Diagnostic Tests and Vaccines for Terrestrial Animals (mammals, birds and bees)*, 5th edn., Office international des épizooties (OIE). pp 727-723.

Arun, S., Neubauer, H., Gürel, A., Ayyildiz, G., Kusçu, B., Yesildere, T., Meyer, H. and Hermanns, W. (1999) Equine glanders in Turkey. *Vet. Rec.* **144**, 255-258.

Gravelat, F. (1997) *Etude de la production d'exoprotéases par les bactéries du genre* Burkholderia. Memoire de DEA, University of Lyons.

Neubauer, H., Sprague, L.D., Joseph, M., Tomaso, H. Al Dohoub, S., Witte, A., Kinne, J, Hensel, A, Wernery, R., Wernery, U and Scholz, H.C. (2006) Development and clinical evaluation of a PCR assay targeting the metalloprotease gene (mprA) of *B. pseudomallei. Zoonoses Public Health* **54**, 44-50.

Neubauer, H., Sprague, L.D., Zacharia, R., Tomaso, H., Al Dahouk, S., Wernery, R., Wernery, U. and Scholz, H.C. (2005) Serodiagnosis of *Burkholderia mallei* infections in horses: state of the art and perspectives. *J. vet. Med. B.* **52**, 201-205.

Scholz, H., Joseph, M., Tomaso, H., Al Dahouk, S., Witte, A., Kinne, J., Hagen, R.M., Wernery, R., Wernery, U. and Neubauer, H. (2006) Detection of the reemerging agent *Burkholderia mallei* in a recent outbreak of glanders in the United Arab Emirates by a newly developed fliP-based polymerase chain reaction assay. *Diagn. Microbiol. Inf. Dis.* **54**, 241-247.

Srinivasan, S., Kraus, C.N., DeShazer, D. Becker, P.M., Dick, J.D., Spacek, L., Bartlett, J.G., Byrne, W.R. and Thomas, D.L. (2001) Glanders in a military research microbiologist. *N. Engl. Med.* **345**, 256-258.

Thepthai, C., Smithtikarn, S., Suksuwan, M., Songsivilai, S. and Dharakul, T. (2005) Serodiagnosis of melioidosis by a competitive enzyme-linked immunosorbent assay using a lipopolysaccharide-specific monoclonal antibody. *Asian Pac. J. Allergy Immunol.* **23**, 127-132.

Verma, R.D. (1981) Glanders in India with special reference to incidence and epidemiology. *Indian vet. J.* **58**, 177-183.

Wattiau, P., Van Hessche, M., Neubauer, H., Zachariah, R., Wernery, U. and Imberechts, H. (2007) Identification of *Burkholderia pseudomallei* and related bacteria by multiple-locus sequence typing-derived PCR and real-time PCR. *J. clin. Microbiol.* **45**, 1045-1048.

Wernery, U., Zachariah R., Wernery R., Joseph, S. and Valsini. L. (2004) Establishment and maintaining the health status of the equine population of the United Arab Emirates for international competition purposes. In: *Proceedings of the 15th International Conference of Racing Analysts and Veterinarians,* R and W Publications, Newmarket. pp 435-438.

Wittig, M.B., Wohlsein, P., Hagen, R.M. Al Dahouk, S., Tomaso, H., Scholz, H.C., Nikolaou, K., Wernery, R., Wernery, U., Kinne, J., Elschner, M. and Neubauer, H. (2006) Ein Übersichtsreferat zur Rotzerkrankung. *Dtsch. Tierärztl Wschrift.* **113**, 323-330.

EQUINE LEPTOSPIROSIS

T. J. Divers

Ithaca, New York, USA.

Keywords: horse; *Leptospira* serovars Pomona and Grippotyphosa; abortion; recurrent uveitis

Summary

Leptospirosis is a proven cause of abortion in horses and is associated with some cases of equine recurrent uveitis. It is an infrequent cause of renal failure in the horse. *Leptospira interrogans* serovar Pomona is responsible for most of the leptospiral-associated disease in North America. *Leptospira kirschneri* serovar Grippotyphosa appears to be most important in Europe. Although there is considerable controversy and conflicting data pertaining to persistent infections of *Leptospira* spp. in the equine eye, there is strong evidence that *Leptospira* infections are at least associated with many cases of equine recurrent uveitis.

Introduction

Leptospirosis is caused by highly invasive, spiral bacteria in the genus *Leptospira*. The infectious agent is capable of infecting man and animals (Sullivan 1974). Leptospirosis occurs worldwide but is most common in temperate or tropical climates. There is less known about leptospirosis in horses than any common domestic animal apart from the cat. The DNA-based genus classification of *Leptospira* includes 8 pathogenic species and 5 nonpathogenic species (Morey *et al.* 2006; Slack *et al.* 2006). Serovars, based upon the older phenotype classification, are sometimes classified as causing host adapted infection or incidental host infection. Host adapted strains seldom cause clinical disease in their maintenance host, infection and shedding are prolonged, and the serological response following infection is relatively low (O'Keefe 2002). Conversely, incidental host serovars are more likely to cause clinical disease in a nonmaintenance host, a marked serological response occurs following infection, and there is only a brief period of shedding. In North American horses, *Leptospira interrogans* serovar Pomona type Kennewicki is the prominent incidental (pathological) serovar, and the skunk is one of the most common maintenance hosts of this serovar (Dwyer *et al.* 1995; Donahue *et al.* 1995). In Europe, important equine strains are *L. kirschneri* serovar Grippotyphosa, strains *duster* (western Europe) and *moskva* (eastern Europe) (Hartskeerl *et al.* 2004). *Leptospira* serovar Bratislava is considered by most researchers to be the host adapted serovar of the horse (Ellis *et al.* 1983; Kitson-Piggot and Prescott 1987; Williams *et al.* 1994). This belief is met with some controversy, as horses may have high equine serum titres to serovar Bratislava and some researchers believe that serovar Bratislava is pathogenic in the horse. The difference in serogroup prevalence between the 2 continents makes comparison of clinical syndromes of leptospirosis between American and European horses difficult.

Clinical diseases

Pathogenic *Leptospira* infections in the horse appear to have organ tropism for either the reproductive tract of the female, kidney or eye (**Fig 1**). Infection may result in placentitis and abortion, acute renal failure, or haematuria and uveitis. Most infected horses do not have obvious clinical signs. Even in experimental studies, fever and mild leg oedema may be the only clinical signs (Girio *et al.* 1999).

Reproductive tract infection

Leptospira interrogans serovar Pomona abortions account for a significant number of bacterial abortions in mares in endemic regions (Donahue and Williams 2000). Serovar Pomona is responsible for most of the *Leptospira* abortions in North America, but serovars Grippotyphosa and Hardjo have also been reported. Most abortions are late term (>9 months), and rarely a live foal may be born ill due to leptospirosis. *Leptospira* organisms are commonly found in the placenta, umbilical cord, kidney and liver of the infected fetus. Pathological damage is present in the

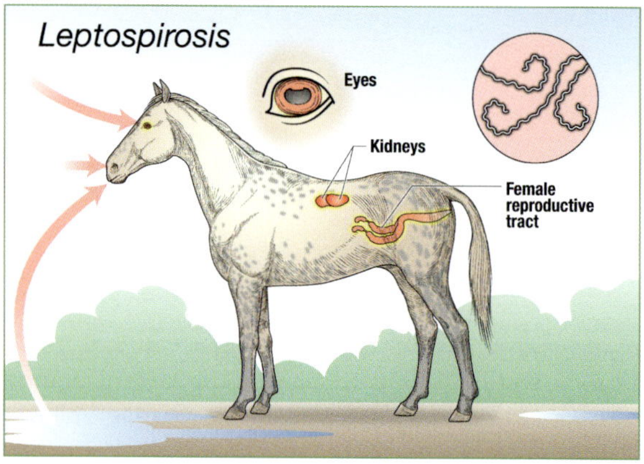

FIGURE 1: Drawing depicting suspected organ tropism for pathogenic Leptospira in the horse.

placenta, resulting in a placentitis (**Fig 2**) not involving the cervical star. Macroscopic lesions include oedema and areas of necrosis in the chorion. Microscopic lesions include necrosis and calcification of the placenta. Macroscopically, the liver may have a yellow discolouration. Liver disease is caused by a combination of multifocal necrosis and giant cell hepatopathy. Tubulonephrosis and interstitial nephritis may be present in the kidney of the aborted fetus. Inflammation of the umbilical cord, funisitis, may be recognised by a diffuse yellowish discolouration (Sebastian *et al.* 2005). It is unknown if the abortion occurs because of the placentitis, funisitis or fetal infection, or all 3. Although more than one mare on a farm may abort due to *Leptospira* infection, it is rare for an epidemic of abortions to occur. Some mares that are infected do not abort. Aborting mares and other recently infected horses are believed to shed serovar Pomona in the urine for approximately 2–3 months (Bernard *et al.* 1993). A small number of horses on the farm experiencing one or more *Leptospira* abortions may develop uveitis weeks later.

Acute renal failure

Occasionally, *Leptospira* serovar Pomona may cause fever and acute renal failure in the adult horse (Divers *et al.* 1992). The kidneys are swollen due to tubulointerstitial nephritis and the urine may have pyuria without visible bacteria. On rare occasions, multiple young horses may be affected with fever and acute renal failure following *Leptospira* infection.

Recurrent uveitis

The most important clinical disease associated with *Leptospira* serovars Pomona or Grippotyphosa infection in the adult horse is equine recurrent uveitis (ERU) or keratitis. The strong association between ERU and serovar Pomona dates back to the early 1950s with a general belief that it was an immune-mediated disease with antibodies (IgG and IgA) against certain *Leptospira* antigens cross-reacting against equine uveal tissue, lens, cornea and possibly retina (Wollanke *et al.* 2001). Since 2000, there have been several scientific publications confirming live *Leptospira* in the uveal tissue, aqueous or vitreous

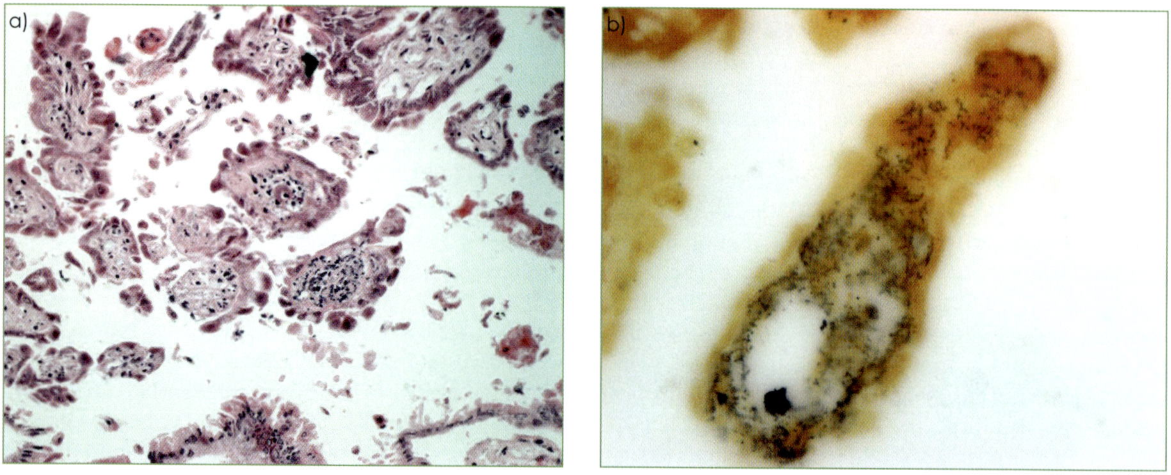

FIGURE 2: a) Microscopic appearance of chronic necrotising equine placentitis caused by leptospirosis. b) Silver stain of placental necrosis demonstrating the Leptospira organism (photos courtesy of Dr Don Schlafer).

fluid of horses with ERU. High antibody concentrations to *Leptospira* serovar Pomona in the aqueous humour compared to serum titres also suggest persistent local antigenic stimulation. Survival of the organism in the face of high ocular antibody indicates an absence of cells/ molecules, e.g. complement, involved in bacterial clearance, suggesting ocular immune privilege similar to the central nervous system.

An additional explanation for *Leptospira* survival in the vitreous may be a protective proteinaceous film that develops around the organism and may inhibit phagocytosis (Brandes *et al.* 2007). The recurrent episodes of the disease may be related to a Th1 response of autoreactivity following mimicry and inter- and/or intramolecular epitope spreading (Deeg *et al.* 2006). Immune reactions in ERU have been found against retinal antigens, lens and ciliary body. Antibody against these sites may cross-react with antibody against leptospiral lipoproteins LruA and LruB (Verma *et al.* 2005). Genetic factors are probably involved in the disease process, helping to explain why only some horses infected with *Leptospira* develop uveitis. Appaloosas are thought to be genetically predisposed (Dwyer *et al.* 1995). ERU is the most common cause of blindness in horses. Prevalence of ERU is unknown, but one estimate is that 1–3% of horses will develop the disease. It is probable that some cases of ERU are not associated with *Leptospira* infection and the association between leptospirosis and ERU probably varies between geographic regions (Hartskeerl *et al.* 2004; Pearce *et al.* 2007). Indeed, some studies have not confirmed any relationship between active *Leptospira* infection and ERU (Pearce *et al.* 2007; Gilger *et al.* 2008). In contrast, in some regions, >50% of ERU cases have been shown to be associated with persistent ocular infections with *Leptospira* (Faber *et al.* 2000; Wollanke *et al.* 2001). It is clear that more research is needed to further confirm or disprove a link between active *Leptospira* infection and ERU! *Leptospira*-associated uveitis may cause corneal, anterior chamber and posterior chamber disease. Therefore, clinical findings may vary from corneal oedema, clinically quiet retinal lesions observed on fundoscopic examination and, most dramatically, recurrent and progressive painful uveitis. The chronic disease of the globe may cause cataracts, retinal degeneration or even glaucoma (**Fig 3**).

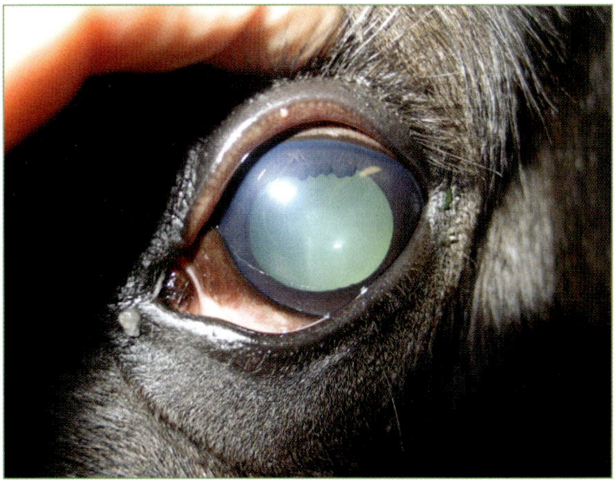

FIGURE 3: Three-year-old horse with bilateral uveitis of several weeks' duration. Retinal detachment has occurred in the left eye; hyperpigmentation and loss of iris detail are evident. Serum antibody to Leptospira *serovar Pomona persisted at 1:1600 and leptospiral organisms were found in the urine on 3 separate samples over a 3 week period (the last sample was positive for leptospiral organisms even following 2 weeks of antibiotic therapy).*

Diagnosis

Diagnosis of *Leptospira* abortion is best accomplished by fluorescent antibody testing (FAT) or immunohistochemistry of the placenta, umbilical cord, or fetal liver and kidney. The sensitivity and specificity of the FAT on those tissues are nearly 100% (Donahue and Williams 2000). Examination of silver stained kidney samples in horses with renal disease does not have a high accuracy, as there may be false negatives and false positives (probably due to nonpathogenic serovars). Marked increases in serum titres (microscopic agglutination test - MAT) often accompany *Leptospira* abortions or acute renal failure, but may be low with recurrent uveitis because of the chronic localised infection (Wollanke *et al.* 2001). Aqueous or vitreous humour fluid antibody titres in horses with *Leptospira* associated RU are generally markedly elevated in comparison to the serum. Acute serovar Pomona infections will often cause marked elevations in antibody titres to several serovars, but the noninfecting serovar titres will decline much more quickly over several weeks than the titres to the actual infecting serovar. Experimentally infected horses seroconverted by 5 days after infection. Serovar specific FAT of a urine sample or dried urine sediment has been recommended as a diagnostic test for infection and determination of continual shedding, but we have found the test on urine to have poor sensitivity. Collection of the second voided urine sample following furosemide administration may improve sensitivity of this test. Dark field microscopy can be used to observe spirochaetes moving in the urine, but requires considerable experience. Serology, culture or PCR of aqueous fluid may be the only way to confirm *Leptospira* associated uveitis.

Treatments

Systemic administration of antibiotics would be indicated for horses with fever and acute renal failure caused by leptospirosis. Ticarcillin was used successfully in one horse with acute renal failure (Divers *et al.* 1992). Other antibiotics that *Leptospira* may be sensitive to include: penicillin, ampicillin, cephalosporins, enrofloxacin, tetracycline and doxycycline (Kim *et al.* 2006). Previous attempts to prevent urine shedding in horses with acute or subacute *Leptospira* infection by using oxytetracycline, penicillin G and streptomycin were not effective (Bernard *et al.* 1993). Fluid therapy would be indicated as supportive treatment of acute renal failure.

There have been a variety of treatments for ERU, e.g. corticosteroids and cyclosporine, used in the hopes of decreasing the inflammatory response, but these have generally provided only temporary relief and many affected horses either become blind or have the eye removed because of intractable and persistent pain (Gilger and Michau 2004). Vitrectomy with inoculation of a gentamicin lavage has been reported to be a successful treatment in Europe (Frühauf *et al.* 1998). The mounting evidence that persistent serovars Pomona or Grippotyphosa infections are present in some horses with ERU may help explain our inability to cure most cases. If *Leptospira* is believed to be associated with a case of ERU, it seems prudent that an effort should be directed towards treating the possible chronic infection. Unfortunately, antibacterial treatment of ocular leptospirosis may not be easy since the blood ocular barrier inhibits movement of antimicrobials from the plasma into the eye. Even with inflammation, some interference may persist. In healthy ponies, doxycycline could not be found (limit of detection <0.3 µg/ml) in the aqueous humour after 21 days of treatment with 10 mg/kg bwt q. 12 h (Gilmour *et al.* 2005). In recent *in vitro* work, enrofloxacin demonstrated low minimal inhibitory and bactericidal concentrations (<0.30 µg/ml) against strains of *Leptospira* serovar Pomona (Kim *et al.* 2006). Peak aqueous levels of enrofloxacin were 0.32 µg/ml in normal horses after repeated i.v. dosing with 7.5 mg/kg bwt (Divers *et al.* 2008). Topical antibiotics may reach adequate levels in the aqueous but typically diffuse poorly into the vitreous.

Prevention

Acutely infected horses and/or mares aborting from *Leptospira* infection should be isolated for 14–16 weeks and/or the urine tested by dark field microscopy, PCR or culture to determine if the mare is shedding the organism. Limiting exposure to stagnant water and to potential maintenance hosts, e.g. skunk, may help in the control of leptospirosis. Vaccination (extralabel use of one of the bovine or porcine multiple serovar killed vaccines) against serovar Pomona is sometimes performed on farms with endemic abortions and/or a high rate of uveitis. A half dose of a 5-way swine vaccine has been used in the horse without noted adverse effects and a serological response was obtained, but protection was not evaluated (Rohrbach *et al.* 2005). Vaccination of infected horses with a whole cell vaccine could theoretically cause ERU, although this has been rarely observed. An effective and safe leptospirosis vaccine, approved for the horse, would be a welcome addition to equine preventative medicine. Several protective antigens have been identified in a hamster model but further studiesw are needed in equids (Palaniappan *et al.* 2006; Chang *et al.* 2007; Faisal *et al.* 2008; Yan *et al.* 2009). There are reports of prophylaxis vaccination, using an autogenous vaccine produced from a stable specific isolate, decreasing the incidence of ERU (Wollanke *et al.* 2004).

References

Bernard, W.V., Bolin, C., Riddle, T., Durando, M., Smith, B.J. and Tramontin, R.R. (1993) Leptospiral abortion and leptospiruria in horses from the same farm. *J. Am. vet. med. Ass.* **202**, 1285-1286.

Brandes, K., Wollanke, B., Niedermaier, G., Brem, S. and Gerhards, H. (2007) Recurrent uveitis in horses: vitreal examinations with ultrastructural detection of leptospires. *J. vet. Med. A Physiol. Pathol. Clin. Med.* **54**, 270-275.

Chang, Y.F., Chen, C.S., Palaniappan, R.U., He, H., McDonough, S.P., Barr, S.C., Yan, W., Faisal, S.M., Pan, M.J. and Chang, C.F. (2007) Immunogenicity of the recombinant leptospiral putative outer membrane proteins as vaccine candidates. *Vaccine* **25**, 8190-8197.

Deeg, C.A., Amann, B., Raith, A.J. and Kaspers, B. (2006) Inter- and intramolecular epitope spreading in equine recurrent uveitis. *Invest. Ophthalmol. Vis. Sci.* **47**, 652-656.

Divers, T.J, Byars, T.D. and Shin, S.J. (1992) Renal dysfunction associated with infection of *Leptospira interrogans* in a horse. *J. Am. vet. med. Ass.* **201**, 1391-1392.

Divers, T.J., Irby, N.L., Mohammed, H.O. and Schwark, W.S. (2008) Ocular penetration of intravenously administered enrofloxacin in the horse. *Equine vet. J.* **40**, 167-170.

Donahue, J.M. and Williams, N.M. (2000) Emerging causes of placentitis and abortion. *Vet. Clin. N. Am.: Equine Pract.* **16**, 443-456.

Donahue, J.M., Smith, B.J., Poonacha, K.B., Donahoe, J.K. and Rigsby, C.L. (1995) Prevalence and serovars of *Leptospira* involved in equine abortions in central Kentucky during the 1991-1993 foaling seasons. *J. vet. diag. Invest.* **7**, 87-91.

Dwyer, A.E., Crockett, R.S. and Kalsow, C.M. (1995) Association of leptospiral seroreactivity and breed with uveitis and blindness in horses: 372 cases (1986-1993). *J. Am. vet. med. Ass.* **207**, 1327-1331.

Ellis, W.A., O'Brien, J.J., Cassells, J.A. and Montgomery, J. (1983) Leptospiral infection in horses in Northern Ireland: serological and microbiological findings. *Equine vet. J.* **15**, 317-320.

Faber, N.A., Crawford, M., LeFebvre, R.B., Buyukmihci, N.C., Madigan, J.E. and Willits, N.H. (2000) Detection of *Leptospira* spp. in the aqueous humor of horses with naturally acquired recurrent uveitis. *J. clin. Microbiol.* **38**, 2731-2733.

Faisal, S.M., Yan, W., Chen, C.S., Palaniappan, R.U., McDonough, S.P. and Chang, Y.F. (2008) Evaluation of protective immunity of *Leptospira* immunoglobulin like protein A (LigA) DNA vaccine against challenge in hamsters. *Vaccine* **26**, 277-287.

Frühauf, B., Ohnesorge, B., Deegen, E. and Boevé, M. (1998) Surgical management of equine recurrent uveitis with single port *pars plana* vitrectomy. *Vet. Ophthalmol.* **1**, 137-151.

Gilger, B.C. and Michau, T.M. (2004) Equine recurrent uveitis: new methods of management. *Vet. Clin. N. Am.: Equine Pract.* **20**, 417-427.

Gilger, B.C., Salmon, J.H., Yi, N.Y., Barden, C.A., Chandler, H.L., Wendt, J.A. and Colitz, C.M. (2008) Role of bacteria in the pathogenesis of recurrent uveitis in horses from the southeastern United States. *Am. J. vet. Res.* **69**, 1329-1335.

Gilmour, M.A., Clarke, C.R., Macallister, C.G., Dedeo, J.M., Caudell, D.L., Morton, R.J. and Pugh, M. (2005) Ocular penetration of oral doxycycline in the horse. *Vet. Ophthalmol.* **8**, 331-335.

Girio, R.J.S., Mathias, L.A., Lacerda Neto, J.C. and Vasconcellos, S.A. (1999) Experimental leptospirosis in horses infected with *Leptospira interrogans* serovar Copenhagenl: clinical and serological aspects. *Arq. Inst. Biol.* **66**, 21-26.

Hartskeerl, R.A., Goris, M.G.A., Brem, S., Meyer, P., Kopp, H., Gerhards, H. and Wollanke, B. (2004) Classification of *Leptospira* from the eyes of horses suffering from recurrent uveitis. *J. vet. med. Series B* **51**, 110-115.

Kim, D., Kordick, D., Divers, T. and Chang, Y.F. (2006) *In vitro* susceptibilities of *Leptospira* spp. and *Borrelia burgdorferi* isolates to amoxicillin, tilmicosin, and enrofloxacin. *J. vet. Sci.* **7**, 355-359.

Kitson-Piggot, A.W. and Prescott, J.F. (1987) Leptospirosis in horses in Ontario. *Can. J. vet. Res.* **51**, 448-451.

Morey, R.E., Galloway, R.L., Bragg, S.L., Steigerwalt, A.G., Mayer, L.W. and Levett, P.N. (2006) Species specific identification of Leptospiraceae by 168-rRNA gene sequencing. *J. clin. Microbiol.* **44**, 3510-3518.

O'Keefe, J.S. (2002) A brief review on the laboratory diagnosis of leptospirosis. *N. Z. vet. J.* **50**, 9-13.

Palaniappan, R.U., McDonough, S.P., Divers, T.J., Chen, C.S., Pan M.J., Matsumoto, M. and Chang, Y.F. (2006) Immunoprotection of recombinant leptospiral immunoglobulin-like protein A against *Leptospira interrogans* serovar Pomona infection. *Infect. Immun.* **74**, 1745-1750.

Pearce, J.W., Galle, L.E., Kleiboeker, S.B., Truk, J.R., Schommer, S.K., Dubielizig, R.R., Mithcell, W.J., Moore, C.P. and Giuliano, E.A. (2007) Detection of *Leptospira interrogans* DNA and antigen in fixed equine eyes affected with end-stage equine recurrent uveitis. *J. vet. diag. Invest.* **19**, 686-690.

Rohrbach, B.W., Ward, D.A., Hendrix, D.V., Cawrse-Foss, M. and Moyres, T.D. (2005) Effect of vaccination against leptospirosis on the frequency, days to recurrence and progression of disease in horses with equine recurrent uveitis. *Vet. Ophthalmol.* **8**, 171-179.

Sebastian, M., Giles, R., Roberts, J., Poonacha, K., Harrison, L., Donahue, J. and Benirschke, K. (2005) Funisitis associated with leptospiral abortion in an equine placenta. *Vet. Pathol.* **42**, 659-662.

Slack, A.T., Symonds, M.L., Dohnt, M.F. and Smythe, L.D. (2006) Identification of pathogenic *Leptospira* species by conventional or real-time PCR and sequencing of the DNA gyrase subunit B encoding gene. *BMC Microbiol.* **6**, 95.

Sullivan, N.D. (1974) Leptospirosis in animals and man. *Aust. vet. J.* **21**, 216-223.

Verma, A., Artiushin, S., Matsunaga, J., Haake, D.A. and Timoney, J.F. (2005) LruA and LruB, novel lipoproteins of pathogenic *Leptospira interrogans* associated with equine recurrent uveitis. *Infect. Immun.* **73**, 7259-7266.

Williams, D.M., Smith, B.J., Donahue, J.M. and Poonacha, K.B. (1994) Serological and microbiological findings on 3 farms with equine leptospiral abortions. *Equine vet. J.* **26**, 105-108.

Wollanke, B., Rohrbach, B.W. and Gerhards, H. (2001) Serum and vitreous humor antibody titers in and isolation of *Leptospira interrogans* from horses with recurrent uveitis. *J. Am. vet. med. Ass.* **219**, 795-800.

Wollanke, B., Brem, S., Meyr, P., Forbrig, T., Grassl, P., Gerhards, H. and Kopp, H. (2004) Prophylaxis of equine recurrent uveitis (ERU): first results with a leptospiral vaccine in horses. *Pferdeheilkunde* **20**, 447-454.

Yan, W., Faisal, S.M., McDonough, S.P., Divers, T.J., Barr, S.C., Chang, C.F., Pan, M.J. and Chang, Y.F. (2009) Immunogenicity and protective efficacy of recombinant *Leptospira* immunoglobulin-like protein B (rLigB) in a hamster challenge model. *Microbes Infect.* **11**, 230-237.

MYCOBACTERIAL INFECTIONS OF HORSES

M. K. Hondalus* and A. S. Rogovskyy

Department of Infectious Diseases, College of Veterinary Medicine, The University of Georgia, Athens, Georgia 30302, USA.

Keywords: horse; equine; mycobacterial infection; mycobacteriosis; mycobacterium; MAC

Summary

Mycobacterium spp. are widespread in the environment, yet disease caused by these organisms is rare in the horse. At present, the species most commonly implicated in equine disease is *Mycobacterium avium* ssp. *avium* (*Maa*). Although localised infections may occur, more typically *Maa* illness manifests as a generalised disseminated granulomatous disease affecting numerous organ systems. Pulmonary and/or intestinal involvement is frequent and is characterised by granulomatous inflammation accompanied by bronchial and/or mesenteric lymph node enlargement. The most commonly observed clinical sign is chronic weight loss, which may or may not be accompanied by diarrhoea. Given the ubiquitous nature of the organism and the apparent natural resistance of horses to mycobacteriosis, it is hypothesised that affected animals may have some cellular immune system deficit that predisposes that particular individual to disease development. Diagnosis is often made *post mortem*, aided by the identification of intracellular acid-fast bacilli located within granuloma macrophages. Treatment of local, well isolated infections that are amenable to surgical debridement may be successful, whereas the prognosis for cases of generalised disease is poor.

Aetiological agents of mycobacterial disease

Mycobacterial infections are caused by members of the genus *Mycobacterium*, the sole genus in the family *Mycobacteriaceae,* encompassing more than 70 individual species (Harmsen *et al.* 2003). These organisms are common inhabitants of soil and water and most are largely innocuous (Tortoli 2003). Although certain *Mycobacterium* spp. represent a significant cause of illness and death in man and a variety of animal species, horses are rarely diagnosed with mycobacterial diseases and on the whole, are considered highly resistant (Larson 2007; Anon 2008; Pavlic *et al.* 2008).

Mycobacteriaceae are aerobic, nonspore-forming and rod- (bacilli) shaped. The bacteria are neither truly Gram-positive nor Gram-negative. The distinct feature that prevents all members of the genus *Mycobacterium* from being conventionally Gram-classified is their waxy lipid-rich cell envelope, which is impermeable to traditional Gram staining techniques. Therefore, to stain these bacteria, a specifically developed Ziehl-Neelsen procedure, which includes a phenol-solubilised dye such as carbol fuchsin and heating to increase dye penetration is used. Following a decolourisation step using acid alcohol, *Mycobacterium* spp. retain the reddish-pink stain and hence are referred to as 'acid fast' (**Fig 1b**) (Pfyffer *et al.* 2003).

Although uncommon, mycobacterial disease in the horse is well-documented. Interestingly though, the aetiology of equine mycobacteriosis has changed in recent history. During the first half of the last century, equine mycobacteriosis was predominantly caused by *M. bovis*, the primary causative agent of bovine tuberculosis. This latter species belongs to the *Mycobacterium tuberculosis* complex (MTC), composed of genetically related human and animal pathogens, namely, *M. tuberculosis*, *M. bovis*, *M. bovis* BCG vaccine strain, *M. africanum*, *M. microti*, *M. canetti*, *M. caprae*, *M. pinnipedii* and the dassie bacillus (Pavlic *et al.* 2004; Alexander and Liu 2006). *M. bovis* is able to cause progressive disease in many warm-blooded vertebrates including man and has the broadest host range of all the *Mycobacterium* species

*Author to whom correspondence should be addressed.

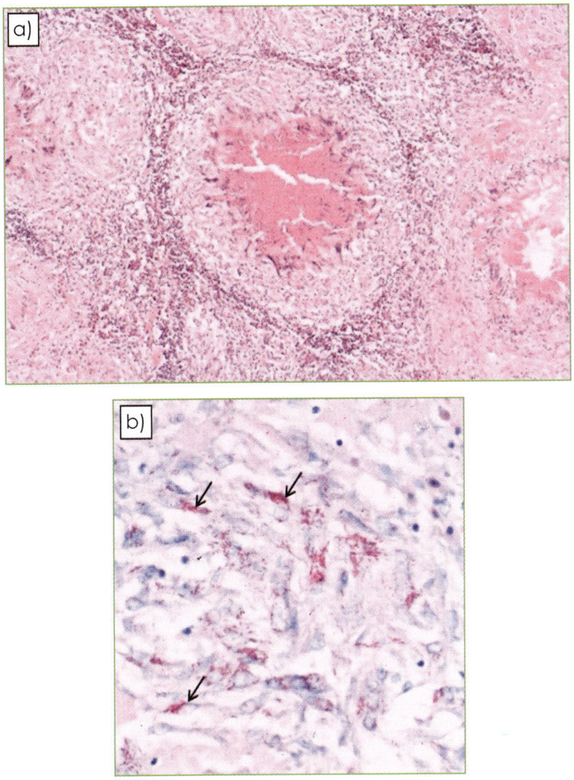

FIGURE 1: Granuloma from the spleen of a horse infected with unidentified mycobacterial species. The spleen sections were processed and stained with haematoxylin and eosin (a) or a Ziehl-Neelsen stain (b). Arrows denote acid-fast bacilli. The photomicrographs were generously provided by Dr Derek A. Mosier.

(Pavlic *et al.* 2004; Pavlic 2006). There is no current evidence that *M. tuberculosis*, the principle aetiological agent of human tuberculosis, causes disease in horses, although the isolation of this human pathogen from horses has been reported (Verge and Senthille 1942; Muser and Nassal 1962).

Presently, equine disease is most often caused by members of the *M. avium-intracellulare* complex (MAC), which includes the closely related organisms *M. avium* and *M. intracellulare*. There are 4 subspecies of *M. avium*: *M. avium* ssp. *avium* (*Maa*), *M. avium* ssp. *hominissuis* (*Mah*), *M. avium* ssp. *paratuberculosis* (*Map*) and *M. avium* ssp. *sylvaticum* (*Mas*). *Maa* is commonly found in the environment and is the causative agent of avian tuberculosis and of sporadic infections of wild mammals, particularly, deer (Alexander and Liu 2006). *Mah* is also a common environmental inhabitant and is frequently identified in immunocompromised human patients and sometimes swine (Matlova *et al.* 2004; Reed *et al.* 2006; Saadeh and Srkalovic 2008). This subspecies is also but less frequently isolated from nonvertebrates, small terrestrial mammals, wild boars and ruminants (Machackova *et al.* 2003, 2004; Fischer *et al.* 2004). *Mas*, also known as wood pigeon bacillus, primarily infects birds. *Map* infects ruminants resulting in Johne's disease, a highly contagious and chronic debilitating enteritis (Alexander and Liu 2006).

Additional species within the *Mycobacterium* genus that have been found to cause infection are *M. kansasii*, *M. chelonae*, *M. fortuitum*, *M. aquae*, *M. cookie*, *M. phlei*, *M. scrofulaceum*, *M. smegmatis* and *M. xenopi*. These soil and water inhabitants may act as wound contaminants and are sometimes referred to as atypical mycobacteria because they are less well-defined and their epidemiology is poorly understood (Littlewood and Heidmann 2006; Radostits *et al.* 2007).

Epidemiology

A correlation between the incidence of infections in horses and mycobacterial disease prevalence in other animals and man has been noted (Mair *et al.* 1986; Monreal *et al.* 2001). In the first half of the 20th century, *M. bovis* was the most frequently isolated *Mycobacterium* from horses (Pavlik *et al.* 2004). Subsequent to the establishment of effective bovine tuberculosis control programmes for cattle, which include testing and removal of affected animals, the incidence of *M. bovis* infection in horses declined dramatically (Larson 2007).

Mycobacterium avium ssp. *avium* infections are now the most frequently diagnosed mycobacterial disease in the equid. *Maa* is acquired from the environment, yet little is known about the specific source in an individual case (Ashford *et al.* 2001; Oaks 2007). Cases have not been diagnosed in horses younger than a year of age, a fact which may reflect a long incubation period for disease development (Oaks 2007). *Maa* disease usually manifests as pulmonary disease or as a generalised disseminated granulomatous disease. Given the ubiquitous nature of MAC and the natural resistance of horses to mycobacterial disease in general, host immunodeficiency is considered a likely predisposing factor to disease development, yet an apparent immunosuppressive condition is generally not recognised. There is no breed or gender predilection to disease susceptibility. In man, generalised *Maa* infections most often occur in severely immunocompromised individuals such as those infected with HIV (Ashford *et al.* 2001). The spread of *Maa* infection from animals to man has not been documented; nonetheless, the possibility of this type of transmission should not be ignored, particularly when affected animals are in contact with persons who are known to be immunosuppressed. There is no evidence to suggest that *Maa* infections are contagious between horses. On occasion localised *Maa* infection may be found, and these cases probably reflect wound contamination following some sort of traumatic event (Littlewood and Heidmann 2006).

Experimental *Map* infection in the horse has been produced (Larsen *et al.* 1972) but natural infection with the Johne's agent most likely does not occur or is exceptionally rare. Localised infections caused by less common species of mycobacteria have been reported including a case of subcutaneous infection caused by *M. smegmatis* (Booth and Wattret 2000) and abortion caused by *M. terrae* (Tasler and Hartley 1981).

Pathogenesis

Given the omnipresent nature of *Mycobacteria* spp., horses are often likely to be exposed to these organisms; yet the infection is adequately controlled and/or efficiently eliminated by the immune system without the development of overt disease. Why the protective response proves ineffective in some animals is not known, but the existence of some deficit in immune function is speculated. The primary routes of infection are ingestion and inhalation and less commonly wound contamination (Littlewood and Heidmann 2006; Oaks 2007). *M. avium* is able to resist the acidic pH (<3) of the stomach, which generally constitutes a formidable barrier to many nonenteric pathogens (Bodmer *et al.* 2000; Sung and Collins 2003). The bacterium transits to the intestine where it traverses the mucosa and infects macrophages in the submucosal layer; entering these cells via ligation of a variety of receptors (complement, mannose, *type A* scavenger receptors) (Fenton *et al.* 2005). *M. avium* also enters the enterocytes and follicle-associated microfold cells (M cells). Once inside macrophages, the bacterium resides in a membrane-bound phagocytic vacuole that fails to fully acidify and does not fuse with lysosomes (Frehel *et al.* 1986; Crowle *et al.* 1991). The bacterium-containing vacuole is thought to interact with endosomal vesicles that transport extracellular material within the mononuclear phagocyte thereby supplying the bacterium with nutrients needed for intracellular survival. In addition, the bacterium produces mycobactins, which are iron-chelating molecules. These siderophores compete with host mechanisms aimed at diminishing the availability of vacuolar iron and function to retain this crucial trace element in the phagosome (Wagner *et al.* 2005). Once acclimatised, the organism starts to multiply within the vacuole and eventually the progeny spread to other cells.

Initially neutrophils are recruited to the site of *M. avium* infection. These short-lived cells of the innate immune system engulf mycobacteria in the course of the first few hours but they ultimately prove to be unsuccessful in clearing the infection (Silva *et al.* 1989). NK (natural killer) cells are also involved in nonspecific immunity probably by secretion of INF-γ, a key activator of macrophages, which leads to partial control of the infection (Florido *et al.* 2003). $\gamma\delta^{+}$T cells, which are commonly found in mucosal and submucosal layers and are thought to participate in the defence against invading pathogens have little or no contribution to the host defence against *M. avium* (Petrofsky and Bermudez 2005). The presence of *M. avium* is signalled by Toll-like receptors (TLRs), which are pattern recognition receptors expressed on the surface of many cell types (macrophages, dendritic and epithelial cells) and recognise conserved motifs common to numerous pathogenic agents. TLR stimulation results in the secretion of multiple chemokines and cytokines (Shiratsuchi *et al.* 1993). A principal mediator of the early innate immune response, interleukin 12 (IL-12), stimulates INF-γ production by T and NK cells and is absolutely essential for restraining mycobacterial infection (Silva *et al.* 2001). Activated by INF-γ, macrophages halt the dissemination of bacteria. In addition, macrophages synthesise TNF-α (tumour necrosis factor α), a key cytokine involved in the formation and maintenance of the granuloma (Smith *et al.* 1997).

As a consequence of ongoing inflammation, lymphocytes (B and T cells) aggregate around the activated macrophages containing intracellular bacteria leading to the creation of a granuloma, also referred to as a tubercle (**Fig 1a**). Granuloma formation is characteristic of mycobacterial disease and is stimulated by the presence of persistent antigen. CD4+ T-helper cells are required for effective adaptive immunity against *M. avium* (Appelberg *et al.* 1994). These cells are also necessary for the induction of effective anti-mycobacterial activity in the macrophage. In the lungs, tubercles contain epithelioid cells, which are large activated macrophages that resemble epithelial cells. Multinucleated giant cells are also present. The outer layer of the granuloma is composed of fibrous tissue produced by fibroblasts. Ultimately, the granuloma serves to protectively wall off the infection from the rest of the host, but it also displaces and destroys healthy parenchyma (Dannenberg and Rook 1994). In cases where the mycobacterial infection affects the intestine, malabsorption frequently occurs. Thus, the clinical symptoms of mycobacterial disease are the result of organ dysfunction.

Clinical syndrome

Clinical signs are variable and reflect the organ system(s) affected and the extent of lesion severity. Chronic progressive loss of weight is the most commonly observed clinical finding in horses. A clinical history ranging from a couple of months to more than a year is commonplace. The weight loss is accelerated by the presence of diarrhoea, a characteristic feature of the granulomatous enteritis that accompanies mycobacterial infection of the small intestine, caecum or colon. The latter is often associated with hypoalbuminaemia derived from malabsorption or protein-losing enteropathy or both. Nonspecific symptoms typical of chronic infection including lethargy, weakness, anorexia and fever are also often observed. Neutrophilia and anaemia may be present in infected animals. In the case of miliary pulmonary disease, a nasal discharge and chronic moist cough with dyspnoea and tachypnoea may occur. Mesenteric and thoracic lymphadenopathy is commonly detected (**Fig 2**). Additional signs including lameness and neck stiffness may be observed and, when present, reflect osteomyelitis of the appendicular skeletal system or involvement of the cervical vertebrae (Zajac 1961; Peel 1983; Brown 2002; Charles 2005; Hewes *et al.* 2005; Radostits *et al.* 2007).

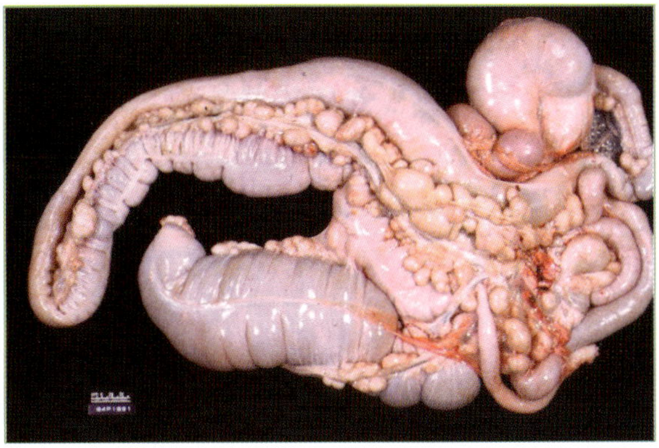

FIGURE 2: Extensive equine colon granulomatous lymphodenitis. The picture was generously provided by Dr Yosiya Niyo.

Cutaneous mycobacteriosis is generally the result of wound contamination following a traumatic injury. The latter typically manifests as hard and painful lumps with draining tracts on the abdomen and medial thighs and is associated with granulomatous or pyogranulomatous inflammation (Littlewood and Heidmann 2006). Abortion caused by *Maa* has been reported (Cline *et al.* 1991). Notably, the infected mares might be asymptomatic both prior to and after abortion (Helie and Higgins 1996). Other clinical manifestations of mycobacterial disease in the horse include ocular disease, guttural pouch infection, oral lesions and mastitis (Mair *et al.* 1986; Buergelt *et al.* 1988; Sills *et al.* 1990; Flores *et al.* 1991; Leifsson *et al.* 1997; Booth and Wattret 2000). The prognosis of highly advanced infections is unfavourable and unfortunately, most cases of *Maa* are well established at the time of diagnosis.

Pathology

Miliary or multifocal nodules are generally present in horses diagnosed with disseminated mycobacterial disease (Gunnes *et al.* 1995). Tubercles are often widespread and typically found in the liver, intestines, spleen, bone marrow and placenta (Mair *et al.* 1986). Occasionally, nodules may be more localised, confined for example to the cervical lymph nodes and cervical vertebrae. Lesions may involve the serosal surface and be associated with copious effusion into the peritoneal or pleural cavity. Lesion size ranges from microscopic to several cm in diameter. Tubercles are generally smooth, firm, solid, greyish and often resemble tumours. Sometimes the nodular lesions are caseous. Calcification is rare.

Intestinal infection is associated with ulceration of the mucosa with the caecum and colon most often affected. If widespread, the lesions may coalesce giving rise to a corrugated appearance to the intestine (**Fig 3**). Mesenteric lymph node enlargement is common (**Fig 2**). Histologically, granulomatous inflammation is apparent and acid fast organisms may be seen within macrophages located in the affected region (Mair *et al.* 1986; Buergelt *et al.* 1988; Lofstedt and Jakowski 1989; Cline *et al.* 1991; Gunnes *et al.* 1995; Helie and Higgins 1996; Hirsh and Biberstein 2004; Cousins *et al.* 2005; Radostits *et al.* 2007).

If involved, the lungs frequently have coarse and confluent nodules and granular thickenings can be found on pulmonary pleura. The enlarged bronchial lymph nodes have a sarcoma-like appearance. In the affected tissue, the alveolar and interalveolar spaces are frequently obliterated by macrophages, epithelioid cells, lymphocytes and giant polynuclear cells (Cousins *et al.* 2005; Pavlik *et al.* 2008).

The skeletal system is occasionally involved and is apparently more often affected in horses than in cattle (Brown 2002). The gross lesions may resemble degenerative joint disease with septic arthritis and granulomatous synovitis. The lesions may be associated with a large amount of fibrin and are characterised by synovial proliferation with minimal cartilage damage. Such pathology is most often caused by members of the *M. avium* complex (Hewes *et al.* 2005).

If affected, the necropsy of a fetus may reveal a creamy white homogeneous material on the chorionic surface of the allantochorion. Reddened and fine granules may be found on the placenta. A few pinpoint whitish foci might be present on the surface and in cut sections of the liver. The amnion and umbilical cord may be unaffected (Cline *et al.* 1991; Helie and Higgins 1996).

Diagnostic methods

Ante mortem diagnosis of mycobacterial infection is complicated by the fact that the range of clinical symptoms displayed are also exhibited by animals affected with other chronic bacterial and fungal infections as well as neoplasia (Pavlik *et al.* 2004; Oaks 2007). Haematological findings are usually characteristic of a chronic inflammatory process, characterised by neutrophilia, hyperfibrinogenaemia and anaemia (Brown 2002).

Horses experiencing weight loss or diarrhoea should undergo a colonic or rectal biopsy in an attempt to confirm the diagnosis of intestinal mycobacteriosis (Pearson and Heidel 1998). Histopathology with Ziehl-Neelsen staining may demonstrate the presence of granulomatous inflammation and acid-fast organisms (**Fig 1b**) (Littlewood and Heidmann 2006). In addition to biopsies, ultrasonography or radiography or both may be helpful in determining the nature and extent of the

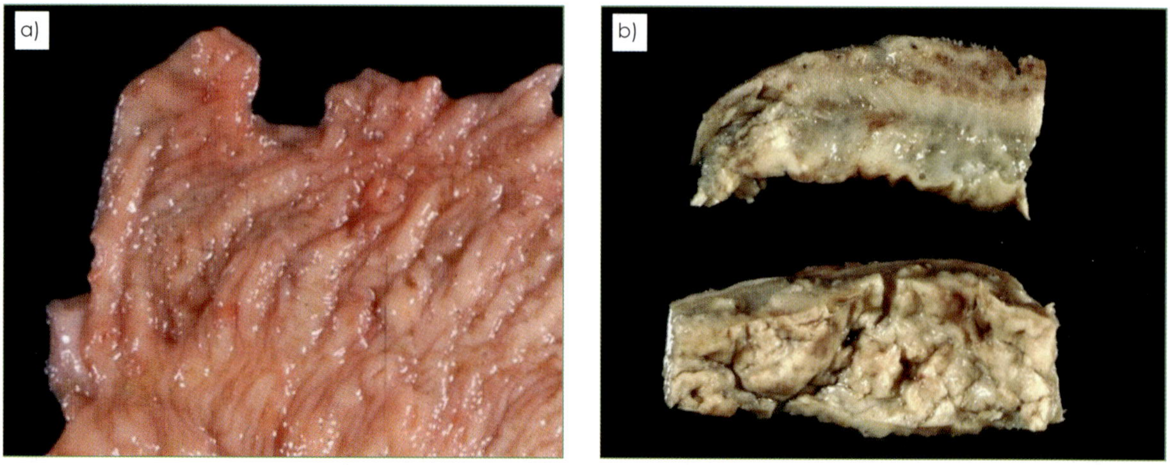

FIGURE 3: Equine granulomatous colitis. Colons show diffuse thickening and corrugation of the mucosa. The pictures were generously provided by Dr Yosiya Niyo (a) and Dr Ron Wilson (b).

disease. In horses with granulomatous enteritis, *M. avium* is often found in the faeces (Peel 1983; Brown 2002; Charles 2005; Oaks 2007; Radostits *et al.* 2007). In cases of pulmonary involvement, identification of acid fast bacilli in exudates taken by means of transtracheal aspiration or bronchoalveolar lavage is suggestive of mycobacterial disease (Brown 2002). Because mycobacterial disease is most often fatal, the opportunity generally exists for a thorough necropsy evaluation. Gross lesions are often suggestive of mycobacterial disease and microscopic analysis may prove definitively diagnostic.

Intradermal tuberculin testing with MAC or *M. bovis* antigens as done in cattle lacks specificity and, therefore is not recommended. In addition to many false positives, tuberculin injection can also induce anaphylaxis (Konyha and Kreier 1971; Brown 2002). The 'gold standard' for detection of mycobacteria is culture of tissue specimens or exudate. Traditional swabbing and transferring to agar plates may not be successful due to the paucity of mycobacteria in the sample and the hydrophobic nature of the organism (Pfyffer *et al.* 2003). Since mycobacterial species can be found in the nasal cavity of normal horses and considering the ubiquitous nature of these pathogens, measures should be taken to prevent the environmental contamination of the specimen being taken (Mair and Jenkins 1990; Pfyffer *et al.* 2003; Tobin-D'Angelo *et al.* 2004). Culture specimens should be stored and shipped to the laboratory at 4°C (Pfyffer *et al.* 2003). The laboratory personnel should also be notified if mycobacterial pathogens are suspected. To grow and successfully isolate *Mycobacteria* spp. specialised media and prolonged incubation times are required.

Growth rate, colony pigmentation and morphology, temperature sensitivity, and biochemical reactions are the phenotypic properties upon which the identification of cultured mycobacteria is based (Anon 1994; Pfyffer *et al.* 2003). The growth rate of mycobacteria varies by species. *M. bovis* and *M. tuberculosis* are slow growing organisms and require from 4–8 weeks of culture, whereas visible growth of *M. avium* can be detected within 7 days. The rapidly growing *M. fortuitum* or *M. smegmatis* require only 2–3 days for recovery from an affected specimen. The optimal temperature for incubation also varies between species. Cultures are generally incubated at 37°C in atmospheres of 5–10% carbon dioxide; however, those cultures derived from wound samples should be incubated at 25–33°C as well (Anon 1997; Pfyffer *et al.* 2003). To stimulate mycobacterial growth, media composed of nitrogen and carbon sources are supplemented with lipids, such as egg yolk, glycerol and oleic acid. Broth media are used to improve recovery rates and decrease the detection time. Middlebrook 7H10 and 7H11 solid formulations are usually utilised for isolation of MAC. These media produce colonies in 2–4 weeks, whereas Middlebrook 7H9 broth may yield the results in 7–14 days (Pfyffer *et al.* 2003). The culture methods are time-consuming and sometimes not definitive for the identification of mycobacteria. Serotyping is another method used to identify and characterise MAC organisms into strains although it has poor interlaboratory reproducibility and autoaglutination issues (Wayne *et al.* 1993). A more useful and rapid diagnostic method for MAC subspeciation is thin-layer, high-performance liquid or gas chromatography. These reliable techniques allow identification of lipids and mycolic acids produced by mycobacterial isolates (Butler *et al.* 1991; Butler and Guthertz 2001; Viader-Salvado and Molina-Torres 2007).

Molecular probing is a reproducible and commercially available method employing sensitive DNA probes that specifically hybridise to unique genomic loci of a particular organism. This technique identifies most common mycobacterial species but it still requires the organism to be first propagated (Chemlal and Portaels 2003). PCR is another powerful diagnostic tool that is widely used by veterinary laboratories to diagnose mycobacterial diseases in many animals (Oaks 2007). PCR may be directly performed on tissue, even on a formalin-fixed, paraffin-embedded clinical specimen. The advantage of this technique is its speed and high specificity, yet it may yield false-negative results (Chemlal and Portaels 2003). A number of PCR methodologies based on amplification of 16S rRNA have been developed not only to detect mycobacteria but also to differentiate them into species and subspecies (Wilton and Cousins 1992; Hews *et al.* 2005; Bartos *et al.* 2006).

Treatment and prevention

Treatment of highly advanced cases of mycobacterial disease particularly those caused by *M. bovis* or *M. tuberculosis* should not be attempted because of poor prognosis and the public health risk associated with these diseases. Infections caused by environmental mycobacteria are more likely to be successfully treated if they are cutaneous in nature or if localised wherein surgical debridement can be applied (Booth and Wattret 2000; Littlewood and Heidmann 2006; Oaks 2007). Given the lack of reports regarding successful therapy for generalised *Maa* disease in horses, if treatment is attempted, the principles used in human treatment could be applied. Whereas ethambutol, isoniazid, rifampin and streptomycin drug combinations are highly effective therapy for human *M. tuberculosis* infections, they are ineffective for treatment of *Maa* disease. The latter may reflect an inherent resistance of *Maa* to antimicrobial agents or may be due to the underlying immune system defect present in individuals with *Maa* disease, and such may prove to be similarly problematic in horses so affected. Newer regimens incorporating the macrolides, azithromycin and clarithromycin together with either ethambutol or rifampicin have been recently successful to treat human MAC infections and might be adaptable to equine cases (Anon 1997; Nuermberger and Grosset 2004).

If attempted, the treatment course will be prolonged (several months to more than a year) and will most probably incur substantial expense. Long term treatment should, therefore, be carefully considered and a recommendation for euthanasia might be appropriate (Booth and Wattret 2000; Brown 2002; Littlewood and Heidmann 2006; Oaks 2007). Prior to any treatment, it is advisable to accurately identify isolates and perform susceptibility tests in order to select appropriate antimicrobials. Nonetheless, the drug regimen will likely be empirically determined (Anon 1997). If possible, it is recommended that regular subculturing and susceptibility testing be performed in the course of the treatment in order to identify the development of resistant strain(s) so that treatment can be adjusted accordingly if necessary (Peel 1983). Preventive measures are generally unsuccessful because of the ubiquitous nature of the environmental mycobacteria.

Potential public health concerns

Mycobacterium bovis and *M. tuberculosis* are zoonotic pathogens and thus diseases caused by these organisms are reportable in most developed countries. However, there are no documented human cases of *M. bovis* or *M. tuberculosis* infection acquired from horses. Nonetheless, there is no reason why this transmission could not occur and so proper precaution including respiratory protection should be used when handling an infected horse (Brown 2002; Pavlik *et al.* 2004). Owners of such animals should be referred to their physicians for routine tuberculosis screening (Kaneene and Thoen 2004; Oaks 2007). Horses infected with *Maa* may constitute a source of infection for immunocompromised human patients (i.e. HIV-infected persons; chemotherapy patients) and, therefore, owners must be made aware of this potential risk if treating such animals.

References

Alexander, D.C. and Liu, J. (2006) Macrobacterial genomes. In: *Bacterial Genomes and Infectious Diseases*, Eds: V.L. Chan, P.M. Sherman and B. Bourke, Humana Press Inc., Totowa. pp 151-174.

Anon (1994) Group 21 - the mycobacteria. In: *Bergey's Manual of Determinative Bacteriology*, 9th edn., Eds: J.G. Holt, N.R. Krieg, P.H.A. Sneath and J.T. Staley, Williams & Wilkins, Baltimore. pp 597-604.

Anon (1997) American Thoracic Society: Diagnosis and treatment of the disease caused by nontuberculous mycobacteria. *Am. J. Respir. crit. care Med.* **156**, S1-S25.

Anon (2008) *Global Tuberculosis Control – Surveillance, Planning, Financing Report.* World Health Organization, Geneva.

Appelberg, R., Castro, A.G., Pedrosa, J., Silva, R.A., Orme, I.M. and Minoprio, P. (1994) Role of gamma interferon and tumor necrosis factor alpha during T-cell-independent and -dependent phases of *Mycobacterium avium* infection. *Infect. Immun.* **62**, 3962-3971.

Ashford, D.A., Whitney, E., Raghunathan, P. and Cosivi, O. (2001) Epidemiology of selected mycobacteria that infect humans and other animals. *Rev. Sci. Tech.* **20**, 325-337.

Bartos, M., Hlozek, P., Svastova, P., Dvorska, L., Bull, T., Matlova, L., Parmova, I., Kuhn, I., Stubbs, J., Moravkova, M., Kintr, J., Beran, V., Melicharek, I., Ocepek, M. and Pavlik, I. (2006) Identification of members of *Mycobacterium avium* species by Accu-Probes, serotyping, and single IS900, IS901, IS1245 and IS901-flanking region PCR with internal standards. *J. Microbiol. Methods* **64**, 333-345.

Bodmer, T., Miltner, E. and Bermudez, L.E. (2000) *Mycobacterium avium* resists exposure to the acidic conditions of the stomach. *FEMS Microbiol. Lett.* **182**, 45-49.

Booth, T.M. and Wattret, A. (2000) Stifle abscess in a pony associated with *Mycobacterium smegmatis*. *Vet. Rec.* **147**, 452-454.

Brown, C.M. (2002) Tuberculosis. In: *The 5-Minute Veterinary Consult Equine*, Ed: D. Troy, Lippincott Williams & Wilkins, Baltimore. pp 1082-1083.

Buergelt, C.D., Green, S.L., Mayhew, I.G., Wilson, J.H. and Merritt, A.M. (1988) Avian mycobacteriosis in three horses. *Cornell Vet.* **78**, 365-380.

Butler, W.R. and Guthertz, L.S. (2001) Mycolic acid analysis by high-performance liquid chromatography for identification of *Mycobacterium* species. *Clin. Microbiol. Rev.* **14**, 704-726.

Butler, W.R., Jost, Jr., K.C. and Kilburn, J.O. (1991) Identification of mycobacteria by high-performance liquid chromatography. *J. clin. Microbiol.* **29**, 2468-2472.

Charles, O.T. (2005) Tuberculosis and other mycobacterial infections. In: *The Merck Veterinary Manual*, 9th edn., Ed: C.M. Kahn, Merck and Co., Whitehouse Station. pp 549-553.

Chemlal, K. and Portaels, F. (2003) Molecular diagnosis of nontuberculous mycobacteria. *Curr. Opin. Infect. Dis.* **16**, 77-83.

Cline, J.M., Schlafer, D.W., Callihan, D.R., Vanderwall, D. and Drazek, F.J. (1991) Abortion and granulomatous colitis due to *Mycobacterium avium* complex infection in a horse. *Vet. Pathol.* **28**, 89-91.

Cousins, D.V., Huchzermeyer, H.F.K.A., Griffin, J.F.T., Brucknek, G.K., van Rensburg, I.B.J. and Kriek, N.P.J. (2005) Tuberculosis. In: *Infectious Diseases of Live Stock*, 3rd edn., Ed: J.A.W. Coetzer and R.C. Tustin, Oxford University Press Southern Africa, Cape Town. pp 1973-1993.

Crowle, A.J., Dahl, R., Ross, E. and May, M.H. (1991) Evidence that vesicles containing living, virulent *Mycobacterium tuberculosis* or *Mycobacterium avium* in cultured human macrophages are not acidic. *Infect. Immun.* **59**, 1823-1831.

Dannenberg, A.M. and Rook, G.A.W. (1994) Pathogenesis of pulmonary tuberculosis: an interplay of tissue-damaging and macrophage-activating immune responses. In: *Tuberculosis: Pathogenesis, Protection, and Control*, 1st edn., Ed: B.R. Bloom, ASM Press, Washington DC. pp 459-484.

Fenton, M.J., Riley, L.W. and Schlesinger, L.S. (2005) Receptor-mediated recognition of *Mycobacterium tuberculosis* by host cells. In: *Tuberculosis and the Tubercle Bacillus*, Ed: S.T. Cole, ASM Press, Washington DC. pp 405-426.

Fischer, O.A., Matlova, L., Dvorska, L., Svastova, P., Peral, D.L., Weston, R.T., Bartos, M. and Pavlik, I. (2004) Beetles as possible vectors of infections caused by *Mycobacterium avium* species. *Vet. Microbiol.* **102**, 247-255.

Flores, J.M., Sanchez, J. and Castano, M. (1991) Avian tuberculosis dermititis in a young horse. *Vet. Rec.* **128**, 407-408.

Florido, M., Correia-Neves, M., Cooper, A.M. and Appelberg, R. (2003) The cytolytic activity of natural killer cells is not involved in the restriction of *Mycobacterium avium* growth. *Infect. Immun.* **62**, 3962-3971.

Frehel, C., de Chastellier, C., Lang, T. and Rastogi, T. (1986) Evidence for inhibition of fusion of lysosomal and prelysosomal compartments with phagosomes in macrophages infected with pathogenic *Mycobacterium avium*. *Infect. Immun.* **52**, 252-262.

Gunnes, G., Nord, K., Vatn, S. and Saxegaard, F. (1995) A case of generalized avian tuberculosis in a horse. *Vet. Rec.* **136**, 565-566.

Harmsen, D., Dostal, S., Roth, A., Niemann, S., Rothgänger, J., Sammeth, M., Albert, J., Frosch, M. and Richter, E. (2003) RIDOM: comprehensive and public sequence database for identification of *Mycobacterium* species. *BMC Infect. Dis.* **3**, 26-36.

Helie, P. and Higgins, R. (1996) *Mycobacterium avium* complex abortion in a mare. *J. vet. diag. Invest.* **8**, 257-258.

Hewes, C.A., Schneider, R.K., Baszler, T.V. and Oaks, J.L. (2005) Septic arthritis and granulomatous synovatis caused by infection with *Mycobacterium avium* complex in a horse. *J. Am. vet. med. Ass.* **12**, 2035-2038.

Hirsh, D.C. and Biberstein, E.L. (2004) Mycobacterium. In: *Veterinary Microbiology*, 2nd edn., Eds: D.C. Hirsh, N.J. MacLachlan and R.L. Walker, Blackwell Publishing, Oxford. pp 223-234.

Kaneene, J.B. and Thoen, C.O. (2004) Tuberculosis. *J. Am. vet. med. Ass.* **224**, 685-691.

Konyha, L.D. and Kreier, J.P. (1971) The significance of tuberculin tests in the horse. *Am. Rev. Respir. Dis.* **103**, 91-99.

Larsen, A.B., Moon, H.V. and Merkal, R.S. (1972) Susceptibility of horses to *Mycobacterium paratuberculosis*. *Am. J. vet. Res.* **33**, 2185-2189.

Larson, J. (2007) Tuberculosis in animals: *Mycobacterium* bacilli that cause devastating zoonotic diseases in many animals. *Animal Welfare Information Center Series No. 2004-01,* Animal Welfare Information Center, U.S. Department of Agriculture.

Leifsson, P.S., Olsen, S.N. and Larsen, S. (1997) Ocular tuberculosis in a horse. *Vet. Rec.* **141**, 651-654.

Littlewood, J.D. and Heidmann, P. (2006) The skin. In: *The Equine Manual*, 2nd edn., Eds: A.J. Higgins and J.R. Snyder, Elsevier Limited, China. pp 305-391.

Lofstedt, J. and Jakowski, R.M. (1989) Diagnosis of avian tuberculosis in a horse by use of a liver biopsy. *J. Am. vet. med. Ass.* **194**, 260-262.

Machackova, M., Svastova, P., Lamka, J., Parmova, I., Liska, V., Smolik, J., Fischer, O.A. and Pavlik, I. (2004) Paratuberculosis in farmed and free-living wild ruminants in the Czech Republic (1999-2001). *Vet. Microbiol.* **101**, 225-234.

Machackova, M., Matlova, L., Lamka, J., Smolik, J., Melicharek, I., Hanzlikova, M., Docekal, J., Cvetnic, Z., Nagy, G., Lipiec, M., Ocepek, M. and Pavlik, I. (2003) Wild boar (*Sus scrofa*) as a possible vector of mycobacterial infections: review of literature and critical analysis of data from Central Europe between 1983 to 2001. *Veterinarni Medicina* **101**, 225-234.

Mair, T.S. and Jenkins, P.A. (1990) Isolation of mycobacteria from the nasal cavity of horses. *Equine vet. J.* **22**, 54-55.

Mair, T.S., Taylor, F.G., Gibbs, C. and Lucke, V.M. (1986) Generalised avian tuberculosis in a horse. *Equine vet. J.* **18**, 226-230.

Matlova, L., Dvorska, L., Palecek, K., Maurenc, L., Bartos, M. and Pavlik, I. (2004) Impact of sawdust and wood shavings in bedding on pig tuberculous lesions in lymph nodes, and IS1245 RFLP analysis of *Mycobacterium avium* subsp. *hominissuis* of serotypes 6 and 8 isolated from pigs and environment. *Vet. Microbiol.* **102**, 227-236.

Monreal, L., Segura, D., Segales, J., Garrido, J.M. and Prades, M. (2001) Diagnosis of *Mycobacterium bovis* infection in a mare. *Vet. Rec.* **149**, 712-714.

Muser, R. and Nassal, J. (1962) Tuberculosis, tuberculin reaction and mycobacteria in horses. *Rindertuberkulose und Brucellose* **11**, 118-126.

Nuermberger, E. and Grosset, J. (2004) Pharmacokinetic and pharmacodynamic issues in the treatment of mycobacterial infections. *Eur. J. Clin. Microbiol. Infect. Dis.* **23**, 243-255.

Oaks, J.L. (2007) Mycobacterial infections. In: *Equine Infectious Diseases*, Eds: D.C. Sellon and M.T. Long, Saunders Elsevier, St Louis. pp 296-300.

Pavlik, I. (2006) The experience of new European Union Member States concerning the control of the bovine tuberculosis. *Vet. Microbiol.* **112**, 221-230.

Pavlik, I., Jahn, P., Dvorska, L., Bartos, M., Novotny, L. and Halouzka, R. (2004) Mycobacterial infections in horses: a review of the literature. *Vet. Med.* **49**, 427-440.

Pavlik, I., Jahn, P., Moravkova, M., Matlova, L., Treml, F., Cizek, A., Nesnalova, E., Dvorska-Bartosova, L. and Halouzka, R. (2008) Lung tuberculosis in a horse caused by *Mycobacterium avium* subsp. *avium* of serotype 2: a case report. *Vet. Med.* **53**, 111-116.

Pearson, E.G. and Heidel, J.R. (1998) Colonic and rectal biopsy as a diagnostic aid in horses. *Comp. cont. Educ. pract. Vet.* **20**, 1354-1359.

Peel, J.E. (1983) Tuberculosis. In: *Current Therapy in Equine Medicine*, Ed: N.E. Robinson, W.B. Saunders, Philadelphia. pp 29-31.

Petrofsky, M. and Bermudez, L.E. (2005) CD4+ T cells but not CD8+ or γδ+T cells lymphocytes are required for host protection against *Mycobacterium avium* infection and dissemination through the intestinal route. *Infect. Immun.* **73**, 2621-2627.

Pfyffer, G.E., Brown-Elliot, B.A. and Wallace, R.J. (2003) Mycobacterium: general characteristics, isolation, and staining procedures. In: *Manual of Clinical Microbiology*, 8th edn., Eds: P.R. Murray, E.J. Baron, J.H. Jorgensen, M.A. Pfaller and R.H. Yolken, ASM Press, Washington DC. pp 532-559.

Radostits, O.M., Gay, C.C., Hinchcliff, K.W., Constable, P.D., Done, S.H., Jacobs, D., Ikede, B., McKenzie, R.A., Colwell, D.D., Osweiter, G. and Bildfell, R. (2007) Mycobacteriosis associated with *Mycobacterium avium-intracellulare* complex and with atypical mycobacteria. In: *Veterinary Medicine: A Textbook of the Diseases of Cattle, Horses, Sheep, Pigs, and Goats*, 10th edn., Eds: O.M. Radostits, C.C. Gay, K.W. Hinchcliff and P.D. Constable, Elsevier Limited, Spain. pp 1014-1017.

Reed, C., Von Reyn, C.F., Chamblee, S., Ellerbrock, T.V., Johnson, J.W., Marsh, B.J., Johnson, J.S., Trenschel, R.J. and Horsburg, C.R. (2006) Environmental risk factors for infection with *Mycobacterium avium* complex. *Am. J. Epidemiol.* **164**, 32-40.

Saadeh, C.E and Srkalovic, G. (2008) *Mycobacterium avium* complex infection after alemtuzumab therapy for chronic lymphocytic leukemia. *Pharmacotherapy* **28**, 281-284.

Shiratsuchi, H., Toossi, Z., Mettler, M.A. and Ellner, J.J. (1993) Colonial morphotype as a determinant of cytokine expression by human monocytes infected with *Mycobacterium avium*. *J. Immunol.* **150**, 2945-2954.

Sills, R.C., Mullaney, T.P., Stickle, R.L., Darien, B.J. and Brown, C.M. (1990) Bilateral granulomatous guttural pouch infection due to *Mycobacterium avium* complex in a horse. *Vet. Pathol.* **27**, 133-135.

Silva, M.T., Silva, M.N.T. and Appelberg, R. (1989) Neutrophil-macrophage cooperation in the host defence against mycobacterial infections. *Microb. Pathogen.* **6**, 369-380.

Silva, R.A., Florido, M. and Appelberg, R. (2001) Interleukine-12 primes CD4+ T cells for interferon-γ production and protective immunity during *Mycobacterium avium* infection. *Immunol.* **103**, 368-374.

Smith, D., Hansh, H., Bancroft, G. and Ehlers, S. (1997) T-cell-independent granuloma formation in response to *Mycobacterium avium*: role of tumour necrosis factor-α and interferon-γ. *Immunol.* **92**, 413-421.

Sung, N. and Collins, M.T. (2003) Variation in resistance of *Mycobacterium paratuberculosis* to acid environments as a function of culture medium. *Appl. Env. Microbiol.* **69**, 6833-6840.

Tasler, G.R. and Hartley, W.J. (1981) Foal abortion associated with *Mycobacterium terrae* infection. *Vet. Pathol.* **18**, 122-125.

Tobin-D'Angelo, M.J., Blass, M.A., del Rio, C., Blumberg, H.M. and Horsburgh, C.R. Jr. (2004) Hospital water as a source of *Mycobacterium avium* complex isolates in respiratory specimens. *J. Infect. Dis.* **189**, 98-104.

Tortoli, E. (2003) Impact of genotypic studies on mycobacterial taxonomy: the new mycobacteria of the 1990s. *Clin. Microbiol. Rev.* **16**, 319-354.

Verge, J. and Senthille, F. (1942) Nouvelles acquisitions sur l'etiologie de la tuberculose des equides. *Bulletin de L'academie Veterinaire de France* **15**, 229-231.

Viader-Salvado, J.M. and Molina-Torres, C.A. (2007) Detection and identification of mycobacteria by mycolic acid analysis of sputum specimens and young cultures. *J. Microbiol. Methods* **70**, 479-483.

Wagner, D., Maser, J., Lai, B., Cai, Z., Barry III, C.E., Honer zu Bentrup, K., Russel, D.G. and Bermudez, L.E. (2005) Elemental analysis of *Mycobacterium avium*-, *Mycobacterium tuberculosis*-, and *Mycobacterium smegmatis*-containing phagosomes indicates pathogen-induced microenvironments within the host cell's endosomal system. *J. Immunol.* **174**, 1491-1500.

Wayne, L.G., Good, R.C., Tsang, A., Butler, R., Dawson, D., Groothuis, D., Gross, W., Hawkins, J., Kilburn, J., Kubin, M., Schroder, K.H., Silcox, V.A., Smith, C., Thorel, M.F., Woodley, C. and Yakrus, M.A. (1993) Serovar determination and molecular taxonomic correlation in *Mycobacterium avium*, *Mycobacterium intracellulare*, and *Mycobacterium scrofulaceum*: a cooperative study of the International Working Group on Mycobacterial Taxonomy. *Int. J. Syst. Bacteriol.* **43**, 482-489.

Wilton, S. and Cousins, D. (1992) Detection and identification of multiple mycobacterial pathogens by DNA amplification in a single tube. *PCR Methods Appl.* **1**, 269-273.

Zajac, R.D. (1961) Tuberculosis in horses. *Can. vet. J.* **2**, 229-230.

BRUCELLOSIS IN THE HORSE

T. S. Mair* and T. J. Divers†

Bell Equine Veterinary Clinic, Mereworth, Maidstone, Kent ME18 5GS, UK; and †Department of Clinical Sciences, College of Veterinary Medicine, Cornell University, Ithaca, New York 14853, USA.

Keywords: horse; *Brucella*; *Brucella abortus*; fistulous withers; poll evil

Summary

Brucellosis is a major disease of domesticated and wild animals worldwide, and is also an important zoonosis. Of the domesticated species, cattle, sheep, pigs and goats are most commonly affected, and reproductive failure is the most common clinical manifestation. Infection in horses is uncommon, but is usually associated with infectious bursitis, arthritis or tenosynovitis. Less commonly, cases of vertebral osteomyelitis, abortion and infertility in stallions have been recorded. Fistulous withers and poll evil are the commonest clinical manifestations in the horse, and infection most frequently involves *Brucella abortus*. Serological surveys indicate that many horses may be exposed to *B. abortus* without developing clinical signs of disease.

Aetiology and epidemiology

Bacteria of the genus *Brucella* are nonmotile, aerobic, intracellular Gram-negative cocci, cocco-bacilli or short rods. *Brucella* spp. are transmissible to a wide range of species, and among the domesticated animals, cattle, sheep, goats and pigs are most commonly affected (**Table 1**) (Godfroid *et al.* 2004). Wild animal species are also occasionally infected (Godfroid 2002). The most important clinical manifestations are reproductive failure (including mid- to late-term abortions and infertility in cows, and orchitis and inflammation of the accessory sex glands in bulls). Chronic infections can result in arthritis. In cattle, the primary sources of infection include fetal membranes and fluids, vaginal discharges, milk and semen. Placental samples from brucellosis-induced abortions in cattle have yielded 10^{10} organisms/g (Alexander *et al.* 1981). Six major *Brucella* species have been classically characterised: *B. abortus*, *B. melitensis*, *B. suis*, *B. canis*, *B. ovis* and *B. neotamae*. Recently, 2 new species, *B. ceti* and *B. pinnipedialis*, have been isolated from marine species (Foster *et al.* 2007). Most *Brucella* spp. have a strong host preference, which is evident in their ability to establish chronic infection in individuals and maintain transmission and infection in populations of specific animal species (Glynn and Lynn 2008).

Brucellosis in cattle is usually caused by biovars of *B. abortus*, although in southern Europe and the Middle East, *B. melitensis* may cause abortion in cattle kept close to infected sheep and goats (Godfroid *et al.* 2004). Brucellosis is an important zoonotic disease; in man, brucellosis (undulant fever) is seen primarily in veterinarians, stock inspectors, abattoir worker, etc. (Anon 1986). Human brucellosis is dependent on the presence of *Brucella* spp. among other animals with which people have direct or indirect contact (Glynn and Lynn 2008). In many areas of the world, animal disease control programmes and occupational safety practices have diminished the impact of brucellosis over the last half century.

None of the *Brucella* spp. are adapted to the horse. Equine infections usually involve the cattle pathogen *B. abortus*, although infection with *B. suis* has been reported (Nicoletti 2007). There are no

TABLE 1: *Brucella* spp. infections among domesticated animals

Brucella species	Disease	Species affected
B. abortus	Brucellosis (contagious abortion)	Sheep
B. ovis	Epididymitis/orchitis	Sheep
B. melitensis	Abortion and orchitis	Sheep and goats
B. suis	Abortion, stillbirth, sterility in sows and orchitis in males	Pigs

*Author to whom correspondence should be addressed.

reports of natural infection of horses with *B. canis* (Hagler *et al.* 1982).

B. abortus infections in domestic animals have been reported worldwide, but have been effectively eradicated from several European countries, Japan and Israel (Nicoletti 2007). There is no apparent age, gender or breed predisposition to infection in horses, although most cases have been reported in horses aged >3 years (Nicoletti 2007).

Brucella spp. are fairly hardy; organisms have been recovered from fetal and manure samples that remained in a cool environment for >2 months. However, exposure to sunlight kills the organisms within a few hours, and the organisms are susceptible to many common disinfectants (Glynn and Lynn 2008).

Pathogenesis and clinical signs

Brucella spp. are facultative intracellular pathogens and establish infection by invading macrophages and evading macrophage-induced host defence mechanisms (Gorvel and Moreno 2002). These characteristics contribute to the clinical signs and therapeutic considerations, including the difficulty in both diagnosis and treatment (Glynn and Lynn 2008). Following ingestion of the organism, the bacteria travel through the oral mucosa to the regional lymph nodes. Infection leads to bacteraemia, which is usually transient; the organisms ultimately settle in the reproductive tissues or musculoskeletal system.

Horses usually become infected by the ingestion of *B. abortus*-contaminated feed, and most reported cases indicate a history of contact with cattle (Duff 1937; McCaughey and Kerr 1967; Denny 1973; O'Sullivan 1981; Ocholi *et al.* 2004). There is no evidence to suggest that horses are a reservoir of brucellosis in endemic areas or that they are an important source of infection for other animals (Acosta-Gonzalez *et al.* 2006).

Serological surveys in endemic areas indicate that many horses can be exposed and infected by *B. abortus* without any clinical signs of disease (Denny 1973; Dawson and Durrant 1975; Dawson 1977; Nicoletti *et al.* 1982; MacMillan and Cockrem 1986). Following experimental infection by instillation of *B. abortus* into the conjunctival sac of horses, an intermittent bacteraemia was detected for up to 2 months, and serum antibodies (measured by serum agglutination, complement fixation, Coombs antiglobulin, 2-mercaptoethanol, Rose Bengal plate and agar gel immunodiffusion tests) became detectable between 7 and 12 days after infection (MacMillan *et al.* 1982). No clinical signs were detected in these horses apart from mild pyrexia. Five of these 7 experimentally infected horses were mares that were subsequently put in foal; they all bred normally, and no organisms were recovered from the horses or from in-contact cattle (MacMillan and Cockrem 1986).

In horses that develop clinical signs of infection the organism usually localises in bursae (causing septic bursitis), tendon sheaths (causing septic tenosynovitis) and joints (causing septic arthritis) (Denny 1972, 1973; Carrigan *et al.* 1987; Ocholi *et al.* 2004). Less commonly, cases of vertebral osteomyelitis (Collins *et al.* 1971), abortion and infertility in stallions have been recorded (Denny 1973). The commonest clinical diseases associated with *Brucella* spp. infection in horses are septic supraspinatous bursitis (fistulous withers) (**Figs 1** and **2**) and septic supra-atlantal bursitis (poll evil) (**Fig 3**). Duff (1937) reported 85 cases of fistulous withers or poll evil, and identified *B. abortus* infection in 80%. Chronic draining sinuses occur in both conditions (Crawford *et al.* 1990). *B. suis* has also been isolated from horses with septic bursitis (Portugal *et al.* 1971; Cook and Kingston 1988), aborted equine fetuses (McNutt and Murray 1924), and the internal organs of a mare with no external signs of disease (Cvetnic *et al.* 2005).

Fistulous withers and poll evil

Fistulous withers is a chronic inflammatory disease of the supraspinatus bursa and associated tissues (Gaughan *et al.* 1988; Rashmir-Raven *et al.* 1990; Cohen *et al.* 1992). Although infection by *B. abortus* has been associated with the condition (Duff 1937; O'Sullivan 1981), other infectious organisms and trauma can also cause the disease. Indeed in geographical areas with a low prevalence of brucellosis in cattle, *B. abortus* is rarely isolated from fistulous withers cases (Gaughan *et al.* 1988; Cohen *et al.* 1992). Infection by multiple bacteria is often present. Other than *B. abortus*, organisms commonly isolated from clinical cases include *Streptococcus zooepidemicus*, *Streptococcus equi*, *Staphylococcus*

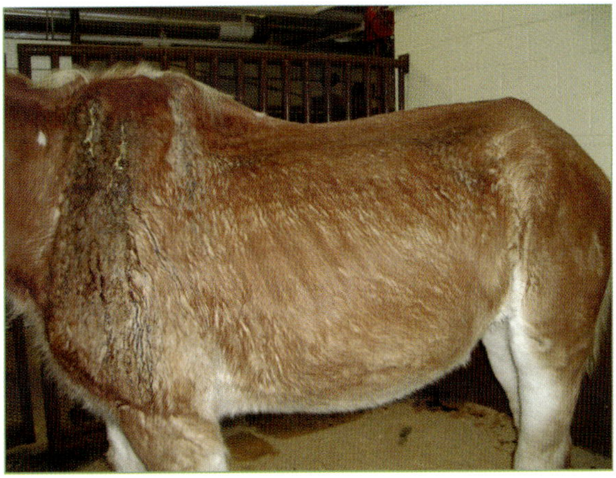

FIGURE 1: Fistulous withers with multiple draining tracts discharging purulent material (courtesy of Ceri Sherlock).

aureus, *Staphylococcus epidermidis*, *Proteus mirablis*, *Actinomyces bovis*, *Bacteroides fragilis*, *Escherichia coli*, *Pasteurella* spp. and *Corynebacterium* spp. (Guard 1932; Gaughan *et al.* 1988; Cohen *et al.* 1992; Hawkins and Fessler 2000). Infection by *Onchocerca cervicalis* has also been incriminated in some cases (Lyons *et al.* 1988; Rashmir-Raven *et al.* 1990; Hawkins and Fessler 2000).

The supraspinous bursa is located between the funicular portion of the nuchal ligament and the dorsal spinous processes of the second to fifth thoracic vertebrae (Hawkins and Fessler 2000). The bursa is approximately 5 cm wide and ranges in length from 5–11 cm, and has a capacity in the normal horse of 30–90 ml. Clinical signs of supraspinous bursitis (fistulous withers) include singular or multiple draining tracts (**Fig 1**) or diffuse swelling of the withers without drainage (**Fig 2**). The onset of clinical signs may be abrupt or insidious. Early signs include localised heat, pain and swelling of the bursa. There may be lethargy and general stiffness. In most cases the bursa ruptures and purulent exudate is discharged from one or more fistulae. These fistulae may heal over, but may subsequently reform. Extensive fibrosis may occur. Horses with fistulous withers that are seropositive to *B. abortus* are significantly more likely than seronegative horses with fistulous withers to have radiographic evidence of osteomyelitis of the underlying dorsal spinous processes (Cohen *et al.* 1992).

Poll evil (septic supra-atlantal bursitis) causes similar clinical signs to fistulous withers in the poll region. There is frequently pain and neck stiffness (**Fig 3**). Swelling of the region occurs which may be followed by discharge of purulent material.

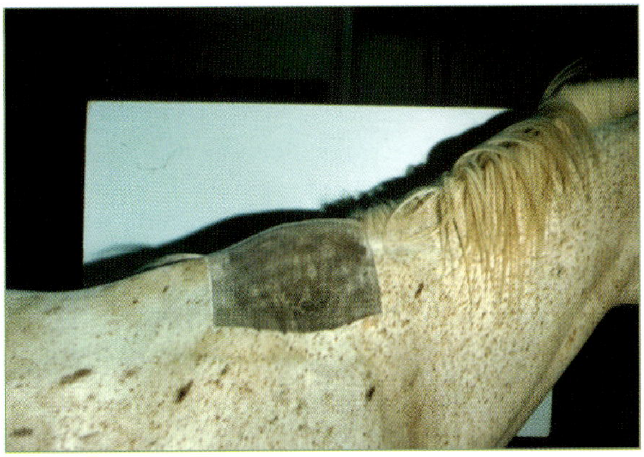

FIGURE 2: Fistulous withers in a 9-year-old mare. There is diffuse swelling of the supraspinous bursa (without drainage in this case).

Abortion

Mid- to late-term abortion in mares has been reported, but this appears to be rare (McNutt and Murray 1924; McCaughey and Kerr 1967; Shortridge 1967; Robertson *et al.* 1973; Hinton *et al.* 1977). *B. abortus* may be isolated from the fetus and fetal membranes, and the affected mares show a

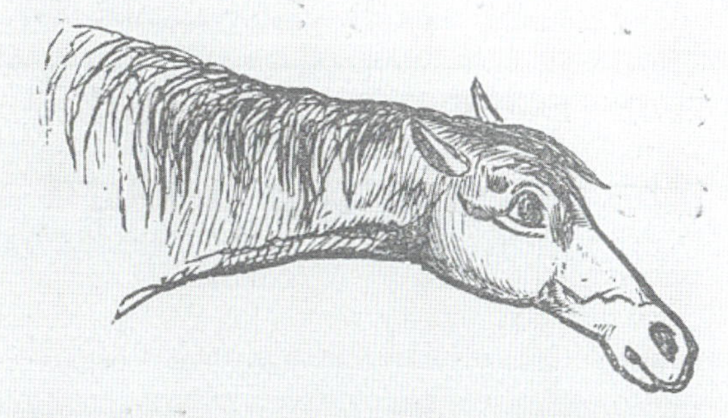

FIG. 229.—*Stiffness previous to external enlargement in Poll Evil.*

FIGURE 3: Neck pain and stiffness associated with poll evil (Armitage 1892).

serological response to infection. Unlike infected cows, excretion of the organism in vaginal discharges appears to be short-lived. In most instances, mares have become infected by co-grazing pastures with infected cattle.

Diagnosis

Brucella spp. require complex media for growth in culture, and many strains require complementary carbon dioxide for optimum growth. Although attempts should always be made to culture *B. abortus* from exudates in cases of fistulous withers and poll evil, overgrowth by other bacteria commonly makes the organism difficult to isolate (Nicoletti 2007).

Serological testing is recommended in suspected cases. The card test that is widely used for screening of *B. abortus* in cattle has poor specificity (Nicoletti 2007). The plate agglutination test is considered to be more sensitive and specific; a titre ≥1:50 is considered positive (Dohoo *et al.* 1986; Nicoletti 2007). Occasionally, false positive results will be obtained, and there are reports or *B. abortus* isolation from seronegative horses (Denny 1973). Other serological tests can be used, including tube agglutination, complement fixation, Coomb's antiglobulin, mercaptoethanol and agar gel diffusion tests. Although a rising titre will establish an acute infection, this might not be seen in long-standing cases; in these circumstances, a high titre in combination with appropriate clinical signs should be considered diagnostic (Nicoletti 2007).

Radiography can be useful in fistulous withers and poll evil cases to assess the extent of bursal distension and associated osseous damage.

Treatment

Treatment of brucellosis in horses generally involves a combination of systemic antimicrobials and local surgical drainage/debridement of infected tissue (see fistulous withers above). Although *Brucella* spp. are generally sensitive to tetracyclines, chloramphenicol, streptomycin and some sulphonamides, there may be insufficient penetration into infected tissues to achieve resolution of the infection (Nicoletti 2007). In addition, polymicrobial infections are common. The successful treatment of 3 horses using clofazimine has been reported (Knottenbelt *et al.* 1989).

Administration of the *Brucella* strain 19 vaccine has been reported in the treatments of horses with brucellosis (Denny 1973; Gardner *et al.* 1983; Cohen *et al.* 1992). In a survey of veterinarians in Florida concerning the treatment of fistulous withers, treatment with antibiotics and strain 19 vaccine was reported to be effective in 37 of 46 horses (80.4%) (Gardner *et al.* 1983). Treatment regimes have varied from a single dose of vaccine to 3 doses at 10 day intervals (Denny 1973; Nicoletti 2007). Local and systemic reactions have been recorded with the use of the vaccine, including death in some horses that received the vaccine intravenously (Cosgrove 1961; Millar 1961; Denny 1973; Cohen *et al.* 1992).

Treatment of fistulous withers and poll evil can be difficult. Medical treatment is directed towards controlling infection and inflammation. Broad-spectrum antibiotics are recommended, pending serological and microbiological findings, and when culture results are unavailable or considered unreliable due to contamination. Lavage of draining

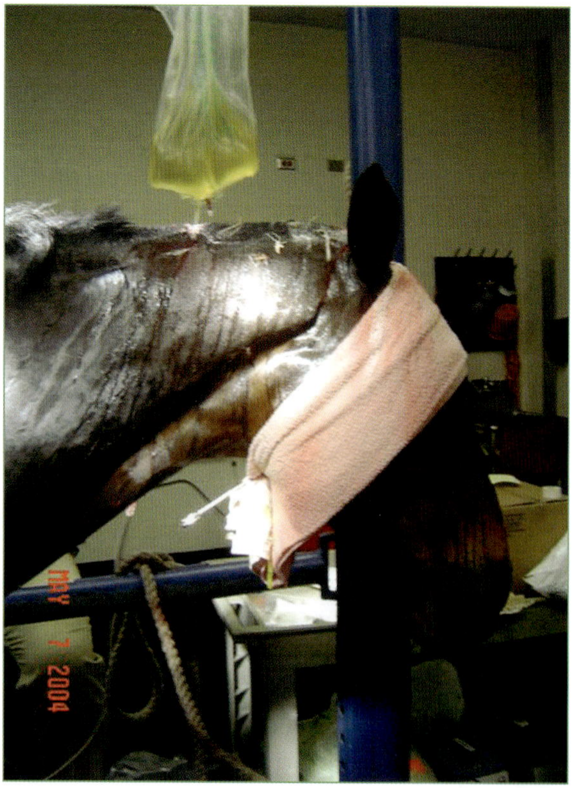

FIGURE 4: Lavage of the supra-atlantal bursa of a horse affected by poll evil.

tracts with antiseptic solutions and dimethyl sulphoxide may be helpful (Cohen *et al.* 1992) (**Fig 4**). Radical surgical debridement of infected bursal tissue, with or without curettage of the dorsal spinous processes in the case of fistulous withers may be necessary in some animals (Gaughan *et al.* 1988; Hawkins and Fessler 2000); the surgery may be performed in the standing horse or under general anaesthesia.

Prevention and public health risk

Since horses usually acquire *B. abortus* infection from cattle (Denny 1973; Cramlet and Bernhanu 1979), they should not be housed or pastured with seropositive cattle. Since trauma is considered to be a predisposing factor for the development of fistulous withers, properly-fitting saddles and tack should always be used. Parasite control measures to reduce the incidence of *Onchocerca* spp. should also be used.

Horses infected by *B. abortus* may represent a source of infection to man (Anon 1986; Acha and Szyfres 1987), although documented cases of this route of infection are rare (Jalil 2008). The organism can enter the body through abraded skin and enter across intact mucous membranes, including the conjunctiva and respiratory mucosa. The number of human cases of brucellosis has declined dramatically over the past 30 years as a result of effective control measures to control the disease in domestic animals (Salata 2000).

B. abortus infection is a reportable disease in many countries, and seropositive horses may require to be quarantined or subjected to euthanasia.

References

Acha, P.N. and Szyfres, B. (1987) *Zoonoses and Communicable Diseases Common to Man and Animals,* 2nd edn., Pan American Health Organization, Washington DC. pp 24-45.

Acosta-Gonzalez, R.I., Gonzalez-Reyes, I. and Flores-Gutierrez, G.H. (2006) Prevalence of *Brucella abortus* antibodies in equines of a tropical region of Mexico. *Can. J. vet. Res.* **70**, 302-304.

Alexander, B., Schnurrenberger, P.R. and Brown, R.R. (1981) Numbers of *Brucella abortus* in the placenta, umbilicus, and fetal fluid of two naturally infected cows. *Vet. Rec.* **108**, 500.

Anon (1986) *Joint FAO/WHO Expert Committee on Brucellosis. World Health Organisation Technical Report Series 740.* World Health Organiztion, Geneva.

Armitage, G.A. (1892) *Every Man his own Horse Doctor*, Frederick Warne & Co., London.

Carrigan, M.J., Cockram, F.A. and Nash, G.V. (1987) *Brucella abortus* biotype 1 arthritis in a horse. *Aust. vet. J.* **64**, 190.

Cohen, N.D., Carter, G.K. and McMullan, W.C. (1992) Fistulous withers in horses: 24 cases (1984-1990). *J. Am. vet. med. Ass.* **201**, 121-124.

Collins, J.D., Kelly, W.R., Twomey, T., Farrelly, B.T. and Witty, B.T. (1971) Brucella-associated vertebral osteomyelitis in a Thoroughbred mare. *Vet. Rec.* **88**, 321-326.

Cook, D.R. and Kingston, G.C. (1988) Isolation of *Brucella suis* biotype 1 from a horse. *Aust. vet. J.* **65**, 162-163.

Cosgrove, J.S.M. (1961) Clinical aspects of equine brucellosis. *Vet. Rec.* **73**, 1377-1382.

Cramlet, S.H. and Berhanu, G. (1979) The relationship of *Brucella abortus* titers to equine fistulous withers in Ethiopia. *Vet. Med. Small Anim. Clin.* **74**, 195-199.

Crawford, R.P., Huber, J.D. and Adams, L.G. (1990) Epidemiology and surveillance. In: *Animal Brucellosis,* Eds: K. Nielsen and L. G. Adams, CRC Press, Orlando. pp 131-151.

Cvetnic, Z., Spicic, S., Curic, S., Jukic, B., Lojkic, M., Albert, D., Thiebaud, M. and Garin-Bastuji, B. (2005) Isolation of *Brucella suis* biovar 3 from horses in Croatia. *Vet. Rec.* **156**, 584-585.

Dawson, F.L.M. and Durrant, D.S. (1975) Some serological reactions to *Brucella* antigen in the horse. *Equine vet. J.* **7**, 137-140.

Dawson, F.L.M. (1977) Further serological reactions to *Brucella* antigen in the horse. *Equine vet. J.* **9**, 158-160.

Denny, H.R. (1972) Brucellosis in the horse. *Vet. Rec.* **90**, 86-90.

Denny, H.R. (1973) A review of brucellosis in the horse. *Equine vet. J.* **5**, 121-125

Dohoo, I.R., Wright, G.M. and Ruckerbauer, B.S. (1986) A comparison of five serologic tests for bovine brucellosis. *Can. vet. J.* **50**, 485-493.

Duff, H.M. (1937) *Brucella abortus* in the horse. *J. comp. Path.* **50**, 151.

Foster, G., Osterman, B.S., Godfroid, J., Jacques, I. and Cloeckaert, A. (2007) *Brucella ceti* sp. nov. and *Brucella pinnipedialis* sp. nov. for *Brucella* strains with cetaceans and seals as their preferred hosts. *Int. J. Syst. Evol. Microbiol.* **57**, 2688-2693.

Gardner, G.R., Nicolleti, P. and Scarratt, W.K. (1983) Treatment for brucellosis in horses by Florida practitioners. *Fla. vet. J.* **12**, 21-23.

Gaughan, E.M., Fubini, S.L. and Dietze, A. (1988) Fistulous withers in horses: 14 cases (1978-1987). *J. Am. vet. med. Ass.* **193**, 964-966

Glynn, M.K. and Lynn, T.V. (2008) Brucellosis. *J. Am. vet. med. Ass.* **233**, 900-908.

Godfroid, J. (2002) Brucellosis in wildlife. *Revue Scientifique et Technique de l'Office des Epizooties* **21**, 277-286.

Godfroid, J., Bosman, P.P. and Bishop, G.C. (2004) Bovine brucellosis. In: *Infectious Diseases of Livestock,* 2nd edn., Eds: J.A.W. Coetzer and R.C. Tustin, Oxford University Press, Cape Town. pp 1510-1527.

Gorvel, J.P. and Moreno, E. (2002) Brucella intracellular life: from invasion to intracellular replication. *Vet. Microbiol.* **90**, 281-297.

Guard, W. (1932) Fistula of the withers. North Am. Vet. **13**, 19-23.

Hagler, D.S., Nicoletti, P.L. and Scarratt, W.K. (1982) Attempt to infect horses with *Brucella canis. Equine vet. Sci.* **2**, 168-169.

Hawkins, J.F. and Fessler, J.F. (2000) Treatment of supraspinous bursitis by use of debridement in standing horses: 10 cases (1968-1999). *J. Am. vet. med. Ass.* **217**, 74-78.

Hinton, M., Barker, G.L. and Morgan, T.L. (1977) Abortion in a mare associated with *Brucella abortus* infection and twins. *Vet. Rec.* **101**, 526.

Jalil, S. (2008) Human brucellosis acquired through horses. *J. Invest. Med.* **56**, 814.

Knottenbelt, D.C., Hill, F.W. and Morton, D.J. (1989) Clofazimine for the treatment of fistulous withers in three horses. *Vet. Rec.* **125**, 509-10.

Lyons, E.T., Drudge, J.H. and Tolliver, S.C. (1988) Verification of ineffectual activity of ivermectin against adult *Onchocerca* spp. in the ligamentum nuchae of horses. *Am. J. vet. Res.* **19**, 16-22.

MacMillan, A.P., Baskerville, A., Hambleton, P. and Corbel, M.J. (1982) Experimental *Brucella abortus* infection in the horse: observations during the three months following inoculation. *Res. vet. Sci.* **33**, 351-359.

MacMillan, A.P. and Cockrem, D.S. (1986) Observations on the long-term effects of *Brucella abortus* infection in the horse, including effects during pregnancy and lactation. *Equine vet. J.* **18**, 388-390.

McCaughey, W.J. and Kerr, W.R. (1967) Abortion due to brucellosis in a Thoroughbred mare. *Vet. Rec.* **80**, 186-187.

McNutt, S.H. and Murray, C. (1924) Bacterium abortion (Bang) isolated from the fetus of an aborting mare. *J. Am. vet. med. Ass.* **97**, 576-580.

Millar, R. (1961) *Brucella abortus* infection in the horse. *Br. vet. J.* **117**, 167-170.

Nicoletti, P.L. (2007) Brucellosis. In: *Equine Infectious Diseases*, Eds: D.C. Sellon and M.T. Long, Saunders Elsevier, Philadelphia. pp 348-350.

Nicoletti, P.L., Mahler, J.R. and Scarratt, W.K. (1982) Study of agglutinins to *Brucella abortus*, *B. canis* and *Actinobacillus equuli* in horses. *Equine vet. J.* **14**, 302-304.

O'Sullivan, B.M. (1981) *Brucella abortus* titres and bursitis in the horse. *Aust. vet. J.* **57**, 103-104.

Ocholi, R.A., Bertu, W.J., Kwaga, J.K., Ajogi, I., Bale, J.O. and Okpara, J. (2004) Carpal bursitis associated with *Brucella abortus* in a horse in Nigeria. *Vet. Rec.* **155**, 566-567.

Portugal, M.A.S.C., Nesti, A., Giorgi, W., Franca, E.N. and De Oliveira, B.S. (1971) Brucelose em equideos determinada por *Brucella suis*. *Arquivas di Instituto Biologica de Sao Paulo* **38**, 125-132.

Rashmir-Raven, A., Gaughan, E.M., Modransky, P. (1990) Fistulous withers. *Comp. cont. Educ. pract. Vet.* **12**, 1633-1641.

Robertson, F.J., Milne, J., Silver, C.L. and Clark, H. (1973) Abortion associated with *Brucella abortus* (biotype 1) in the T.B. mare. *Vet. Rec.* **92**, 480-481.

Salata, R.A. (2000) Brucellosis. In: *Cecil Textbook of Medicine*. Eds: L. Goldman and J.C. Bennett, W.B. Saunders, Philadelphia. pp 1717-1719.

Shortridge, E.H. (1967) Two cases of suspected *Brucella abortus* abortion in mares. *N.Z. vet. J.* **15**, 33-34.

ANTHRAX IN THE HORSE

T. S. Mair* and G. R. Pearson†

Bell Equine Veterinary Clinic, Mereworth, Maidstone, Kent ME18 5GS; and †Department of Clinical Veterinary Science, School of Veterinary Science, Bristol University, Langford House, Langford, Bristol BS40 5DU, UK.

Keywords: horse; anthrax; *Bacillus anthracis*

Summary

Anthrax is a highly contagious disease of domestic animals, wild animals and man caused by *Bacillus anthracis*. In most animals it results in a rapidly fatal septicaemia and 'sudden death'. The organism exists in vegetative and spore states. Sporulation occurs during exposure to air, and the spores can survive in the environment for many years. The source of *B. anthracis* spores in infections is usually the soil, but spores have also been found in hay and feed. Infection usually occurs by ingestion, although inhalation and cutaneous penetration can also occur. Although peracute infection and 'sudden death' may occur, many horses develop an acute infection resulting in signs of colic, fever, dyspnoea and subcutaneous oedema. The disease typically progresses rapidly, with death within 24–48 h. Treatment with i.v. penicillin or oxytetracycline can be effective so long as it is initiated early.

Introduction

Anthrax (German: *milzbrand*; French: *charbon*) is an important peracute, acute or sub-acute highly contagious disease of domestic animals, wild animals and man caused by *Bacillus anthracis* (de Vas and Turnbull 2004; Long 2007). In most animals it results in a rapidly fatal septicaemia and 'sudden death'. Anthrax most commonly develops in domestic and wild herbivores, such as cattle, sheep, goats, antelope and deer (Shadomy and Smith 2008). Anthrax is of particular topical importance because of its bioterrorist potential (Crupi *et al.* 2003).

*Author to whom correspondence should be addressed.

Aetiology and epidemiology

Bacillus anthracis is a large, spore-producing, Gram-positive rod (approximately 1 µm in diameter and 3–6 µm long) that can be cultured under both aerobic and nonaerobic conditions on most laboratory media. Optimum growth occurs at 37°C. On agar plates, the anthrax organisms form surface colonies with a ground glass appearance, and the margins of the colonies are irregular under low magnification ('Medusa-head colonies').

The bacillus was first isolated from animals that died of anthrax in 1877 by Robert Koch (Koch 1877); he was able to infect mice with the spores, thus demonstrating Koch's postulates for the first time (Shadomy and Smith 2008). The bacillus is nonhaemolytic, has a capsule, and is nonmotile. In infected tissues, the large bacilli occur individually or grow in chains (2–6 organisms) and the characteristic capsule is visible when stained with polychrome methylene blue (McFadyean reaction) (Parry *et al.* 1983; Quinn and Turnbull 1998). The capsule stains pink, in contrast to the body of the organism, which stains blue. *B. anthracis* can be differentiated from other bacilli on the basis of the presence of a capsule, susceptibility to penicillin, lack of motility, absence or delayed haemolysis when cultured on blood agar, and susceptibility to γ phage (Shadomy and Smith 2008). The organism exists in vegetative and spore states. The organism sporulates during nutrient deprivation and exposure to air, as occurs during *in vitro* cultivation or when an infected carcase is disrupted by scavengers or during necropsy. Sporulation allows the organism to survive in the environment for many years, and spores are highly resistant to extremes of temperature, UV light and many chemical disinfectants. Spores can survive the tanning and processing of hides, and have been shown to remain viable for more than 50 years (Umeno and Nobata 1938). Spores germinate when exposed to 65°C for 15 min, and change into the vegetative bacillary form. In contrast to spores, the vegetative bacilli are susceptible to desiccation, high temperatures and chemical disinfectants. Anthrax has a worldwide distribution, but it is most common in agricultural regions of South and Central America, sub-Saharan Africa, central and southwestern Asia, and southern and eastern Europe (Hugh-Jones 1999).

The source of *B. anthracis* spores in infections is usually the soil, which is considered to be the natural reservoir of *B. anthracis*, but spores have also been found in hay and feed (e.g. from contaminated bone meal and vegetable proteins such as groundnut). Wool and hair wastes, cleanings used in fertilisers, and tannery effluents can also be sources of infection (Timoney *et al.* 1988). Outbreaks typically occur in the summer during periods of hot, dry weather that follow heavy rain and flooding. Additionally, outbreaks may be triggered by disruption of the soil in areas where anthrax-infected carcases have been buried (Shadomy and Smith 2008). Natural outbreaks often occur in cycles, with the primary infection involving one or more animals that have recently been introduced into an area. After they die, the infected carcases contaminate the soil with *B. anthracis*. The next cycle of infection may involve multiple animals that are exposed to the contaminated soil (or carcases). Most natural cases of anthrax in horses are associated with disease in cattle.

Outbreaks of anthrax in animals are often associated with low-lying areas with soil that has high moisture and organic contents, and alkaline pH (Dragon and Rennie 1995). Such areas have been described as 'incubator areas', indicating favourable conditions that permit spore germination and vegetative multiplication (van Ness and Stein 1956). As the area dries out, resporulation occurs. Grazing animals become infected when they ingest *B. anthracis* spores on vegetation. Vegetative bacilli are shed in blood and other discharges from infected animals that are dying or dead; the bacilli then sporulate and contaminate the surrounding soil and water sources (Shadomy and Smith 2008). Within the intact carcases of animals that have died of anthrax, the vegetative bacilli cannot compete with anaerobic bacteria, and they usually die within 2–3 days because of the putrefactive processes in the decomposing carcases (Hugh-Jones and de Vos 2002). Thus, only if the carcase is disrupted, or discharges are released, will the vegetative bacilli be able to reach an aerobic environment and sporulate.

In man, anthrax primarily develops following exposure to infected animals, tissues or products from infected animals (Brachman *et al.* 1996). Anthrax exposure can be divided into either agricultural (nonindustrial) or industrial routes (Shadomy and Smith 2008). Agricultural exposure occurs among people with direct contact with sick or dying *B. anthracis*-infected animals or through handling the carcases or tissues of such animals. Industrial exposure results from cutaneous inoculation or inhalation of particles containing anthrax spores that are generated during the processing of contaminated hides, hair or wool.

Pathogenesis

Infection usually occurs by ingestion, although inhalation and cutaneous penetration can also occur. Infection by biting flies may also be possible (Cousineau and McClenaghan 1965). Following entry into a host by ingestion, inhalation or introduction through the skin, the spores are triggered to germinate.

Susceptibility to the disease varies among different species with herbivores being most susceptible. Pigs are susceptible, but unlike other species they may survive the disease. When spores are ingested, germination and production of vegetative bacilli occurs either in the mucosa of the pharynx or in the intestinal tract. The organisms multiply in an oedematous focus near the site of primary invasion, and then spread via lymphatic channels to lymph nodes. Replication and multiplication continues in the regional lymph nodes, followed by spread to the bloodstream, with resultant bacteraemia, septicaemia and dissemination to multiple organs. The organism is filtered out by the spleen until splenic clearance capacity is overwhelmed. Uncontrolled multiplication continues in the blood until the animal dies. At death, 80% of the organisms are in the blood and 20% are in the spleen, which is often greatly enlarged (Timoney *et al.* 1988).

Proliferation of lethal toxin is the usual cause of death. The bacterium has 3 main virulence factors: the poly-D-glutamic acid capsule and 2 protein exotoxins (oedema toxin, ET, and lethal toxin, LT). The 3 virulence factors are encoded on 2 plasmids, pXO1 and pXO2. The poly-D-glutamic acid capsule protects it against complement and phagocytosis. The pXO1 plasmid encodes for 3 components that comprise the 2 exotoxins: protective antigen, lethal factor and oedema factor. Protective antigen (PA) allows the toxin to bind to cell surfaces and is responsible for inducing protective immunity against *B. anthracis* infection. PA combines with either oedema factor or lethal factor to form ET or LT respectively. Lethal toxin mediates the lethal effects of the toxin by virtue of hypoxic tissue injury, liver failure and shock. Oedema toxin causes the extravasation of intercellular fluids into subcutaneous, peritoneal and tissue spaces; it also impairs host defences, including inhibition of neutrophil function and phagocytosis. The pOX2 plasmid contains genes for the capsule, which is weakly antigenic and protects vegetative bacilli from phagocytosis by host macrophages.

Clinical features

Nonhuman animals most often develop anthrax following ingestion of spore-contaminated foodstuffs. Herbivores (e.g. cattle, sheep and goats) are considered to be most susceptible. Horses are susceptible, and in some outbreaks, the infection rate has been reported to be higher in horses than in cattle (Fox *et al.* 1977). It has been suggested that horses may either be more susceptible than cattle to anthrax, or they may graze in a manner that results in the greater ingestion of contaminated soil (Fox *et al.* 1977).

The clinical manifestations of the disease depend on the manner of infection. When it occurs through the respiratory or gastrointestinal tract with no visible evidence of localisation, its principal character is its sudden onset and rapidly fatal course (Timoney *et al.* 1988). Three different forms of anthrax are recognised in man and animals (Turnbull 2002; Shadomy and Smith 2008). Cutaneous disease is seen most commonly in people working with animal hides (this form is unusual in domestic animals); it results in localised gelatinous oedema leading to a 'malignant pustule'. The organism can then disseminate from the necrotic ulcer to cause septicaemia and death. Pulmonary anthracic disease occurs in man and animals following the inhalation of spores. This results in a fatal acute haemorrhagic mediastinitis. Gastrointestinal disease follows oral ingestion of the organism; following penetration of the mucosa, local pustule formation and ulceration is followed by systemic dissemination.

The incubation period following exposure to *B. anthracis* spores typically ranges from 3–7 days (range <1 day–14 days). Peracute infection may occur in horses and other herbivores, and results in 'sudden death' (death within 1–2 h). Alternatively, horses can develop an acute infection resulting in signs of depression, colic, fever, dyspnoea, congested mucosae and tachycardia. Subcutaneous oedema of the ventral neck, thorax and abdomen may occur, and there may be haemorrhagic discharges from body orifices. The disease typically progresses rapidly, with death within 24–48 h.

In swine and dogs, anthrax generally assumes a localised form with pharyngeal involvement and gastroenteritis (Timoney *et al.* 1988). There is often severe inflammatory oedema of the tissues of the head and neck, which can cause suffocation as a result of severe oedema of the glottis.

The principle lesions in animals dying from anthrax include widespread oedema, necrosis, haemorrhage and haemorrhagic discharges from the orifices. Rapid *post mortem* decomposition follows with bloating and incomplete development of *rigor mortis*, often with petechiae and ecchymoses (Gleiser 1967). If anthrax is suspected as the cause of death in any animal, the carcase should not be incised so as to prevent sporulation and dissemination of the spores (Shadomy and Smith 2008).

Diagnosis

Necropsy of suspected anthrax cases should not be performed. Diagnosis should be attempted by methods that release a minimum number of anthrax organisms into the environment. Exposure to atmospheric oxygen will allow the formation of spores, which will be extremely difficult to destroy. Blood samples or dried blood smears should be obtained from a peripheral vessel such as an ear vein. Since fulminant anthrax is usually associated with an overwhelming bacteraemia, *B. anthracis* can usually be identified in blood smears. Swabs or smears of local oedematous lesions can also be examined. Samples should if possible be obtained within a few hours of death. Polychrome methylene blue (McFadyean reaction) or Giemsa stains should be used. Laboratory personnel should be aware that anthrax spores are not necessarily killed by the heat required to fix smears on microscope slides (Timoney *et al.* 1988). A fluorescent antibody test, agar-gel precipitin technique or PCR can also be used. The organism is readily isolated in culture if antimicrobial therapy has not been initiated. However, in view of the public health risk, culture of *B. anthracis* should only be performed by suitably specialised state laboratories.

Treatment

Prompt and aggressive treatment of infected animals is necessary because of the rapidly progressive, and often fatal nature of the disease (Shadomy and Smith 2008). Penicillin has generally been considered the treatment of choice for many years, but variable penicillin resistance and inducible β–lactamase production by *B. anthracis* isolates have been reported (Lightfoot *et al.* 1990). Failure of penicillin treatment in animals has been reported (Bailey 1954). However, high doses of penicillin administered i.v. (44,000 iu/kg bwt q. 6 h) would be expected to be efficacious in most cases. Oxytetracycline administered i.v. (6.6 mg/kg bwt q. 12 h) is also likely be effective. Antimicrobial treatment should be continued for at least 5 days.

In many countries, anthrax is considered to be a notifiable or reportable disease, and the state veterinary services should be informed of all suspect or confirmed cases. Affected premises should be quarantined, and all infected carcases, as well as contaminated bedding, soil etc., should be incinerated. If incineration is not feasible, infected carcases should be buried at least 2 m deep with a covering of quick lime (calcium oxide) or chloride of lime (calcium hydroxide, calcium chloride, and calcium hypochlorite, with 25% active chlorine) and soil. All items that become contaminated with *B. anthracis* should undergo decontamination. The spores resist steaming or boiling at 100°C for 5 min, but can be destroyed by steam sterilisation under pressure at 121°C for 30 min (i.e. autoclaving) or by ethylene oxide sterilisation with a contact time of at least 18 h (Shadomy and Smith 2008). The spores are also resistant to disinfectants such as 5% phenol or mercuric chloride. A 2–3% solution of formalin is effective if applied at a temperature of 40°C, and a 0.25% solution is effective when applied for 6 h at 60°C (Timoney *et al.* 1988).

Vaccination

The Sterne vaccine (Sterne 1937) is produced by growing virulent anthrax strains on 50% serum agar in an atmosphere of 10–30% CO_2. The vaccine is used to prevent anthrax in cattle but is not recommended for use in horses. It is not available in many countries. Injection site reactions and severe oedema have been reported following the use of this vaccine in horses (Mongoh *et al.* 2008).

References

Bailey, W.W. (1954) Antibiotic therapy in anthrax. *J. Am. vet. med. Ass.* **124**, 296-300.

Brachman, P.S., Kaufman, A.F. and Dalldorf, F.G. (1996) Industrial inhalation of anthrax. *Bacteriol. Rev.* **30**, 646-659.

Cousineau, S.G. and McClenaghan, R.J. (1965) Anthrax in bison in the northwest territories. *Can. vet. J.* **6**, 22-24

Crupi, R.S., Asnis, D.S., Lee, C.C., Santucci, T., Marino, M.J. and Flanz, B.J. (2003) Meeting the challenge of bioterrorism: lessons learned from West Nile virus and anthrax. *Am. J. emerg. Med.* **21**, 77-79.

De Vas, V. and Turnbull, P.C. (2004) Anthrax. In: *Infectious Diseases of Livestock*, 2nd edn., Eds: J.A.W. Coetzer and R.C. Tustin, Oxford University Press, Cape Town. pp 1788-1818.

Dragon, D.C. and Rennie, R.P. (1995) The ecology of anthrax spores: tough but not invincible. *Can. vet. J.* **36**, 295-301.

Hugh-Jones, M. (1999) 1996-1997 global anthrax report. *J. appl. Microbiol.* **87**, 189-191.

Hugh-Jones, M. and de Vos, V. (2002) Anthrax and wildlife. *Rev. Sci. Tech.* **21**, 359-383.

Fox, M.D., Boyce, J.M., Kaufman, A.F., Young, J.B. and Whitford, H.W. (1977) An epizootiologic study of anthrax in Falls County, Texas. *J. Am. vet. med. Ass.* **170**, 327-333.

Gleiser, C.A. (1967) Pathology of anthrax infection in animal hosts. *Fed. Proc.* **26**, 1518-1521

Koch, R. (1877) The aetiology of anthrax based on the ontogeny of the anthrax bacillus. *Med. Classics* (1937) **2**, 787-820. Originally published in German in: *Beitrage zur Biologie der Pflanzen* **2**, 277-282.

Lightfoot, N.F., Scott, R.J.D. and Turnbull, P.C.B. (1990) Antimicrobial susceptibility of *Bacillus anthracis. Salisbury Med. Bull., Suppl.* **68**, 95-98.

Long, M.T. (2007) Anthrax. In: *Equine Infectious Diseases*, Eds: D.C. Sellon and M.T. Long, Saunders Elsevier, Philadelphia. pp 273-275.

Mongoh, M.N., Dyer, N.W., Stoltenow, C.L. and Khaitsa, M.L. (2008) Risk factors associated with anthrax outbreak in animals in North Dakota, 2005: a retrospective case-control study. *Public Health Rep.* **123**, 352-359.

Parry, J.A., Turnbull, P.C.B. and Gibson, J.R. (1983) *A Colour Atlas of* Bacillus *Species,* Wolfe Medical Publications, London.

Quinn, C. and Turnbull, P. (1998) Anthrax. In: *Topley and Wilson's Microbiology and Microbial Infection,* Eds: W.J. Hausler and M. Sussman, Edward Arnold, London. pp 799-818.

Shadomy, S.V. and Smith, T.L. (2008) Anthrax. *J. Am. vet. med. Ass.* **233**, 63-72.

Timoney, J.F., Gillespie, J.H., Scott, F.W. and Barlough, J.E. (1988) *Bacillus anthracis.* In: *Hagan and Bruner's Microbiology and Infectious Diseases of Domestic Animals,* 8th edn., Comstock Publishing Associates, Ithaca. pp 206-211.

Turnbull, P.C. (2002) Introduction: anthrax history, disease and ecology. *Curr. Top. Microbiol. Immunol.* **271**, 1-19.

Umeno, S. and Nobata, R. (1938) On viability of anthrax spores. *J. Jpn. Soc. vet. Sci.* **17**, 221-223.

Van Ness, G. and Stein, C.D. (1956) Soils of the United States favourable for anthrax. *J. Am. vet. med. Ass.* **128**, 7-9.

LYME DISEASE IN HORSES

T. J. Divers*, T. S. Mair† and Y. F. Chang

College of Veterinary Medicine, Cornell University, Ithaca, New York, USA; and †Bell Equine Veterinary Clinic, Mereworth, Maidstone, Kent, UK.

Keywords: horse; Lyme disease; *Borrelia burgdorferi*; tick; *Ixodes*

Summary

Lyme disease is a tick-borne infectious disease caused by the spirochete *Borrelia burgdorferi*. Infection in most horses appears to be subclinical. Clinical signs most commonly attributed to Lyme disease in horses include low-grade fever, stiffness and lameness in more than one limb, muscle tenderness, hyperaesthesia, swollen joints, lethargy and behavioural changes. Diagnosis is made on the basis of the horse being housed in an endemic area, compatible clinical signs, ruling out other causes for these signs and a high titre using kinetic enzyme-linked immunosorbent assay, other serological tests or positive western blot (WB) test results for anti-*B. burgdorferi* antibodies. Treatments include oral doxycycline, i.v. oxytetracycline or i.m. ceftiofur.

Introduction

Lyme disease is a global health concern in man and has been associated with numerous neurological, rheumatological and psychiatric manifestations (Cameron 2008). It is a tick-borne infectious disease that occurs in parts of North America, Europe and Asia (Hovius *et al.* 2007). Although *Borrelia* spp. have been associated with human diseases (such as louse-borne relapsing fever and tick-borne relapsing fever) for many years, scant attention was directed toward the study of these organisms in the latter half of the 20th century until an epidemic of arthritis was described in Lyme, Connecticut (Steere *et al.* 1977). In sequential fashion, this condition was associated with a typical rash previously described in Europe as *erythema migrans* and the bite of the blacklegged tick, *Ixodes scapularis* (Steere *et al.* 1978; Steere and Malawista 1979). In 1982, Burgdorfer *et al.* (1982) reported the discovery of a spirochete in *Ixodes scapularis*, and a few months later in *Ixodes ricinus* (Burgdorfer *et al.* 1983), that proved to be the aetiological agent of Lyme disease or Lyme borreliosis. This spirochete was subsequently named *Borrelia burgdorferi* (Johnson *et al.* 1984).

Aetiology and epidemiology

Borrelia burgdorferi, the cause of Lyme disease, is a helical shaped gram negative spirochete (Burdorfer 1984). In Europe and Asia, 3 major *Borrelia* genospecies (*burgdorferi* sensu stricto, garinii and afzelii) can be the causative agents of Lyme disease (Hovius *et al.* 2007), whereas in North America only, *B. burgdorferi* sensu stricto causes the disease (Lo Re III *et al.* 2004). *B. burgdorferi* is maintained in a 2-year enzootic cycle involving *Ixodes* spp. ticks and mammals (Rosa 1997). *Ixodes scapularis*, *Ixodes ricinus* and *Ixodes persulacatus* are the most important vectors in North America, Europe and Asia respectively (Hovius *et al.* 2007). Deer and the white-footed mouse (*Peromyscus leucopus*) are the most common mammals involved in maintaining the life cycle in North America. *I. ricinus* feeds on an extraordinarily broad array of hosts, from small, medium and large-sized mammals to birds and reptiles (Anderson 1991) and is the tick species that most frequently bites human subjects in Europe. Several species of mice, voles, rats and shrews have been shown to be competent reservoirs of *B. burgdorferi* in Europe (Gern *et al.* 1998).

Infection in mammals generally results from larval or nymph bites in the spring and summer, or adult female ticks feeding in the summer, autumn or winter. In horses, it is not known whether larval and nymph bites play an important role in Lyme infection. In most instances, the ticks must be attached to the mammal for at least 24 h for

*Author to whom correspondence should be addressed.

B. burgdorferi transmission (Norman *et al.* 1996). Once tick feeding begins, the *Borrelia* organism begins both up and down regulation of certain genes to allow transmission and survival. OspA may be down-regulated, while other surface proteins (OspE, OspF and Vis-E/C6) that are in low concentration in the tick gut are up-regulated during transmission to enhance immune evasion in mammals (Pal *et al.* 2001; Kraiczy *et al.* 2002).

The organism may also live in the host by residing in connective tissue and collagen, and having no requirement for iron (Nanagara *et al.* 1996; Posey and Gherardini 2000). A large percentage of adult horses in the more eastern parts of the northeast and mid-Atlantic USA are or have been infected with *B. burgdorferi* (Magnarelli *et al.* 2000; Divers 2007). Infection is also common in Wisconsin and Minnesota (Burgess 1988). Prevalence is confirmed by serological surveys up to 75% of adult horses in some of these areas are believed to be seropositive (Divers 2007). Seroprevalence in horses in many other parts of the USA has not been reported, but would be expected to fluctuate in a manner similar to that seen with the human form of the disease. In the USA, the geographic area of human Lyme disease appears to be increasing based upon the Center for Disease Control (CDC) maps from 2002 and 2006 (**Fig 1**). In horses, high seroprevalence is more widespread than reflected by the 2002 CDC map, as horses in northern and central Virginia are commonly seropositive. Infection in Central and South America appears rare with only one report of infection in a small number of horses in northeast Mexico (Salinas-Mélendez *et al.* 2001).

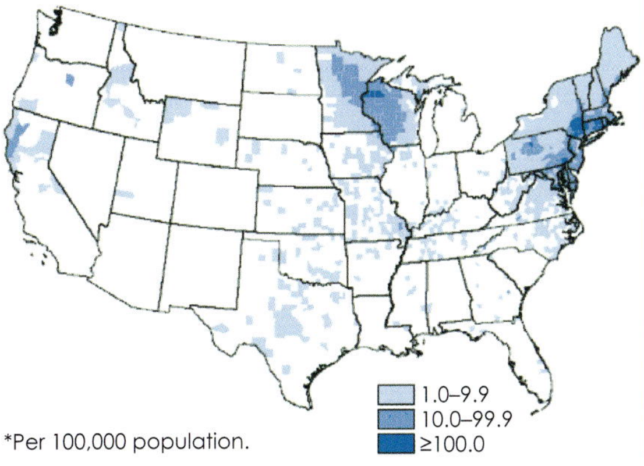

FIGURE 1: High-risk areas for Lyme Disease in the United States. From MMWR Surveill Summ. 2008 Oct 3;57 (10):1-9. Surveillance for Lyme disease-United States, 1992–2006. R.M. Bacon, K.J. Kugeler, P.S. Mead; Centers for Disease Control and Prevention (CDC).

Seroprevalence of infection in horses is reported in Sweden (Egenvall *et al.* 2001), Poland (Stefanciková *et al.* 2008), Austria (Müller *et al.* 2002), Japan and Turkey (Bhide *et al.* 2008), all having lower seroprevalence than in the northeast USA. Seropositive horses are also known to occur in the UK and Germany (Carter *et al.* 1994; Gerhards and Wollanke 1996). There are probably other areas of Europe and elsewhere in the world where seroprevalence may be moderately high. The incidence of human Lyme disease in Europe is unknown, but based on rates of serodiagnosis (and taking the limitations of seroprevalence methods into account) it is clear that Lyme disease shows a gradient of increasing incidence from west to east with the highest incidences in central-eastern Europe (**Table 1**). A gradient of decreasing incidence from south to north in Scandinavia and north to south in Italy, Spain and Greece has also been noted.

Clinical signs

A broad spectrum of clinical signs has been attributed to *Borrelia* infection in horses, but cause and effect have been difficult to document (Divers 2007). In fact, there is little doubt that most infected horses do not show obvious clinical signs. This seems to be agreed upon by most veterinarians regardless of the country

TABLE 1: Estimated human Lyme disease annual incidence in selected European countries (Anon 1995)

Country	Incidence per 100,000 population	Annual number of cases
UK*	0.3	200
Ireland	0.6	30
France	16.0	7,200
Germany*	25.0	20,000
Switzerland*	30.4	2,000
Czech Republic*	39.0	3,500
Bulgaria	55.0	3,500
Sweden (south)	69.0	7,120
Slovenia	120.0	2,000
Austria	130.0	14,000

* No published figures available.

of practice. Clinical signs most commonly attributed to Lyme disease in horses include low-grade fever, stiffness and lameness in more than one limb, muscle tenderness, hyperesthesia, swollen joints, lethargy and behavioural changes (Magnarelli *et al.* 2000). Neurological dysfunction and panuveitis have been reported in a horse and a pony (Burgess *et al.* 1986; Hahn *et al.* 1996).

Recently, one author (T.D.) has helped in the evaluation of 2 horses with ataxia, neck stiffness and behavioural changes that were attributed to Lyme infection. In one case, marked lymphocytic pleocytosis was found in the CSF and, upon necropsy, a marked cervical lymphocytic meningitis with thickened dura and nerve root involvement were found. Lymphocytes were of mixed size and type, ruling out lymphoma. In the other horse, there was a high CSF *Borrelia* antibody titre (ELISA of 393 units; 412 in the serum). Using the same samples, comparison of serum to CSF antibody to EHV1 (1:32 vs. 1:4), antibody to EPM (positive serum, negative CSF), and IgG (32 g/l serum vs. <2 g/l CSF) strongly suggested intrathecal production of *Borrelia* antibodies. The horse responded favourably to oxytetracycline and doxycycline treatments. The neurological signs, absence of other causes for the CNS signs, strong evidence of intrathecal antibody production, and response to therapy would meet the criteria for diagnosing neuroborreliosis in man (Lanska *et al.* 2008). Nine months after infection, one pony experimentally-infected with *Borrelia* had lymphocytic neuritis of the facial, tibial and fibular nerves only on the side that the infected ticks had been attached, suggesting that peripheral neuritis could be a possible clinical consequence of infection (Chang *et al.* 2000a).

Even more recently, an adult horse with bilateral uveitis was shown to have large numbers of *Borrelia* organisms in the ocular fluids of both eyes (observed on cytology and confirmed by PCR). Ocular involvement with *Borrelia* may be a rare occurrence as we have not seen this before and, in a study from Germany involving 79 horses with recurrent uveitis and controls, no association was found between seropositivity to *Borrelia* and the presence of ocular disease (Gerhards and Wollanke 1996). Why only a small number of horses might have clinical signs following infection is unknown, but could be related to an individual horse immune response to the infection. Fever and limb oedema frequently reported in association with recent *Borrelia* infection (proven by seroconversion) are most often the result of *Anaplasma phagocytophilum* infection, as many ticks are dually infected with both *Borrelia* and *A. phagocytophilum* in Lyme endemic areas in both the USA and Europe (Chang *et al.* 2000b; Engvall and Egenvall 2002).

Two retrospective clinical studies with control groups have been published in which an attempt was made to correlate seropositivity for *Borrelia* with commonly incriminated clinical signs. In one report from Connecticut, *Borrelia* infection, confirmed by serology, spirochetaemia or both was more common in horses with lameness or behavioural changes than in horses in the same region that did not have these clinical signs (Manion *et al.* 1998). A differently designed study (retrospective identification of seropositive horses examined for any illness followed up by owner questionnaire) was conducted in Sweden. In that study, no association was found between *Borrelia* seropositivity and the clinical signs commonly attributed to Lyme disease (Egenvall *et al.* 2001). Experimental infection in ponies causes disease in the skin, muscle, peripheral nerves and both perisynovial nerves and blood vessels, but clinical signs were not obvious (Chang *et al.* 2000a). After experimentally attaching infected ticks for 7 days followed by 9 months observation, *Borrelia* was consistently found in all synovial membranes and in skin and fascia near the site of previous tick attachment. There does seem to be a predilection for persistence of infection at these sites (Chang *et al.* 2000a).

The anatomical predilection for persistent infection and mild lymphocytic response in the synovial membranes may help explain the dramatic response to either doxycycline and/or oxytetetracycline observed in many suspect field cases (strongly seropositive horses with multiple limb stiffness/lameness that was not explained by other diseases) (Divers 2007). Oxytetracycline and doxycycline have their primary matrix metalloproteinase anti-inflammatory effect on the synovium as opposed to articular cartilage cells (L.A. Fortier, unpublished data). The common finding of *Borrelia* in the fascia of experimentally infected horses may explain the hyperaesthesia reported in many suspect cases and may give a clue as to potential movement and persistence of the organism (skin, fascia, nerves and synovial membranes).

Diagnosis

Lyme disease is diagnosed on the basis of the horse being housed in an endemic area, compatible clinical signs, ruling out other causes for these signs, and a high kinetic enzyme-linked immunosorbent assay (ELISA) (KELA) titre (generally >300 KELA units), other serological test or positive western blot (WB) test results for anti-*B. burgdorferi* antibodies (Divers 2007). If the ELISA titre is >300, there is a 99% probability that WB results will be positive (Divers 2007). The WB is most useful in horses with moderate ELISA titres (200–300) or when there is suspicion that the horse may have received a commercial canine Lyme disease vaccine. Time from infection to seroconversion appears to be 3–10 weeks (Chang *et al.* 2000a). One potential limitation of serological tests is that they do not distinguish between active infection and previous exposure. For this reason, tests that detect the spirochete directly are more conclusive of current infection.

Detection of *B. burgdorferi* DNA in a synovial membrane of a painful joint via polymerase chain reaction (PCR) assay is strongly indicative of infection. The sensitivity of PCR amplification of *Borrelia* in a synovial membrane biopsy specimen in the horse is currently unknown. It is also possible that many infected horses may be infected for a prolonged duration, even life, or are repeatedly re-infected since prior infection may not produce protective antibody. These possibilities are supported by the fact that field horses with high ELISA values rarely have a substantial numerical decline in ELISA titre when monitored for months or even years. Treatment of naturally-occurring cases may result in a decline in titre compared to nontreated horses but the mean magnitude of decline is small (20–30 KELA units). The small titre decline in field cases is quite different from the decline seen in treated experimentally infected ponies (experimentally infected ponies had dramatic decline in serum antibody to *Borrelia* immediately after 4 weeks of treatment with either oral doxycycline i.v. oxytetetracycline or i.m. ceftiofur). Antibodies rose again within another 4 weeks in ponies that were not cured of the infection (3/4 in both the doxycycline and ceftiofur treated ponies, while one in each group and all 4 in the oxytetetracycline treated group had continual decline of antibody to <110 KELA units and absence of organism on *post mortem* examination [both culture and PCR] [Chang *et al.* 2005]).

More recently, an on-site C-6 ELISA Snap test marketed for detection of *Borrelia*, heartworm, *Ehrlichia canis* and *Anaplasma phagocytophilum* infection in dogs was evaluated for detection of *Borrelia* infection in horses; sensitivity of the test is lower than that of ELISA performed at referral laboratories. It does not appear to detect antibodies during infection any earlier than the ELISA (when 110 is used as a cut off for positive) nor did it become negative more rapidly after successful treatment in the experimental ponies (Johnson *et al.* 2008). Evaluation of this assay in treated field cases has not been reported. An advantage of the C-6 snap test and WB test (in most cases) is that vaccination with OSPA antigen or whole cell does not cause positive results. Most infections do not cause a strong reaction of the P32 WB band (associated with OSPA antigen), but a small number of horses will produce antibody to this antigen following natural infection. A luminex assay is currently under evaluation and it may be further helpful in determining the infection status of seropositive horses (B. Wagner, personal communication).

Common disorders that may be confused with Lyme disease and should be ruled out include osteoarthritis of the hock, osteochondrosis, polysaccharide storage myopathy and other chronic myopathies, polysynovitis (suspect Lyme cases rarely have dramatic synovial effusion), thoracic spinous process osteoarthritis and equine protozoal myelitis. Diagnostic tests that may be useful in ruling out these diseases include thorough lameness and neurological examinations, radiography, scintigraphy, muscle biopsy, cerebrospinal fluid collection and appropriate testing and serum analysis for concentrations of muscle enzymes (both before and after exercise). Lyme disease seems to be most commonly diagnosed in nonracing performance horses such as dressage, stadium jumping and 3-day event horses. We are not sure why this may be the case but, if true, it could be explained by: 1) more turnout into pasture and woods, and therefore increased tick exposure in sport horses; and 2) trainer/rider ability to detect subtle gait or behavioural changes in those horses.

Treatment

The 2 most commonly used antibiotics for treating Lyme disease in horses are oxytetracycline, given i.v., and doxycycline, given *per os* (Divers 2007). Horses with what are often believed to be more typical signs of Lyme disease (e.g. chronic stiffness, lameness and hyperesthesia) are most frequently treated with doxycycline (10 mg/kg bwt, *per os*, every 12 h). Duration of treatment is often 1 month, but this duration is only empirical. Horses treated with doxycycline should be observed for a change in stool consistency, as diarrhoea develops in a low percentage of treated horses. A clinical response of less stiffness or lameness is often reported following doxycycline treatment, but this could be a nonspecific anti-inflammatory response because doxycycline inhibits metalloproteinase activity (Fortier *et al.* 2008).

Oxytetracycline (6.6–11.0 mg/kg bwt, i.v., every 24 h) may be more efficacious because of higher blood concentration and, therefore, higher tissue concentrations of i.v. oxytetracycline as opposed to poorly absorbed doxycycline given *per os*. In the experimental infection studies, oxytetracycline given i.v. was superior to doxycycline given *per os* (Chang *et al.* 2005). Oxytetracycline should not be administered in high doses or for prolonged periods if dehydration is present or there is pre-existing renal dysfunction. Acute renal failure may occur in those horses if oxytetracycline is administered. Ceftiofur (2–4 mg/kg bwt, i.v. or i.m. administration, every 12 h) has also been used in the treatment of horses with Lyme disease. Although antibody titres decreased in experimentally-infected ponies given the antibiotic treatments, similar declines in titre in association with those same treatments have been rare in naturally-infected horses. The reasons for this may be a longer duration of infection before beginning treatment in horses with naturally-occurring disease (which would decrease the effectiveness of the antimicrobials in clearing the infection), reinfection or antibody mimicry.

Because horses do not develop *erythema migrans* (a characteristic cutaneous manifestation of human Lyme disease [Mullegger and Glatz 2008]), recognition of early infection is nearly impossible except in cases when firmly attached infected female *Ixodes* ticks are removed. In the experimentally-infected ponies, the organism was eliminated from the body only in ponies that maintained ELISA titres below 110 units for 2 months after treatment was completed (Chang *et al.* 2005). Other treatments that can be considered supportive include chondroprotective agents, nonsteroidal anti-inflammatory agents, and acupuncture. Acupuncture may be especially valuable for management of hyperaesthesia-perineuritis syndromes that are often poorly responsive to treatment with nonsteroidal anti-inflammatory drugs.

Prevention

Prevention of Lyme disease in endemic areas would involve preventing tick exposure or prolonged (more than 24 h) attachment and/or early antimicrobial treatment after *Ixodes* exposure; however the efficacy of these techniques is unproven. Decreased tick infection may be accomplished by clipping tall grasses, clearing shrubs and bushes, and preventing the horse from entering forest and woodlands. Topical sprays could be used when exposure to ticks is expected. We are not aware of adverse effects from use of the more common canine tick sprays (e.g. fipronil)[1] in the horse. Spraying is most commonly used when adult ticks are noticeable in the late summer, autumn and the early part of winter, but infection with larval or nymphal stages earlier in the year should also be considered. If ticks are found on the horse, they should be identified to determine whether they are *Ixodes* spp., which is the only species of tick in North America known to transmit *B. burgdorferi*. Ponies have been protected by vaccination with a OPSA vaccine (Chang *et al.* 1999), but a vaccine approved for use in equids is not commercially available at present. Efficacy of administration of the canine vaccine in the horse is unknown, but based upon the experimental study, efficacy might be expected. Re-infection can occur following natural infection, so vaccination during antibiotic treatment is used by some veterinarians. In the future, vaccines that deter tick attachment may be feasible in the horse.

Manufacturer's address

[1]FrontLine, Merial Limited, Iselin, New Jersey, USA.

References

Anderson, J.F. (1991) Epizootiology of Lyme borreliosis. *Scand. J. Inf. Dis. Suppl.* **77**, 23-34.

Anon (1995) Report of WHO workshop on Lyme Borreliosis Diagnosis and Surveillance, Warsaw, Poland, 20–22 June, 1995, WHO/CDS/VPH/95. [1996] 141-1.

Bhide, M., Yilmaz, Z., Golcu, E., Torun, S. and Mikula, I. (2008) Seroprevalence of anti-*Borrelia burgdorferi* antibodies in dogs and horses in Turkey. *Ann. Agric. Environ. Med.* **15**, 85-90.

Burdorfer, W. (1984) Discovery of the Lyme disease spirochete and its relation to tick vectors. *Yale J. Biol. Med.* **57**, 515-520.

Burgdorfer, W., Barbour, A.G., Hayes, S.F., Benach J.L., Grunwaldt, E. and Davis, J.P. (1982) Lyme disease. A tick-borne spirochetosis? *Science* **216**, 1317-1319.

Burgdorfer, W., Barbour, A.G., Hayes, S.F., Peter, O. and Aeschlimann, A. (1983) *Erythema migrans* – A tick-borne spirochetosis. *Acta. Tropica.* **40**, 79-83.

Burgess, E.C. (1988) *Borrelia burgdorferi* infection in Wisconsin horses and cows. *Ann. NY Acad. Sci.* **539**, 235-243.

Burgess, E.C., Gillette, D. and Pickett, J.P. (1986) Arthritis and panuveitis as manifestations of *Borrelia burgdorferi* infection in a Wisconsin pony. *J. Am. vet. med. Ass.* **189**, 1340-1342.

Cameron, D. (2008) Severity of Lyme disease with persistent symptoms. Insights from a double-blind placebo-controlled clinical trial. *Minerva Med.* **99**, 489-496.

Carter, S.D., May, C., Barnes, A. and Bennett, D. (1994) *Borrelia burgdorferi* infection in UK horses. *Equine vet. J.* **26**, 187-190.

Chang, Y., Novosol, V. and McDonough, S.P. (1999) Vaccination against Lyme disease with recombinant *Borrelia burgdorferi* outer-surface protein A (rOspA) in horses. *Vaccine* **18**, 540-548.

Chang, Y.F., Novosol, V. and McDonough, S.P. (2000a) Experimental infection of ponies with *Borrelia burgdorferi* by exposure to Ixodid ticks. *Vet. Pathol.* **37**, 68-76.

Chang, Y.F., McDonough, S.P., Chang, C.F., Shin, K.S., Yen, W. and Divers, T. (2000b) Human granulocytic ehrilichiosis agent infection in a pony vaccinated with a *Borrelia burgdorferi* recombinant OspA vaccine and challenged by exposure to naturally infected ticks. *Clin. Diagn. Lab. Immunol.* **7**, 68-71.

Chang, Y.F., Ku, Y.W., Chang, C.F. , Chang, C.D., McDonough, S.P., Divers, T., Pough, M. and Torres, A. (2005) Antibiotic treatment of experimentally *Borrelia burgdorferi*-infected ponies. *Vet. Microbiol.* **107**, 285-294.

Divers, T.J. (2007) Lyme disease. In: *Equine Infectious Diseases*, Eds: D.C. Sellon and M.T. Long, W.B. Saunders, St Louis. pp 310-312.

Egenvall, A., Franzén, P., Gunnarsson, A., Engvall, E.O., Vågsholm, I., Wikström, U.B. and Artursson, K. (2001) Cross-sectional study of the seroprevalence to *Borrelia burgdorferi* sensu lato and granulocytic *Ehrlichia* spp. and demographic, clinical and tick-exposure factors in Swedish horses. *Prev. vet. Med.* **49**, 191-208.

Engvall, E.O. and Egenvall, A. (2002) Granulocytic ehrlichiosis in Swedish dogs and horses. *Int. J. Med. Microbiol.* **291**, 100-103.

Gern, L., Estrada-Pena, A., Frandsen, F., Gray, J. S., Jaenson, T.G. T., Jongejan, F., Kahl, O., Korenberg, E., Mehl, R. and Nuttall, P.A. (1998) European reservoir hosts of *Borrelia burgdorferi* sensu lato. *Zentralblatt Bakteriologie* **287**, 196-204.

Gerhards, H. and Wollanke, B. (1996) Antibody titers against *Borrelia* in horses in serum and in eyes and occurrence of equine recurrent uveitis. *Berl. Munch. Tierarztl. Wochenschr.* **109**, 273-278.

Hahn, C.N., Mayhew, I.G., Whitwell, K.E., Smith, K.C., Carey, D., Carter, S.D. and Read, R.A. (1996) A possible case of Lyme borreliosis in a horse in the UK. *Equine vet. J.* **28**, 84-88.

Hovius, J., van Dam, A. and Fikrig, E. (2007) Tick-host-pathogen interactions in Lyme borreliosis. *Trends Parasitol.* **23**, 434-438.

Johnson, R.C., Schmid, G.P., Hyde, F.W., Stiegerwalt, A.G. and Brenner, D.J. (1984) *Borrelia burgdorferi* sp. nov.: Etiologic agent of Lyme disease. *Int. J. Syst. Bacteriolog.* **34**, 496-497.

Johnson, A.L., Divers, T.J. and Chang, Y.F. (2008) Validation of an in-clinic enzyme-linked immunosorbent assay kit for diagnosis of *Borrelia burgdorferi* infection in horses. *J. vet. Diagn. Invest.* **20**, 321-324.

Kraiczy, P., Skerka, C., Kirschfink, M., Zipfel, P.F. and Brade, V. (2002) Immune evasion of *Borrelia burgdorferi*: insufficient kill of the pathogens by complement and antibody. *Int. J. Med. Microbiol.* **291**, 141-146.

Lanska, D.J., Blanc, F., Jaulhac, B., Fleury, M., de Seze, J., de Martino, S.J., Blaison, G., Hansmann, Y., Christmann, D. and Tranchant, C. (2008) Relevance of the antibody index to diagnose Lyme neuroborreliosis among seropositive patients. *Neurol.* **71**, 150-151.

Lo Re, V III., Occi, J.L. and MacGregor, R.R. (2004) Identifying the vector of Lyme disease. *Am. Fam. Physician* **69**, 1935-1937.

Magnarelli, L.A., Ijdo, J.W., van Andel, A.E., Wu, C., Padula, S.J. and Fikrig, E. (2000) Serologic confirmation of *Ehrlichia equi* and *Borrelia burgdorferi* infections in horses from the northeastern United States. *J. Am. vet. med. Ass.* **217**, 1045-1050.

Manion, T.B., Bushmich, S.L., Mittel, L., Laurendeau, M., Werner, H. and Reilly, M. (1998) Lyme disease in horses: serological and antigen testing differences. *Proc. Am. Ass. equine Practnrs.* **44**, 144-145.

Mullegger, R.R. and Glatz, M. (2008) Skin manifestations of lyme *borreliosis*: diagnosis and management. *Am. J. Clin. Dermatol.* **9**, 355-368.

Müller, I., Khanakah, G., Kundi, M. and Stanek, G. (2002) Horses and *Borrelia*: Immunoblot patterns with five *Borrelia burgdorferi* sensu lato strains and sera from horses of various stud farms in Austria and from the Spanish Riding School in Vienna. *Int. J. Med. Microbiol.* **291**, 80-87.

Nanagara, R., Duray, P.H. and Schumacher, H.R. Jr. (1996) Ultrastructural demonstration of spirochetal antigens in synovial fluid and synovial membrane in chronic Lyme disease: possible factors contributing to persistence of organisms. *Hum. Pathol.* **27**, 1025-1034.

Norman, G.L., Antig, J.M., Bigaignon, G. and Hogrefe, W.R. (1996) Serodiagnosis of Lyme borreliosis by *Borrelia burgdorferi* sensu strict, *B. garinii,* and *B. afzelii* western blots (immunoblots). *J. Clin. Microbiol.* **34**, 1732-1738.

Pal, U., Montgomery, R.R., Lusitani, D., Voet, P., Weynants, V., Malawista, S.E., Lobet, Y. and Fikrig, E. (2001) Inhibition of *Borrelia burgdorferi* – tick interactions *in vivo* by outer surface protein A antibody. *J. Immunol.* **166**, 7398-7403.

Posey, J.E. and Gherardini, F.C. (2000) Lack of a role for iron in Lyme disease pathogen. *Science* **288**, 1651-1653.

Rosa, P.A. (1997) Microbiology of *Borrelia burgdorferi. Semin. Neurol.* **17**, 5-10.

Salinas-Mélendez, J.A., Galván de la Garza, S., Riojas-Valdés, V.M., Wong, Gonzàlez, A. and Avalos-Ramírez, R. (2001) Antibody detection against *Borrelia burgdorferi* in horses located in the suburban areas of Monterrey, Nuevo León. *Rev. Latinoam. Microbiol.* **43**, 161-164.

Steere, A.C., Broderick, T.F. and Malawista, S.E. (1978) *Erythema chronicum migrans* and Lyme arthritis: epidemiologic evidence for a tick vector. *Am. J. Epidemiol.* **108**, 312-321.

Steere, A.C. and Malawista, S.E. (1979) Cases of Lyme disease in the United States: locations correlated with distribution of *Ixodes dammini. Ann. Int. Med.* **91**, 730-733.

Steere, A.C., Malawista, S.E., Snydman, D.R., Shope, R.E., Andiman, W.A., Ross, M.R. and Steele, F.M. (1977) Lyme arthritis: an epidemic of oligoarticular arthritis in children and adults in three Connecticut communities. *Arthritis Rheumatol.* **20**, 7-17.

Stefanciková, A., Adaszek, L., Pet'ko, B., Winiarczyk, S. and Dudinák, V. (2008) Serological evidence of *Borrelia burgdorferi* sensu lato in horses and cattle from Poland and diagnostic problems of Lyme borreliosis. *Ann. Agric. Environ. Med.* **15**, 37-43.

TYZZER'S DISEASE

S. F. Peek

Department of Medical Sciences, School of Veterinary Medicine, 2015 Linden Drive West, University of Wisconsin, Madison, Wisconsin 53706, USA.

Keywords: horse; Tyzzer's disease; foal; *Clostridium piliforme*; hepatic failure

Summary

Tyzzer's disease is a sporadic, but rare, cause of hepatic failure in foals aged 1–6 weeks. The majority of cases are sporadic, although farm outbreaks have been occasionally recorded. The disease is caused by *Clostridium piliforme* infection, and appears to have a worldwide distribution. The disease is often peracute with the time between the onset of signs to death being as short as 2 h; many affected foals are found dead. Affected foals (whether they are dead or alive) are typically jaundiced. Other signs that are commonly present include tachycardia, tachypnoea and seizures. Diagnosis can currently be achieved by demonstrating the organism histologically in liver tissue obtained at *post mortem* or by identifying the organism in liver tissue using PCR. Treatment should be aimed at aggressive antimicrobial therapy combined with intensive supportive management of hepatic failure.

History of the disease and aetiology

The first descriptions of Tyzzer's disease as a cause of acute, fatal, enterohepatic disease were reported in mice as long ago as 1917 (Tyzzer 1917), but the disease does not appear to have been characterised in horses until the 1970s. Occasional farm outbreaks and clusters of cases have been reported to occur on some breeding farms (Swerczek *et al.* 1973; Swerczek, 1977; Peek *et al.* 1994), but the majority of cases appear to be sporadic. The list of mammalian and avian species in which Tyzzer's disease has now been described is lengthy and includes rodents (Tyzzer 1917; Feldman *et al.* 2006), lagomorphs (Peeters *et al.* 1985; Feldman *et al.* 2006), red pandas (Langan *et al.* 2000), lorikeets (Raymond *et al.* 2001), farm raised deer (Brooks *et al.* 2006), cattle (Ikegami *et al.* 1999), immunocompromised human patients (Smith *et al.* 1996), dogs (Young *et al.* 1995) and tamarins (Sasseville *et al.* 2007). In many affected species, excluding horses, the predominant manifestations of clinical disease relate to the gastrointestinal tract, with colitis being particularly common in species in which the condition is more prevalent, such as rodents and rabbits (Feldman *et al.* 2006). Following the original description of the disease in the early 20th century, the causative organism was initially classified as *Bacillus piliformis*, but was taxonomically reclassified in the 1990s as *Clostridium piliforme* on the basis of 16s ribosomal RNA sequence analysis (Duncan *et al.* 1993). Reports of the disease in foals have been forthcoming from the USA, UK (Whitwell 1976), Germany (Paar *et al.* 1993), Canada (Thomson *et al.* 1977; St Denis *et al.* 2000), Australia (Carrigan *et al.* 1984; Copland *et al.* 1984), New Zealand (Dickinson 1980) and South Africa (van der Lugt *et al.* 1985), such that it is likely that the disease has a worldwide distribution in horses.

Anamnesis and clinical signs

The peracute nature of the disease means that affected foals may be found moribund or dead with very little in the way of premonitory signs. Indeed, veterinarians should include Tyzzer's disease as a differential for foals that are found dead in a field or stall since the elapsed time from the onset of signs to death can be as short as 2 h (Turk *et al.* 1981). Whether dead or alive, affected foals will typically be jaundiced and this can add a higher index of suspicion on examination of the body if the foal died peracutely. Petechiation or other clinical evidence of a haemorrhagic diathesis may also be observed in foals with this disease (Turk *et al.* 1981; Humber *et al.* 1988). Other clinical signs that have been repeatedly encountered include severe depression and reluctance to nurse, pyrexia, diarrhoea and recumbency with seizure activity (Swerczek *et al.* 1973; Humber *et al.* 1988; Peek *et al.* 1994; Borchers *et al.* 2006). Seizures are quite common in foals with Tyzzer's disease and are probably triggered by either hypoglycaemia and/or hyperammonaemia accompanying liver failure. A recently published retrospective review (Borchers *et al.* 2006) identified tachycardia, tachypnoea, icterus and seizures as the most common presenting clinical signs at one referral centre.

Although one of the retrospective case series in the literature identified 2 out of 21 proven cases as occurring in Arabian foals with combined immunodeficiency (Turk *et al.* 1981) it seems that the majority of foals with the condition demonstrate no known immunodeficiency and have been completely healthy in the preceding neonatal period. Indeed, several other retrospective publications have documented that most affected foals have had adequacy of passive transfer (Humber *et al.* 1988; Peek *et al.* 1994), normal age appropriate protein (Borchers *et al.* 2006) or globulin levels (Brown *et al.* 1983; St Denis *et al.* 2001), and normal total lymphocyte counts (Brown *et al.* 1983). Other environmental factors may therefore play important roles in the development of disease. Literature from rodents suggests that the organism can persist in the spore form for at least a year in bedding (Tyzzer 1917) such that persistence in the environment from breeding season to breeding season may occur on some farms. Clinical experience alongside some of the original literature on the disease in foals from central Kentucky (Swerczek *et al.* 1973) and more recently from California (Fosgate *et al.* 2002) suggest that some farms experience multiple cases over consecutive breeding seasons.

Differential diagnosis

The most commonly encountered clinical signs and the typical age at presentation potentially create an extensive differential diagnosis list based on physical examination findings alone, although this list can be significantly shortened once baseline bloodwork is performed identifying hepatic failure and the peracute nature of the foal's clinical course becomes manifest. The common presenting clinical signs of depression, icterus, diarrhoea and seizures cover a wide range of primary gastrointestinal, infectious and neurological conditions of foals. The age at onset typically rules out neonatal isoerythrolyis and other primary haemolytic diseases are also very rare in foals of this age. Typical haematological abnormalities documented in affected foals include haemoconcentration, leucopenia (usually a neutropenia with a degenerative left shift) and hyperfibrinogenaemia indicative of peracute bacterial infection (Brown *et al.* 1983; Humber *et al.* 1988; Borchers *et al.* 2006). Biochemical analysis usually documents severe hepatic disease with marked hypoglycaemia, metabolic acidaemia, and unconjugated hyperbilirubinaemia alongside profound elevations in the hepatocellular enzymes aminoaspartate transferase (AST) and sorbitol dehydrogenase (SDH). More modest elevations are also seen in the biliary enzymes gamma glutamyltranspeptidase (GGT) and alkaline phosphatase (AP) (Brown *et al.* 1983; Humber *et al.* 1988; Borchers *et al.* 2006). Creatine phosphokinase activity is often mildly elevated due to recumbency and hypovolaemia (Brown *et al.* 1983; Borchers *et al.* 2006) but may become more markedly elevated with seizure activity. Although rarely performed in first opinion practice, coagulation profiles may be remarkably abnormal in affected foals (Borchers *et al.* 2006). A more refined differential diagnosis list subsequent to bloodwork would therefore include those diseases causing fulminant hepatic failure in young foals. Candidate differentials subsequent to performing blood work therefore include equine herpes virus 1 infection, iron overload due to administration of iron fumarate or repeated transfusion, and sepsis probably associated with enterohepatic infection with other bacterial organisms such as *Salmonella* or *Clostridium* spp.

Definitive diagnosis

Historically, a definitive diagnosis was reached by demonstrating the organism histologically in liver tissue obtained at *post mortem* examination. More recently, the development of specific PCR primers based on the 16s ribosomal RNA gene of *Clostridium piliforme* has allowed the organism to be identified in faeces (Furukawa *et al.* 2002) and liver tissue (Goto and Itoh 1994; Borchers *et al.* 2006). This technique has been applied to detect the organism *post mortem* and liver biopsy tissue from suspect foals (Borchers *et al.* 2006) but has yet to be reported using faeces from horses. The fulminant liver failure associated with

C. piliforme carries with it a substantial risk of iatrogenic haemorrhage from a biopsy site, such that it is unlikely that the *ante mortem* diagnosis of Tyzzer's disease in foals will be frequently justifiable via demonstration of the organism by silver stains or PCR in liver tissue. One of the surviving foals in the literature (Borchers *et al.* 2006) did, however, undergo a diagnostic liver biopsy with no complications being reported. It is to be hoped that the sensitivity of PCR on faecal samples of infected horses will be adequate to safely confirm the diagnosis in clinically affected foals as well as potentially identify asymptomatic adult horses, especially broodmares, which may be shedding the organism.

Gross *post mortem* changes of note include marked heptomegaly with areas of focal pallor associated with hepatic necrosis. Histologically, intrahepatocellular filamentous bacteria can be seen using Warthin-Starry silver stains. Histological evidence of enteritis, myocarditis and lymphofollicular and splenic necrosis are also commonly reported (Turk *et al.* 1981; Borchers *et al.* 2006). Readers are directed to the following website for excellent gross and histological *post mortem* images of the disease: http://w3.vet.cornell.edu/nst/nst.asp.

Treatment

Unfortunately the exceptionally high mortality rate provides little opportunity for treatment and most attempts at therapy in the published literature document treatment failure even within referral centres. However, the disease should not be viewed as 100% fatal as there are 2 cases of either confirmed (Borchers *et al.* 2006) or presumptive Tyzzer's disease (Peek *et al.* 1994) that survived following hospital based therapy. Treatment should be aimed at aggressive antimicrobial therapy combined with intensive supportive management of hepatic failure. *C. piliforme* typically demonstrates sensitivity to beta lactams, macrolides and aminoglycosides in laboratory studies (Ganaway *et al.* 1971), and the 2 successfully treated foals in the literature received i.v. sodium penicillin and sulphamethoxazole-trimethoprim and i.v. ampicillin and gentamicin respectively. From pathological reports in horses it is evident that the organism can be found within organs other than the liver, including the heart (van der Lugt *et al.* 1985; Humber *et al.* 1988), suggesting that the disease can initiate a true bacteraemia and that treatment efforts should mirror those of the most critical septicaemic neonate. Perhaps of note is the fact that both survivors also received partial parenteral nutrition underscoring the value of i.v. nutritional support of foals with liver failure. Undoubtedly, suspect Tyzzer's cases should be hospitalised because there will be an intensive need to monitor glucose, acid base status and electrolyte levels as well as to provide antiseizure medication should the need arise. Plasma may also be of benefit in affected foals as a source of globulin, albumin, acute phase proteins and clotting factors.

Because the majority of cases reported have died within 48 h of presentation, survival of a presumed or confirmed Tyzzer's disease case beyond the first few days of therapy should be taken as a very encouraging sign. Several cases in the literature experienced transient improvement with correction of glucose, acid-base status and hypovolaemia but died nonetheless within this short time frame (Humber *et al.* 1988; Borchers *et al.* 2006).

Epidemiology, risk factors and prevention

Although the majority of the literature on Tyzzer's disease focuses on retrospective clinical case material there is confirmation from the study by Swerczek (1977) that the disease can be reproduced by oral inoculation of foals with the organism recovered from faeces of experimentally infected adult horses. This, alongside clinical observations and experience on problem farms in high density breeding areas would suggest that foals become infected by consuming the organism from their environment, probably in faeces of mares. The case control study by Fosgate *et al.* (2002) identified several significant risk factors for *C. piliforme* infection in foals on one large California breeding farm. Specifically, foals born between mid-March and mid-April were >7 times more likely to be infected compared to foals born at other times, foals from nonresident mares were >3 times more likely and foals born to mares aged <6 years were also approximately 3 times more likely to be infected. The fact that foals born to younger mares or to mares transported onto the farm specifically for breeding purposes are at higher risk would suggest that both quantity and specificity of colostral antibody may be important in protecting foals against this disease.

Further evidence that specificity of protection is important is suggested by work showing that horses can be infected with multiple strains of *C. piliforme* including those that are more typically associated with rodent infection, and that there is no cross protection between these strains (Hook *et al.* 1995). This same study from the central USA revealed that approximately 25% of healthy adult horses sampled had detectable antibody to an equine strain suggesting quite widespread infection in the adult horse population (Hook *et al.* 1995). One other study from the north-western USA did not document any breed or sex predilection to the disease when 21 cases were reviewed retrospectively (Turk *et al.* 1981).

Due to the sporadic nature of the disease it is unnecessary for most farms to implement control measures specific to Tyzzer's disease. Furthermore it is highly unlikely that there will be an equine vaccine available for the disease in the future. Instead, nonspecific advice about hygiene and minimising risk for faeco-oral exposure of foals to adults may be made but are largely impractical because of the coprophagic behaviour of nursing foals. Within the environment the organism persists in spore form, the vegetative organism being much more labile and short-lived, and the spores are reported to be sensitive to disinfection with 0.3% sodium hypochlorite (Ganaway *et al.* 1971). The study by Fosgate *et al.* (2002) would suggest that problem farms may be able to reduce the risk of infection by minimising the numbers of younger and nonresident broodmares in the breeding programme. As with other infectious diseases in the neonatal period, ensuring adequacy of passive transfer using colostrum from the foal's own mare or perhaps mares maintained on the problem farm in question may help increase both the volume and specificity of colostral antibody against the strains of *C. piliforme* endemic at that location. Foals born on problem farms should be monitored closely for early behavioural and clinical signs consistent with Tyzzer's disease, and promptly moved into a hospital setting for intensive treatment should their value justify.

References

Borchers, A., Magdesian, K.G., Halland, S., Pusterla, N. and Wilson, D.W. (2006) Successful treatment and polymerase chain reaction confirmation of Tyzzer's disease in a foal and clinical and pathologic characteristics of 6 additional foals (1986-2005). *J. vet. intern. Med.* **20**, 1212-1218.

Brooks, J.W., Whary, M.T., Hattel, A.L., Shaw, D.P., Ge, Z., Fox, J.G. and Poppenga, R.H. (2006) *Clostridium piliforme* infection in two farm raised white-tailed deer fawns (*Odocoileus vriginianus*) and association with copper toxicosis. *Vet. Pathol.* **43**, 765-768.

Brown, C.M., Ainsworth, D.M., Personett, L.A. and Derksen, F.J. (1983) Serum biochemical and hematological findings in two foals with focal bacterial hepatitis (Tyzzer's disease). *Equine vet. J.* **15**, 375-376.

Carrigan, M.J., Pedrana, R.G. and McKibbin, A.W. (1984) Tyzzer's disease in foals. *Aust. vet. J.* **61**, 199-200.

Copland, M.D., Robertson, C.W., Fry, J. and Wilson, G. (1984) Tyzzer's disease in a foal. *Aust. vet. J.* **61**, 302-304.

Dickinson, L.A. (1980) Tyzzer's disease in foals (Letter to Editor). *N.Z. vet. J.* **28**, 60.

Duncan, A.J., Carman, R.J., Olsen, G.J. and Wilson, K.H. (1993) Assignment of the agent of Tyzzer's disease to *Clostridium piliforme* comb. Nov. on the basis of 16s rRNA sequence analysis. *Int. J. Syst. Bacteriol.* **43**, 314-318.

Feldman, S.H., Kiavand, A., Seidelin, M. and Rieske, H.R. (2006) Ribosomal RNA sequences of *Clostridium piliforme* isolated from rodent and rabbit: re-examining the phylogeny of the Tyzzer's disease agent and development of a diagnostic polymerase chain reaction assay. *J. Am. Ass. Lab. Anim. Sci.* **45**, 65-73.

Fosgate, G.T., Hird, D.W., Read, D.H. and Walker, R.L. (2002) Risk factors for *Clostridium piliforme* infection in foals. *J. Am. vet. med. Ass.* **220**, 785-790.

Furukawa, T., Furmoto, K., Mitsuhiro, F. and Okada, E. (2002) Detection by PCR of the Tyzzer's disease organism (*Clostridium piliforme*) in feces. *Exp. Anim.* **51**, 513-516.

Ganaway, J.R., Allen, A.M. and Moore, T.D. (1971) Tyzzer's disease. *Am. J. Pathol.* **64**, 717-732.

Goto, K. and Itoh, T. (1994) Detection of *Bacillus piliformis* by specific amplification of ribosomal sequences. *Jikken Dobutsu.* **43**, 389-394.

Hook, R.R., Riley, L.K., Franklin, C.L. and Besch-Williford, C.L. (1995) Seroanalysis of Tyzzer's disease in horses: implications that multiple strains can infect *Equidae*. *Equine vet. J.* **27**, 8-12.

Humber, K.A., Sweeney, R.W., Saik, J.E., Hansen, T.O. and Morris, C.F. (1988) Clinical and clinicopathologic findings in two foals infected with *Bacillus piliformis*. *J. Am. vet. med. Ass.* **193**, 1425-1428.

Ikegami, T., Shirota, K., Une, Y., Nomura, Y., Wda, Y., Goto, A., Takakura, A., Itoh, T. and Fujiwara, K. (1999) Naturally occurring Tyzzer's disease in a calf. *Vet. Pathol.* **36**, 253-255.

Langan, J., Bemis, D., Harbo, S., Pollock, C. and Schumacher, J. (2000) Tyzzer's disease in a red panda (*Ailurus fulgens fulgens*) *J. Zoo. Wildl. Med.* **31**, 558-562.

Paar, M., Stockhofe-Zurweiden, N., Pohlmeyer, G., Gerhards, H., and Pohlenz, J. (1993) Infection with *Bacillus piliformis* (Tyzzer's disease) in foals. *Schweiz Arch. Tierheilkd.* **135**, 79-88.

Peek, S.F., Byars, T.D. and Rueve, E. (1994) Neonatal hepatic failure in a Thoroughbred foal: Successful treatment of a case of presumptive Tyzzer's disease. *Equine. vet. Educ.* **6**, 307-309.

Peeters, J.E., Charlier, G., Halen, P., Geeroms, R. and Raeymaekers, R. (1985) Naturally occurring Tyzzer's disease in commercial rabbits: a clinical and pathological study. *Ann. Rech. vet.* **16**, 69-79.

Raymond, J.T., Topham, K., Shirota, K., Ikeda, T. and Garner, M.M. (2001) Tyzzer's disease in a neonatal rainbow lorikeet (*Trichoglossus haematodus*). *Vet. Pathol.* **38**, 326-327.

Sasseville, V.G., Simon, M.A., Chalifoux, L.V., Lin, K.C. and Mansfield, K.G. (2007) Naturally occurring Tyzzer's disease in cotton top tamarins (*Saguinus oedipus*). *Comp. Med.* **57**, 125-127.

Smith, K.J., Skelton, H.G., Hilyard, E.J., Hadfield, T., Moeller, R.S., Tuur, S., Decker, C., Wagner, K.F. and Angritt, P. (1996) *Bacillus piliformis* infection (Tyzzer's disease) in a patient infected with HIV-1; confirmation with 16s ribosomal RNA sequence analysis. *J. Am. Acad. Dermatol.* **34**, 343-348.

St. Denis, K.A., Waddell-Parks, N. and Belanger, M. (2000) Tyzzer's disease in an 11-day old foal. *Can. vet. J.* **41**, 491-492.

Swerczek, T.W., Crowe, M.W. and Prockett, M.E. (1973) Focal bacterial hepatitis in foals: preliminary report. *Mod. vet. Pract.* **54**, 66-67.

Swerczek, T.W. (1977) Multifocal hepatic necrosis and hepatitis in foals caused by *Bacillus piliformis* (Tyzzer's disease). *Vet. Ann.* **17**, 130-132.

Thomson, G.W., Wilson, R.W., Hall, E.A. and Physick-Sheard, P. (1977) Tyzzer's disease in the foal. Case reports and review. *Can. vet. J.* **18**, 41-43.

Turk, M.A., Gallina, A.M. and Perryman, L.E. (1981) *Bacillus piliformis* infection (Tyzzer's disease) in foals in north western United States. A retrospective study of 21 cases. *J. Am. vet. med. Ass.* **178**, 279-281.

Tyzzer, E.E. (1917) A fatal disease of the Japanese waltzing mouse caused by a spore-bearing bacillus (*Bacillus piliformis*, n sp) *J. med. Res.* **37**, 307-338.

Van der Lugt, J.J., Coetzer, J.A., Jordaan, P. and Marlow, C.H. (1985) Suspected Tyzzer's disease in two foals. *J. S. Afr. vet. Ass.* **56**, 1017-108.

Whitwell, K.E. (1976) Four cases of Tyzzer's disease in foals in England. *Equine vet. J.* **8**, 118-122.

Young, J.K., Baker, D.C. and Burney, D.P. (1995) Naturally occurring Tyzzer's disease in a puppy. *Vet. Pathol.* **32**, 53-65.

TETANUS

A. L. Johnson

Large Animal Internal Medicine, New Bolton Center, 382 West Street Road, Kennett Square, Pennsylvania 19348, USA.

Keywords: horse; tetanus; *Clostridium tetani*; vaccination; exotoxin; anti-toxin; stiff gait; muscle rigidity; *risus sardonicus*

Summary

Horses with wounds are at risk of developing tetanus if they have not been appropriately vaccinated. This often fatal disease is caused by *Clostridium tetani*, a bacterium that produces 3 exotoxins, one of which blocks the release of inhibitory neurotransmitters in the central nervous system. This loss of inhibition leads to sustained contraction of muscles, manifested clinically by abnormal facial expression ('*risus sardonicus*'), stiff gait and posture, and extensor rigidity. Diagnosis of tetanus relies upon identification of these clinical signs and not on ancillary testing. Although anti-toxin is available and treatment is possible, the prolonged supportive care required for a good outcome is labour-intensive and expensive. Therefore, vaccination, which is highly efficacious in preventing disease, is strongly recommended.

Introduction

Although tetanus is technically defined as sustained contraction of muscles without relaxation, the word is generally used to refer to the disease caused by infection with the bacterium *Clostridium tetani*. Tetanus has a worldwide distribution and may occur in any domestic animal or human being. Horses appear to be most susceptible to developing tetanus, while dogs and cats are least susceptible, and the disease is commonly fatal in horses (de Lahunta and Glass 2009). Herd outbreaks of tetanus after tail docking or castration have been described in ruminant species, but tetanus is usually a disease of individual horses (Smith 2002).

Aetiology

Clostridium tetani is a spore-forming, Gram-positive, anaerobic rod that produces 3 exotoxins: tetanospasmin, tetanolysin and nonspasmogenic toxin. The functions of tetanolysin and nonspasmogenic toxin are less fully described than that of tetanospasmin, which is the neurotoxin responsible for the clinical signs. The spores are very resistant to degradation and persist for long periods of time in the environment. They are widely distributed in soil and in the intestines and faeces of many species, including horses, cattle, sheep, dogs, cats, rats and chickens (Anon 2008). Manure-treated soil may contain high numbers of spores. For animal infection to occur, an anaerobic environment must be present. The most common cause of infection in the horse is a puncture wound, but other types of wounds – including surgical or superficial wounds – may also provide appropriate conditions for *C. tetani* growth.

Pathophysiology

After spores contaminate damaged tissue in an anaerobic environment, they begin to germinate. Within 4–8 h, the spores may convert to their vegetative form and produce neurotoxin, which is disseminated throughout the body via blood and lymphatics. This toxin binds to axonal gangliosides at the telodendrons of peripheral motor neurons and is internalised. Retrograde transport of toxin to the grey matter of the spinal cord occurs within a few hours; in the spinal cord the toxin exits the neuronal cell bodies and binds to adjacent Renshaw cells, which are inhibitory interneurons that predominantly influence motor neurons of anti-gravity (extensor) muscles. The toxin is a zinc endopeptidase that cleaves cell membrane proteins required for the release of inhibitory neurotransmitters (glycine in the spinal cord and gamma-aminobutyric acid in the brainstem). Therefore, the bound toxin blocks release of inhibitory neurotransmitters, and this loss of inhibition causes

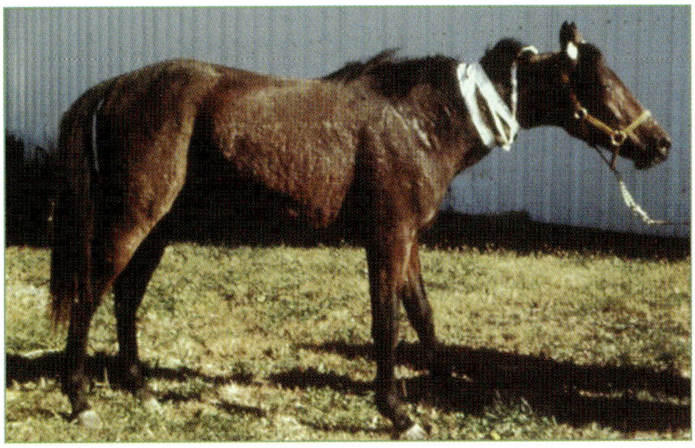

FIGURE 1: Adult horse with tetanus showing typical 'sawhorse' stance. Photo courtesy of Dr Raymond Sweeney.

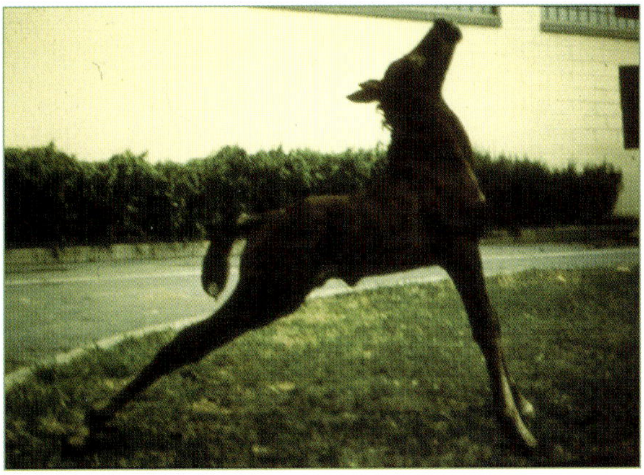

FIGURE 2: Foal with tetanus displaying 'sawhorse' stance and opisthotonus. Photo courtesy of Dr Raymond Sweeney.

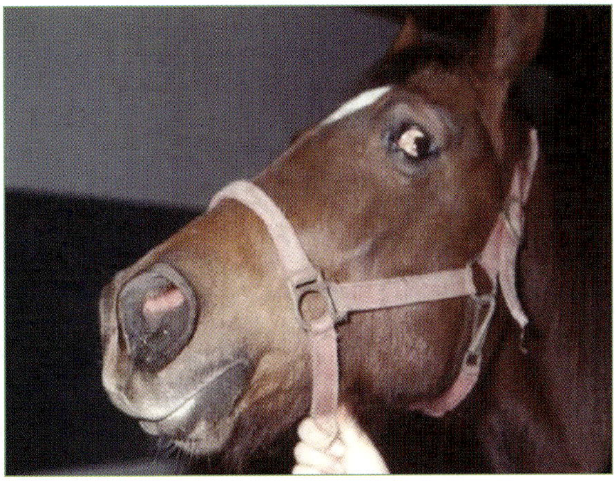

FIGURE 3: Adult horse with tetanus. Note flared nostrils, protruding third eyelid, elevated upper eyelid and erect ears. Photo courtesy of Dr Robert Whitlock.

sustained contraction of the extensor muscles. Although extensor muscle rigidity is the most common result of intoxication, tetanus neurotoxin may also affect the brain and autonomic nervous system, causing seizures and autonomic nervous system dysfunction. Toxin may remain bound for >3 weeks (de Lahunta and Glass 2009).

Clinical signs

Generally, signs occur within 5–10 days of a wound becoming infected (de Lahunta and Glass 2009). However, a recent retrospective study found that the time between wound acquisition and first signs of tetanus ranged from 2 days to 2 months (van Galen *et al.* 2008), whereas a second study showed a range of 2–21 days (Green *et al.* 1994). It was noted that the horse affected 2 months after castration was administered tetanus antitoxin at the time of surgery, which may have delayed development of clinical signs. Mild signs include a stiff gait and posture, elevated tail, and an altered facial expression known as '*risus sardonicus*', or 'scornful laughter' (de Lahunta and Glass 2009). **Figures 1** and **2** illustrate the characteristic posture, also known as a 'sawhorse stance', and **Figures 3** and **4** illustrate '*risus sardonicus*'. This facial expression results from contraction of all the facial muscles, including the extraocular muscles, and includes retracted lips, flared nostrils, elevated upper eyelid, a spasmodically protruding third eyelid, and erect or caudally directed ears. The jaws may be clamped shut and difficult or impossible to open (trismus or 'lockjaw'). In one report

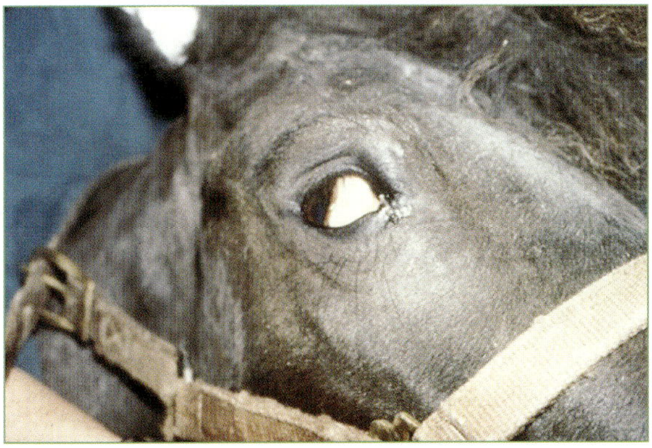

FIGURE 4: Adult horse with tetanus. Note severe protrusion of third eyelid. Photo courtesy of Dr Raymond Sweeney.

of 20 cases, hyperaesthesia and protrusion of the third eyelid were the most common clinical signs (Green *et al.* 1994). Horses may develop signs of intractable abdominal pain during the first 24 h (Smith 2002). More severely affected animals are unable to walk and may become recumbent with extensor rigidity of all limbs, opisthotonus, severe trismus and, possibly, seizures. The most severely affected animals are unable to stand or eat, and die from respiratory failure (hypoxaemia) due to involvement of the diaphragm and intercostal muscles (Smith 2002).

Severely affected horses may develop complications secondary to recumbency, such as pressure sores, myopathy, pneumonia, urine retention and cystitis, or ileus and gastrointestinal impaction. Difficulty chewing and swallowing may cause aspiration pneumonia. The muscle hyperactivity causes pyrexia, and horses sweat profusely, causing dehydration and electrolyte derangements. Affected horses appear to be at significant risk of falling in the stall and have been reported to suffer fatal injuries such as pelvic, skull, tibial and femoral fractures (Green *et al.* 1994; Sedrish *et al.* 1996).

Horses that survive usually begin to show some improvement within about 2 weeks, but clinical signs may persist for a month, and on occasion lameness may be permanent (Smith 2002).

Diagnosis

The diagnosis of tetanus in horses is entirely based on clinical signs and does not require bacteriological or toxin confirmation. In human cases of tetanus, *C. tetani* is cultured from the wound in only 30% of cases and can also be isolated from patients who do not have tetanus (Anon 2008). The same is probably true for horses. Therefore, wound culturing is not necessary for diagnosis, although it may be warranted for other reasons. Signs may be subtle in early or mild cases, and diagnosis may be aided by attempting to elicit muscle spasms by auditory, ocular or tactile stimulation. Performing a menacing gesture towards the horse's head or slapping the horse on the neck often causes retraction of the eye and rapid flashing of the third eyelid over the cornea. There are no characteristic *post mortem* lesions associated with tetanus.

Differential diagnoses include electrolyte abnormalities such as hypocalcaemia, hyperkalaemia or hypomagnesaemia. These derangements can be easily excluded with serum biochemistry. If the affected horse is possibly a descendant of 'Impressive' (Quarter Horse, Appaloosa or Paint lineage), consider hyperkalaemic periodic paralysis, particularly if the serum potassium is elevated. Horses with acute laminitis, myopathies (polysaccharide storage myopathy, immune-mediated myositis, nutritional rhabdomyolysis, exertional rhabdomyolysis) or meningitis may have a stiff gait similar to that of horses with tetanus. Lateral radiographs of the third phalangeal bones, analysis of serum muscle enzyme activities, and/or cerebrospinal fluid collection and analysis can be performed if there is any suspicion of these conditions. Occasionally horses with tetanus may present for evaluation of colic. Other conditions that may look like tetanus include equine motor neuron disease, shivers, severe neck pain or acquired myotonias such as occur with ear tick (*Otobius megnini*) infestation.

Treatment

The mainstays of treatment include providing excellent supportive care, aiding in muscular relaxation, treating the infection, neutralising unbound toxin and establishing immunity.

Supportive care

Signs are exacerbated by activity or excitement, and increased activity may actually increase the rate of axonal transport of toxin (de Lahunta 1983). Therefore, one of the most important aspects of treatment is providing a quiet environment where the horse can rest. Caretakers should avoid stimulating the patient as much as possible. Darkened lighting, stuffing the ears with cotton and sedation may be beneficial. Good footing is essential to allow the horse to remain ambulatory, as muscular hypertonicity makes it difficult for horses to rise and stand. Deep bedding and meticulous care are required to prevent pressure sores in recumbent patients. Sling support may aid horses that cannot stand on their own but should not be used if the horse becomes nervous or agitated in the sling. Rarely, horses may require tracheostomy to aid respiration. Hydration status should be closely monitored and i.v. fluids administered if dehydration or electrolyte derangements develop. Finally, acupuncture may be used as an adjunctive treatment for tetanus (White and Christie 1985).

Nutritional support should also be considered. Mildly affected horses may be able to eat and sustain an adequate plane of nutrition as long as feed is elevated for easier access. However, more severely affected cases should receive supplementary nutrition via nasogastric intubation or parenteral administration. Parenteral administration may be preferable if the horse does not tolerate nasogastric intubation well. Commercial liquid enteral diets are available for horses, but patients may easily be maintained for 2 weeks or more with alfalfa meal gruel (1.8 kg alfalfa meal with 8–12 l of water administered twice daily via nasogastric tube). Alternatively, the horse's daily maintenance requirement of a complete pelleted feed (i.e. a 'senior' feed) may be divided into 2–4 feedings, dissolved into 6–12 l of water, and administered via nasogastric tube. If the horse's temperament or stress level precludes repeated nasogastric intubation, partial or total parenteral nutrition (TPN) may be utilised. Full maintenance requirements can be met using 10 g/kg bwt/day dextrose, 2 g/kg bwt/day amino acids and 1 g/kg bwt/day lipids. However, full maintenance with TPN is extraordinarily expensive for adult horses, and quarter- or half-maintenance rates may be more reasonable.

Muscular relaxation

As aforementioned, a quiet, nonstressful environment will aid in muscular relaxation. Sedatives are also useful to relax the horse; acepromazine, barbiturates, and chloral hydrate have been used. Muscle relaxants such as methocarbamol and diazepam may also be helpful. One of the most effective protocols appears to be using acepromazine initially and adding diazepam with or without xylazine if necessary. Approximate dosages are as follows (Hackett *et al.* 2008):

Acepromazine: 0.02–0.05 mg/kg bwt q. 6–8 h i.v. or i.m.

Chloral hydrate: 20–60 mg/kg bwt as a 12% solution by slow i.v. infusion (low end of dose range provides moderate sedation; high end provides profound sedation).

Diazepam: 0.05–0.44 mg/kg bwt i.v. (respiratory depression may occur at high end of dose range).

Methocarbamol: 40–60 mg/kg bwt *per os* or 10–50 mg/kg bwt i.v. q. 12–24 h.

Phenobarbital: 2–10 mg/kg bwt *per os* or i.v. slowly q. 12 h (respiratory depression may occur at high end of dose range).

Xylazine: 0.2–1.1 mg/kg bwt q. 8–12 h i.v. or i.m.

Treating the infection

The horse should be examined carefully for an infected wound, which should be debrided and lavaged if identified. Procaine penicillin may be infiltrated locally or used to lavage the wound. Penicillin (or another antibiotic effective against *C. tetani*) should also be administered systemically to prevent additional bacterial proliferation. Intravenous potassium penicillin G (22,000 iu/kg bwt q. 6 h) or i.m. procaine penicillin G (22,000 iu/kg bwt q. 12 h) is typically used.

Neutralising unbound toxin

Antitoxin should be administered as soon as clinical signs are recognised. The dosing regimen for horses is not standardised. Four equine-origin tetanus antitoxin products manufactured in the USA are listed in the Compendium of Veterinary Products (http://bayerall.naccvp.com/). The manufacturers' instructions for treatment of tetanus vary as follows:

Durvet: 10,000–50,000 iu i.m. or subcut.;

Fort Dodge: 30,000–100,000 iu i.v., subcut. or intraperitoneally;

Colorado Serum: 10,000–50,000 iu i.m. or subcut.;

Professional Biological: 10,000–50,000 iu i.m. or subcut.

Other protocols have been described in the literature; a few examples follow:

1. 3000 iu for an adult horse, route not specified (Neily 1954);
2. 5000–30,000 iu i.v. or i.m. for an adult horse, with the suggestion that i.v. administration followed by 2500 iu subcut. for 5 consecutive days may be beneficial (Green *et al.* 1994);
3. 3000–9,000 iu infiltrated locally; wide dose range of 2–5000 iu/kg bwt, route not specified (Smith 2002);
4. 50–150 iu/kg bwt i.v., i.m. or subcut. (van Galen *et al.* 2008).

Although antitoxin does not significantly affect bound toxin, it should prevent additional toxin from being transported to the spinal cord and binding. If the wound site is known, antitoxin can be injected around and proximal to it.

Intrathecal administration of tetanus antitoxin has been described (Muylle *et al.* 1975; Green *et al.* 1994), but benefit has not been clearly demonstrated in horses. In one report, 5 horses administered tetanus antitoxin intrathecally did not survive the disease, and one had seizures as a complication of treatment (Green *et al.* 1994). However, an older study reported an improved survival rate with subarachnoid injection of tetanus antitoxin (Muylle *et al.* 1975). If intrathecal administration is attempted, the described protocol involves slow injection of 50 ml antitoxin (1000 iu/ml; only use 30 ml for foals) into the subarachnoid space at the atlanto-occipital or lumbosacral space after removal of a similar volume of CSF (Muylle *et al.* 1975; Green *et al.* 1994). Intrathecal administration has been more fully evaluated in human patients; a recent meta-analysis that included 942 patients in 12 trials (484 in intrathecal group and 458 in i.m. group) showed that intrathecal administration of tetanus antitoxin was more beneficial, with a combined relative risk of mortality of 0.71 for intrathecal vs. i.m. administration (Kabura *et al.* 2006).

Establishing immunity

Due to the extreme potency of tetanus toxin, natural infection does NOT result in adequate immunity to tetanus (Anon 2008). Therefore, active immunisation (via vaccination with tetanus toxoid) should begin immediately. If tetanus antitoxin has been administered, tetanus toxoid should be given in a distant site. Vaccine protocols are included later in this chapter under 'Prevention'.

Prognosis

With conscientious supportive care, affected horses may survive. However, published survival rates are relatively low. The most recent retrospective study, involving 31 equids diagnosed with tetanus in Belgium between 1991 and 2006, yielded a survival rate of 32% (van Galen *et al.* 2008). None of these cases were appropriately vaccinated, and most were aged ≤5 years. Nonsurvivors were significantly younger than survivors and more likely to show dysphagia, dyspnoea and recumbency. All nonsurvivors died within 8 days of developing signs. A study performed in Morocco on equine cases of tetanus admitted in 2003–2004 yielded a survival rate of 41% (Kay and Knottenbelt 2007). A slightly older retrospective study of 20 horses with tetanus in Canada between 1970 and 1990 showed a survival rate of 25% (Green *et al.* 1994). Previously vaccinated horses were much more likely to survive than nonvaccinated horses. Favourable prognostic indicators also included a response to phenothiazine tranquilisers and the absence of rapid (24–48 h) progression to recumbency. The highest survival rate reported was 72.5% (Muylle *et al.* 1975) in a group of horses treated with intrathecal injection of tetanus antitoxin. However, this improved survival has not been documented by other groups that have attempted intrathecal treatment. It has been proposed for horses, and has been stated for man, that the shorter the incubation period, the higher the chance of death, and *vice versa* (Dawley 1960; Anon 2008).

Prevention

Prevention strategies focus on adequate vaccination and appropriate wound care. Current American Association of Equine Practitioners vaccination guidelines list tetanus as one of the 'core' vaccines, defined by the American Veterinary Medical Association as vaccines "that protect from diseases that are endemic to a region, those with potential public health significance, required by law, virulent/highly infectious, and/or those posing a risk of severe disease. Core vaccines have clearly demonstrated efficacy and safety, and thus exhibit a high enough level of patient benefit and low enough level of risk to justify their use in the majority of patients" (http://www.aaep.org/core_vaccinations.htm). The vaccines available are formalin-inactivated, adjuvanted toxoids. Full text of the recommended vaccination schedule can be found at http://www.aaep.org/tetanus.htm. In brief:

1. Foals born to vaccinated mares should receive an initial 3-dose series beginning at age 6 months, with a 4–6 week period between the first and second doses and the third dose administered at age 10–12 months. NOTE: although the AAEP recommendations say "beginning at 4–6 months

of age", recent research shows that maternal antibodies exert a significant inhibitory effect on the response of these foals to tetanus toxoid, and that primary immunisation should not begin before age 6 months (Wilson *et al.* 2001).

2. Foals born to nonvaccinated mares (or mares of unknown vaccinal status) should receive an initial 3-dose series beginning at age 1–4 months, with 4 weeks between each dose.
3. Adult horses that have been previously vaccinated should be re-vaccinated annually. If the horse is wounded or has surgery 6 or more months after its most recent vaccination, it should be immediately re-vaccinated.
4. Adult horses that have not been vaccinated or that have an unknown vaccinal status should receive an initial 2-dose series with 4–6 weeks between doses and then annual re-vaccination.
5. Pregnant mares that have been previously vaccinated should be re-vaccinated annually, 4–6 weeks prior to foaling.
6. Pregnant mares that have not been vaccinated or have an unknown vaccinal status should receive an initial 2-dose series with 4–6 weeks between doses and be re-vaccinated 4–6 weeks prior to foaling.

The use of tetanus antitoxin to provide passive immunity is recommended in situations where the foal or horse is at risk of tetanus infection and has not been adequately immunised. Examples include an unvaccinated horse that sustains a wound or a foal that needs surgery and was born to an unvaccinated mare. The recommended dose of tetanus antitoxin is 1500 iu subcut. or i.m. for prevention of infection. Although tetanus antitoxin historically was administered routinely to periparturient mares, this practice is now discouraged (Messer and Johnson 1994a). There is a much more significant risk of complications following tetanus antitoxin administration as compared to tetanus toxoid; several reports have associated hepatic disease ('Theiler's disease') with administration of tetanus antitoxin (Messer and Johnson 1994a; Guglick *et al.* 1995). Clinical or subclinical hepatitis may occur from 48–120 days after administration of tetanus antitoxin, and affected horses may display depression, lethargy, anorexia, icterus, photodermatitis, subcutaneous oedema, high serum activities of liver-specific enzymes and/or encephalopathic signs (Messer and Johnson 1994b; Guglick *et al.* 1995). If tetanus antitoxin administration is indicated, it should be administered in one i.m. site and the first dose of an initial series of tetanus toxoid vaccinations should be administered in a separate, distant muscular site.

Conclusion

As discussed, tetanus is a serious infectious disease that sporadically affects horses. The disease is generally preventable through vaccination but is likely to be fatal in nonvaccinated horses. Diagnosis is based entirely on clinical signs, which include a stiff gait and posture, extensor muscle rigidity, and an altered facial expression characterised by flared nostrils, retracted lips, protruding third eyelids and caudally directed ears. Affected horses may be successfully treated with significant supportive care, antimicrobials effective against *C. tetani*, tetanus antitoxin, muscle relaxants and immunisation. Poor prognostic indicators for survival include dysphagia, dyspnoea and recumbency.

References

Anon (2008) *Epidemiology and Prevention of Vaccine-Preventable Diseases,* 10th edn. 2nd printing, Centers for Disease Control and Prevention, Eds: W. Atkinson, J. Hamborsky, L. McIntyre and S. Wolfe, Washington DC: Public Health Foundation.

Dawley, S.W. (1960) Tranquilizers in the treatment of tetanus in the horse. *Can vet. J.* **1**, 563-564.

de Lahunta, A. (1983) Tetanus. Upper Motor Neuron System. In: *Veterinary Neuroanatomy and Clinical Neurology,* 2nd edn. Ed: A. de Lahunta, Philadelphia: W.B. Saunders Company, Chapter 7, pp 141-142.

de Lahunta, A. and Glass, E. (2009) Tetanus. Upper Motor Neuron. In: *Veterinary Neuroanatomy and Clinical Neurology*, 3rd edn. Eds: A. de Lahunta and E. Glass, Saunders Elsevier, St. Louis, Chapter 8. pp 209-210.

Green, S.L., Little, C.B., Baird, J.D., Tremblay, R.R. and Smith-Maxie, L.L. (1994) Tetanus in the horse: a review of 20 cases (1970–1990). *J. vet. intern. Med.* **8**, 128-132.

Guglick, M.A., MacAllister, C.G., Ely, R.W. and Edwards, W.C. (1995) Hepatic disease associated with administration of tetanus antitoxin in eight horses. *J. Am. vet. med. Ass.* **206**, 1737-1740.

Hackett, E.S., Orsini, J.A. and Divers, T.J. (2008) Equine emergency drugs: Approximate dosages and adverse drug reactions. In: *Equine Emergencies: Treatment and Procedures,* 3rd edn., Eds: J.A. Orsini and T.J. Divers, Saunders Elsevier, St. Louis. 739-752.

Kabura, L., Ilibagiza, D., Menten, J. and van den Ende, J. (2006) Intrathecal vs. intramuscular administration of human antitetanus immunoglobulin or equine tetanus antitoxin in the treatment of tetanus: a meta-analysis. *Trop. Med. Int. Health.* **11**, 1075-1081.

Kay, G. and Knottenbelt, D.C. (2007) Tetanus in equids: A report of 56 cases. *Equine vet. Educ.* **2**, 107-112.

Messer, N.T. and Johnson, P.J. (1994a) Idiopathic acute hepatic disease in horses: 12 cases (1982-1992). *J. Am. vet. med. Ass.* **204**, 1934-1937.

Messer, N.T. and Johnson, P.J. (1994b) Serum hepatitis in two brood mares. *J. Am. vet. med. Ass.* **204**, 1790-1792.

Muylle, E., Oyaert, W., Ooms, L. and Decraemere, H. (1975) Treatment of tetanus in the horse by injections of tetanus antitoxin into the subarachnoid space. *J. Am. vet. med. Ass.* **167**, 47-48.

Neily, L.G. (1954) Tetanus in the horse. *Can. J. comp. Med.* **18**, 338-339.

Sedrish, S.A., Seahorn, T.L. and Martin, G. (1996) What is your neurologic diagnosis? Tetanus. *J. Am. vet. med. Ass.* **209**, 57-58.

Smith, M.O. (2002) Tetanus (lockjaw). Diseases of the nervous system. In: *Large Animal Internal Medicine*, 3rd edn., Ed: B.P. Smith, Mosby, St Louis. pp 995-998.

Van Galen, G., Delguste, C., Sandersen, C., Verwilghen, D., Grulke, S. and Amory, H. (2008) Tetanus in the equine species: a retrospective study of 31 cases. *Tijdschr. Diergeneeskd.* **133**, 512-517.

White, S.S. and Christie, M.P. (1985) Acupuncture used as an adjunct in the treatment of a horse with tetanus. *Aust. vet. J.* **62**, 25-26.

Wilson, W.D., Mihalyi, J.E., Hussey, S. and Lunn, D.P. (2001) Passive transfer of maternal immunoglobulin isotype antibodies against tetanus and influenza and their effect on the response of foals to vaccination. *Equine vet. J.* **33**, 644-650.

EQUINE BOTULISM

B. Barr

Rood and Riddle Equine Hospital, PO Box 12070, 2150 Georgetown Road, Lexington, Kentucky 40580, USA.

Keywords: horse; weakness; dysphagia; neuromuscular; muscle fasciculations; acetylcholine; antitoxin

Summary

Botulism causes a flaccid neuromuscular paralysis in horses and has classically been termed 'forage poisoning' in adults and 'shaker foal syndrome' in foals. Toxins produced by the Gram-positive spore forming anaerobic bacterium *Clostridium botulinum* cause botulism. Clinical signs frequently observed include generalised muscle weakness, dysphagia and muscle fasciculations. Exposure of the horse to botulinum toxin may occur from ingesting preformed toxin (forage poisoning), ingestion of spores, which vegetate and form toxin (toxicoinfectious), or contamination of a wound with spores. Diagnosis is often a clinical diagnosis. Treatment includes administration of antitoxin and appropriate supportive care. The best chance for recovery is administration of antitoxin early in the course of the disease. Prevention involves common sense approaches to feeding and care of the horse and use of vaccination in endemic areas.

Introduction

Botulism is a rapidly progressive neuromuscular disease that may be fatal to horses. *Clostridium botulinum* is an anaerobic bacterium that is responsible for producing the toxin that causes botulism. Two other clostridial species, *Clostridium barati* and *Clostridium butyricum*, also produce botulinum toxin (Mohanty *et al.* 2001; Gupta *et al.* 2005). The first published reports of botulism in the horse were from the 1950s. Botulinum toxin is one of the most potent biological toxins known and can cause neuromuscular weakness in most mammals, birds, and fish. *Clostridium botulinum* is a Gram-positive, spore forming anaerobic rod-shaped bacterium. Eight different botulinum toxins are produced and designated as Types A, B, Ca, Cb, D, E, F and G with each being produced by a different serogroup (A through G). The distribution in the environment of the different types of toxin varies, although all produce identical clinical disease. In general, Types A, B, E, F and G principally inhabit soil and seawater or freshwater, whereas Types C and D seem to be obligate parasites in animals and birds (Galey 2001). Type B makes up a majority of the cases in horses (>85%) in the USA with Types A and C causing the rest (Whitlock and Buckley 1997) (**Table 1**). Botulism toxin Type A is used for medicinal purposes.

Epidemiology

Clostridium botulinum is found in soils and organic matter worldwide but is most commonly observed in Kentucky and the mid-Atlantic region of the USA. The spores are found in the soil of 18.5% of the USA with variability in the distribution (Johnston and Whitlock 1987). *Clostridium botulinum* Type A spores are more common in the western part of the USA, whereas *C. botulinum* Type B spores are more uniformly distributed throughout the USA, with the highest concentration northeast of the Mississippi River. Type C is found most commonly in Europe, although cases have been reported from Florida, California, New England, Arizona and Canada

TABLE 1: Species affected by each type of Botulinum toxin

Species	Botulinum toxin
Horses	A, B, C, D
Man	A, B, E, F
Cattle	B, C, D
Sheep	C, D
Dog	C, D
Avian	C, E
Mink/ferret	A, C, E

(MacKay and Berkhoff 1982; Heath *et al.* 1988; Kinde *et al.* 1991). In Australia the most common types are C and D (Hutchins 1994). *Clostridium botulinum* is an obligate anaerobic bacterium that produces spores when stressed. In an alkaline pH with increasing temperature spores may germinate with production of toxin. The spores are highly resistant to heat, light and drying. The toxin is rapidly destroyed by heat and changes in pH.

Pathogenesis

There are 3 modes of botulism intoxication. Botulism can occur following the ingestion of preformed toxin present in feed materials or the environment. This is termed forage poisoning and is the most common source of intoxication in the adult horse. Type B botulism in horses is usually caused by direct proliferation of *C. botulinum* and production of toxin in decaying vegetable matter and rarely by consumption of feed contaminated by decomposing animal carcasses (Whitlock and Buckley 1997). In contrast, Type C botulism is typically associated with contamination of feed materials by carcasses, which are excellent anaerobic incubators for botulism spores present in the intestinal tract of the animal or bird (Whitlock and Buckley 1997). Once toxin is formed in the carcass, it leaches out and contaminates the hay or other feed material.

Toxicoinfectious botulism is the most common route of intoxication for foals aged 2 weeks to 8 months (Swerczek 1980a). The spores are ingested, then vegetate and produce toxin within the gastrointestinal tract. It has been suggested that inflammatory lesions such as gastric ulcers may be potential sites for toxin production (Swerczek 1980a, b). Toxicoinfection with *Clostridium botulinum* Type C has been hypothesised as the cause of grass sickness in Europe.

The final mode of intoxication is wound botulism. Wound botulism may result from deep contamination of wounds with the anaerobic germination of spores within the tissues of the host. Lacerations, castration sites, other surgery sites and infected umbilical stumps are possible areas of contamination.

Botulism toxin acts primarily presynaptically at the peripheral cholinergic neuromuscular junction. The botulinum toxin is a 2-chain metalloproteinase with a 100-kDa heavy chain joined by a disulphide bond to a 50-kDa light chain. The toxin first binds to polysialogangliosides on the nerve terminal and is then internalised into the nerve terminus via a specific protein receptor. The light chain is an enzymatic protease that attacks one of the SNARE proteins involved in fusion of the synaptic vesicles with the plasma membrane at the neuromuscular junction. By attacking the SNARE proteins the toxin prevents the synaptic vesicle from releasing acetylcholine (**Fig 1**). The prevention of the release of acetylcholine results in a flaccid paralysis. The one exception is Type Cb toxin, which causes a change in the membrane permeability (Galey 2001; Wilkins 2007). The type of SNARE protein involved depends on the serotype. Botulism toxin Types A and E cleave SNAP-25, Types B, D, F and G inactivate VAMP (synaptobrevin) and Type C inactivates syntaxin (Humeau *et al.* 2000; Turton *et al.* 2002). Once the toxin is bound at the motor end plates of the neuromuscular junction, improvement is achieved only by the regeneration of new motor end plates, explaining the usual delay of 4–10 days before noticeable clinical improvements even after treatment with antitoxin.

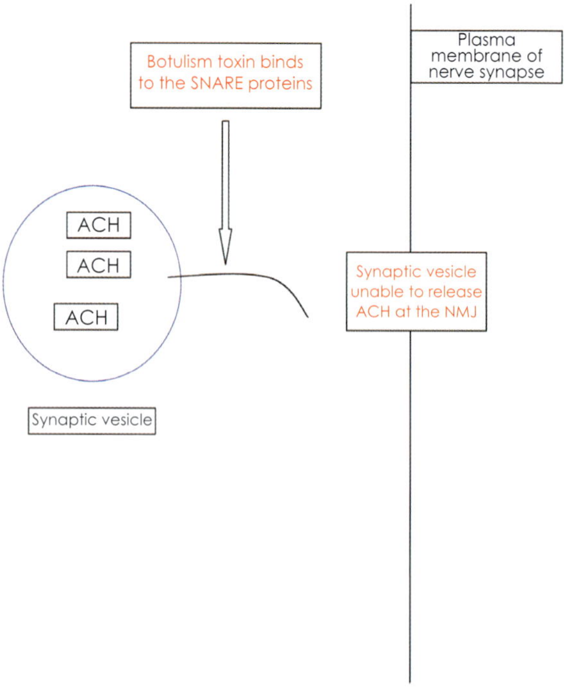

FIGURE 1: Botulinum toxin mechanism of action at the neuromuscular junction. ACH = acetylcholine; NMJ = neuromuscular junction.

Clinical features

Clinical signs are the same regardless of the route of infection and can vary from subtle signs to horses found dead. The severity of clinical signs and the rapidity of progression depend upon the amount of toxin ingested, which cannot be determined other than a horse that progresses to recumbency quickly is assumed to have a large toxin load. The first clinical signs can be seen from 12 h to 10 days following ingestion of the toxin (Critchley 1991; Whitlock and Buckley 1997). Early in the clinical course of botulism mydriasis and ptosis can be observed along with generalised muscle weakness, slow eating and a shuffling gait with toe dragging. In some cases a sluggish pupillary light response is detected within 6–18 h after toxin ingestion. Oftentimes eyelid tone is weak but in an experimental model of Types A and C botulism in horses, the clinician's ability to detect decreased eyelid tone was found to be subjective and often inaccurate (Whitlock 1995, 1996). Tail tone is often decreased in clinical cases of botulism, but in an experimentally induced disease model it was reported to be variable (Whitlock 1995, 1996). Often, before the onset of obvious muscle weakness, reduced tongue tone and slow tongue retraction occur. Normal horses retract their tongue very quickly when it is pulled gently from the commissure of the lips; horses with botulism will retract the tongue very slowly and in the more advanced cases not at all. Prehension of food and the ability to swallow are commonly affected in horses with botulism. In experimental cases the time to consume a standard amount of grain was prolonged. A normal horse should consume 250 ml of grain in less than 2 min, whereas in those with botulism consumption is longer, the grain is mixed with more saliva and some grain falls from the horse's lips during eating (Whitlock and Buckley 1997). Hay will be found in quidded balls on the ground or in the mouth/checks. The inability to swallow water occurs after the loss of the ability to swallow hay. Horses that are unable to swallow water will refuse to drink or will immerse their entire muzzle under water in an attempt to drink. Secondary aspiration pneumonia may be present because of the inability to swallow normally. Horses with botulism walk with a stiff, stilted gait and short, choppy strides. Botulism causes weakness not ataxia. Stumbling and tripping may occur due to weakness not proprioceptive deficits. Muscle fasciculations initially are observed over the triceps and then progress to larger muscle groups. Head carriage is typically lower, which may result in oedema of the head and respiratory stridor. Some horses may spend more time lying down than normal and thus colic may be the initial complaint (Ricketts *et al.* 1984; Heath *et al.* 1988; Whitlock and Buckley 1997). The clinical signs of botulism are always symmetric and gradually progress to recumbency. Early in the course of the disease vital signs are normal. Over time the horse may become dehydrated because of the inability to drink. Recumbent horses will frequently be tachycardic and tachypnoeic as they struggle to stand. In more severe cases an exaggerated respiratory effort is noted with a decreased or normal rate. Constipation, ileus, bladder distension and urine dribbling may be seen in affected horses. Death is caused by respiratory paralysis.

In foals the most common clinical signs include dysphagia, excessive recumbency and muscle fasciculations. The term 'shaker foal syndrome' was given to this disease in the 1980s when foals were dying from this disease. After the foal stands for 2–5 min, there is typically a sudden onset of weakness, with tremors of the muscles of the limbs. The foal will drop abruptly to the ground, landing on the sternum, and roll to its side. While lying down, the foal appears bright and alert, and the muscular tremors cease. The pupils are dilated, and there is decreased pupillary response to light. If the foal is assisted to stand after 30–60 min, the clinical signs recur. Standing time decreases as the disease progresses. Dysphagia is common with milk spilling from the mouth when nursing is attempted. The other clinical signs described above can also be seen in foals.

Diagnosis

A presumptive diagnosis of botulism is based on history and physical examination findings. The abrupt onset of diffuse, symmetrical weakness that gradually progresses to recumbency in 1–4 days with normal mentation and the presence of dysphagia and decreased tongue tone should put botulism at the top of the differential diagnosis list. A diagnosis of botulism is reached by excluding other diseases that cause profound muscular weakness, dysphagia or muscle fasciculations (**Table 2**). Diseases to rule-out include other neurological diseases (equine protozoal myeloencephalitis, equine motor neuron disease, equine herpesvirus 1 myeloencephalopathy, eastern and western equine encephalitis and rabies), white muscle disease, hyperkalaemic periodic paralysis (HYPP), electrolyte abnormalities, guttural pouch mycosis, leucoencephalomalacia, ionophore toxicosis, yew poisoning, white snake root poisoning, organochlorine toxicosis and pharyngeal ulcerations. A cerebrospinal fluid sample may be helpful in differentiating botulism from other central nervous system disorders. The absence of systemic signs of illness usually helps to rule-out sepsis and other generalised infectious diseases. Endoscopy of the upper airway and guttural pouches can rule-out pharyngeal ulcerations and guttural pouch mycosis. Signs of HYPP are episodic and often associated with increased serum potassium concentrations. Electrolyte abnormalities that result in weakness and muscle fasciculations include hypocalcaemia, hyponatraemia and hypokalaemia. Electromyography has been used to diagnose human botulism, but in horses it is not practical and some suggest it to be of minimal value.

Laboratory diagnosis of botulism is based on identification of preformed toxin in serum, feed, gastrointestinal contents or wounds, or *C. botulinum* spores in gastrointestinal contents or feed. Detection of an antibody response in a recovered patient will further support the diagnosis of botulism. The most sensitive test for detection of botulinum toxin is the mouse bioassay. Serum from an affected horse is administered via intraperitoneal injection into mice and the mice are monitored for clinical signs of botulism. If clinical signs of botulism develop additional mice are pretreated with polyvalent antitoxin and then injected with the serum. The presence of botulism toxin is confirmed if the antitoxin treated mice survive. Individual groups are treated with separate antitoxin specific to the different toxin types to determine the type of botulism that is present. The mouse bioassay is often negative because horses are extremely susceptible to botulinum toxin and the level of circulating toxin is below the threshold for detection. There are 2 additional tests that have been developed to determine the presence of specific types of botulinum toxin. An enzyme-linked immunosorbent assay was developed to determine the presence of Types C and D botulinum toxin and a polymerase chain reaction test for detection of the botulinum neurotoxin B gene (Szabo *et al.* 1994). Both tests have only been used in the research setting and may not be as specific as the mouse bioassay.

A diagnosis of botulism can be reached if spores are detected in the faeces or feed of horses showing clinical signs of botulism. Botulism spores have been detected in 70% of shaker foals but are rarely found in normal foals or adults (Whitlock and Buckley 1997). Gross and histopathological findings are often unremarkable. Samples must be sent to a specialised laboratory because selective media and culture procedures are required (e.g. Botulism Laboratory,

TABLE 2: Differential diagnoses for botulism based on common clinical signs

Dysphagia
- Pharyngeal ulcers, abscess
- Guttural pouch mycosis, infection, tympany
- Yellow star thistle
- White muscle disease
- Lead toxicity
- Rabies
- Tick paralysis
- Encephalitis, meningitis
- White snakeroot toxicity
- Mouldy corn poisoning (leucoencephalomalacia)

Weakness
- White muscle disease
- Electrolyte abnormalities
- Equine degenerative myeloencephalopathy
- Equine motor neuron disease
- Hyperkalaemic periodic paralysis
- Encephalitis, myelitis
- Equine protozoal myeloencephalitis
- Rabies
- West Nile virus
- Tick paralysis
- White snakeroot toxicity
- Heavy metal toxicity
- Equine herpes virus-1 myeloencephalopathy
- Mouldy corn poisoning (leucoencephalomalacia)
- Ionophore toxicity
- Yew toxicity

Muscle fasciculations
- Hyperkalaemic periodic paralysis
- Hypocalcaemia
- Organochlorine toxicity

New Bolton Center)[1]. If multiple samples are submitted there is a higher possibility of isolation of toxin or spores. Representative sampling should be done from various portions of the feed because toxins are not evenly distributed in feed. Samples should be handled appropriately because toxin is inactivated by environmental conditions. If necropsy is performed, liver tissue, gastrointestinal tract contents and/or faeces should be frozen and transported to the laboratory immediately. It is best to contact the laboratory for the appropriate protocol for handling and shipping of samples.

Treatment

The fundamental principle of treating botulism in horses is the neutralisation of circulating toxin with specific or multivalent antiserum. Botulism is generally fatal unless treated promptly with the antitoxin. Occasionally horses with mild, slowly progressive disease survive without receiving antitoxin. Prior to the availability of polyvalent antitoxin, the mortality rate was higher than 90% (Whitlock and Buckley 1997). If antitoxin is administered to adult horses with botulism before recumbency, the likelihood of survival approached 70% (Johnston and Whitlock 1987; Whitlock and Buckley 1997; Wilkins 2007). A polyvalent antitoxin can be obtained from the Botulism Laboratory[1] or a monovalent antitoxin for Types B and C is available from Veterinary Diagnostics[2]. Each product has a recommended foal and adult dose. In the author's experience one treatment is adequate. It is important to remember that clinical signs may progress for 12–24 h after antitoxin treatment because the antitoxin has no effect after the toxin has been internalised into the neuron. Therefore it is important that the antitoxin be administered early in the course of the disease.

In the case of wound botulism, tissue debridement of the wound and disruption of the anaerobic environment should be performed. Antimicrobial drugs may be used in cases of wound botulism and to treat secondary complications such as aspiration pneumonia. Types of antimicrobials that can be administered include cephalosporins, fluoroquinolones and sulphonamides. Antimicrobial drugs that potentate neuromuscular weakness, including aminoglycosides, tetracyclines and procaine penicillin, should be avoided (Whitlock 1996). Antimicrobial treatment does not eliminate the organism from the gastrointestinal tract and for this reason its use cannot be justified. Neostigmine and 4-aminopyridine have been used in human patients and animals to treat botulism because these compounds will increase acetylcholine release in the neuromuscular junction (NMJ). In horses, treatment with these compounds is not recommended because overall mortality is higher in horses treated with these compounds, as they exhaust the acetylcholine (ACH) that is present (Johnston and Whitlock 1987; Whitlock and Buckley 1997).

Another very important aspect of treatment is appropriate nursing care. Affected horses should be maintained in a quiet environment so that they can conserve energy. Since most horses cannot swallow, they should be muzzled to prevent aspiration of food or bedding. Hydration status can be maintained through oral or i.v. fluids. Periodically feeding a slurry through a nasogastric tube, or more effectively using i.v. nutrition, provides adequate nutrition. Foals can be fed mare's milk or milk replacer frequently (every 2 h) by an indwelling nasogastric tube. Mineral oil should be administered periodically to prevent constipation and impaction in horses with ileus. Manual evacuation of the rectum and catheterisation of the bladder are sometimes necessary. Recumbent horses and foals should be turned frequently to prevent decubital sores and hypostatic congestion of the lungs. Ocular lubricants are useful as some horses develop dry-eye and to help prevent corneal ulcers. Medication to prevent gastric ulcers may be warranted.

Approximately 50% of foals will require some form of ventilatory support, ranging from intranasal oxygen to mechanical ventilation (Wilkins 2007). Improvement in neuromuscular function is achieved in up to 10 days, which is the time required for regeneration of new end plates at the neuromuscular junction. Return to full strength may take up to one month (Whitlock and Buckley 1997). The more severe the weakness, the longer recovery takes. Dysphagic horses that are able to stand gradually regain the ability to swallow over 3–7 days, but sometimes it takes more than 2 weeks (Whitlock and Buckley 1997). Most adult horses are able to eat hay and swallow grain and water by 7–10 days following treatment with antitoxin (Whitlock and Buckley 1997). Horses that are recumbent and unable to rise

TABLE 3: Vaccination recommendations as per the AAEP

Adults
Initial series of 3 doses one month apart, then annual booster
Pregnant mares: initial series of 3 doses one month apart with the last one given 2–4 weeks prior to parturition, then annual booster 2–4 weeks prior to parturition.

Foals
Born to properly vaccinated mare: begin the series at age 8–10 weeks, give 3 doses one month apart, then booster annually.
Born to improperly vaccinated mare or no history of vaccination: begin series as early as age 2 weeks, give 3 doses one month apart, then booster annually.

Modified protocol in cases of an outbreak (nonvaccinated horses)
Initial series of 3 given 7–10 days apart, followed by additional dose one month after the last of the series of 3, then annual booster.

carry a grave prognosis for recovery. After 7–10 days of intensive nursing care, recumbent foals are usually able to stand (Vaala 1991). The most common complications of recumbency are aspiration pneumonia and decubital ulcers. The greater the amount of toxin present at the neuromuscular junction, the more rapidly progressive the clinical signs and the poorer the prognosis for survival.

Prevention

A vaccine against Type B botulism is available in North America (BotVax B)[3]. The vaccine is highly effective against Type B botulism, but infection with other serotypes can occur. Horses that reside in endemic areas should be vaccinated. The current AAEP recommendations are as shown in **Table 3**. Adults should be immunised with an initial series of 3 doses given one month apart, then one dose yearly. Pregnant mare should be vaccinated with an initial series of 3 doses one month apart with the last dose being administered 2–4 weeks prior to parturition. Then revaccinate annually with one dose 2–4 weeks prior to parturition. Foals from properly vaccinated mares are protected through colostral antibodies thus vaccination should begin at age 8–10 weeks. The foal should receive a series of 3 doses one month apart. Foals from nonimmunised mares should receive an initial series of 3 doses as early as 2 weeks following birth. In the case of an outbreak in nonimmunised horses, the protocol can be modified to allow for quicker protection. This protocol would include the initial 3 doses give 7–10 days apart followed by an additional dose one month after the last of the series of 3 doses. European researchers have developed an alternative recombinant vaccine for *Clostridium botulinum* Type C, which appears to stimulate an adequate neutralising antibody response, but further testing is warranted (Frey *et al.* 2007).

Additional preventative measures involve good husbandry. Grain and hay should be examined closely for parts of dead animals or decayed vegetation. Numerous reports worldwide have documented round bales as the source of botulinum toxin intoxication (Ricketts *et al.* 1984; Hunter *et al.* 2002). If round bales are fed, the should be properly processed and stored. Educate clients to protect hay stored outdoors by stacking it on palates or rubber tires to keep it off the ground. In addition hay stored outdoors should be covered not wrapped in plastic to protect it from rain and snow. Strict control of rodents and birds should be provided and surrounding premises should be clear of rotting carcasses and decaying vegetation.

Manufacturers' addresses

[1]University of Pennsylvania, Kennett Square, Pennsylvania, USA.
[2]Veterinary Diagnostics, Templeton, California, USA.
[3]Neogen Corporation, Lexington, Kentucky, USA.

References

Critchley, E.M.R. (1991) A comparison of human and animal botulism: a review. *J. R. Soc. Med.* **84**, 295-298.

Frey, J., Eberle, S., Stahl, C., Mazuet, C., Popoff, M., Schatzmann, M., Gerber, V., Dungu, B. and Straub, R. (2007) Alternate vaccination against equine botulism (BoNT/C). *Equine vet. J.* **39**, 516-520.

Galey, F.D. (2001) Botulism in horses. *Vet. Clin. N. Am.: Equine Pract.* **17**, 579-588.

Gupta, A., Sumner, C.J., Caster, M., Maslanka, S. and Sobel, J. (2005) Adult botulism type F in the United States, 1981-2002. *Neurology* **65**, 1694-1700.

Heath, S.E., Bell, R.J. and Harland R.J. (1988) Botulinum type C intoxication in a mare. *Can. vet. J.* **29**, 530-531.

Humeau, Y., Doussau, R., Grant, N.J. and Poulain, B. (2000) How botulinum and tetanus neurotoxins block neurotransmitter release. *Biochimie* **82**, 427-446.

Hunter, J.M., Rohrbach, B.W., Andrews, F.M. and Whitlock, R.H. (2002) Round bale grass hay: a risk factor for botulism in horses. *Compend.* **24**, 166-171.

Hutchins, R. (1994) Preliminary report on an out-break of botulism. *Aust. equine Vet.* **12**, 54-55.

Johnston, J. and Whitlock, R.H. (1987) Botulism. In: *Current Therapy in Equine Medicine 2*, Ed: N.E. Robinson, W.B. Saunders, Philadelphia. pp 367-370.

Kinde, H., Bettey, R.L., Ardans, A., Galey, F.D., Daft, B.M., Walker, R.L., Eklund, M.W. and Byrd, J.W. (1991) *Clostridium botulinum* type-C intoxication associated with consumption of processed alfalfa hay cubes in horses. *J. Am. vet. med. Ass.* **199**, 742-746.

MacKay, R.J. and Berkhoff, G.A. (1982) Type C toxicoinfectious botulism in a foal. *J. Am. vet. med. Ass.* **180**,163-164.

Mohanty, S., Dhawan, B. and Chaudhry, R. (2001) Botulism: an update. *Indian J. Med. Microbiol.* **19**, 35-43.

Ricketts, S.W., Greet, T.R.C., Glyn, P.J., Ginnett, C.D.R., McAllister, E.P., McCaig, J., Skinner, P.H., Webbon, P.M., Frape, D.L., Smith, G.R. and Murry, L.G. (1984) Thirteen cases of botulism in horses fed big bale silage. *Equine vet. J.* **16**, 515-518.

Swerczek, T.W. (1980a) Toxicoinfectious botulism in foals and adult horses. *J. Am. vet. med. Ass.* **176**, 217-220.

Swerczek, T.W. (1980b) Experimentally induced toxicoinfectious botulism in horses and foals. *Am. J. vet. Res.* **41**, 348-350.

Szabo, E.A., Pemberton, J.M., Gibson, A.M., Thomas, R.J., Pascoe, R.R. and Desmarchelier, P.M. (1994) Application of PCR to a clinical and environmental investigation of a case of equine botulism. *J. Clin. Micro.* **32**, 1986-1991.

Turton, K., Chaddock, J.A. and Acharya, K.R. (2002) Botulinum and tetanus neurotoxins: structure, function and therapeutic utility. *Trends Biochem Sci.* **27**, 552-558.

Vaala, W.E. (1991) Diagnosis and treatment of *Clostridium botulinum* infection in foals: a review of fifty-three cases. *Proceedings of the 9th Annual Meeting of the American College of Veterinary Internal Medicine* **9**, 379-381.

Whitlock, R.H. (1995) Botulism type C experimental and field cases in the horse. In: *Proceedings of the 13th Annual Meeting of the American College of Veterinary Internal Medicine* **13**, 720-723.

Whitlock, R.H. (1996) Botulism, type C experimental and field cases in horses. *Equine Pract.* **18**, 11-17.

Whitlock, R.H. and Buckley, C. (1997) Botulism. *Vet. Clin. N. Am.: Equine Pract.* **13**,107-128.

Wilkins, P.A. (2007) Botulism. In: *Equine Infectious Diseases*, Eds: D.C. Sellon and M.T. Long, Saunders Elsevier, St Louis. pp 372-376.

POTOMAC HORSE FEVER

J. Madigan*, B. Toth and N. Pusterla

The Department of Medicine and Epidemiology, School of Veterinary Medicine, University of California-Davis, California, USA.

Keywords: horse; EME; PHF; *Neorickettsia*; enterocolitis; abortion; laminitis

Summary

Neorickettsia risticii is the causative agent of Potomac horse fever (PHF) which may manifest as enterocolitis, laminitis and the so called '7 month abortion'. This rickettsial organism is found in nature in a complex life cycle involving trematodes, freshwater snails and aquatic insects. Horses become infected and part of the lifecycle when accidently consuming the infected adult insects, such as caddis flies, which harbour *N. risticii* in a metacercarial phase of a fluke. Leading clinical features include depression, anorexia, diarrhoea, fever, colic, dehydration, laminitis and abortion. Diagnosis is based on clinical signs and available real-time TaqMan PCR on blood and/or faeces. Treatment consists of antibiotics (tetracyclines) and in severely affected cases supportive therapy including i.v. polyionic fluids, anti-inflammatory medications, anti-endotoxic medications, gastroprotectants, analgesics, nutritional support and strategies for laminitis prevention. Prevention is the key in avoiding the disease and includes reduction of snail populations in adjacent creeks and ditches, drainage of ditches, application of insect traps and avoiding stable lights in endemic areas.

Introduction

Neorickettsia risticii (formerly *Ehrlichia risticii*) (Dumler *et al.* 2001) was first isolated from monocytes of a horse with a clinical diagnosis of colitis over 25 years ago (Knowles *et al.* 1983). Due to the extensive research on the organism, the natural hosts have been found, the life cycle has been determined and recently the mode of transmission has been experimentally reproduced. The purpose of this review is to provide an outline on the most recent developments of aetiology, epizootiology, pathogenesis and describe diagnostic methods, treatment and control measures for Potomac horse fever (PHF).

*Author to whom correspondence should be addressed. Professor Madigan's present address: UC Davis, VMTH, One Shields Ave Davis, California 95616, USA.

Epizootiology

Horses with clinical symptoms of fever, colic, and diarrhoea followed by laminitis were first recognised by veterinarians as being a distinct syndrome along the Potomac River in Maryland (Knowles *et al.* 1983). Blood transmission from an affected clinical case to a control horse reproduced the syndrome and eventually led to isolation of a rickettsial agent initially called *Ehrlichia risticii* and now renamed *Neorickettsia risticii*. *N. risticii* is the aetiological agent of PHF, also called equine monocytic ehrlichiosis (EME), equine ehrlichial colitis and Shasta River Crud. Genetic analysis has recently led to reclassification based on relatedness among three other species, which are *N. sennetsu* (human agent of Sennetsu fever), *N. helminthoeca* (agent of salmon poisoning in the dog) and an ehrlichia-like bacterium present in the metacercarial stage of the fluke *Stellantchasmus falcatus* (SF agent) (Dumler *et al.* 2001).

Neorickettsia risticii is a Gram-negative coccus that stains dark blue to purple with Giemsa and Romanowsky's stains but cannot be visualised on blood films in monocytes or other cells. The agent grows in cell culture but cannot be isolated in conventional bacterial media.

Following isolation of *N. risticii* from the blood of horses along the Potomac River, horses with similar clinical signs were believed to be suffering from PHF. Serological surveys of horses were conducted to determine antibodies to *N. risticii*. Based on the indirect fluorescence antibody (IFA) test PHF has been suggested to occur in 43 states of the USA, Canada, Europe (Netherlands, France and Italy),

Australia, South America (Uruguay, Brazil, Venezuela) and India. Later work showed that the indirect fluorescence antibody test IFA test produces over 30% false positives (Madigan *et al.* 1995). Using the criteria of isolation or detection of the causative agent from clinical cases of the disease using conventional cell culture or PCR assay narrows the geographic location of the disease to 14 states, Canada, Uruguay and Brazil to date. Antibody titres to *N. risticii* have been found in domestic and wild animals such as dogs, cats, coyotes, pigs and goats from endemic regions (Perry *et al.* 1989). Moreover a variety of mammalian species, such as mice, dogs, cats and cattle, have been shown to be susceptible to *N. risticii* (Dawson *et al.* 1988; Ristic *et al.* 1988; Pusterla *et al.* 2001).

Defining the epizootiology of *N. risticii* has been the subject of intensive research efforts for >25 years. Initially the organism was classified as an *Ehrlichia* and since all members of that species were believed to be tick transmitted, a long unrewarding hunt for the vector of PHF took place for 2 decades (Hahn *et al.* 1990). Evidence of the DNA homologies of the agent to members of the *Neorickettsia* group provided new fundamental information (Pretzman *et al.* 1995). Since PHF was reported in close proximity of freshwater streams, creeks, rivers and irrigated pastures mainly during midsummer to late summer (May to November) investigation of the role of freshwater snails in the epidemiology of PHF was begun. Development of reliable PCR tests for the detection of *N. risticii* DNA in materials from aquatic environments aided further discoveries. DNA evidence of *N. risticii* in operculate snails (*Pleuroceridae*: *Juga* spp.) of *N. risticii* was found as well as the determination that these snails also contained trematodes, which also tested positive for *N. risticii* DNA (Barlough *et al.* 1998; Reubel *et al.* 1998).

Based on *N. risticii* DNA sequence detection in blood, liver or spleen of bats and swallows, it is speculated that these insectivores may act as both definitive host of the helminth vector and natural reservoir of *N. risticii* (Chae *et al.* 2000; Pusterla *et al.* 2003; Gibson *et al.* 2005).

The means of natural transmission was investigated in several ways. *N. risticii* DNA found in nature was correlated with the clinical disease manifestations of PHF in horses. Horses injected subcutaneously with *N. risticii* PCR positive trematode stages collected from *Juga yrekaensis* snails, developed clinical signs of colic and diarrhoea and hematological changes consistent with PHF (Pusterla *et al.* 2001). Furthermore, *N. risticii* was transmitted to mice using PCR positive metacercariae isolated from caddis fly larvae (*Dicosmoecus* spp.) (Chae *et al.* 2000). The final proof of insect ingestion transmission came from collection of caddis fly larvae from the endemic areas for PHF, allowing hatching into mature flies and placing the flies in the feed of an experimental horse that 10 days later developed the full spectrum of clinical signs of PHF and related haematological changes (Madigan *et al.* 2003). Cell culture isolation, PCR detection, gene sequence identification and reinoculation of the isolate into additional horses produced the same syndrome, fulfilling Koch's postulates (Madigan *et al.* 2003). This work was repeated by others in a different geographic location, using caddis fly species and again confirmed the natural transmission by oral ingestion of insects harbouring *N. risticii* in metacercariae (Mott *et al.* 2002). It is concluded that aquatic insects, such as caddis flies and mayflies, represent a likely source of infection due to their abundance in the natural environment, their high infection rate with *N. risticii* determined by PCR, and the mass hatches regularly observed during summer-autumn. Under natural conditions, horses grazing near rivers/creeks will ingest adult insects along with grass (adults live near water and so are likely to die there) or consume adult insects trapped on the water surface, or possibly, those that are attracted by stable lights and subsequently accumulate in feed and water.

Pathogenesis

The organism can be reisolated from the peripheral blood monocytes 6–11 days after intravenous infection and ehrlichaemia may persist up to 1–2 weeks after clinical signs have abated (Mott *et al.* 2002). The organism has great affinity for blood monocytes and infects intestinal tissue macrophages especially those in the colon. It probably enters the macrophages and monocytes through the Fc receptors. The organism may persist for 1–2 months in the intestinal wall and up to 4 months in the pregnant mare-fetus system (Long *et al.* 1995a). Infected epithelial cells loose their microvilli, which leads to malabsorbtive diarrhoea and loss of $Na+$ and $Cl-$ into the intestinal lumen. Unlike other Gram-negative organisms, Rickettsial organisms do not possess the lipopolysaccharide cell wall component, as an important facilitator of the inflammatory cascade. Therefore the organism alone does not induce severe cytokine release except for IL-1 and TNFα, which may be the key of the pathogenesis of this disease (van Heckeeren *et al.* 1993). The organism can survive and multiply in the macrophages by inhibiting the production of reactive oxygen metabolites and by preventing phagosome-lysosome fusion (Williams and Timoney 1993).

Neorickettsia risticii also has fetotropic properties. Transplacental transmission of the agent may occur in pregnant mares and has been seen in natural and experimental infections (Long *et al.* 1995a,b). In mares experimentally infected at 90–120 days of gestation, abortion occurred at 65–111 days post inoculation (Long *et al.* 1995b). There are reports of pregnant mares developing clinical signs of PHF and subsequently aborting around 7 months of gestation, regardless of the severity of infection (Long *et al.* 1995a; Coffman *et al.* 2008).

Clinical findings

The incubation period for *N. risticii* infection is approximately 1–3 weeks. Naturally occurring cases of PHF are initially characterised by an acute onset of mild-moderate depression, anorexia, malaise and decreased borborygmi followed by a biphasic increase in body temperature ranging from 38.9–41.7°C (Dutta *et al.* 1998). Within 24–48 h, moderate to severe diarrhoea ranging from 'cowpat' to watery consistency develops in approximately 60% of affected horses. Mild colic signs are often concurrently present. Certain horses develop severe endotoxaemia, systemic inflammatory response syndrome (SIRS), which result in haemoconcentration, metabolic acidosis and cardiovascular compromise characterised by elevated heart rate and respiratory rate, congested mucous membranes and cold extremities. Subcutaneous oedema along the ventral abdomen may be observed due to colitis and resultant protein losing enteropathy. Laminitis is reported in 15–25% of affected cases. The associated laminitis may progress, despite resolution of other clinical signs. Interestingly, laminitis has only been reported in naturally infected horses and probably reflects as yet unknown pathophysiological mechanisms which are related exclusively to the natural route of transmission. PHF may present with all or any combination of the aforementioned clinical signs. Mortality rates vary from 5–30% and may depend on the strain involved and the host response. Long-term problems all appear to be mostly related to sequelae especially laminitis. Abortions are spontaneous with a fetus appearing in fresh condition. The organism may also induce resorption of the fetus (maceration, mummification, and petrification) or produce weak foals.

To date, no evidence exists that *N. risticii* infection results in chronic disease, and many attempts to isolate *N. risticii* by culture or PCR after clinical signs resolved, failed to be successful.

Haematological findings vary in the early stage of PHF and are not useful in making a definitive diagnosis. Findings vary from leucopenia (white blood cell count <5.0 x 10^9/l), characterised by a neutropenia with left shift and a lymphopenia, to a normal haemogram (Ziemer *et al.* 1987). Other cases of PHF develop leucocytosis (>14.0 x 10^9/l), which is normally observed within a few days of onset of the disease.

A transient nonregenerative anaemia and thrombocytopenia may develop. Increases in both packed cell volume and plasma protein concentration secondary to dehydration and haemoconcentration can occur. Electrolyte derangements may be seen secondary to diarrhoea and metabolic acidosis. Hypoproteinaemia may be present in chronic cases of diarrhoea attributable to the increased albumin loss. Azotaemia is often present and usually prerenal in origin however less frequently severe complicated cases, showing signs of DIC (disseminated intravascular coagulopathy) or MODS (multi organ dysfunction syndrome), may develop primary renal insult.

Diagnosis

Serology

A presumptive diagnosis of PHF often is based on the presence of typical clinical signs and the seasonal and geographical occurrence of the disease in an endemic area. A definitive diagnosis of PHF, however, should be based on the isolation or detection of *N. risticii* from the blood and/or the faeces of infected horses. Serological testing using the indirect fluorescent antibody or enzyme-linked immunosorbent assay test are of limited value as a diagnostic tool in a clinical case. Antibody levels to *N. risticii* have unpredictable patterns in individual horses at the time of onset of clinical disease. Antibodies may not reach detectable levels for some period of time after infection or conversely long incubations may allow the titre to peak at the time of initial presentation. Paired serum titres may not show 4-fold rises because the titre may be elevated at the time of initial presentation. While elevated single titres have been attempted to be used for diagnosis this should be considered unreliable as they may overlap with levels found in healthy horses with no evidence of disease. Additionally, the reliability of the indirect immunofluorescence technique for antibody detection has been questioned, since the test yields a high percentage of false-positive results and does not allow distinction between natural- and vaccine-derived antibody responses (Madigan *et al.* 1995). Isolation of the agent in cell culture from the peripheral blood of affected patients, though possible, can take from several days to weeks of culturing before detection is successful and is not routinely available in many diagnostic laboratories.

Polymerase chain reaction

The recent development of *N. risticii*-specific PCR assays has greatly facilitated the diagnosis of PHF (Biswas *et al.* 1991; Barlough *et al.* 1997). In experimentally and naturally infected animals, PCR performed on faeces and peripheral blood was more sensitive than was culture (Mott *et al.* 1997). Real-time PCR platforms associated with automated nucleic acid extraction allow the detection of *N. risticii* DNA within the same day of sample receipt, making this technology a much more feasible test for routine diagnostic examination (Pusterla *et al.* 2000a). To enhance the chances of detection of *N. risticii*, the assay should be performed on blood as well as on a fecal sample, since the presence of the organism in blood and feces may not necessarily coincide. PCR is also used in the detection of *N. risticii* DNA in fresh or formalin-fixed and paraffin-embedded colon tissue, allowing *post mortem* diagnosis.

Differential diagnosis should include any cause of enterocolitis, including salmonellosis, clostridial diarrhoea and parasitosis, intestinal ileus secondary to displacement or obstruction, and peritonitis. Diagnostic tests specific to ruling out these diseases should be concurrently pursued.

Treatment

Since rickettsial organisms are obligatory intracellular bacteria, antibiotics that penetrate through cell walls and reach high intracellular concentrations should be the drugs of choice. *N. risticii* is highly susceptible to tetracyclines including doxycycline, chlortetracycline and oxytetracycline. Macrolides also reach high concentrations in macrophages but are of limited value because of the high likelihood of exacerbating antibiotic induced colitis in adult horses. In most clinical settings, oxytetracycline is the easiest and safest choice. However one should be careful when administering it as a rapid i.v. injection as it may chelate ionised calcium in the blood and can manifest adverse reactions including collapse, seizure, asystolia and death. Enterally formulated oxytetracycline has been associated with individual case reports of serious or fatal antibiotic induced colitis. Other factors to be considered with the administration of tetracyclines include dose-dependent nephrotoxicity. Clinical experiences with severe cases of PHF suggest that many horses may remain azotaemic for several days despite aggressive fluid therapy. Administration of oxytetracycline is still recommended in the lowest effective dose after definitive diagnosis is established and primary renal origin of azotaemia is ruled out. Therefore prompt treatment of PHF cases with oxytetracycline 7 mg/kg bwt i.v. b.i.d. is imperative and can reduce the morbidity and mortality of the disease. Delay in treatment with oxytetracycline may lessen the therapeutic value of the antibiotic. The duration of therapy is suggested to be 5–7 days. Alternatively, doxycycline can be given orally at 10 mg/kg bwt b.i.d.

Supportive treatment as needed for enterocolitis cases may include i.v. polyionic fluids as dehydration occurs rapidly and fluid and electrolyte balance must be maintained. NSAIDs may be beneficial to diminish the effects of endotoxaemia, although one should be careful about using them for a prolonged time as they inhibit PGE2 mediated mucosal repair mechanisms and also may aggravate azotemia. Analgesics (α2-agonists, opioids) and spasmolytics (butyl-scopolamine) may be used to reduce pain associated with colonic inflammation and increased abdominal pressure. Anti-endotoxic medications (Polymyxin-B, J5-plasma) are advantageous in patients suffering from the effects of endotoxaemia. Gastro- and entero-protectants (omeprazole, sucralfate, misoprostol) are recommended in animals exhibiting anorexia and diarrhoea. Nutritional support is usually not indicated other than for patients showing profound anorexia and depression for more than 24–48 h. Gastrointestinal absorbents have been suggested to be useful for toxin absorption and for decreasing enteral fluid losses. Prevention strategies for laminitis are also indicated and should include measures to alleviate signs of SIRS, to decrease enzymatic activity in the laminae (cryotherapy) and to provide deep, soft bedding. One should be aware of that laminitis may progress, despite the resolution of other clinical signs.

Prevention

Aquatic insects, such as caddis flies and mayflies, represent a likely source of infection due to their abundance in the natural environment, their high infection rate with *N. risticii* determined by PCR and the mass hatches regularly observed during summer-autumn. Under natural conditions, horses grazing near rivers/creeks will ingest adult insects along with grass or consume adult insects trapped on the water surface, or possibly, those that are attracted by stable lights and subsequently accumulate in feed and water. Therefore in local environments where PHF is a problem, consideration can be given to methods to reduce snail numbers in adjacent creeks, ditches or other bodies of water. Mayfly hatch alert systems or horse owners could decrease the risk by keeping the light off for the critical periods of the night or there may be alternative types of lights in which the polarity or frequency of light is less attractive to the mayfly species (Wilson *et al.* 2006).

The question of whether vaccination protects against the naturally occurring disease is unknown. Horses have only been challenged by the intravenous route following immunisation with available vaccines and not by the oral route. Additionally, the presence of antibodies does not always correlate with clearance of Neorickettsial organisms and presence of protective immunity. This has been shown with horses that have been vaccinated with a killed *N. risticii* vaccine and subsequently developed clinical disease after natural exposure (Dutta *et al.* 1998). Antibodies induced by a killed vaccine may not be effective, because protective antigens may only be expressed during cell invasion or replication. It is likely that cell-mediated immunity plays a dominant role in protecting the host from *N. risticii* infection as shown for other rickettsial infections. However, animals recovered from experimental infection have been reported to be resistant to reinfection or relapse for at least 20 months (Palmer *et al.* 1990). It is the subjective impression of the authors that vaccinated horses, although still susceptible to the disease, display a lesser form of disease than unvaccinated animals. In particular, the severe complication of laminitis is often not seen in previously vaccinated animals. The routine use of vaccine has been anecdotally reported to lessen the clinical signs and prevent the complications of PHF (Wilson *et al.* 2006). Until new vaccines become available, more strategic vaccination to target peak antibody production in horses with the highest likelihood of exposure to *N. risticii* may be the most useful tool for reducing disease mortality in endemic areas (Wilson *et al.* 2006).

References

Barlough, J.E., Rikihisa, Y. and Madigan, J.E. (1997) Nested polymerase chain reaction for detection of *Ehrlichia risticii* genomic DNA in infected horses. *Vet. Parasitol.* **68**, 367.

Barlough, J.E., Reubel, G.H., Madigan, J.E., Vredevoe, L.K., Miller, P.E. and Rikihisa, Y. (1998) Detection of *Ehrlichia risticii*, the agent of Potomac horse fever, in freshwater stream snails (*Pleuroceridae*: *Juga* spp.) from northern California. *Appl. Environ. Microbiol.* **64**, 2888.

Biswas, B., Mukherjee, D., Mattingly-Napier, B.L. and Dutta, S.K. (1991) Diagnostic application of polymerase chain reaction for detection of *Ehrlichia risticii* in equine monocytic ehrlichiosis (Potomac horse fever). *J. clin. Microbiol.* **29**, 2228.

Chae, J.S., Pusterla, N., Johnson, E., Derock, E., Lawler, S.P. and Madigan, J.E. (2000) Infection of aquatic insects with trematode metacercariae carrying *Ehrlichia risticii*, the cause of Potomac horse fever. *J. med. Entomol.* **37**, 619-625.

Coffman, E.A., Abd-Eldaim, M. and Craig, L.E. (2008) Abortion in a horse following *Neorickettsia risticii* infection. *J. vet. diagn. Invest.* **20**, 827-830.

Dawson, J.E., Abeygunawardena, I., Holland, C.J., Buese, M.M., and Ristic, M. (1988) Susceptibility of cats to infection with *Ehrlichia risticii*, causative agent of equine monocytic ehrlichiosis. *Am. J. vet. Res.* **49**, 2096-2100.

Dumler, J.S., Barbet, A.F., Bekker, C.P., Dasch, G.A., Palmer, G.H., Ray, S.C., Rikihisa, Y. and Rurangirwa, F.R. (2001) Reorganization of genera in the families *Rickettsiaceae* and *Anaplasmataceae* in the order *Rickettsiales*: unification of some species of *Ehrlichia* with *Anaplasma*, *Cowdria* with *Ehrlichia* and *Ehrlichia* with *Neorickettsia*, descriptions of six new species combinations and designation of *Ehrlichia equi* and 'HGE agent' as subjective synonyms of *Ehrlichia phagocytophila. Int. J. syst. evol. Microbiol.* **51**, 2145-2165.

Dutta, S.K., Vemulapalli, R. and Biswas, B. (1998) Association of deficiency in antibody response to vaccine and heterogeneity of *Ehrlichia risticii* strains with Potomac horse fever vaccine failure in horses. *J. clin. Microbiol.* **36**, 506.

Gibson, K.E., Rikihisa, Y., Zhang, C. and Martin, C. (2005) *Neorickettsia risticii* is vertically transmitted in the trematode *Acanthatrium oregonense* and horizontally transmitted to bats. *Environ. Microbiol.* **7**, 203.

Hahn, N.E., Fletcher, M., Rice, R.M., Kocan, K.M., Hansen, J.W., Hair, J.A., Barker, R.W. and Perry, B.D. (1990) Attempted transmission of *Ehrlichia risticii*, causative agent of Potomac horse fever, by the ticks, *Dermacentor variabilis, Rhipicephalus sanguineus, Ixodes scapularis* and *Amblyomma americanum. Exp. appl. Acarol.* **8**, 41-50.

Knowles, R.C., Anderson, C.W., Shipley, W.D., Whitlock, R.H., Perry, B.D. and Davidson, J.P. (1983) Acute equine diarrhea syndrome (AEDS): a preliminary report. *Proc. Am. Ass. equine Practnrs.* **29**, 353.

Long, M.T., Goetz, T.E., Whiteley, H.E., Kakoma, I. and Lock, T.E. (1995a) Identification of *Ehrlichia risticii* as the causative agent of two equine abortions following natural maternal infection. *J. vet. Diagn. Invest.* **7**, 201-205.

Long, M.T., Goetz, T.E., Kakoma, I., Whiteley, H.E., Lock, T.E., Holland, C.J., Foreman, J.H. and Baker, G.J. (1995b) Evaluation of fetal infection and abortion in pregnant ponies experimentally infected with *Ehrlichia risticii. Am. J. vet. Res.* **56**, 1307-1316.

Madigan, J.E., Rikihisa, Y., Palmer, J.E., DeRock, E. and Mott, J. (1995) Evidence for a high rate of false-positive results with the indirect fluorescent antibody test for *Ehrlichia risticii* antibody in horses. *J. Am. vet. med. Ass.* **207**, 1448-1453.

Madigan, J.E., Pusterla, N., Johnson, E., Chae, J.S., Pusterla, J.B., Derock, E. and Lawler, S.P. (2000) Transmission of *Ehrlichia risticii*, the agent of Potomac horse fever, using naturally infected aquatic insects and helminth vectors: preliminary report. *Equine vet. J.* **32**, 275-279.

Mott, J., Rikihisa, Y., Zhang, Y., Reed, S.M. and Yu, C.Y. (1997) Comparison of PCR and culture to the indirect fluorescent-antibody test for diagnosis of Potomac horse fever. *J. clin. Microbiol.* **35**, 2215-2219.

Mott, J., Muramatsu, Y., Seaton, E., Martin, C., Reed, S. and Rikihisa, Y. (2002) Molecular analysis of *Neorickettsia risticii* in adult aquatic insects in Pennsylvania, in horses infected by ingestion of insects, and isolated in cell culture. *J. clin. Microbiol.* **40**, 690-693.

Palmer, J.E., Benson, C.E. and Whitlock, R.H. (1990) Resistance to Development to equine ehrichial colitis in experimentally inoculated horses and ponies. *Am. J. vet. Res.* **51**, 763-765.

Perry, B.D., Schmidtmann, E.T., Rice, R.M., Hansen, J.W., Fletcher, M., Turner, E.C., Robl, M.G. and Hahn, N.E. (1989) Epidemiology of Potomac horse fever: an investigation into the possible role of non-equine mammals. *Vet. Rec.* **125**, 83-86.

Pretzman, C., Ralph, D., Stothard, D.R., Fuerst, P.A. and Rikihisa, Y. (1995) 16S RNA sequence of *Neorickettsial helminthoeca* and the its phylogenetic alignment with members of the genus *Ehrlichia. Int. J. Syst. Bacteriol* **45**, 207-211.

Pusterla, N., Leutenegger, C.M., Sigrist, B., Chae, J.S., Lutz, H. and Madigan, J.E. (2000a) Detection and quantitation of *Ehrlichia risticii* genomic DNA by real-time PCR in infected horses and snails. *Vet. Parasitol.* **90**, 129-135.

Pusterla, N., Madigan, J.E., Chae, J.S., DeRock, E., Johnson, E., and Pusterla, J.B. (2000b) Helminthic transmission and isolation of *Ehrlichia risticii*, the causative agent of Potomac horse fever, by using trematode stages from freshwater stream snails. *J. clin. Microbiol.* **38**,1293-1297.

Pusterla, N., Berger, Pusterla, J., DeRock, E. and Madigan, J.E. (2001) Susceptibility of cattle to *Ehrlichia risticii*, the causative agent of Potomac horse fever. *Vet. Rec.* **148**, 86-87.

Pusterla, N., Johnson, E.M., Chae, J.S. and Madigan, J.E. (2003) Digenetic trematodes, *Acanthatrium* sp. and *Lecithodendrium* sp., as vectors of *Neorickettsia risticii*, the agent of Potomac horse fever. *J. Helminthol.* **77**, 335-339.

Reubel, G.H., Barlough, J.E., Madigan, J.E. (1998) Production and characterization of *Ehrlichia risticii*, the agent of Potomac horse fever, from snails (*Pleuroceridae*: *Juga* spp.) in aquarium culture and genetic comparison to equine strains. *J. clin. Microbiol.* **36**, 1501-1511.

Ristic, M., Dawson, J., Holland, C.J. and Jenny, A. (1988) Susceptibility of dogs to infection with *Ehrlichia risticii*, causative agent of equine monocytic ehrlichiosis (Potomac horse fever). *Am. J. vet. Res.* **49**, 1497-1500.

van Heckeeren, A., Rikihisa, Y., Park, J. and Fertel, R. (1993) Tumor necrosis factor-α interleukin 1α and prostaglandin E2 production in murine peritoneal macrophages infected with *Ehrlichia risticii. Infect. Immun.* **61**, 4333.

Williams, N.M. and Timoney, P.J. (1993) *In vitro* killing of *Ehrlichia risticii* by activated and immune-mouse peritioneal macrophages. *Infect. Immun.* **61**, 861-867.

Wilson, J.H., Pusterla, N., Bengfort, J.M. and Arney, L. (2006) Incrimination of mayflies as a vector of Potomac horse fever in an outbreak in minnesota. *Proc. Am. Ass. equine Practnrs.* **52**, 53-56.

Ziemer, E.L., Whitlock, R.H., Palmer, J.E. and Spencer, P.A. (1987) Clinical and hematologic variables in ponies with experimentally induced equine ehrlichial colitis (Potomac horse fever). *Am. J. vet. Res.* **48**, 63.

EQUINE PROTOZOAL MYELOENCEPHALITIS

L. H. Javsicas* and R. J. MacKay

University of Florida College of Veterinary Medicine, Large Animal Clinical Sciences, PO Box 100136, Gainesville, Florida 32610-0136, USA.

Keywords: horse; internal medicine; neurology; equine protozoal myeloencephalopathy; *Sarcocystis neurona*

Summary

Equine protozoal myeloencephalitis (EPM) is a common infectious neurological disease of horses. Endemic EPM occurs primarily in North and South America and is caused by the apicomplexan protozoan *Sarcocystis neurona*. *Neospora hughesi* causes a rare sporadic form of EPM. The life cycle of *S. neurona* involves reciprocal passage between an opossum definitive host (*Didelphis* spp.) and an intermediate host. Horses with EPM most commonly have abnormalities of gait, but also may present with signs of brain disease. The disease ranges in severity from mild lameness to sudden recumbency, and clinical signs are usually progressive. Current treatments available for EPM include the folate inhibitor sulphadiazine/pyrimethamine, the triazinetrione ponazuril, and the nitrothiazole nitazoxanide. On the basis of published results of clinical efficacy studies, it is reasonable to expect that about 60% of horses with moderate to severe EPM will improve after treatment with any of the approved medications, with 10–20% recovering completely.

Aetiology and pathogenesis

Sarcocystis neurona is the most common aetiological agent of equine protozoal myeloencephalitis (EPM), with sporadic cases caused by *Neospora hughesi* (Marsh *et al.* 1996a, 1998, 1999; Hamir *et al.* 1998; Dubey *et al.* 2001a; Finno *et al.* 2007a). We will use EPM to refer to disease caused by *S. neurona* except where noted.

Life cycle

Species of *Sarcocystis* have an obligatory predator-prey 2-host life cycle (Dubey *et al.* 2001b). Sexual reproduction occurs in the definitive host, the opossum (*Didelphis virginiana* and *D. albiventris*; Fenger *et al.* 1995), while asexual reproduction occurs in the intermediate host. Several intermediate hosts including the 9-banded armadillo (*Dasypus novemcinctus*), the striped skunk (*Mephitis mephitis*) and the raccoon (*Prylon locor*), and a variety of incidental hosts have been identified (Cheadle *et al.* 2001a,b; Dubey *et al.* 2001c). Their combined geographic range includes the areas where EPM occurs most commonly. The domestic cat (*Felis catus*) also can support the life cycle in a laboratory setting but it is not clear whether cats are important hosts in nature. The hosts for *N. hughesi* are not known.

Sarcocysts of *S. neurona* are usually embedded in striated muscle of the intermediate host. The sarcocyst is the only developmental stage that is infectious for the definitive host. Ingestion of sarcocysts by the flesh-eating opossum results in invasion of the small intestinal epithelium of the opossum and sexual proliferation and differentiation to produce oocysts. Each oocyst contains 2 sporocysts that usually are released from the thin-walled oocysts before they are passed with faeces. Sporocysts are immediately infectious for the intermediate host. They are quite persistent in the environment and may survive for months, even during extremes of heat and cold (Dubey *et al.* 1991). Intermediate hosts are infected by ingestion of food or water contaminated with sporocysts. Although *S. neurona* muscle sarcocysts were identified in one 4-month-old filly (Mullaney *et al.* 2005), only precystic stages (merozoites and schizonts) have been found in the central nervous system (CNS) of horses with EPM (**Fig 1**) and it is assumed that the horse is most often an aberrant dead-end host for *S. neurona*.

*Author to whom correspondence should be addressed. Present address: Upstate Equine Medical Center, 362 Rugg Road, Schuylerville, New York 12871, USA.

Pathogenesis

The pathophysiology and immunology of *S. neurona* infection in horses is not completely understood. Horses ingest the infective sporocyst stage of *S. neurona* in food and water that has been contaminated by opossum faeces. Following experimental infection of ponies with extremely large numbers of *S. neurona* sporocysts, the parasite was isolated from mesenteric lymph nodes by one day, liver by 2 days, and lung by 5 days post infection, suggesting rapid lymphatic and haematogenous spread (Elitsur *et al.* 2007). The mechanism of entry of *S. neurona* into the CNS of the horse is unknown but may be via blood mononuclear cells (Lindsay *et al.* 2006). Once in the CNS, *S. neurona* can localise and replicate in any region, from cerebrum to spinal cord. Peripheral nerves and nerve roots are not infected. The location and extent of the lesions determine the character and severity of clinical signs. Histologically, protozoa are usually associated with mixed inflammatory cellular responses and neuronal destruction. Schizonts, in various stages of maturation, or free merozoites are seen commonly in the cytoplasm of neurons or mononuclear phagocytes and rarely in other inflammatory or CNS cells (**Fig 1**).

Both cellular and humoural immune responses are thought to be important for control of infection by *S. neurona*. Horses seroconvert within 32 days after experimental infection (Cutler *et al.* 2001), and more rapidly if they are first stressed by transport (Saville *et al.* 2001). Antibodies directed against cell surface proteins of *S. neurona* have been shown to prevent penetration of cells by the parasite *in vitro* (Liang *et al.* 1998). However, it is not known if such antibodies are protective against parasitic invasion of the CNS *in vivo*. Because of the intracellular location of the parasite, competent cell-mediated adaptive immune responses are considered essential for its elimination. Murine models of EPM have shown CD8+ T lymphocytes (cytotoxic T lymphocytes) and interferon gamma to be critical for protection against *S. neurona* encephalitis and elimination of the parasite (Dubey *et al.* 1998; Witonsky *et al.* 2005).

Epidemiology

Equine protozoal myeloencephalitis is considered a disease of horses that have spent time in North or South America. There are isolated reports of horses diagnosed with EPM elsewhere that have no travel history to the Americas and the nature of infection in these cases remains unclear (Goehring and Sloet van Oldruitenborgh-Oosterbaan 2001; Pitel *et al.* 2002). Horses of all breeds can be affected by EPM and there is no gender bias. Some studies suggest that Thoroughbreds and Standardbreds are over-represented (Fayer *et al.* 1990). The age of onset of reported cases ranges from 2 months (Gray *et al.* 2001) to 24 years (MacKay *et al.* 1992), with an average age around 4 years (Mayhew *et al.* 1977). Horses aged >2 years are at an increased risk of developing EPM in some studies (Duarte *et al.* 2004a; Cohen *et al.* 2007), while another study identified an increased risk in horses aged 1–4 years and horses aged >14 years (Saville *et al.* 2000). Equine protozoal myeloencephalitis typically occurs sporadically as individual cases, but clusters of cases have occasionally been reported (Granstrom *et al.* 1992; Fenger *et al.* 1997).

The seroprevalence of *S. neurona* infection as evidenced by *S. neurona* antibodies in horses in various locations throughout the USA varies from 10–60% (Bentz *et al.* 2003; Blythe *et al.* 1997; Rossano *et al.* 2001; Saville *et al.* 1997). The geographic variation in prevalence is accounted for by the range of the definitive host, the opossum. Less information is available for *N. hughesi*. Reported seroprevalence of antibodies to *N. hughesi* is 37% in California, 20% in Montana and 5% in New Zealand (Vardeleon *et al.*

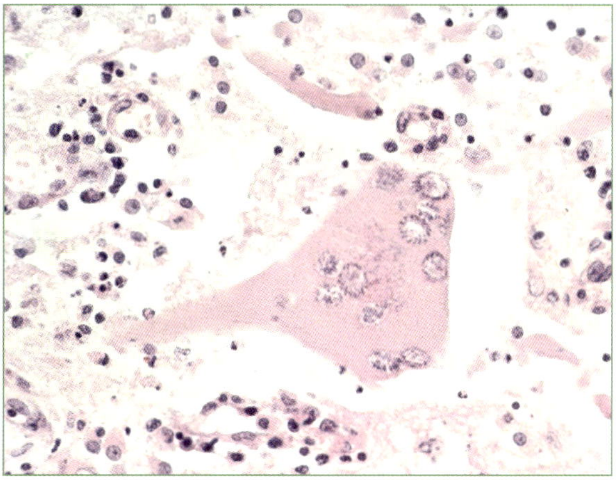

FIGURE 1: Sarcocystis neurona schizonts in a neuronal cell body from a horse with EPM. Note the radial arrangement or the individual merozoites comprising each.

2001). The seroprevalence of antibodies to either *S. neurona* or *N. hughesi* has been shown to increase with age (Duarte *et al.* 2004a). Although there is a high rate of infection by *S. neurona*, only a small percentage of exposed horses develop clinical disease, suggesting clearance of the organism by the immune system in most cases (Dubey *et al.* 2001b). There is an annual incidence of EPM of 0.14% in US horses not used for racing based on owner-reported information (Anon 1998). The factors that influence the relationship between infection with *S. neurona* and development of neurological disease are not fully understood. Genetic variability in *S. neurona* surface antigens (SnSAGs) among different strains has recently been shown (Crowdus *et al.* 2008; Howe *et al.* 2008). Such polymorphisms may result in differences among strains in pathogenicity and immunogenicity for horses (Crowdus *et al.* 2008). Further work is needed in this area because variability in SnSAGs may affect sensitivity of antigen-based diagnostic tests as well as pathogenicity.

Results of risk factor analysis for EPM vary by study, but factors likely to increase exposure to opossums, their environment and their faeces are consistently identified. Other risk factors include previous diagnosis of EPM on the premises, primary use of the horse, with show horses and race horses at increased risk, recent transport, and recent adverse health events, including medical problems, parturition, and management changes. This suggests that physiological stress may play an important role in the onset of EPM (Saville *et al.* 2000; Cohen *et al.* 2007; Morley *et al.* 2008).

Diagnosis

Definitive *ante mortem* diagnosis of EPM remains challenging. Criteria for diagnosis include finding clinical signs consistent with EPM, ruling out other differential diagnoses, and confirming the presence of *S. neurona*-specific antibodies through immunodiagnostic testing (Furr *et al.* 2002; Furr 2008). Proof of diagnosis *post mortem* is demonstration of protozoa in CNS lesions, often done with immunohistochemical staining. Even when the organism is not seen, the diagnosis frequently is made presumptively if characteristic inflammatory changes are found (Fayer *et al.* 1990).

Immunodiagnostic testing

Interpretation of immunodiagnostic testing for EPM is based partly on the premise that the presence of *S. neurona*-specific antibodies in serum indicates exposure to the parasite but does not confirm infection of the CNS, while presence of antibodies in CSF indicates local antibody production in the CNS due to active infection, since no antibodies should cross the blood-brain barrier. Unfortunately, it has become clear that there is some movement of antibodies into the CSF in healthy animals, resulting in false-positive results and making the

TABLE 1: Summary of commercially available diagnostic tests for EPM. Modified from Furr (2008)

Test type	Source	Test principle	Sensitivity/specificity (%)	Comments
WB	EBI[5]	Detects the presence of antibodies to surface proteins.	89/90 (Furr *et al.* 2002)	Nonquantitative test
WB (modified)	Michigan State[2]	Detects the presence of antibodies to surface proteins after blocking with *Sarcocystis cruzi* antibodies.	100/98 (Rossano *et al.* 2000)	Nonquantitative test
WB	Neogen[1]	Detects the presence of antibodies to surface proteins.	86–69 (Duarte *et al.* 2003)	Semiquantitative report (RQ) provided
IFAT	University of California-Davis[6]	Detects the presence of antibodies to surface proteins.	89/100	Quantitative method
SAG-1 ELISA	Antech[3]	Detects the presence of antibodies to a single *Sarcocystis neurona* surface protein.	Not reported	Quantitative

WB = western blot; RQ = relative quotient; IFAT = indirect fluorescent antibody test; SAG-1 ELISA = surface antigen-1 enzyme-linked immunosorbent assay.

interpretation of CSF antibody tests difficult (Furr 2008). **Table 1** provides a summary of currently available diagnostic tests.

Western blot (WB), the traditional diagnostic test for EPM, detects the presence of *S. neurona*-specific antibodies in serum or CSF. A positive serum result indicates previous or current infection by *S. neurona*. Initial evaluation of the serum WB from horses with neurological signs and histologically-confirmed lesions showed a sensitivity for diagnosis of EPM of 91% but specificity of only 70% (Granstrom 1995). Results of a more recent study using immunohistochemical staining of organisms in the CNS as the gold standard for diagnosis of EPM showed a sensitivity of 88% and specificity of only 38% in horses with neurological signs (Daft *et al.* 2002). On the basis of these results, a negative serum test is useful to help rule out EPM (i.e., false-negative results are uncommon) but has little value in confirming the disease (false-positive results are very common).

Compared to the serum test, WB testing of undiluted CSF has a better specificity for EPM in some studies, with a reported specificity and sensitivity of 89% (Granstrom 1997). When compared to immunohistochemical staining of *post mortem* CNS samples as the gold standard for diagnosis of EPM, CSF WB had a sensitivity and specificity of 87% and 44% respectively, in horses with neurological signs, and 88% and 60% respectively, in horses without neurological signs (Daft *et al.* 2002). There are numerous causes of contamination of the CSF by plasma *S. neurona* antibodies. Plasma proteins may enter CSF: 1) by accidental blood contamination during CSF collection; 2) as a result of disruption of the blood-CNS barrier (e.g. West Nile encephalomyelitis, trauma); or 3) by 'leakage' of antibody across normal blood-CNS barrier in horses with high serum titre of *S. neurona* IgG. It has been shown that very low-level contamination of CSF with blood (equivalent to 10 RBC/μl) can turn a sample positive (Miller *et al.* 1999). Any sample that has a RBC count >50/μl should therefore not be submitted. Notwithstanding the problems outlined above, the CSF WB, when used in horses that do have abnormal neurological signs, appears to correlate well with *S. neurona* infection of the CNS (Furr *et al.* 2002). Because the significance of positive CSF WB in clinically normal horses is unclear, the WB should not be used as a screening test in neurologically normal horses.

Modifications of the WB have been developed in attempts to improve specificity or quantify the *S. neurona* antibody. Identifying the fraction of *S. neurona* antibody that is CNS-derived, rather than plasma-derived, would improve the specificity of tests that rely on the presence of antibody in the CSF. An *S. neurona* antibody index (AI) for paired CSF and plasma samples has recently been reported (Heskett and MacKay 2008). The AI is calculated by using an enzyme-linked immunosorbent assay (ELISA) to quantify *S. neurona*-specific IgG in plasma and CSF. The AI relates *S. neurona*-specific IgG titre to total IgG concentration. Therefore, the AI should not be affected by movement of specific antibody into the CSF as a result of passive diffusion across an intact blood-CSF barrier, leakage across a porous barrier, or blood contamination during sample collection. Following experimental inoculation of horses with sporocysts, the AI did not change, suggesting that *S. neurona*-specific IgG in the CSF was of systemic origin (Heskett and MacKay 2008). This raises the possibility that experimental inoculation of horses with *S. neurona* does not reliably result in CNS infection but the results do support a role for AI calculation in interpreting WB results. Further investigation is required to determine the value of AI in the diagnosis of naturally occurring EPM.

A test routinely performed by one commercial diagnostic laboratory (Neogen)[1] is the relative quantity CSF (RQ). This test semi-quantifies the amount of CSF antibody directed against a 17 kDa antigen on *S. neurona*. Values range from 0–100, with higher values within this range considered more supportive of a diagnosis of EPM than are lower values. Another laboratory (Michigan State)[2] has modified the WB by blocking reaction to *S. cruzi*, which they consider to be a cross-reacting antigen (Rossano *et al.* 2000). Evaluation of the test in 6 horses with EPM found a specificity of 100% and sensitivity of 98% (Rossano *et al.* 2000), but further investigation in a larger number of horses found a sensitivity and specificity of 89 and 69%, respectively (Duarte *et al.* 2003).

An indirect fluorescent antibody test (IFAT) for detection of *S. neurona*-specific antibodies has been developed and tested in naturally and experimentally infected horses (Duarte *et al.* 2004b, 2006). When tested against a small panel of 'gold standard' samples from EPM-negative and -positive horses, a sensitivity of 83.3% and specificity of 96.9% was reported for IFAT testing of serum and 100% and 99% for CSF (Duarte *et al.* 2003, 2004b). A serum titre >1:100 and a CSF titre >1:5 are considered positive. The superiority of this test compared to WB has been questioned (Furr 2008) and further work is needed since the IFAT is unable to differentiate between antibodies against *S. neurona* and *S. fayeri* (a nonpathogenic species; Saville *et al.* 2004). A comparative study of available diagnostic tests is needed, although the lack of a gold standard for diagnosis in horses that are not subjected to necropsy makes this challenging. An IFAT for *N. hughesi* is available commercially and has been shown to be able to differentiate experimentally infected from noninfected horses using a serum cut-off of 1:640 (Packham *et al.* 2002). Cerebrospinal fluid IFAT results for *S. neurona* and *N. hughesi* have been shown to be reliable in the face of blood contamination up to 10,000 RBC/µl (Finno *et al.* 2007b).

An ELISA test for antibodies to the *S. neurona* surface antigen SnSAG-1 is commercially available (Antech[3]; Ellison *et al.* 2003). A serum titre >1:100 is considered indicative of active infection EPM (Ellison *et al.* 2003). Concerns have been expressed about the accuracy of this test (Furr 2008) because the cut-off value is arbitrary and the test has apparently not been evaluated in clinical cases for sensitivity and specificity. Furthermore, SnSAG-1 is not found in all *S. neurona* isolates (Hyun *et al.* 2003), creating the potential for false-negative results (Furr 2008; Hoane *et al.* 2005).

Polymerase chain reaction

Polymerase chain reaction testing of CSF has a high specificity but a very low sensitivity for the diagnosis of EPM (Fenger *et al.* 1994; Marsh *et al.* 1996). False-negatives are common because free parasitic DNA is destroyed by enzymes in the CSF and merozoites rarely enter the CSF (Fenger *et al.* 1994; Marsh *et al.* 1996a). Testing by PCR of tissue samples may be helpful for *post mortem* diagnosis (Pusterla *et al.* 2006).

Ancillary aids to diagnosis

Ancillary procedures, including survey cervical radiographs, lameness examination and serology, may be required to rule out competing differential diagnoses. In horses with signs of brain involvement, suggestive lesions may be seen with advanced imaging techniques (**Fig 2**; Javsicas *et al.* 2008). Consistent abnormalities are not found in complete and differential white blood cell counts and serum chemistry values in horses with EPM. Abnormal CSF values occur in some horses with EPM. It has been reported that as many as 35% of horses at a referral hospital have increased protein concentration (>65 mg/dl) or nucleated cell count (>7 cells/µl) (Reed *et al.* 1994). In the authors' experience, in horses with mild clinical signs of EPM (i.e. those that typically are encountered in practice), a very low percentage have any abnormality on routine CSF analysis. Creatine kinase (CK) activity may be high in CSF, reflecting diffusion of the BB isoenzyme from damaged CNS gray matter (Furr and Tyler 1990). Unfortunately, inadvertent inclusion of a small plug of epidural fat or dura during CSF collection can dramatically elevate CK activity, thus reducing the specificity of the test (Jackson *et al.* 1995).

Clinical signs

Protozoa may infect any part of the CNS, making almost any neurological sign possible. The disease usually begins insidiously but also may present acutely and be severe at onset. Signs of spinal cord involvement are seen much more commonly than signs of brain disease. Horses with EPM involving the spinal cord have asymmetric or symmetric truncal and limb weakness and ataxia (**Fig 3**). If all lesions are behind the second thoracic spinal cord segment (T2), only the pelvic limbs are affected. If a lesion (or lesions) is located in front of T3, all 4 limbs may be affected. Rarely, when the spinal cord behind the second sacral spinal cord segment (S2) is involved, there are signs of *cauda equina* syndrome, which may include degrees of rectal, anal, bladder and penile paralysis, and hypalgesia of the skin of the tail and perineum. If gray matter of the ventral horn of the spinal cord is damaged for more than 1–2 weeks, there may be obvious muscle atrophy (**Fig 4**) (usually asymmetric) and electromyographic changes in denervated muscle. Common locations for atrophy in horses with EPM are the gluteal, *biceps femoris*, *infraspinatus/supraspinatus* and *serratus ventralis* muscles. Lesions in the spinal cord also may result in

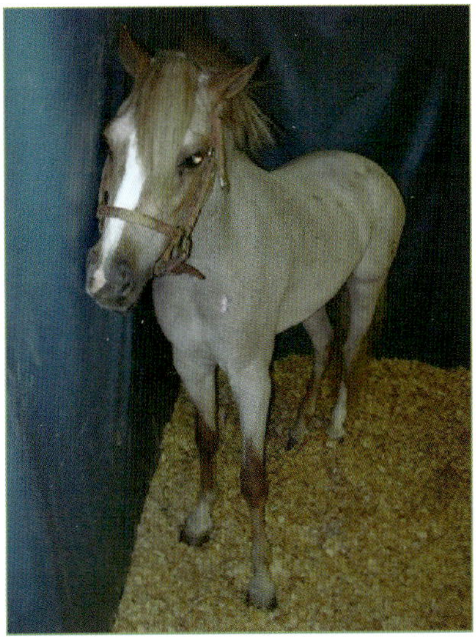

FIGURE 2a: An 8-year-old mixed breed hunter pony that presented for acute onset of neurological signs. Neurological examination revealed abnormalities consistent with paradoxical vestibular syndrome, circling to the right, consisting of a head tilt to the left, head and neck turn to the right, and right CN VII facial paralysis, dorsal deviation of the right pupil and ventral deviation of the left pupil. Physiological nystagmus was apparently normal to the right side, but absent to the left side. The mandible was deviated to the right. Results of CSF western blot analysis identified antibodies against S. neurona (relative quantity, 35).

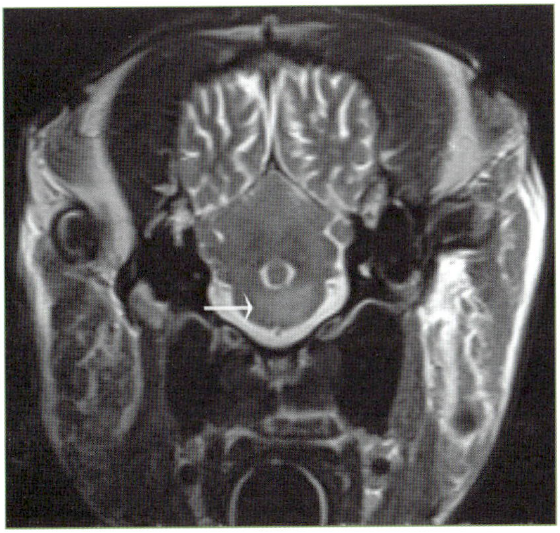

FIGURE 2b: Transverse T2-weighted magnetic resonance image of the pony's brain. The pony's right side is to the left in the image; dorsal is toward the top of the image. Notice an area of increased signal intensity (arrow) located slightly to the left of midline in the caudal brainstem.

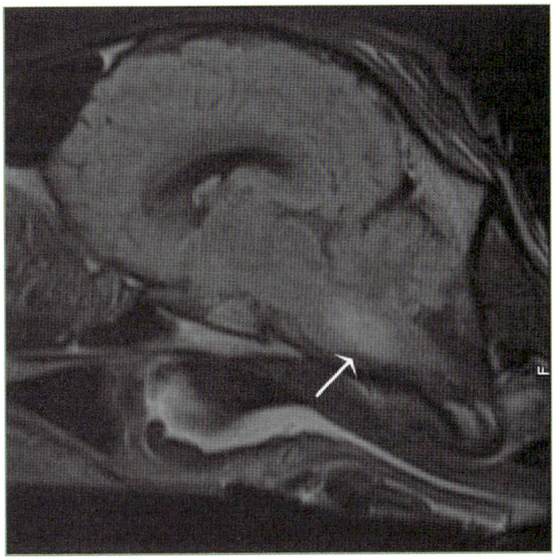

FIGURE 2c: Sagittal fluid-attenuated inversion recovery (FLAIR) image of the brain of the pony. Rostral is toward the left and dorsal is toward the top of the image. An ovoid focus of increased signal intensity (arrow) is present in the brainstem.

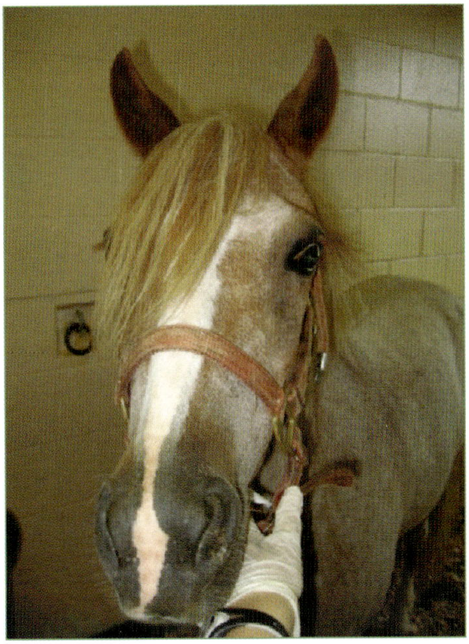

FIGURE 2d: The pony following one month of treatment with pyrimethamine (1 mg/kg bwt, per os, q. 24 h), sulphadiazine (20 mg/kg bwt, per os, q. 24 h) and ponazuril (5 mg/kg bwt, per os, q. 24 h). No head tilt, neck tilt or circling were evident and apparently normal physiological nystagmus could be elicited. The cranial nerve VII deficits had improved but there was a mild left ear droop and muzzle deviation to the right.

demarcated areas of spontaneous sweating or loss of reflexes and cutaneous sensation.

Neurological signs noticed at the walk or during neurological examination include any to all of the following: asymmetric stride length, toe dragging, circumduction of hindlimbs and hypometria (also described as floating or marching) of forelimbs. Other signs may be noted only during breaking or training (Fenger 1996). There may be frequent bucking, head tossing, excessively high head carriage, difficulty maintaining a specific lead, cross cantering or cross galloping, and difficulty negotiating turns. Some signs that usually are attributed to primary musculoskeletal disease, such as back soreness or upward fixation of the patella(s), can be caused by weak or asymmetric use of muscle groups in horses with EPM that are in training.

The most common manifestation of brain disease in horses with EPM is a brain stem syndrome with signs of obtundation and asymmetric vestibular (VIII) nerve dysfunction (**Fig 2**). There may also be facial paralysis (VII), dysphagia (X), tongue paralysis (XII), laryngeal paralysis (X), strabismus (III, IV, IV), failure of globe retraction (VI) and weak jaw tone (V) (**Fig 5**). With involvement of the rostral brain stem or cerebrum, EPM may manifest as seizures, visual deficit/abnormal menace response and behavioural abnormality.

Without treatment, EPM usually progresses. Progression to recumbency occurs over hours to years and may occur steadily or in a stop-start manner.

Treatment

Since 2000, the folate inhibitors sulphadiazine/pyrimethamine (SDZ/PYR), the triazinetrione ponazuril (PNZ), and the nitrothiazole nitazoxanide (NTZ) have all been licensed by the Federal Drug Administration (FDA) for the treatment of EPM. The production of nitazoxanide was recently discontinued (personal communication, IDEXX pharmaceuticals). The triazinedione diclazuril (DCZ) has been approved, but a commercial product has not been launched. Approved and pending treatments including protocols are summarised in **Table 2**. Because of differences in techniques and

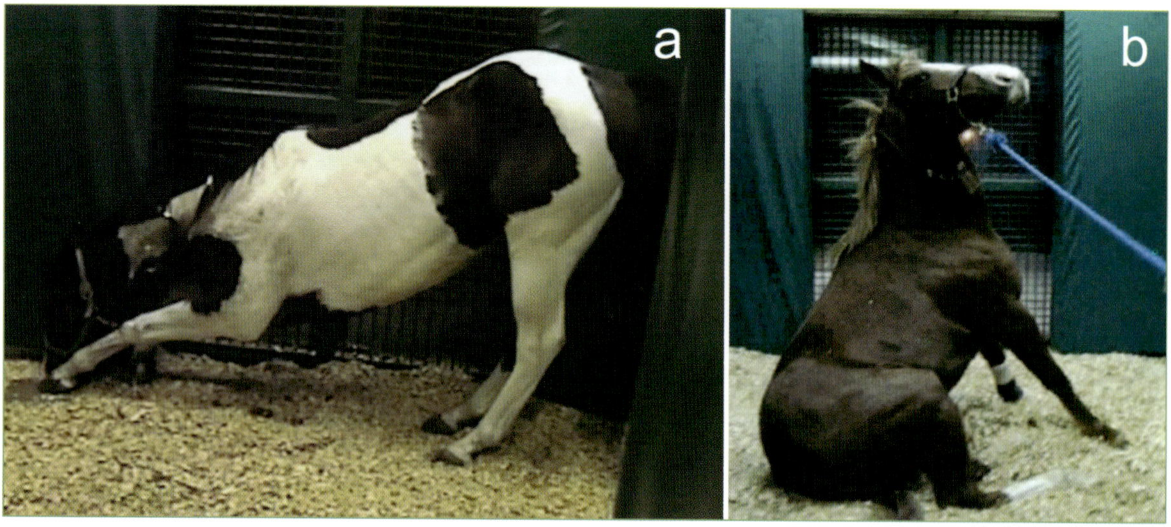

FIGURE 3: The 4-year-old Paint gelding in panel A (capture from video) began stumbling and tripping in the thoracic limbs on the day before presentation. At the time of examination, there was profound (grade 4/5) weakness in both thoracic limbs and slight weakness and ataxia (grade 1/5) in the pelvic limbs. These signs are consistent with extensive involvement of the ventral horns of the gray matter in spinal cord segments giving rise to the motor nerves of the brachial plexus (C6-T2), without substantial involvement of the white matter long tracts to and from the pelvic limbs. The 3-year-old Standardbred in panel B (capture from video) acutely became weak and ataxic in the pelvic limbs 2 days before presentation. By the time of examination, the horse was unable to stand on his pelvic limbs but was judged to have normal strength in the thoracic limbs. These signs are consistent with at least one lesion within the T2 to S3 range of spinal cord segments.

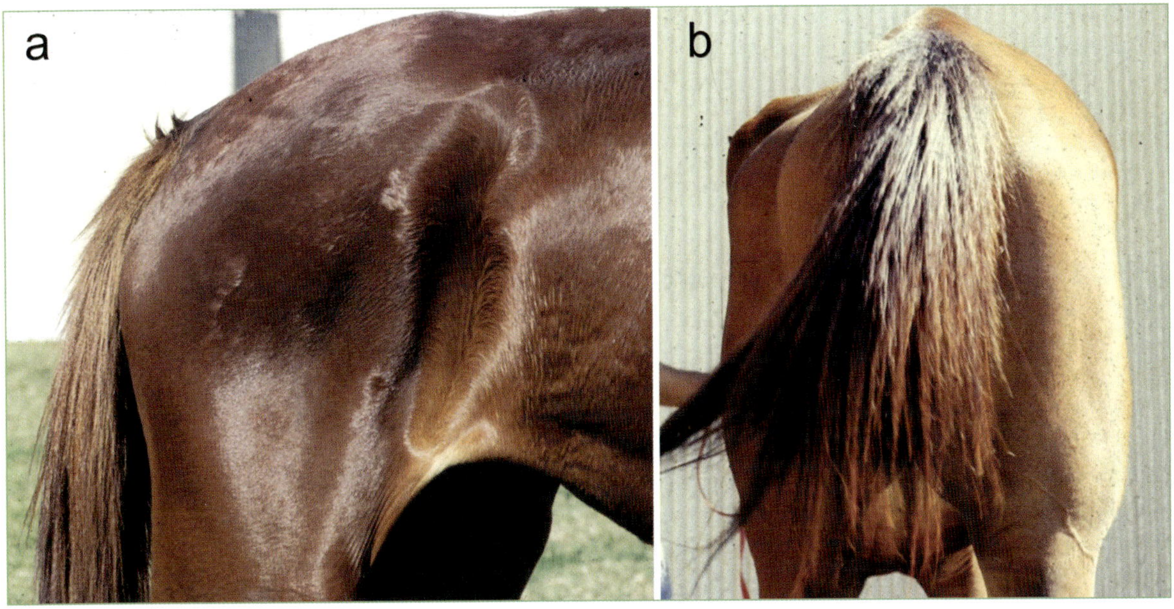

FIGURE 4: Neurogenic muscle atrophy in 2 horses with EPM. There is severe atrophy of the right quadriceps and biceps femoris muscles (panel A) and left gluteal muscles (panel B) reflecting damage to the cell bodies of lower motor neurons in the ventral horn of the gray matter within spinal cord segments L3 to S2.

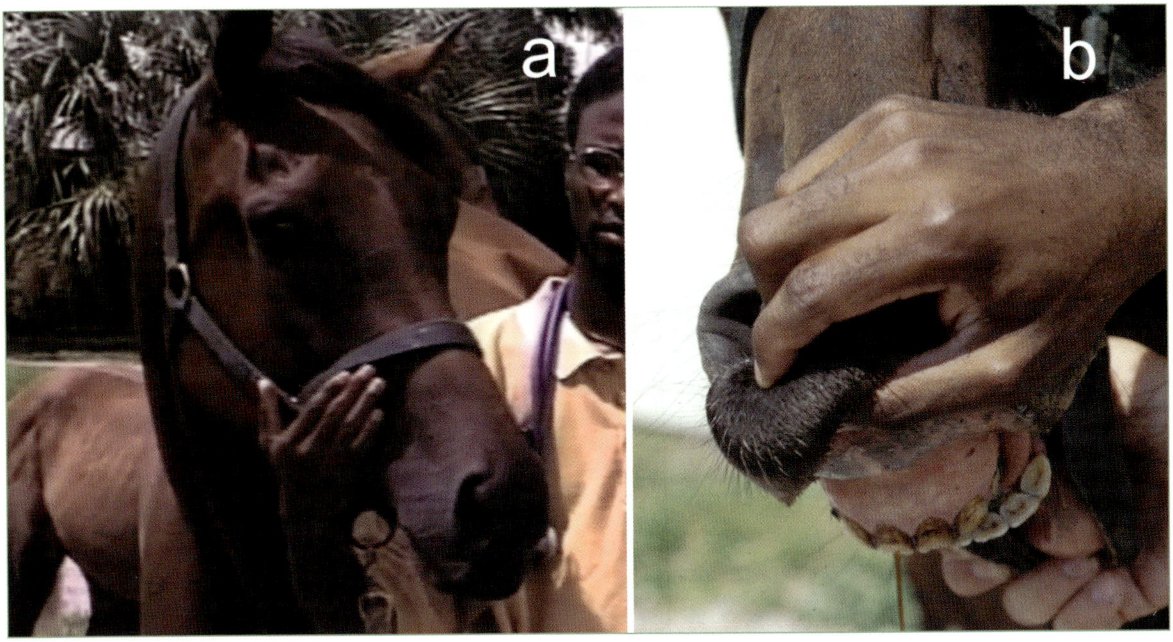

FIGURE 5: This 12-year-old Thoroughbred mare had a sudden onset of limb weakness and ataxia 5 weeks after foaling, diagnosed as EPM. Four weeks later, at the time of examination, there was also left-sided facial paralysis and the poll was rotated to the right. As shown in Panel A (capture from video), there was atrophy of the right masseter and temporal muscles, indicating involvement of the ipsilateral (right) motor nucleus of cranial nerve V. The asymmetric actions of the masticatory muscles in this mare have caused deviation of the mandible to the left (Panel B).

experimental design among studies performed for each of these drugs, objective comparison of different treatments is not yet possible. Quantitative data of any kind are not yet available for the efficacy of anti-EPM treatments against *N. hughesi*, although clinical improvement was observed in 3 horses treated with ponazuril (Finno *et al.* 2007a).

Clinical efficacy testing

Multi-centre studies of SDZ/PYR, PNZ, NTZ and DCZ have been performed as part of the process of application for approval for licensing by the FDA (Anon , 2001, 2003, 2004, 2005). A summary of these studies is given in **Table 3**. By necessity, these efficacy trials lacked a placebo control group. Despite substantive differences in protocols among the studies, the basic designs were similar. Horses were treated according to the protocols intended for subsequent commercial products. Treatment success in these trials was defined as improvement by one grade or, for the SDZ/PYR study (number 5, **Table 3**), 2 grades if the WB remained positive, according to neurological examinations made by a single experienced examiner before and at some point after treatment. Video recordings of the examinations were used as a further parameter of treatment success.

Reported success rates for 5 of the 6 studies (numbers 1, 3-6, **Table 3**) were strikingly similar (57.1– 61.5%, mean 58.9%). These 5 trials were of similar design, involving relatively small numbers of trained examiners, and all required a positive CSF WB result for enrolment. The second NTZ study (number 2, **Table 3**) reported a success rate of 81.2%; however, the design of this trial was quite different from the others in that positive CSF WB results were not required for enrolment, 150 different practitioners were involved in extremely variable field conditions, and examinations were not videotaped.

TABLE 2: FDA-approved treatments for EPM

Drug	Trade name	Manufacturer	Form	FDA approval	Dose (mg/kg bwt)	Duration	Considerations
PNZ	Marquis	Bayer[4]	15% paste	2000	5	28	oil[a]
NTZ[c]	Navigator	Idexx[7]	32% paste	2004	50	28	oil[a]
SDZ/PYR	ReBalance	Phoenix[8]	25%/1% suspension	2005	20/1	90–270	empty stomach[b]
DCZ[c]	Protazil	Schering-Plough[9]	1.56% pellet	2007	1	28	

NTZ = nitazoxanide; PNZ = ponazuril; SDZ = sulphadiazine; PYR = pyrimethamine; DCZ = diclazuril. [a]Addition of 30 ml corn oil increases absorption; [b]Should not be administered within 1 h of hay or concentrate feeding; [c]Commercial product not currently available.

TABLE 3: Results of clinical efficacy trials for anti-EPM drugs

Study	Drug	Form	*N1*	*N2*	Dose (mg/kg bwt)	Duration (days)	End[a] (days)	Success Real-Time[b]	Success (%) video[c]	WB[d]
1	NTZ[g]	32% paste	96	49	25/50[e]	28	85	57.1	44.9	14.3
2	NTZ	32% paste	419	250	25/50[e]	28	85	81.2		20.0
3	PNZ	15% paste	53	47	5	28	118	59.6	44.7	10.1[f]
4	PNZ	15% paste	60	55	10	28	118	58.0	32.5	10.1[f]
5	SDZ/PYR	25% SDZ, 1.25% PYR	48	26	20/1	90–270	various	61.5	53.8	19.2
6	DCZ[g]	1.56% pellets	72	49	1	28	48	58.0	31.0	6.3

[a]Time of final evaluation; [b]Clinical improvement and/or reversion to WB-negative; [c]Clinical improvement as determined by viewers masked as to examination order. Only horses deemed real-time successes were examined on video. [d]Reversion to western blot-negative. [e]25 mg/kg bwt for 5 days, then 50 mg/kg bwt. [f]Combined result for 5 and 10 mg/kg bwt dosage groups as reported in ref 14. [g]Commercial product not currently available. *N1* = number enrolled; *N2* = number that completed study; NTZ = nitazoxanide; PNZ = ponazuril; SDZ = sulphadiazine; PYR = pyrimethamine; DCZ = diclazuril.

Formulation, dosage and duration of treatments

The treatment protocols for approved drugs shown in **Table 2** are reasonable guidelines based on cost, convenience, *in vitro* potency against *S. neurona*, pharmacokinetic/pharmacodynamic considerations, safety and the results of clinical efficacy studies. Many dosage permutations and combinations of these products and the use of pharmacologically similar products occur in clinical practice although their use is untested. Some veterinarians have routinely given the total recommended course of PNZ as 4 or 5 large doses over several days to weeks, e.g. one syringe of Marquis (Bayer[4]) per treatment. A sodium salt formulation of diclazuril has been shown to have good oral bioavailability and may have potential as a feed additive (Dirikolu *et al.* 2006). There also is anecdotal support for the use of a compounded i.v. form of diclazuril, usually given daily for 6 days at dosage of 1 mg/kg bwt/day (L. Bauslaugh, personal communication 2005). There is experimental support for the combination of PYR with either DCZ or PNZ in treatment of other coccidian infections (Lindsay and Dubey 1999; Sisson *et al.* 2002). For this reason, the authors routinely use both PNZ and SDZ/PYR when treating horses diagnosed with EPM for clients with the necessary financial resources. Such treatments constitute unapproved and/or extra-label use and cannot be recommended here since there are FDA-approved products available for treating EPM.

Treatment of relapses

Horses may relapse soon after the initial course of treatment is discontinued (Furr *et al.* 2001), or up to several years after improvement or apparent resolution of signs (Fenger 1998). An estimated 10–25% of horses successfully treated with modern protocols subsequently relapse (Fenger 1998; MacKay 2006). It is presumed that relapses represent recrudescence of lingering infections rather than new infections. Continuing treatment until the CSF WB result became negative has been recommended (Fenger 1998). Because the positive predictive value of a positive WB for EPM is poor and <20% of treated horses become CSF-antibody negative after treatment (**Table 2**), this criterion is seldom followed. To minimise the frequency of relapses, the authors prefer to use PNZ for 2 successive treatments (56 days) and/or SDZ/PYR for at least 180 days. Twelve horses that completed the PNZ trials but had incomplete responses were re-enrolled as part of a separate protocol for an additional round of treatment (Bayer Corporation 2001). All of these horses improved at least one additional grade, lending support to the idea that longer treatment durations can have salutary effects on the clinical disease. Although there is no consensus on how to treat relapses, the authors prefer to change (e.g. from Marquis[4] to Navigator[7]) or add products. If a horse relapses twice, the authors usually recommend indefinite intermittent therapy with SDZ/PYR, 2 days/week at the standard dose. A similar rationale can be used to treat horses only around stressful events that may predispose to relapses (MacKay *et al.* 2008).

Toxicity

Sulphadiazine/pyrimethamine

The toxic effects of these drugs reflect inhibition of mammalian dihydrofolate reductase by PYR, inducing folate deficiency. Signs include reproductive and neonatal disorders, and bone marrow suppression, including anaemia, leucopenia, neutropenia, and thrombocytopenia, in decreasing frequency (Anon 2004). SDZ/PRY is believed to induce abortions in pregnant mares although data on this point are lacking. SDZ/PRY showed no effect on pregnancy rates, early embryonic death, or semen quality (Brendemuehl *et al.* 1998; Bedford and McDonnell 1999). Mares treated with SDZ/PYR during pregnancy have given birth to foals with multiple congenital abnormalities (Toribio *et al.* 1998) and there are rare reports of glossitis and dysphagia in adult horses (Piercy *et al.* 2002).

Horses treated with SDZ/PYR should be kept on good quality green forage (e.g. alfalfa hay or pasture), which is likely to be rich in folate. There is no advantage to supplementation with folic acid during treatment, and some evidence from other species indicate that this practice could increase the possibility of toxicity (Chung *et al.* 1993; Toribio *et al.* 1998). Most cases of bone marrow suppression resolve if treatment is suspended for 1–2 weeks. If signs are severe, treatment with folinic acid (100 mg *per os* s.i.d. for one month, then EOD for one month) is indicated (MacKay *et al.* 2000).

Ponazuril

Ponazuril appears to be safe when administered at the recommended dose. During the efficacy trial, ulceration of skin on the lower lip adjacent to the site of oral administration was seen in a few horses (Anon 2001). During the toxicity study, moderate oedema of uterine tissues was detected in mares given 30 mg/kg bwt (6 x dose) for at least 28 days but not in mares given 10 mg/kg bwt. Clinical experience and the results of a small study in healthy mares (T.J. Kennedy, unpublished data 2005) suggests that the label dose of PNZ (5 mg/kg bwt/day) is safe to use in pregnant mares.

Diclazuril

No adverse events attributable to the drug were reported during the efficacy or pharmacokinetic studies (Anon 2005a; Dirikolu *et al.* 2006). The results of target animal safety studies have not yet been reported. Like PNZ, DCZ is expected to be safe when used at the recommended dose. An i.v. formulation of DCZ has also commonly been used for treatment of EPM, although it never has been formally evaluated for safety and efficacy (L. Bauslaugh, personal communication 2005). During >7 years clinical experience with this agent, toxicity problems have not been reported.

Nitazoxanide

Nitazoxanide has a narrow therapeutic index. At 2.5 x the recommended dose, 3/8 horses died with signs of acute typhlocolitis (Anon 2003). During the field efficacy study, fever, lethargy, and reduced appetite were seen singly or together in 10–14% of treated horses. Other signs included diarrhoea, colic, dependent oedema and laminitis. Five out of 419 horses in study number 2 (**Table 3**) died with signs possibly attributable to NTZ. The adverse effects of NTZ probably are due to disturbance of intestinal flora and signs appear similar to those of other antibiotic-associated enterocolitides. The frequency of adverse reactions appears to have been reduced by the practice of giving a 0.5 x dose for the first 5 days of treatment. Abnormal signs resolve quickly if horses are promptly removed from treatment and these signs do not usually recur when treatment is resumed. Administration of probiotics for prevention of antibiotic-associated enterocolitis is rational but unproved.

Ancillary therapy

Products and suggested regimens for ancillary therapies are listed in **Table 4**. In mild acute cases of EPM (grade 1), additional therapy is unnecessary. In horses with moderate or severe disease, anti-inflammatory and antioxidant treatment is usually provided for the first 1–2 weeks. If the horse is grade 3 or worse, a glucocorticoid (e.g. dexamethasone) and dimethyl sulphoxide may be added. Vitamin E is often given empirically throughout the period of antiprotozoal treatment for additional antioxidant effect. Oral administration of vitamin E has been shown to result in increased concentrations of alpha-tocopherol in serum and CSF (Higgins *et al.* 2008); however, it is not known if orally administered vitamin E has effects on absorption and elimination of anti-EPM drugs.

TABLE 4: Ancillary treatments for EPM

Active component	Product and source	Suggested regimen
Dimethyl sulphoxide	Generic	1 g/kg bwt i.v. b.i.d. for 1–3 days.
Vitamin E	Generic	20 iu/kg bwt *per os* daily.
Flunixin	Generic	1.1 mg/kg bwt i.v. b.i.d. for one week, then s.i.d. for an additional week.
Dexamethasone	Generic	0.05 mg/kg bwt i.v. s.i.d. for 1–3 days.
Levamisole	Levasole injectable 13.65%, Schering Plough[9]	1–2 mg/kg bwt/day *per os.*
Killed *Proprioibacterium acnes*	EqStim, Neogen[1]	4 ml i.m. 3 times/week in a 450 kg horse, repeated monthly.
Mycobacterial wall extract	Equimune i.v., Bioniche Animal Health[10]	1.5 ml i.v., repeated q. 2 weeks.
Killed *parapox ovis* virus	Zylexis, Pfizer Animal Health[11]	2 ml i.m. on Days 0, 2, and 9 then during relapses or prior to stress-inducing events.
Cimetidine	Generic	2.5 mg/kg bwt *per os* q. 8 h.

Several lines of evidence suggest that immunosuppression is key in allowing subclinical *S. neurona* infection to progress to clinical EPM (Saville *et al.* 2001; Witonsky *et al.* 2008). As a relatively crude way to address putative immunodeficiency and 'boost' cellular immunity, immune stimulants (**Table 4**) are sometimes given to horses with EPM.

Prognosis

On the basis of drug efficacy studies and clinical experience, it is reasonable to expect that about 60% of moderately or severely affected horses will improve at least one grade after treatment. Only 10–20% of such horses will completely recover and 10–20% of successfully treated horses will suffer at least one relapse. The outlook for mildly affected horses (grade 1) is considerably better, particularly if treatment is begun promptly. Although there are no published data for the latter, more common class of treated horse, at least 80% of such cases can be expected to improve and at least 50% should recover completely, with low possibility of recurrence.

Prevention

Vaccination

A vaccine made from killed, cultured *S. neurona* merozoites in MetaStim[12] adjuvant has been produced (Anon 2005b). The vaccine was marketed under conditional approval by the USDA. The conditional license lapsed in March 2008 and the vaccine is no longer available (Fort Dodge Animal Health, personal communication). Vaccinated horses at least transiently became WB-positive in CSF (Witonsky *et al.* 2004) and in the event that EPM is suspected in a vaccinated horse, WB results will be even more difficult to interpret.

Antiprotozoal agents

Prevention of EPM by antiprotozoal agents is probably effective but likely to be cost-prohibitive. Prevention of infection by *S. neurona* may be possible by daily administration of a drug such as DCZ, as has been shown in mice (Dubey *et al.* 2001d). Ponazuril given at 5 mg/kg bwt once daily to horses prior to experimental challenge with infective sporocysts reduced the incidence of clinical EPM but did not eliminate it (Furr *et al.* 2006). The disadvantage of this approach is that normal, possibly protective, immune responses to the organism may be prevented. An alternative approach is metaphylaxis, wherein intermittent doses of drug are given which allow extraneural schizogony and normal immune responses to take place, but prevent invasion of the CNS. Ponazuril given at 20 mg/kg bwt every 7 days but not every 14 days significantly reduced *S. neurona* antibody in the CSF of *S. neurona*-challenged horses, suggesting the potential utility of such an approach (MacKay *et al.* 2008).

Management

Common-sense measures can be instituted to prevent contamination of feed with *S. neurona* sporocysts. Opossums can be trapped and removed or kept away by free-ranging dogs. Spilled grain, fallen fruit and animal or bird feed should be removed, and horse food sources should be monitored and secured. The utility of controlling intermediate hosts in an effort to reduce environmental sporocyst load is doubtful; however, if there are heavy populations of host animals on a problem premise, then such animals should be trapped and removed. Products useful for cleaning of areas potentially contaminated with sporocysts have been described (Dubey *et al.* 2002; Dwyer 2004).

Manufacturers' addresses

[1]Neogen Corporation, Lansing, Michigan, USA.
[2]Michigan State University, Diagnostic Center for Population and Animal Health, Lansing, Michigan, USA.
[3]Antech Diagnostics, Los Angeles, California, USA.
[4]Bayer HealthCare Animal Health Division, Shawnee Mission, Kansas, USA.
[5]EBI, IDEXX, Lexington, Kentucky, USA.
[6]University of California-Davis, V.M.T.H., Immunology/Virology Laboratory, Davis, California, USA.
[7]IDEXX Pharmaceuticals, Westbrook, Maine, USA.
[8]Phoenix Scientific, St. Joseph, Missouri, USA.
[9]Schering-Plough Animal Health, Summit, New Jersey, USA.
[10]Bioniche Animal Health, Belleville, Ontario, Canada.
[11]Pfizer Animal Health, New York, USA.
[12]Fort Dodge Animal Health, Fort Dodge, Iowa, USA.

References

Anon (1998) Equine protozoal myeloencephalitis (EPM) in the U.S. *USDA:APHIS:VS, CEAH*, National Animal Health Monitoring System, Fort Collins. #N312. 0501.

Anon (2001) Freedom of information summary. *NADA* 141-188. Marquis™ (15% w/w ponazuril) antiprotozoal oral paste for treatment of equine protozoal myeloencephalitis caused by *Sarcocystis neurona*. Bayer Corporation. pp 1-18.

Anon (2003) Freedom of information summary. NADA 141-178. NAVIGATOR (32% nitazoxanide). Antiprotozoal oral paste for the treatment of horses with equine protozoal myeloencephalitis (EPM) caused by *Sarcocystis neurona*. IDEXX Pharmaceuticals

Anon (2004) Freedom of information summary. NADA 141-240. REBALANCE Antiprotozoal oral suspension (sulfadiazine and pyrimethamine) for the treatment of horses with equine protozoal myeloencephalitis (EPM) caused by *Sarcocystis neurona*. Animal Health Pharmaceuticals. p 1.

Anon (2005a) Freedom of information summary (draft). PROTAZIL (1.56% diclazuril) Antiprotozoal Pellets for the treatment of horses with equine protozoal myeloencephalitis (EPM) caused by *Sarcocystis neurona*. Schering-Plough Animal Health.

Anon (2005b) Equine protozoal myeloencephalitis. http://www.epmvaccine.com/ Fort Dodge Animal Health.

Bedford, S.J. and McDonnell, S.M. (1999) Measurements of reproductive function in stallions treated with trimethoprim-sulfamethoxazole and pyrimethamine. *J. Am. vet. med. Ass.* **215**, 1317-1319.

Bentz, B.G., Ealey, K.A., Morrow, J., Claypool, P.L. and Saliki, J.T. (2003) Seroprevalence of antibodies to *Sarcocystis neurona* in equids residing in Oklahoma. *J. vet. diagn. Invest.* **15**, 597-600.

Blythe, L.L., Granstrom, D.E., Hansen, D.E., Walker, L.L., Bartlett, J., and Stamper, S. (1997) Seroprevalence of antibodies to *Sarcocystis neurona* in horses residing in Oregon. *J. Am. vet. med. Ass.* **210**, 525-527.

Brendemuehl, J.P., Waldridge, B.M. and Bridges, E.R. (1998) Effects of sulfadiazine and pyrimethamine and concurrent folic acid supplementation on pregnancy and embryonic loss rates in mares. *Proc. Am. Ass. equine Practnrs.* **44**, 142-143.

Cheadle, M.A., Tanhauser, S.M., Dame, J.B., Sellon, D.C., Hines, M., Ginn, P.E., MacKay, R.J. and Greiner, E.C. (2001a) The nine-banded armadillo (*Dasypus novemcinctus*) is an intermediate host for *Sarcocystis neurona*. *Int. J. Parasitol.* **31**, 330-335.

Cheadle, M.A., Yowell, C.A., Sellon, D.C., Hines, M., Ginn, P.E., Marsh, A.E., MacKay, R.J., Dame, J.B. and Greiner, E.C. (2001b) The striped skunk (*Mephitis mephitis*) is an intermediate host for *Sarcocystis neurona*. *Int. J. Parasitol.* **31**, 843-849.

Chung, M.K., Han, S.S. and Roh, J.K. (1993) Synergistic embryotoxicity of combination pyrimethamine and folic acid in rats. *Reprod. Toxicol.* **7**, 463-468.

Cohen, N.D., MacKay, R.J., Toby, E., Andrews, F.M., Barr, B.S., Beech, J., Bernard, W.V., Clark, C.K., Divers, T.J., Furr, M.O., Kohn, C.W., Levy, M., Reed, S.M., Seahorn, T.L. and Slovis, N.M. (2007) A multicenter case-control study of risk factors for equine protozoal myeloencephalitis. *J. Am. vet. med. Ass.* **231**, 1857-1863.

Crowdus, C.A., Marsh, A.E., Saville, W.J., Lindsay, D.S., Dubey, J.P., Granstrom, D.E. and Howe, D.K. (2008) SnSAG5 is an alternative surface antigen of *Sarcocystis neurona* strains that is mutually exclusive to SnSAG1. *Vet. Parasitol.* **158**, 36-43.

Cutler, T.J., MacKay, R.J., Ginn, P.E., Gillis, K., Tanhauser, S.M., LeRay, E.V., Dame, J.B. and Greiner, E.C. (2001) Immunoconversion against *Sarcocystis neurona* in normal and dexamethasone-treated horses challenged with *S. neurona* sporocysts. *Vet. Parasitol.* **95**, 197-210.

Daft, B.M., Barr, B.C., Gardner, I.A., Read, D., Bell, W., Peyser, K.G., Ardans, A., Kinde, H. and Morrow, J.K. (2002) Sensitivity and specificity of western blot testing of cerebrospinal fluid and serum for diagnosis of equine protozoal myeloencephalitis in horses with and without neurologic abnormalities. *J. Am. vet. med. Ass.* **221**, 1007-1013.

Dirikolu, L., Karpiesiuk, W., Lehner, A.F., Hughes, C., Woods, W.E., Harkins, J.D., Boyles, J., Atkinson, A., Granstrom, D.E. and Tobin, T. (2006) New therapeutic approaches for equine protozoal myeloencephalitis: pharmacokinetics of diclazuril sodium salts in horses. *Vet. Ther.* **7**, 52-63.

Duarte, P.C., Daft, B.M., Conrad, P.A., Packham, A.E. and Gardner, I.A. (2003) Comparison of a serum indirect fluorescent antibody test with two Western blot tests for the diagnosis of equine protozoal myeloencephalitis. *J. vet. diagn. Invest.* **15**, 8-13.

Duarte, P.C., Ebel, E.D., Traub-Dargatz, J., Wilson, W.D., Conrad, P.A. and Gardner, I.A. (2006) Indirect fluorescent antibody testing of cerebrospinal fluid for diagnosis of equine protozoal myeloencephalitis. *Am. J. vet. Res.* **67**, 869-876.

Duarte, P.C., Conrad, P.A., Barr, B.C., Wilson, W.D., Ferraro, G.L., Packham, A.E., Carpenter, T.E. and Gardner, I.A. (2004a) Risk of transplacental transmission of *Sarcocystis neurona* and Neospora hughesi in California horses. *J. Parasitol.* **90**, 1345-1351.

Duarte, P.C., Daft, B.M., Conrad, P.A., Packham, A.E., Saville, W.J., MacKay, R.J., Barr, B.C., Wilson, W.D., Ng, T., Reed, S.M. and Gardner, I.A. (2004b) Evaluation and comparison of an indirect fluorescent antibody test for detection of antibodies to *Sarcocystis neurona*, using serum and cerebrospinal fluid of naturally and experimentally infected, and vaccinated horses. *J. Parasitol.* **90**, 379-386.

Dubey, J.P., Speer, C.A. and Lindsay, D.S. (1998) Isolation of a third species of Sarcocystis in immunodeficient mice fed feces from opossums (*Didelphis virginiana*) and its differentiation from *Sarcocystis falcatula* and *Sarcocystis neurona*. *J. Parasitol.* **84**, 1158-1164.

Dubey, J.P., Liddell, S., Mattson, D., Speert, C.A., Howe, D.K. and Jenkins, M.C. (2001a) Characterization of the Oregon isolate of *Neospora hughesi* from a horse. *J. Parasitol.* **87**, 345-353.

Dubey, J.P., Lindsay, D.S., Saville, W.J., Reed, S.M., Granstrom, D.E., and Speer, C.A. (2001b) A review of *Sarcocystis neurona* and equine protozoal myeloencephalitis (EPM). *Vet. Parasitol.* **95**, 89-131.

Dubey, J.P., Saville, W.J., Stanek, J.F., Lindsay, D.S., Rosenthal, B.M., Oglesbee, M.J., Rosypal, A.C., Njoku, C.J., Stich, R.W., Kwok, O.C., Shen, S.K., Hamir, A.N. and Reed, S.M. (2001c) *Sarcocystis neurona* infections in raccoons (*Procyon lotor*): evidence for natural infection with sarcocysts, transmission of infection to opossums (*Didelphis virginiana*), and experimental induction of neurologic disease in raccoons. *Vet. Parasitol.* **100**, 117-129.

Dubey, J.P., Fritz, D., Lindsay, D.S., Shen, S.K., Kwok, O.C., and Thompson, K.C. (2001d) Diclazuril preventive therapy of gamma interferon knockout mice fed *Sarcocystis neurona* sporocysts. *Vet. Parasitol.* **94**, 257-264.

Dubey, J.P., Saville, W.J., Sreekumar, C., Shen, S.K., Lindsay, O.S., Pena, H.F., Vianna, M.C., Gennari, S.M. and Reed, S.M. (2002) Effects of high temperature and disinfectants on the viability of *Sarcocystis neurona* sporocysts. *J. Parasitol.* **88**, 1252-1254.

Dubey, J.P., Davis, S.W., Speer, C.A., Bowman, D.D., de Lahunta, A., Granstrom, D.E., Topper, M.J., Hamir, A.N., Cummings, J.F. and Suter, M.M. (1991) *Sarcocystis neurona* n. sp. (Protozoa: Apicomplexa), the etiologic agent of equine protozoal myeloencephalitis. *J. Parasitol.* **77**, 212-218.

Dwyer, R.M. (2004) Environmental disinfection to control equine infectious diseases. *Vet Clin. N. Am.: Equine Pract.* **20**, 531-542.

Elitsur, E., Marsh, A.E., Reed, S.M., Dubey, J.P., Oglesbee, M.J., Murphy, J.E. and Saville, W.J. (2007) Early migration of *Sarcocystis neurona* in ponies fed sporocysts. *J. Parasitol.* **93**, 1222-1225.

Ellison, S.P., Kennedy T. and Brown K.K. (2003) Development of an ELISA to detect antibodies to rSG1 in the horse. *J. appl. Res. vet. Med.* **1**, 318-327.

Fayer, R., Mayhew, I.G., Baird, J.D., Dill, S.G., Foreman, J.H., Fox, J.C., Higgins, R.J., Reed, S.M., Ruoff, W.W. and Sweeney, R.W. (1990) Epidemiology of equine protozoal myeloencephalitis in North America based on histologically confirmed cases. A report. *J. vet. Intern. Med.* **4**, 54-57.

Fenger, C.K. (1996) Equine protozoal myeloencephalitis, In: *Current Therapy in Equine Medicine* 4, Ed: N. E. Robinson, W.B. Saunders, Philadelphia. pp. 329-332.

Fenger, C.K. (1998) Treatment of equine protozoal myeloencephalitis. *Comp. cont. Ed. pract. Vet.* **20**, 1154-1157.

Fenger, C.K., Granstrom, D.E., Langemeier, J.L. and Stamper, S. (1997) Epizootic of equine protozoal myeloencephalitis on a farm. *J. Am. vet. med. Ass.* **210**, 923-927.

Fenger, C.K., Granstrom, D.E., Langemeier, J.L., Gajadhar, A., Cothran, G., Tramontin, R.R., Stamper, S. and Dubey, J.P. (1994) Phylogenetic relationship of *Sarcocystis neurona* to other members of the family Sarcocystidae based on small subunit ribosomal RNA gene sequence. *J. Parasitol.* **80**, 966-975.

Fenger, C.K., Granstrom, D.E., Langemeier, J.L., Stamper, S., Donahue, J.M., Patterson, J.S., Gajadhar, A.A., Marteniuk, J.V., Xiaomin, Z. and Dubey, J.P. (1995) Identification of opossums (*Didelphis virginiana*) as the putative definitive host of *Sarcocystis neurona*. *J. Parasitol.* **81**, 916-919.

Finno, C.J., Aleman, M. and Pusterla, N. (2007a) Equine protozoal myeloencephalitis associated with neosporosis in 3 horses. *J. vet. Intern. Med.* **21**, 1405-1408.

Finno, C.J., Packham, A.E., David, W.W., Gardner, I.A., Conrad, P.A. and Pusterla, N. (2007b) Effects of blood contamination of cerebrospinal fluid on results of indirect fluorescent antibody tests for detection of antibodies against *Sarcocystis neurona* and *Neospora hughesi*. *J. vet. diagn. Invest.* **19**, 286-289.

Furr, M., MacKay, R., Granstrom, D., Schott, H. and Andrews, F. (2002) Clinical diagnosis of equine protozoal myeloencephalitis (EPM). *J. vet. Intern. Med.* **16**, 618-621.

Furr, M., McKenzie, H., Saville, W.J., Dubey, J.P., Reed, S.M. and Davis, W. (2006) Prophylactic administration of ponazuril reduces clinical signs and delays seroconversion in horses challenged with *Sarcocystis neurona*. *J. Parasitol.* **92**, 637-643.

Furr, M.O. (2008) Equine protozoal myeloencephalitis, In: *Equine Neurology*, Ed: M. O. Furr and S. M. Reed, Blackwell Publishing, Ames. pp. 197-212.

Furr, M.O., Kennedy, T.J., MacKay, R.J., Reed, S.M., Andrews, F.M., Bernard, B., Bain, F.T. and Byars, T.D. (2001) Efficacy of ponazuril 15% oral paste as a treatment for equine protozoal myeloencephalitis. *Vet. Ther.* **2**, 215-222.

Furr, M.O. and Tyler, R.D. (1990) Cerebrospinal fluid creatine kinase activity in horses with central nervous system disease: 69 cases (1984-1989). *J. Am. vet. med. Ass.* **197**, 245-248.

Goehring, L.S. and Sloet van Oldruitenborgh-Oosterbaan, M.M. (2001) Equine protozoal myeloencephalitis in the Netherlands? An overview. *Tijdschr. Diergeneeskd.* **126**, 346-351.

Granstrom, D. E. (1995) EPM Seminar. *The Horse* **14**.

Granstrom, D.E. (1997) Equine protozoal myeloencephalitis: parasite biology, experimental disease and laboratory diagnosis, In: *Proceedings of the International Equine Neurology Conference,* Ithaca. pp. 4-6.

Granstrom, D.E., Alvarez, O., Jr., Dubey, J.P., Comer, P.F., and Williams, N.M. (1992) Equine protozoal myelitis in Panamanian horses and isolation of *Sarcocystis neurona*. *J. Parasitol.* **78**, 909-912.

Gray, L.C., Magdesian, K.G., Sturges, B.K. and Madigan, J.E. (2001) Suspected protozoal myeloencephalitis in a two-month-old colt. *Vet. Rec.* **149**, 269-273.

Hamir, A.N., Tornquist, S.J., Gerros, T.C., Topper, M.J. and Dubey, J.P. (1998) Neospora caninum-associated equine protozoal myeloencephalitis. *Vet. Parasitol.* **79**, 269-274.

Heskett, K.A. and MacKay, R.J. (2008) Antibody index and specific antibody quotient in horses after intragastric administration of *Sarcocystis neurona* sporocysts. *Am. J. vet. Res.* **69**, 403-409.

Higgins, J.K., Puschner, B., Kass, P.H. and Pusterla, N. (2008) Assessment of vitamin E concentrations in serum and cerebrospinal fluid of horses following oral administration of vitamin E. *Am. J. vet. Res.* **69**, 785-790.

Hoane, J.S., Morrow, J.K., Saville, W.J., Dubey, J.P., Granstrom, D.E. and Howe, D.K. (2005) Enzyme-linked immunosorbent assays for detection of equine antibodies specific to *Sarcocystis neurona* surface antigens. *Clin. Diagn. Lab. Immunol.* **12**, 1050-1056.

Howe, D.K., Gaji, R.Y., Marsh, A.E., Patil, B.A., Saville, W.J., Lindsay, D.S., Dubey, J.P. and Granstrom, D.E. (2008) Strains of *Sarcocystis neurona* exhibit differences in their surface antigens, including the absence of the major surface antigen SnSAG1. *Int. J. Parasitol.* **38**, 623-631.

Hyun, C., Gupta, G.D. and Marsh, A.E. (2003) Sequence comparison of *Sarcocystis neurona* surface antigen from multiple isolates. *Vet. Parasitol.* **112**, 11-20.

Jackson C., De Lahunta A., Divers, T.J., and *et al.* (1995) Diagnostic significance and variables affecting spinal fluid creatine kinase activity in the horse [abstr 116], In: *Proceedings of the 13th Annual Veterinary Medical Forum of the American College of Veterinary Internal Medicine,* Lake Buena Vista. p 1023.

Javsicas, L.H., Watson, E. and MacKay, R.J. (2008) What is your neurologic diagnosis? Equine protozoal myeloencephalitis. *J. Am. vet. med. Ass.* **232**, 201-204.

Liang, F.T., Granstrom, D.E., Zhao, X.M. and Timoney, J.F. (1998) Evidence that surface proteins Sn14 and Sn16 of *Sarcocystis neurona* merozoites are involved in infection and immunity. *Infect. Immun.* **66**, 1834-1838.

Lindsay, D.S. and Dubey, J.P. (1999) Determination of the activity of pyrimethamine, trimethoprim, sulfonamides, and combinations of pyrimethamine and sulfonamides against *Sarcocystis neurona* in cell cultures. *Vet. Parasitol.* **82**, 205-210.

Lindsay, D.S., Mitchell, S.M., Yang, J., Dubey, J.P., Gogal, R.M., Jr. and Witonsky, S.G. (2006) Penetration of equine leukocytes by merozoites of *Sarcocystis neurona*. *Vet. Parasitol.* **138**, 371-376.

MacKay, R.J. (2006) Equine protozoal myeloencephalitis: treatment, prognosis and prevention. *Clin. Tech. Equine. Pract.* **5**, 9-16.

MacKay, R.J., Davis, S.W. and Dubey, J.P. (1992) Equine protozoal myeloencephalitis. *Comp. cont. Educ. pract. Vet.* **14**, 1367.

MacKay, R.J., Granstrom, D.E., Saville, W.J. and Reed, S.M. (2000) Equine protozoal myeloencephalitis. *Vet. Clin. N.Am.: Equine Pract.* **16**, 405-425.

MacKay, R.J., Tanhauser, S.T., Gillis, K.D., Mayhew, I.G. and Kennedy, T.J. (2008) Effect of intermittent oral administration of ponazuril on experimental *Sarcocystis neurona* infection of horses. *Am. J. vet. Res.* **69**, 396-402.

Marsh, A.E., Barr, B.C., Packham, A.E. and Conrad, P.A. (1998) Description of a new *Neospora species* (Protozoa: Apicomplexa: Sarcocystidae). *J. Parasitol.* **84**, 983-991.

Marsh, A.E., Barr, B.C., Madigan, J., Lakritz, J. and Conrad, P.A. (1996a) Sequence analysis and polymerase chain reaction amplification of small subunit ribosomal DNA from *Sarcocystis neurona*. *Am. J. vet. Res.* **57**, 975-981.

Marsh, A.E., Barr, B.C., Madigan, J., Lakritz, J., Nordhausen, R. and Conrad, P.A. (1996b) Neosporosis as a cause of equine protozoal myeloencephalitis. *J. Am. vet. med. Ass.* **209**, 1907-1913.

Marsh, A.E., Howe, D.K., Wang, G., Barr, B.C., Cannon, N. and Conrad, P.A. (1999) Differentiation of *Neospora hughesi* from *Neospora caninum* based on their immunodominant surface antigen, SAG1 and SRS2. *Int. J. Parasitol.* **29**, 1575-1582.

Mayhew, I.G., De Lahunta, A. and Whitlock, R.H. (1977) Equine protozoal myeloencephalitis, *Proc. Am. Ass. equine Practnrs.* **23**, 107-114.

Miller, M.M., Sweeney, C.R., Russell, G.E., Sheetz, R.M. and Morrow, J.K. (1999) Effects of blood contamination of cerebrospinal fluid on western blot analysis for detection of antibodies against *Sarcocystis neurona* and on albumin quotient and immunoglobulin G index in horses. *J. Am. vet. med. Ass.* **215**, 67-71.

Morley, P.S., Traub-Dargatz, J.L., Benedict, K.M., Saville, W.J., Voelker, L.D. and Wagner, B.A. (2008) Risk factors for owner-reported occurrence of equine protozoal myeloencephalitis in the US equine population. *J. vet. intern. Med.* **22**, 616-629.

Mullaney, T., Murphy, A.J., Kiupel, M., Bell, J.A., Rossano, M.G. and Mansfield, L.S. (2005) Evidence to support horses as natural intermediate hosts for *Sarcocystis neurona*. *Vet. Parasitol.* **133**, 27-36.

Packham, A.E., Conrad, P.A., Wilson, W.D., Jeanes, L.V., Sverlow, K.W., Gardner, I.A., Daft, B.M., Marsh, A.E., Blagburn, B.L., Ferraro, G.L. and Barr, B.C. (2002) Qualitative evaluation of selective tests for detection of *Neospora hughesi* antibodies in serum and cerebrospinal fluid of experimentally infected horses. *J. Parasitol.* **88**, 1239-1246.

Piercy, R.J., Hinchcliff, K.W. and Reed, S.M. (2002) Folate deficiency during treatment with orally administered folic acid, sulphadiazine and pyrimethamine in a horse with suspected equine protozoal myeloencephalitis (EPM). *Equine vet. J.* **34**, 311-316.

Pitel, P.H., Pronost, S., Gargala, G., Anrioud, D., Toquet, M.P., Foucher, N., Collobert-Laugier, C., Fortier, G. and Ballet, J.J. (2002) Detection of *Sarcocystis neurona* antibodies in French horses with neurological signs. *Int. J. Parasitol.* **32**, 481-485.

Pusterla, N., Wilson, W.D., Conrad, P.A., Barr, B.C., Ferraro, G.L., Daft, B.M. and Leutenegger, C.M. (2006) Cytokine gene signatures in neural tissue of horses with equine protozoal myeloencephalitis or equine herpes type 1 myeloencephalopathy. *Vet. Rec.* **159**, 341-346.

Reed, S.M., Granstrom, D.E., Rivas, L.J. *et al.* (1994) Results of cerebrospinal fluid analysis in 119 horses testing positive to the Western blot test on serum and CSF to equine protozoal encephalomyelitis. *Proc. Am. Ass. equine Practnrs.* **41**, 199.

Rossano, M.G., Kaneene, J.B., Marteniuk, J.V., Banks, B.D., Schott, H.C. and Mansfield, L.S. (2001) The seroprevalence of antibodies to *Sarcocystis neurona* in Michigan equids. *Prev. vet. Med.* **48**, 113-128.

Rossano, M.G., Mansfield, L.S., Kaneene, J.B., Murphy, A.J., Brown, C.M., Schott, H.C. and Fox, J.C. (2000) Improvement of western blot test specificity for detecting equine serum antibodies to *Sarcocystis neurona*. *J. vet. diagn. Invest.* **12**, 28-32.

Saville, W.J., Dubey, J.P., Oglesbee, M.J., Sofaly, C.D., Marsh, A.E., Elitsur, E., Vianna, M.C., Lindsay, D.S. and Reed, S.M. (2004) Experimental infection of ponies with *Sarcocystis fayeri* and differentiation from *Sarcocystis neurona* infections in horses. *J. Parasitol.* **90**, 1487-1491.

Saville, W.J., Reed, S.M., Granstrom, D.E., Hinchcliff, K.W., Kohn, C.W., Wittum, T.E. and Stamper, S. (1997) Seroprevalence of antibodies to *Sarcocystis neurona* in horses residing in Ohio. *J. Am. vet. med. Ass.* **210**, 519-524.

Saville, W.J., Reed, S.M., Morley, P.S., Granstrom, D.E., Kohn, C.W., Hinchcliff, K.W. and Wittum, T.E. (2000) Analysis of risk factors for the development of equine protozoal myeloencephalitis in horses. *J. Am. vet. med. Ass.* **217**, 1174-1180.

Saville, W.J., Stich, R.W., Reed, S.M., Njoku, C.J., Oglesbee, M.J., Wunschmann, A., Grover, D.L., Larew-Naugle, A.L., Stanek, J.F., Granstrom, D.E. and Dubey, J.P. (2001) Utilization of stress in the development of an equine model for equine protozoal myeloencephalitis. *Vet. Parasitol.* **95**, 211-222.

Sisson, G., Goodwin, A., Raudonikiene, A., Hughes, N.J., Mukhopadhyay, A.K., Berg, D.E. and Hoffman, P.S. (2002) Enzymes associated with reductive activation and action of nitazoxanide, nitrofurans, and metronidazole in *Helicobacter pylori*. *Antimicrob. Agents Chemother.* **46**, 2116-2123.

Toribio, R.E., Bain, F.T., Mrad, D.R., Messer, N.T., Sellers, R.S. and Hinchcliff, K.W. (1998) Congenital defects in newborn foals of mares treated for equine protozoal myeloencephalitis during pregnancy. *J. Am. vet. med. Ass.* **212**, 697-701.

Vardeleon, D., Marsh, A.E., Thorne, J.G., Loch, W., Young, R. and Johnson, P.J. (2001) Prevalence of *Neospora hughesi* and *Sarcocystis neurona* antibodies in horses from various geographical locations. *Vet. Parasitol.* **95**, 273-282.

Witonsky, S., Ellison, S., Yang, J., Gogal, R., Lawler, H., Suzuki, Y., Sriranganathan, N., Andrews, F., Ward, D. and Lindsay, D. (2008) *In vitro* suppressed immune response in horses experimentally infected with *Sarcocystis neurona*. *J. Parasitol.* In press.

Witonsky, S., Morrow, J.K., Leger, C., Dascanio, J., Buechner-Maxwell, V., Palmer, W., Kline, K. and Cook, A. (2004) *Sarcocystis neurona*-specific immunoglobulin G in the serum and cerebrospinal fluid of horses administered *S. neurona* vaccine. *J. vet. intern. Med.* **18**, 98-103.

Witonsky, S.G., Gogal, R.M., Jr., Duncan, R.B., Jr., Norton, H., Ward, D. and Lindsay, D.S. (2005) Prevention of meningo/encephalomyelitis due to *Sarcocystis neurona* infection in mice is mediated by CD8 cells. *Int. J. Parasitol.* **35**, 113-123.

EQUINE PIROPLASMOSIS

C. M. B. Donnellan and H. J. Marais*

Department of Companion Animal Clinical Studies, Faculty of Veterinary Science, University of Pretoria, South Africa.

Keywords: horse; piroplasmosis; *Theileria equi*; *Babesai caballi*; imidocarb

Summary

Theileria equi and *Babesia caballi* are the causative agents of equine piroplasmosis. These tick-transmitted piroplasms cause haemolytic anaemia in the acute phase of the disease. Clinical signs include fever, anorexia, pale to icteric mucous membranes, tachycardia and weakness. Transplacental transmission can lead to abortions or neonatal piroplasmosis, which is invariably fatal. Diagnosis in acute disease is based on microscopic detection of parasites in red blood cells by thorough examination of Wright-Giemsa stained blood smears. Serology is used for detection of carriers. PCR is currently the most sensitive diagnostic technique. Imidocarb and diminazene are the most frequently used babesiacides for the treatment of clinical disease.

Introduction

The causative agents of equine piroplasmosis are the intra-erythrocytic tick transmitted protozoan parasites: *Theileria equi* and *Babesia caballi*. *T. equi* was previously named *Babesia equi*. Horses, donkeys, mules and zebras are susceptible to infection with these protozoa; however, clinical disease rarely occurs in donkeys, mules or zebras.

Epidemiology

Equine piroplasmosis is characterised by a narrow range of parasite-insect vector-host system. The geographical distribution is dependant upon the presence or absence of appropriate insect vectors whose ecology determines the basic epidemiological pattern. The disease is widespread occurring in most tropical and subtropical areas. Piroplasmosis is endemic in Africa, Central and South America, the Caribbean (including Puerto Rico), Middle East, Asia except Japan, southern Europe in coastal countries of the Mediterranean (Portugal, Spain, France, Italy and the Balkan peninsula), and countries of the Commonwealth of Independent States. In endemic areas the prevalence of *T. equi* tends to be higher than *B. caballi* (de Waal 1995; Boldbaatar *et al.* 2005; Camacho *et al.* 2005; Sevinc *et al.* 2008)

The USA, Canada, Iceland, Greenland, UK, Ireland, Northern Europe, Singapore, Japan, New Zealand and Australia are not considered endemic areas for piroplasmosis (Tenter and Friedhoff 1986; Friedhoff *et al.* 1990). Equine piroplasmosis was introduced into Florida, USA with the importation of Cuban horses in 1959, and was eradicated by 1988. In 2008, 20 horses on 7 separate premises in Florida tested positive for *T. equi*. These 20 horses were all closely epidemiologically linked to 2 horses that entered Florida from Mexico. All 19 horses were destroyed. There was no evidence of tick transmission in these cases, and transmission was associated with poor management practices with needle sharing between horses.

Transmission

The natural method for transmission of piroplasmosis is by ticks. Ticks of the genera *Dermacentor*, *Hyalomma*, *Rhipicephalus* and *Boophilus* are the vectors of piroplasmosis in horses. The following are the reported tick vectors of piroplasmosis in horses (de Waal 1995; Stiller and Coan 1995; Mehlhorn and Schein 1998; Ikadai *et al.* 2007): *Boophilus microplus*, the southern cattle tick; *Dermacentor albipictus*, the winter tick (*B. caballi* experimentally transovarially only); *D. marginatus*, the ornate sheep tick; *D. nitens*, the tropical horse tick (*B. caballi* only); *D. nuttalli*; *D. pictus*; *D. reticulatus*, the ornate cow tick (*B. caballi*

*Author to whom correspondence should be addressed. Dr Marais's present address: Private Bag X04, Onderstepoort, 0110, South Africa.

transovarially only); *D. silvarum* (*B. caballi* only); *D. variabilis*, the American dog tick; *Hyalomma anatolicum*; *H. dromedari*, the camel tick; *H. marginatum*, the Mediterranean tick; *H. truncatum*, the small smooth bont-legged tick (*B. caballi* transovarially only); *H. uralense* (*B. equi* transstadially only); *H. volgense* (*B. caballi* transovarially only); *Rhipicephalus bursa*; *R. evertsi evertsi*, red-legged tick; *R. evertsi mimeticus*, south-west African red-legged tick (*T. equi* transstadially only); *R. pulchellus* (*B. equi* transstadially only); *R. sanguineus* or *turanicus*, the brown dog tick; and *Haemaphysalis longicornis* (experimentally).

After horses become infected with *T. equi* or *B. caballi*, the horses become carriers with parasites being found for years within the red blood cells. Carrier status after *T. equi* infection may be life-long (Mehlhorn and Schein 1998). The length of persistence of *B. caballi* in the horse has not been established but animals may remain carriers for up to 4 years (de Waal and van Heerden 1994; Knowles 1996). These carrier animals provide a reservoir of infection for the tick vectors. Carrier horses with very low parasitaemias are capable of transmitting the infection to tick vectors and transmission of infection by the tick vectors only requires a small number of infected ticks feeding on susceptible horses (Ueti *et al.* 2005). Sexual reproduction occurs within the tick, and asexual division occurs within the mammalian host (Mehlhorn and Schein 1998).

Theileria equi transmission in the tick is transstadial (from larval to nymphal stage or from nymph to adult stage). Recently, transovarial transmission of *T. equi* has been suggested to occur in: *Haemaphysalis longicornis*, the bush tick; *Boophilus microplus*, the southern cattle tick; and *Dermacentor nuttalli* (Battsetseg *et al.* 2002a,b; Ikadai *et al.* 2007). The larvae or nymph become infected by ingesting red blood cells containing the piroplasm while feeding on the host. Larvae are not preinfected from ova. The next stage of the tick life cycle, i.e. the nymph or adult tick, transmit the infection by injecting the infective sporozoites into the host together with the tick saliva. The nymph or adult tick transmitting the infection is

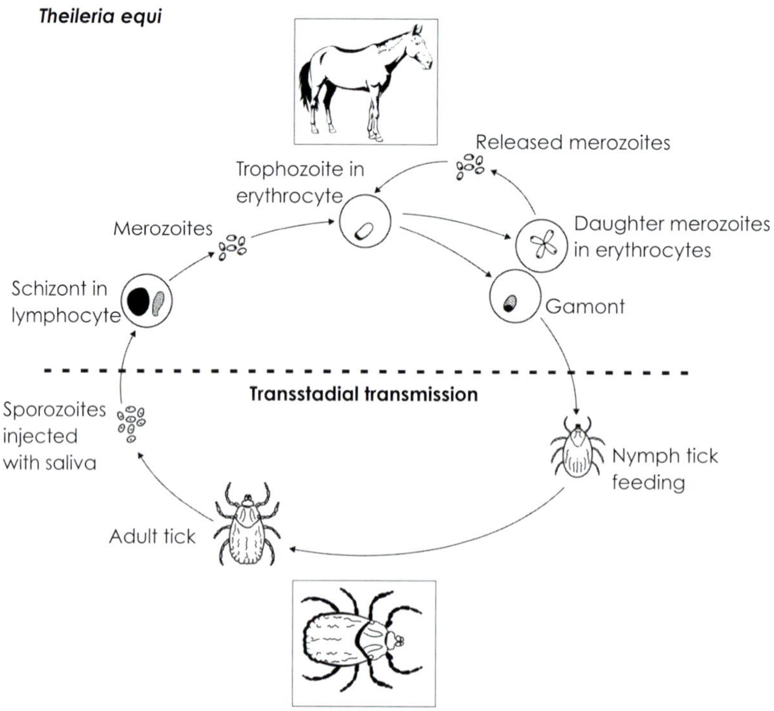

FIGURE 1: The life cycle of Theileria equi.

not immediately infective to the host as maturation of the infective sporozoites in the salivary gland, which takes 2–5 days after attachment, has to take place before transmission to the mammalian host can occur. The tick loses the infection after having transmitted it (Mehlhorn and Schein 1998; Uilenberg 2006).

In the mammalian host, the sporozoites penetrate lymphocytes, developing into schizonts. Merozoites are released from the lymphocytes after 9 days to invade erythrocytes. The merozoites in the erythrocytes transform into trophozoites, and divide to form daughter merozoites; frequently 4 daughter merozoites with the typical maltese cross formation. The rapid multiplication leads to rupture of the red blood cells and release of the merozoites to infect other red cells. Some trophozoites do not divide but become spherical/ovoid gamonts within the red blood cell. The gamonts in red blood cells are ingested by the tick and develop further within the tick (Mehlhorn and Schein 1998) (**Fig 1**).

With *Babesia caballi* both transstadial and transovarial (from one tick generation to the next via the egg) tick transmission occurs. With transovarial transmission the female tick becomes infected by ingesting red blood cells containing the protozoa. The infection passes through the ovary and the egg to the next tick generation. The sporozoites are injected into the mammalian host with the tick saliva and directly infect red blood cells. Multiplication occurs in the red blood cells to produce 2 pear-shaped daughter merozoites, which are released, rupturing the red blood cell and enter other red cells. *B. caballi* infection may persist in ticks over several generations, without new infections, acting as a reservoir of infection for *B. caballi* (Friedhoff *et al.* 1990) (**Fig 2**).

Piroplasmosis may also be transmitted mechanically through subcutaneous, i.m. or i.v. injections. Carrier horses may transmit piroplasmosis when used as blood donors. Transplacental transmission of *T. equi* occurs. This transplacental transmission may occur across a normal placenta as early as the first trimester of pregnancy and has been suggested to be a relatively normal occurrence in carrier mares with the birth of healthy carrier foals. Abortions and neonatal piroplasmosis may occur subsequent to transplacental transmission of *T. equi*

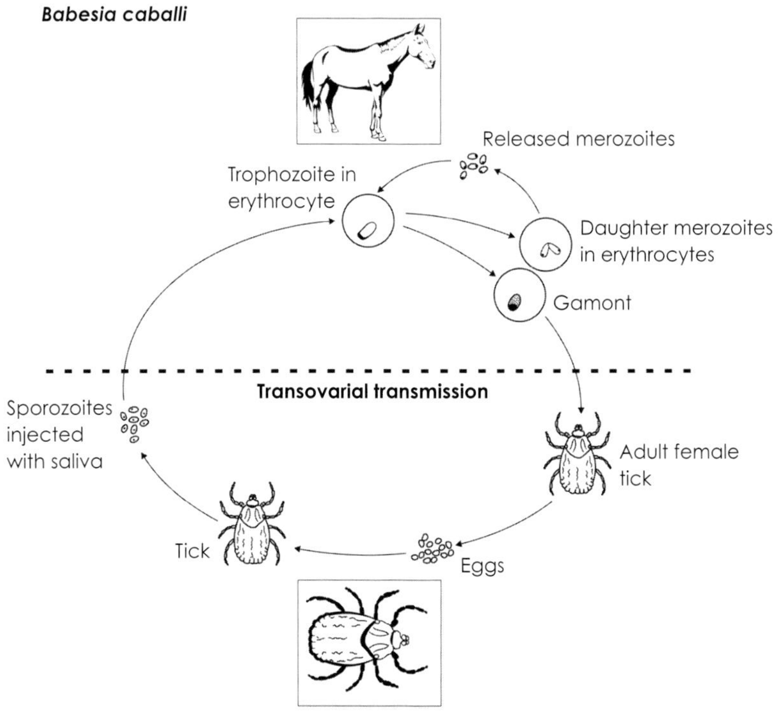

FIGURE 2: The life cycle of Babesia caballi.

when the number of parasites infecting the fetus is high. In naturally occurring *T. equi* abortions and neonatal piroplasmosis, parasitaemias of >50% of red blood cells infected with parasites are frequently observed (Allsopp *et al.* 2007).

Immunity

Following acute infection, the continued presence of the organism in red blood cells confers a level of active immunity from acute disease; premunity. Foals born of pre-immune mares (carrier mares with an active immunity) are naïve at birth but acquire passive immunity through colostrum with antibodies for *T. equi* and *B. caballi* lasting 1–5 months (de Waal 1995; Heuchert *et al.* 1999). Foals may be protected from piroplasmosis infection by passively acquired and nonspecific factors during the first 6–9 months of life. Such foals will develop immunity without developing clinical disease (de Waal and van Heerden 1994). After initial infection, a carrier state develops and this low grade persistent infection maintains the immunity protecting the animal from further clinical disease with re-infection. Relapses of *T. equi* infection may occur when these equids are exposed to stressful situations including concurrent disease such as African horse sickness, strenuous exercise, and emergency or elective surgeries. There is no cross immunity between *B. caballi* and *T. equi* (Mehlhorn and Schein 1998) and horses may carry a mixed infection of *T. equi* and *B. caballi* (Boldbaatar *et al.* 2005; Heim *et al.* 2007).

Pathogenesis

The pathogenesis of equine piroplasmosis is not well described, but may consist of both a haemolytic process leading to anaemia and an inflammatory process, as described in canine babesiosis (Matijatko *et al.* 2007). The haemolytic anaemia may be caused by direct red cell damage with intraerythrocytic multiplication, and immune mediated haemolysis with autoantibodies directed against the membranes of infected and uninfected erythrocytes leading to extra- and intravascular haemolysis (Boozer and Macintire 2003).

Clinical signs

Clinical disease is usually as a result of *T. equi* infection. When *B. caballi* is responsible for clinical disease the signs are milder. Clinical cases may occur throughout the year in endemic areas, although most cases are seen during the warmer summer months when the activity of the tick vectors is at its peak. The incubation period varies from 5–30 days; 12–19 days for *T. equi* and 10–30 days for *B. caballi*.

Horses with acute *T. equi* infection usually have a fever (40–42°C), depression and reduced appetite leading to weight loss. Signs of haemolytic anaemia including pale to icteric mucous membranes, tachycardia, tachypnoea, systolic heart murmur, weakness, haemoglobinuria or bilirubinuria may be evident. Petechiation or ecchymosis, most notable on the third eyelid, is usually present. Horses may show signs of mild colic including pawing, looking at the flanks and lying down with constipation, decreased borborygmi and passage of small dry faeces. This may be followed by diarrhoea. Oedema of the distal limbs, head and eyelids can occur. Myalgia, asthaenia and back pain have also been reported (Zobba *et al.* 2008). Acute piroplasmosis may be fatal. A rare peracute form resulting in horses being found dead or moribund has been reported in South Africa (de Waal and van Heerden 1994).

Complications that can occur with *T. equi* infection include acute renal failure, disseminated intravascular coagulation (DIC), arrhythmias with myocardial damage, pulmonary oedema or pneumonia, immune mediated haemolytic anaemia, laminitis and temporary or permanent partial or complete loss in fertility in stallions (Diana *et al.* 2007). Neurological signs are rarely seen but have been reported in young foals with *T. equi* and high fever showing ataxia, trembling and tonic-clonic spasms (de Waal and van Heerden 1994).

A chronic form of piroplasmosis has been described leading to poor performance, decreased appetite, weight loss, anaemia and splenomegaly (de Waal and van Heerden 1994).

Transplacental infection of *T. equi* can cause abortions, still births or neonatal piroplasmosis. Eleven percent of abortions occurring in South Africa are due to *T. equi* (Lewis *et al.* 1999). Abortions usually occur in the last trimester and the carrier mares are usually clinically healthy at the time of abortion. Carrier mares can produce more than one infected fetus during their breeding life. Foals born with neonatal piroplasmosis have severe haemolysis with marked icterus and anaemia. The parasitaemias in these foals are high. Neonatal piroplasmosis is usually fatal. Some foals with neonatal babesiosis are apparently normal at birth, but develop symptoms only 2–3 days after birth (de Waal and van Heerden 1994; Allsopp *et al.* 2007).

Clinical signs noted after *B. caballi* infection include transient fever, icterus and reduced appetite (de Waal *et al.* 1987).

Clinicopathological findings that can occur with piroplasmosis include anaemia with decreased packed cell volume (PCV), decreased red blood cell count and decreased haemoglobin concentrations. The mean corpuscular haemoglobin (MCH) and mean corpuscular haemoglobin concentrations (MCHC) may be decreased and mean corpuscular volume (MCV) increased in *T. equi* with regenerative anaemia and more immature erythrocytes in circulation. Reticulocytes are not found in the peripheral blood of horses even with regenerative anaemia. Increases in MCH and MCHC may be seen with intravascular haemolysis. Thrombocytopenia is a common finding. The cause of the thrombocytopenia is not known but may involve sequestration of platelets within the spleen, immune-mediated destruction and local or systemic disseminated intravascular coagulation (DIC) (Boozer and Macintire 2003). Both leucopenia with neutropenia and leucocytosis can occur with acute piroplasmosis. Proteins may be increased with dehydration or decreased with hypoalbuminaemia. Mild to marked (7 g/l) increases in fibrinogen may occur (de Waal *et al.* 1987; Diana *et al.* 2007). Hyperbilirubinaemia from haemolysis is frequently seen. Increases and decreases in phosphorous have been reported. Liver enzymes including aspartate transaminase (AST), alkaline phosphatase (ALP) and gammaglutamyltransferase (GGT) may be elevated with anaemic hypoxia and centrilobular degeneration and necrosis of hepatocytes. Increases in creatine kinase (CK) and AST with muscle damage are also reported (de Waal and van Heerden 1994; Hailat *et al.* 1997; Camacho *et al.* 2005; Zobba *et al.* 2008). Increases in urea and creatinine may be from dehydration (Camacho *et al.* 2005). The increase in urea may be more marked than that of creatinine. This increase in urea may be from catabolism of lysed erythrocytes (Jacobson and Clark 1994).

Diagnosis

Diagnosis of clinical cases of acute piroplasmosis is made on by the identification of parasites within erythrocytes in Romanovsky-type stained blood such as Giemsa, Wright's or Diff-Quick (Kyroquick)[1]. As the parasitaemia may be low even in acute clinical disease, careful and thorough examination of the blood smear is required to confirm or exclude the diagnosis. *T. equi* trophozoites can be identified as predominantly oval, organisms up to 3 μm, while the merozoites usually occur as 4 piriform parasites, 1.5 μm long, in the characteristic Maltese cross formation (**Figs 3** and **4**). The percentage of erythrocytes parasitised is usually around 1–5% in clinically diseased animals, but may exceed 20%. *B. caballi* is the larger species. Trophozoites are usually oval or elliptical, with the pear-shaped merozoites occurring in pairs (**Fig 5**). The

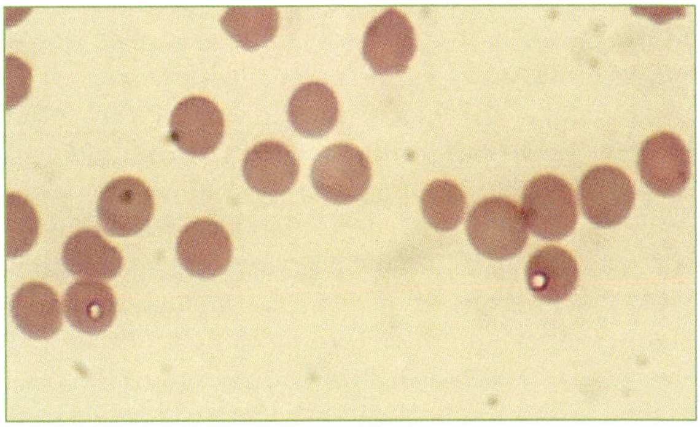

FIGURE 3: Trophozoites of T. equi in erythrocytes.

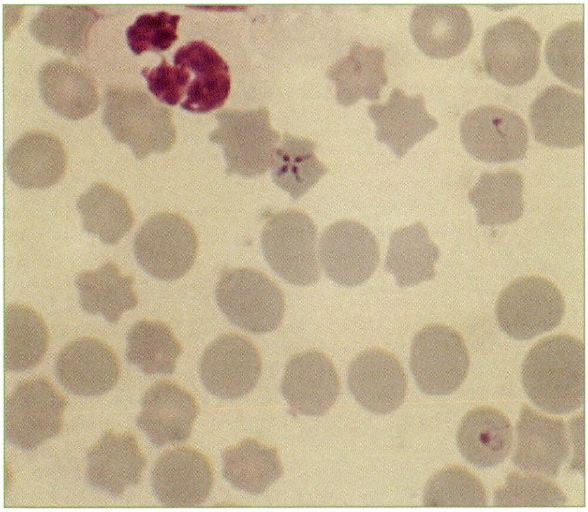

FIGURE 4: Trophozoites and merozoites in Maltese cross formation of T. equi.

percentage of erythrocytes parasitised is usually low, <0.1%. Thick blood smears can be used to increase the sensitivity of detection of parasitised erythrocytes (de Waal and van Heerden 1994).

In carrier animals, parasitaemias are too low for microscopic detection of infection. Serological testing is recommended for the detection of carrier animals. The indirect fluorescent antibody (IFA) and competition inhibition enzyme-linked immunosorbent assays (ELISAs) are the prescribed tests of the OIE for international trade. These tests have high concordance, and are more sensitive than the complement fixation test (CFT). Carrier animals, especially those that have recently been treated, may have false negative CFT titres, and still be infective to ticks (Tenter and Friedhoff 1986).

Polymerase chain reaction (PCR) assays are highly sensitive for the diagnosis of piroplasmosis, accurately differentiating between *T. equi* and *B. caballi* infections. PCR can be used for the detection of infection in clinically affected horses, carrier horses with low parasitaemias and in the tick vector (Battsetseg *et al.* 2002b).

Treatment

In endemic countries the aim of treating is to eliminate clinical signs, while in countries free of piroplasmosis chemosterilisation of infection is required. Sterilisation of infection in not warranted in endemic areas as the individual will lose premunity and become susceptible to re-infection. *T. equi* is more refractory to babesiacidal drugs than *Babesia caballi*. The drugs most commonly used for the treatment of piroplasmosis in horses are imidocarb and diminazene. Amicarbalide isothionate and euflavine that historically have been recommended for the treatment of babesiosis are no longer readily available (Vial and Gorenflot 2006). Tetracyclines have been used for the treatment of *T. equi* at 5–6 mg/kg bwt once a day i.v. for up to 7 days, but appear to be less effective than imidocarb (Zobba *et al.* 2008). Tetracyclines are not effective against *B. caballi*. Antitherilerial compounds including paravquone and buparvaquone may be effective against the parasitaemia of the initial infection, but fail to sterilise *T. equi* infections. Horses with marked tachycardia, tachypnoea, weakness, collapse or anaemia or PCV <15% may require blood transfusion. Fluid therapy should be given to dehydrated and hypovolaemic animals. Nonsteroidal anti-inflammatory drugs (NSAIDs) may be required in horses with prolonged pyrexia. Kidney function should be monitored and azotaemia addressed as renal failure is a concern in dehydrated horses with haemolytic anaemia and haemoglobinuria. Prolonged rest and adequate nutrition are required for horses recovering from anaemia.

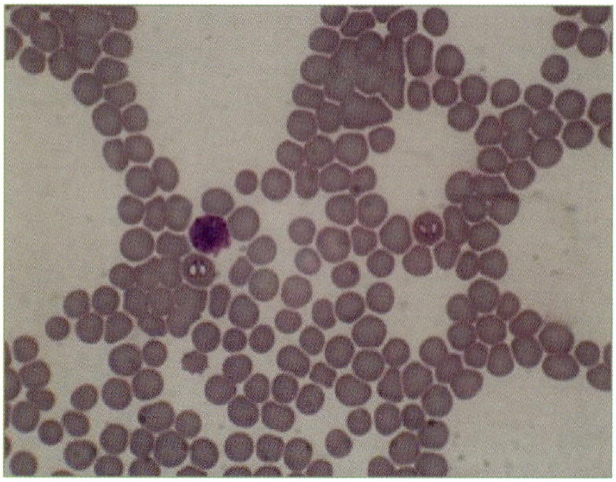

FIGURE 5: Pear-shaped merozoites of B. caballi.

Imidocarb is the most effective of the available therapeutic agents. A dose of 2.4 mg/kg bwt i.m. is recommended for the treatment of piroplasmosis. This dose may need to be repeated after 24 h for successful treatment of *T. equi. Imidocarb* causes a dose dependant hepatotoxicity and nephrotoxicity. Higher doses of 4 mg/kg bwt q. 72 h i.m. for 4 treatments in healthy horses had no detectable effect on liver function and a mild transient effect on renal function. However, clinical cases may have dehydration together with renal hypoxia, haemoglobinuria and altered drug disposition kinetics potentiating the negative effect of imidocarb (Meyer *et al.* 2005). It is important to ensure adequate hydration status in horses treated with imidocarb. A lower dose of 1.7 mg/kg bwt q. 24 h given twice recently proved very effective for the treatment of *T. equi* (Zobba *et al.* 2008). Donkeys are more susceptible to the toxic effects of imidocarb and a dose of 2 mg/kg bwt at q. 24 h for 4 treatments is lethal in donkeys (Frerichs *et al.* 1973). Imidocarb causes cholinesterase inhibition leading to signs of colic and diarrhoea. Pretreating with glycopyrrolate at 0.0025 mg/kg bwt i.v. will alleviate the colic signs without a detrimental inhibition of gastrointestinal motility. While atropine 0.2 mg/kg bwt i.v. may also be used to reduce these cholinergic effects, its prolonged effect on gastrointestinal motility is disadvantageous. Splitting the drug dose and administering half the drug dose at 30 min intervals, may also reduce these untoward effects. The diproprionate salt of imidocarb causes less muscle irritation than the dihydrochloride salt.

A dose of 2 mg/kg bwt imidocarb q. 24 h twice has been reported to be extremely effective in sterilisation of *B. caballi*, while imidocarb 4 mg/kg bwt q. 72 h for 4 treatments may sterilise *T. equi* infections. This drug regime is not always effective in the sterilisation of *T. equi* carrier state. It has been recently reported that higher doses of 4.7 mg/kg bwt q. 72 h for 5 treatments was not effective in eliminating either *B. caballi* or *T. equi* carrier states (Butler *et al.* 2008), demonstrating the importance of using sensitive diagnostic techniques such as PCR to ensure that negative carrier status is maintained.

Diminazene is an effective treatment of *T. equi* at a dose of 3.5 mg/kg bwt i.m. repeated after 48 h (Rashid *et al.* 2008), but does not lead to chemosterilisation of the infection. Diminazene is only 50–70% effective after one dose, with increasing effectivity of 80–90% when a second dose is administered after 48 h. Diminazene aceturate is more effective than diminazene diaceturate. Diminazene may cause severe muscle irritation or abscess development at the site of injection with diminazene diaceturate being more irritant than diminazene aceturate. The myonecrosis can be reduced by subdividing the dose and administering it at more than one intramuscular site (Rashid *et al.* 2008).

Control

There is no vaccine currently available. Contact between the tick vector and the equine host should be eliminated by regular application of an acaricide specifically concentrating on the back of the pasterns, inner thighs, udder, prepuce, perianal area and umbilical regions. However, keep in mind that foals need a certain amount of tick exposure to allow them to develop immunity early in life in enzootic areas.

There is the risk of introducing piroplasmosis into disease free countries with the international movement of infected horses. Disease-free countries have populations of horses that are presumably susceptible to infection and may have tick vectors or a climate suitable for foreign tick vectors capable of transmitting *T. equi* and *B. caballi*. Countries that restrict the entrance of horses that are serologically positive for piroplasmosis and require testing of animals for importation purposes include: Canada, USA, Hong Kong, Singapore, Malaysia, Australia and New Zealand.

In endemic countries, blood donors should be tested for equine piroplasmosis. In the recent outbreak in the USA the disease was spread by poor management practices including sharing of needles and not tick vectors. Good veterinary practices to prevent iatrogenic spread of piroplasmosis through hypodermic needles are of vital importance.

Manufacturer's address

[1]Kyroquick, Kyron laboratories, Johannesburg, South Africa.

References

Allsopp, M.T., Lewis, B.D. and Penzhorn, B.L. (2007) Molecular evidence for transplacental transmission of *Theileria equi* from carrier mares to their apparently healthy foals. *Vet. Parasitol.* **148**, 130-136.

Battsetseg, B., Lucero, S., Xuan, X., Claveria, F., Byambaa, B., Battur, B., Boldbaatar, D., Batsukh, Z., Khaliunaa, T., Battsetseg, G., Igarashi, I., Nagasawa, H. and Fujisaki, K. (2002a) Detection of equine *Babesia spp.* gene fragments in *Dermacentor nuttalli* Olenev 1929 infesting mongolian horses, and their amplification in egg and larval progenies. *J. vet. med. Sci.* **64**, 727-730.

Battsetseg, B., Lucero, S., Xuan, X., Claveria, F.G., Inoue, N., Alhassan, A., Kanno, T., Igarashi, I., Nagasawa, H., Mikami, T. and Fujisaki, K. (2002b) Detection of natural infection of *Boophilus microplus* with *Babesia equi* and *Babesia caballi* in Brazilian horses using nested polymerase chain reaction. *Vet. Parasitol.* **107**, 351-357.

Boldbaatar, D., Xuan, X., Battsetseg, B., Igarashi, I., Battur, B., Batsukh, Z., Bayambaa, B. and Fujisaki, K. (2005) Epidemiological study of equine piroplasmosis in Mongolia. *Vet. Parasitol.* **127**, 29-32.

Boozer, A.L. and Macintire, D.K. (2003) Canine babesiosis. *Vet. Clin. N. Am.: Small Anim. Pract.* **33**, 885-904, viii.

Butler, C.M., Nijhof, A.M., van der Kolk, J.H., de Haseth, O.B., Taoufik, A., Jongejan, F. and Houwers, D.J. (2008) Repeated high dose imidocarb dipropionate treatment did not eliminate *Babesia caballi* from naturally infected horses as determined by PCR-reverse line blot hybridization. *Vet. Parasitol.* **151**, 320-322.

Camacho, A.T., Guitian, F.J., Pallas, E., Gestal, J.J., Olmeda, A.S., Habela, M.A., Telford, S.R. 3rd and Spielman, A. (2005) *Theileria (Babesia) equi* and *Babesia caballi* infections in horses in Galicia, Spain. *Trop. anim. Health Prod.* **37**, 293-302.

de Waal, D.T. (1995) *Distribution, Transmission and Serodiagnosis of Babesia equi and Babesia caballi in South Africa.* PhD Thesis, Faculty of Veterinary Science, University of Pretoria, Pretoria, South Africa.

de Waal, D.T. and van Heerden, J. (1994) *Equine babesiosis. In: Infectious Diseases of Livestock with Special Reference to Southern Africa*, 1st edn., Eds: J.A.W. Coetzer, G.R. Thomson and R.C. Tustin, Oxford University Press, Cape Town. pp 295-304.

de Waal, D.T., van Heerden, J. and Potgieter, F.T. (1987) An investigation into the clinical pathological changes and serological response in horses experimentally infected with *Babesia equi* and *Babesia caballi. Onderstepoort J. vet. Res.* **54**, 561-568.

Diana, A., Guglielmini, C., Candini, D., Pietra, M. and Cipone, M. (2007) Cardiac arrhythmias associated with piroplasmosis in the horse: a case report. *Vet. J.* **174**, 193-195.

Frerichs, W.M., Allen, P.C. and Holbrook, A.A. (1973) Equine piroplasmosis (*Babesia equi*): therapeutic trials of imidocarb dihydrochloride in horses and donkeys. *Vet. Rec.* **93**, 73-75.

Friedhoff, K.T., Tenter, A.M. and Muller, I. (1990) Haemoparasites of equines: impact on international trade of horses. *Rev. Sci. Tech.* **9**, 1187-1194.

Hailat, N.Q., Lafi, S.Q., al-Darraji, A.M. and al-Ani, F.K. (1997) Equine babesiosis associated with strenuous exercise: clinical and pathological studies in Jordan. *Vet. Parasitol.* **69**, 1-8.

Heim, A., Passos, L.M., Ribeiro, M.F., Costa-Junior, L.M., Bastos, C. V., Cabral, D.D., Hirzmann, J. and Pfister, K. (2007) Detection and molecular characterization of *Babesia caballi* and *Theileria equi* isolates from endemic areas of Brazil. *Parasitol. Res.* **102**, 63-68.

Heuchert, C.M., de Giulli, V.,Jr, de Athaide, D.F., Bose, R. and Friedhoff, K.T. (1999) Seroepidemiologic studies on *Babesia equi* and *Babesia caballi* infections in Brazil. *Vet. Parasitol.* **85**, 1-11.

Ikadai, H., Sasaki, M., Ishida, H., Matsuu, A., Igarashi, I., Fujisaki, K. and Oyamada, T. (2007) Molecular evidence of *Babesia equi* transmission in *Haemaphysalis longicornis. Am. J. Trop. Med. Hyg.* **76**, 694-697.

Jacobson, L.S. and Clark, I.A. (1994) The pathophysiology of canine babesiosis: new approaches to an old puzzle. *J. S. Afr. vet. Ass.* **65**, 134-145.

Knowles, D.,Jr. (1996) Equine babesiosis (piroplasmosis): a problem in the international movement of horses. *Br. vet. J.* **152**, 123-126.

Lewis, B.D., Penzhorn, B.L. and Volkmann, D.H. (1999) Could treatment of pregnant mares prevent abortions due to equine piroplasmosis?. *J. S. Afr. vet. Ass.* **70**, 90-91.

Matijatko, V., Mrljak, V., Kis, I., Kucer, N., Forsek, J., Zivicnjak, T., Romic, Z., Simec, Z. and Ceron, J.J. (2007) Evidence of an acute phase response in dogs naturally infected with *Babesia canis. Vet. Parasitol.* **144**, 242-250.

Mehlhorn, H. and Schein, E. (1998) Redescription of *Babesia equi* Laveran, 1901 as *Theileria equi* Mehlhorn, Schein 1998. *Parasitol. Res.* **84**, 467-475.

Meyer, C., Guthrie, A.J. and Stevens, K.B. (2005) Clinical and clinicopathological changes in 6 healthy ponies following intramuscular administration of multiple doses of imidocarb dipropionate. *J. S. Afr. vet. Ass.* **76**, 26-32.

Rashid, H.B., Chaudhry, M., Rashid, H., Pervez, K., Khan, M.A. and Mahmood, A.K. (2008) Comparative efficacy of dimiazene diaceturate and diminazene aceturate for the treatment of babesiosis in horses. *Trop. anim. Health Prod.* **40**, 463-467.

Sevinc, F., Maden, M., Kumas, C., Sevinc, M. and Ekici, O.D. (2008) A comparative study on the prevalence of *Theileria equi* and *Babesia caballi* infections in horse sub-populations in Turkey. *Vet. Parasitol.* **156**, 173-177.

Stiller, D. and Coan, M.E. (1995) Recent developments in elucidating tick vector relationships for anaplasmosis and equine piroplasmosis. *Vet. Parasitol.* **57**, 97-108.

Tenter, A.M. and Friedhoff, K.T. (1986) Serodiagnosis of experimental and natural *Babesia equi* and *B. caballi* infections. *Vet. Parasitol.* **20**, 49-61.

Ueti, M.W., Palmer, G.H., Kappmeyer, L.S., Statdfield, M., Scoles, G. A. and Knowles, D.P. (2005) Ability of the vector tick *Boophilus microplus* to acquire and transmit *Babesia equi* following feeding on chronically infected horses with low-level parasitemia. *J. clin. Microbiol.* **43**, 3755-3759.

Uilenberg, G. (2006) Babesia-a historical overview. *Vet. Parasitol.* **138**, 3-10.

Vial, H.J. and Gorenflot, A. (2006) Chemotherapy against babesiosis. *Vet. Parasitol.* **138**, 147-160.

Zobba, R., Ardu, M., Niccoline, S., Chessa, B., Manna, L., Cocco, R. and Parpaglia, M.L.P. (2008) Clinical and laboratory findings in equine piroplasmosis. *J. equine vet. sci.* **28**, 301-308.

EQUINE GRANULOCYTIC EHRLICHIOSIS

N. Pusterla* and J. E. Madigan

The Department of Medicine and Epidemiology, School of Veterinary Medicine, University of California, Davis, California 95616, USA.

Keywords: horse; equine granulocytic ehrlichiosis; *Anaplasma phagocytophilum*

Summary

Equine granulocytic ehrlichiosis (EGE) is a rickettsial disease of horses first reported in the late 1960s in the foothills of California. The causative agent is *Anaplasma phagocytophilum*, a coccobacillary Gram-negative organism with a tropism for neutrophils. Clinical manifestations include fever, lethargy, anorexia, limb oedema and petechial haemorrhage. The vector of EGE is *Ixodes* spp. ticks. Diagnosis is based on awareness of geographic area for infection, typical clinical signs, abnormal laboratory findings, and visualising characteristic morulae in the cytoplasm of neutrophils and eosinophils in a peripheral blood smear. Treatment consists of the i.v. administration of oxytetracycline. The disease is being diagnosed with increasing frequency in the USA, Canada, Brazil and northern Europe.

Aetiology

Anaplasma phagocytophilum (formerly *Ehrlichia equi*) is the aetiological agent of equine granulocytic ehrlichiosis (EGE). *A. phagocytophilum* has recently been classified based on genetic analysis in the genera *Anaplasma*, along with *A. marginale*, which causes infectious anaemia in cattle by infecting erythrocytes, and *A. platys*, which causes canine cyclic thrombocytopenia by infecting platelets (Dumler *et al.* 2001). Because 16S rRNA gene sequences differ in only up to 3 bases (99.1% homology) among former *E. equi*, *E. phagocytophila* (cause of tick-borne fever in Europe) and the recently discovered human granulocytic ehrlichiosis (HGE) agent, these organisms are now all considered strains of *A. phagocytophilum*. Each of *E. equi*, *E. phagocytophila* and the HGE agent is also closely related on the basis of morphology, host cell tropism and antigen analysis by indirect fluorescent antibody tests (Dumler *et al.* 1995). The DNA sequences of the 16S rRNA gene from the peripheral blood of naturally infected horses in Connecticut and California are identical to that of the HGE agent (Madigan *et al.* 1996). Moreover, infective human blood from HGE patients injected into horses causes typical EGE, which can be transmitted to other horses. It induces protection in horses to subsequent challenge with *E. equi* (Barlough *et al.* 1995; Madigan *et al.* 1995). These data suggest that the agent of EGE and HGE are conspecific. *A. phagocytophilum* has been cultured *in vitro* using the tick-embryo cell line IDE8 and a human promyelocytic leukaemia cell line HL60 (Goodman *et al.* 1996; Munderloh *et al.* 1996).

A. phagocytophilum is found in membrane-lined vacuoles within the cytoplasm of infected eukaryotic host cells, primarily neutrophilic and eosinophilic granulocytes. These inclusion bodies consist of one or more coccoid or cocco-bacillary organisms approximately 0.2 µm in diameter to large granular aggregates called morulae, which are approximately 5 µm in diameter. Organisms are visible under high power, dry or oil emersion with light microscopy. They stain deep blue to pale blue grey with Giemsa or Wright-Leishman stains. By electron microscopy, several loosely packed ovoid to round *A. phagocytophilum* organisms are seen in several membrane-lined vacuoles of equine granulocytes. The size of vacuoles ranges from 1.5–5 µm in diameter.

Epidemiology

EGE occurs during late autumn, winter and spring. The horse represents an aberrant host and it seems unlikely that infected horses could serve as effective reservoirs of *A. phagocytophilum* since the presence of the organism in an affected animal is limited to the

*Author to whom correspondence should be addressed.

acute phase of the disease. Horses of any age are susceptible, but the clinical manifestations are less severe in horses aged <4 years (Madigan and Gribble 1987). Horses from endemic areas have a higher seroprevalence of antibody to *A. phagocytophilum* than horses from nonendemic areas, suggesting the occurrence of subclinical infection in some animals (Madigan *et al.* 1990). Further, horses introduced into an endemic area are more likely to develop EGE than native horses. Persistence of *A. phagocytophilum* has not been demonstrated in naturally or experimentally infected horses. The disease is not contagious, but infection can be transferred readily to susceptible horses with transfusion of as little as 20 ml of blood from horses with active infection. Most often, one infected horse is observed in a group of horses in the same pasture. The disease, first reported in the late 1960s in the foothills of northern California, has since been reported in horses in Washington, Oregon, New Jersey, New York, Colorado, Illinois, Minnesota, Connecticut, Florida and Wisconsin, and in Canada, Brazil, northern Europe, Japan, Korea and China.

In recent years, EGE has been experimentally transmitted by the western black-legged tick (*Ixodes pacificus*) and the deer tick (*I. scapularis*) (Reubel *et al.* 1998; Pusterla *et al.* 2002). Further, an epidemiological study in California showed that the spatial and temporal pattern of EGE cases closely paralleled the well-characterised life history and distribution of *I. pacificus*, but not other ticks commonly associated with horses (Vredevoe *et al.* 1999). In the east and midwest of the USA, *I. scapularis* is the vector of granulocytic ehrlichiosis and small rodents such as white-footed mice, chipmunks and voles, as well as the white-tailed deer, are potentially important reservoirs (Walls *et al.* 1997). In California, white-footed mice, dusky-footed wood rats, cervids, lizards and birds have been proposed as reservoirs (Castro *et al.* 2001; Foley *et al.* 2008). In Europe, where granulocytic ehrlichiosis is transmitted by the sheep tick (*Ixodes ricinus*), the reported reservoir hosts are wild rodents, deer and sheep (Ogden *et al.* 1998).

Pathogenesis

The pathogenesis of granulocytic ehrlichiosis is poorly understood. Clearly, after entering the dermis via tick bite inoculation and spread, presumably via lymphatics or blood, ehrlichiae invade target cells of the haematopoietic and lymphoreticular systems. The *in vivo* target cells of ehrlichiae are professional phagocytes, where they replicate within vacuoles of the host cell. Whether or how these granulocytic ehrlichiae directly injure cells is not known despite clear evidence of cytolytic activity *in vitro* (Goodman *et al.* 1996). Granulocytic ehrlichiae are suspected to initiate a cascade of localised pathological inflammatory events after invading organs such as spleen, liver and lungs. Subsequent tissue injury is thought to be mediated locally by accumulating inflammatory cells and systematically by induction of proinflammatory responses (Lepidi *et al.* 2000). The mechanism by which sufficient cells are removed to cause pancytopenia is unknown. However, the presence of normal cellularity or diffuse hyperplasia of bone marrow, combined with the presence of haemophagocytosis in spleen and lymph node, and the presence of infected granulocytes in spleen and lung support peripheral sequestration, consumption or destruction of normal blood elements as the major mechanisms for ehrlichia-induced pancytopenia (Lepidi *et al.* 2000).

Granulocytic ehrlichiosis caused by *A. phagocytophilum* is disease that triggers dysfunction or suppression of host defences. It is well established that horses infected with *A. phagocytophilum* are predisposed, like man and sheep, to develop opportunistic infections and secondary infections with bacteria, fungi and viruses (Gribble 1969). These animals develop defects in both humoural and T-cell-mediated immunity and abnormalities in normal neutrophil phagocytic and migratory functions (Garyu *et al.* 2005).

Immunological studies with *A. phagocytophilum* indicate both a cell-mediated and humoural immune response to clinical infection. Horses that recover from experimental infections develop humoural and cell-mediated immune responses by 21 days post infection (Artursson *et al.* 1999). In naturally infected horses, antibody titres peak 19–81 days after the onset of clinical signs. Immunity persists for at least 2 years and does not appear to be dependent on a latent infection or carrier status (Nyindo *et al.* 1978; van Andel *et al.* 1998).

Clinical findings

The prepatent period following experimental exposure of horses to infected ticks is 8–12 days and

3–10 days after needle inoculation of infectious blood. Inoculation period of the natural infection is believed to be <14 days. This is based on the time of onset of clinical signs in horses that had presumptive exposure to ticks while on a trail ride before returning to a nonendemic area for EGE.

The severity of clinical signs of EGE is a function of the age of the horse and the duration of the illness (Madigan and Gribble 1987). This can make clinical recognition of EGE difficult at the time of the first examination. Adult horses aged >4 years generally develop the characteristic progressive signs, which are fever, depression, partial anorexia, limb oedema, petechiation, icterus, ataxia and reluctance to move.

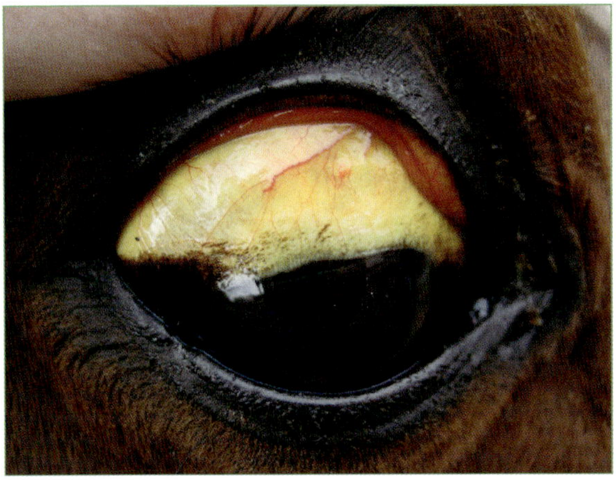

FIGURE 1: Horse infected with Anaplasma phagocytophilum *showing icteric sclera.*

Clinically and experimentally, it appears that horses aged <4 years tend to develop milder signs, including moderate fever, depression, moderate limb oedema and ataxia. In horses aged <1 year, clinical signs may be difficult to recognise, with only a fever present. During the first 1–2 days of infection, fever is generally high, fluctuating from 39.4–41.3°C. Initial clinical signs are reluctance to move, ataxia, depression, icterus (**Fig 1**) and mucosal petechiation (**Fig 2**). Weakness and ataxia can be severe to the point that horses will sustain fractures after falling. Staggering is seen commonly and the tendency to assume a base-wide stance leads one to suspect proprioceptive deficits. Partial anorexia develops in most cases. Limb oedema (**Fig 3**) and more severe signs of disease develop by Day 3–5, with fever and illness lasting 10–14 days in untreated horses. Heart rate is often modestly high (50–60 beats/min). Rarely, there is cardiac involvement with development of cardiac arrhythmias. Ventricular tachycardia and premature ventricular contractions have been observed with the usually recognised clinical signs. The clinical course of the disease ranges from 3–16 days. The disease is normally self-limiting in untreated horses; fatalities can occur due to secondary infection and to injury secondary to trauma caused by incoordination. Abortion has not been observed in pregnant mares nor has laminitis been a reported feature of the clinical syndrome.

The initial stage of the disease is characterised by the development of a fever and may be mistaken for

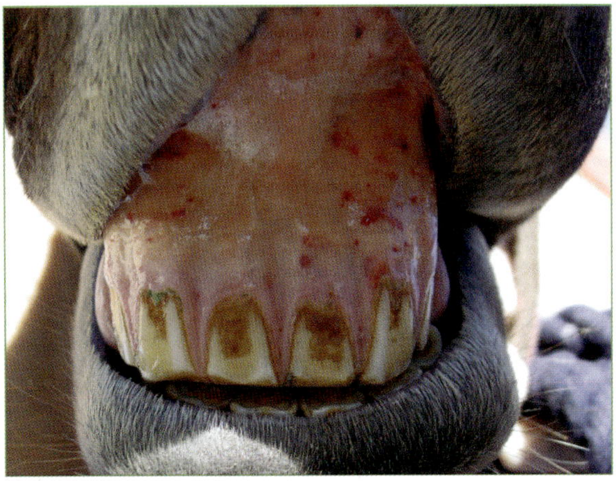

FIGURE 2: Horse infected with Anaplasma phagocytophilum *showing mucosal petechiation.*

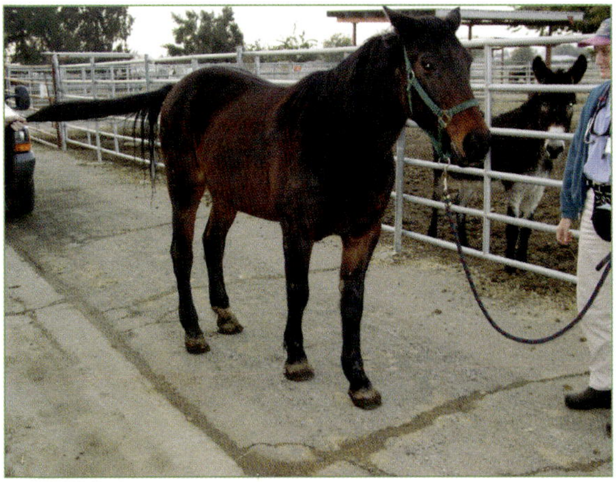

FIGURE 3: Horse infected with Anaplasma phagocytophilum *showing distal limb oedema.*

a viral infection. The differential diagnoses for EGE include purpura haemorrhagica, liver disease, equine infectious anaemia, equine viral arteritis and encephalitis.

Laboratory abnormalities in horses affected by EGE consist of leucopenia, thrombocytopenia, anaemia, icterus and characteristic inclusion bodies (morulae) in neutrophils and eosinophils. The morulae are pleomorphic, blue-grey to dark blue in colour, and often have a spoke-wheel appearance.

Diagnosis

Diagnosis is based on awareness of geographic areas for infection, typical clinical signs, abnormal laboratory findings and visualising characteristic morulae in the cytoplasm of neutrophils and eosinophils in a peripheral blood smear stained with Giemsa or Wright stain (**Fig 4**). Because affected horses are leucopenic, a greater percentage of neutrophils can be examined by use of the buffy coat preparation and subsequent staining. The number of cells containing morulae varies from <1% of cells initially, to 20–50% of the neutrophils by Day 3–5 of infection. However, >3 ehrlichial inclusion bodies need to be seen on a blood smear to consider the diagnosis definitive. Culture is rarely attempted for horses infected with *A. phagocytophilum*. Alternatively, an indirect fluorescent antibody test is available, and paired titre testing with a significant (≥4-fold) rise in antibody titre to *A. phagocytophilum* can be performed to retrospectively confirm recent exposure (Madigan *et al.* 1990). However, because inclusion bodies are always visible during the mid-stage of the febrile period, antibody testing is not usually required to make a definitive diagnosis. Recently, several polymerase chain reaction (PCR) assays have been developed for members of the *A. phagocytophilum* genogroup and are found to be highly sensitive and specific (Barlough *et al.* 1996; Pusterla *et al.* 1999). The detection through PCR analysis is useful for the diagnosis of EGE, particularly during early and late stages, when the number of organisms may be too small for diagnosis by microscopy.

Pathological findings

The characteristic gross lesions observed in experimentally infected horses are haemorrhages, usually petechiae and ecchymoses, and oedema. Oedema is found in the legs, ventral abdominal wall and prepuce. Haemorrhages are most common in the subcutaneous tissues, fascia and epimysium of the distal limbs. Histologically, there is inflammation of the small arteries and veins primarily those in the subcutis, fascia and nerves of the legs, and in the ovaries, testes and pampiniform plexus (Gribble 1969). Vascular lesions may be proliferative and necrotising, with swelling of the endothelial and smooth muscle cells, cellular thromboses, and perivascular accumulations primarily of monocytes and lymphocytes, and to a lesser extent of neutrophils and eosinophils. Mild inflammatory vascular or interstitial lesions have also been reported in the kidneys, heart, brain and lungs of animals necropsied during the course of the disease (Lepidi *et al.* 2000). The ventricular tachycardia and premature ventricular contractions occasionally observed in affected horses are thought to be associated with myocardial vasculitis. Further, horses with a chronic bacterial infection may develop an exacerbation of the pre-existing lesion (bronchopneumonia, arthritis, pericarditis, lymphadenitis, cellulitis) (Gribble 1969).

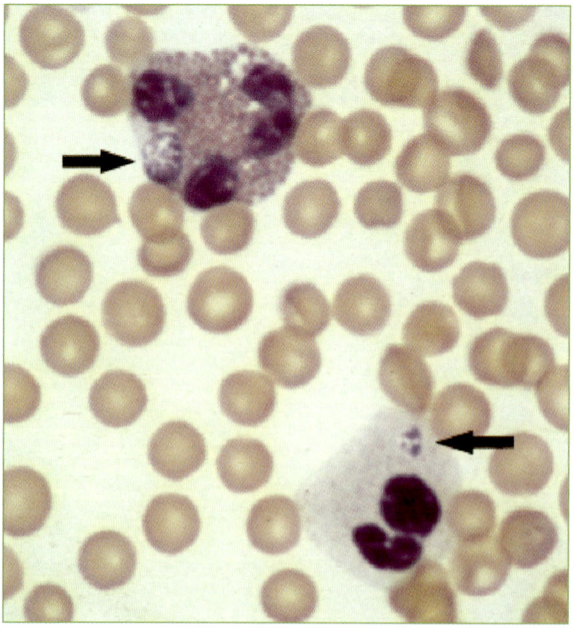

*FIGURE 4: **Anaplasma phagocytophilum** inclusions (arrow) in a neutrophilic and an eosinophilic granulocyte of a horse with EGE (buffy coat smear, Giemsa stain, magnification x1000).*

Therapy

The i.v. administration of oxytetracycline at a rate of 7 mg/kg bwt once daily for 5–7 days has been an effective treatment for EGE (Madigan and Gribble 1987). Prompt improvement in clinical appearance and appetite and drop in fever are noticed within 12 h of treatment. Indeed a failure of defervescence within 24 h would strongly point to another cause for illness. On rare occasions, horses treated for <7 days relapse within the following 30 days. When untreated, the disease can be self-limiting in 2–3 weeks when no concurrent infection is present, but weight loss, oedema, and ataxia are of increased severity and duration. In treated horses, ataxia will persist for 2–3 days, and limb oedema may persist for several days. Inclusion bodies generally are difficult to find after the first day of treatment and are no longer present within 48–72 h. Supportive measures are recommended in severe cases, including fluid and electrolyte therapy, supportive limb wraps, and stall confinement of severely ataxic horses in order to prevent secondary injury. The prognosis in EGE is considered excellent in uncomplicated cases. This is in sharp contrast to some of the other diseases on the list of differential diagnostic considerations.

Prevention

At present, there is no vaccine available against EGE and so, prevention is limited to the practice of tick control measures, such as the use of permethrin repellant products (Blagburn *et al.* 2004).

Acknowledgement

This article was published in a similar form as Madigan, J.E. and Pusterla, N. (2000) Ehrlichial diseases. *Veterinary Clinics of North America: Equine Practice,* **16**, 487-499, Copyright Elsevier (2000).

References

Artursson, K., Gunnarsson, A., Wikstrom, U.B. and Engvall, E.O. (1999) A serological and clinical follow-up in horses with confirmed equine granulocytic ehrlichiosis. *Equine vet. J.* **31**, 473-477.

Barlough, J.E., Madigan, J.E., DeRock, E., Dumler, J.S. and Bakken, J.S. (1995) Protection against *Ehrlichia equi* is conferred by prior infection with the human granulocytotropic *Ehrlichia* (HGE agent). *J. clin. Microbiol.* **33**, 3333-3334.

Barlough, J.E., Madigan, J.E., DeRock, E. and Bigornia, L. (1996) Nested polymerase chain reaction for detection of *Ehrlichia equi* genomic DNA in horses and ticks (*Ixodes pacificus*). *Vet. Parasitol.* **63**, 319-329.

Blagburn, B.L., Spencer, J.A., Billeter, S.A., Drazenovich, N.L., Butler, J.M., Land, T.M., Dykstra, C.C., Stafford, K.C., Pough, M.B., Levy, S.A. and Bledsoe D.L. (2004) Use of imidacloprid-permethrin to prevent transmission of *Anaplasma phagocytophilum* from naturally infected *Ixodes scapularis* ticks to dogs. *Vet. Ther.* **5**, 212-217.

Castro, M.B., Nicholson, W.L., Kramer, V.L. and Childs, J.E. (2001) Persistent infection in *Neotoma fuscipes* (Muridae: Sigmodontinae) with *Ehrlichia phagocytophila* sensu lato. *Am. J. Trop. Med. Hyg.* **65**, 261-267.

Dumler, J.S., Asanovich, K.M., Bakken, J.S., Richter, P., Kimsey, R., and Madigan, J. (1995) Serologic cross-reactions among *Ehrlichia equi*, *Ehrlichia phagocytophila*, and human granulocytic *Ehrlichia*. *J. clin. Microbiol.* **33**, 1098-1103.

Dumler, J.S., Barbet, A.F., Bekker, C.P., Dasch, G.A., Palmer, G.H., Ray, S.C., Rikihisa, Y. and Rurangirwa, F.R. (2001) Reorganization of genera in the families *Rickettsiaceae* and *Anaplasmataceae* in the order Rickettsiales: unification of some species of *Ehrlichia* with *Anaplasma*, *Cowdria* with *Ehrlichia* and *Ehrlichia* with *Neorickettsia*, descriptions of six new species combinations and designation of *Ehrlichia equi* and 'HGE agent' as subjective synonyms of *Ehrlichia phagocytophila*. *Int. J. Syst. Evol. Microbiol.* **51**, 2145-2165.

Foley, J.E., Clueit, S.B. and Brown, R.N. (2008) Differential exposure to *Anaplasma phagocytophilum* in rodent species in northern California. *Vector Borne Zoonotic Dis.* **8**, 49-55.

Garyu, J.W., Choi, K.S., Grab, D.J. and Dumler, J.S. (2005) Defective phagocytosis in *Anaplasma phagocytophilum*-infected neutrophils. *Infect. Immun.* **73**, 1187-1190.

Goodman, J.L., Nelson, C., Vitale, B., Madigan, J.E., Dumler, J.S., Kurtti, T.J. and Munderloh, U.G. (1996) Direct cultivation of the causative agent of human granulocytic ehrlichiosis. *N. Engl. J. Med.* **334**, 209-215.

Gribble, D.H. (1969) Equine ehrlichiosis. *J. Am. vet. med. Ass.* **155**, 462-469.

Lepidi, H., Bunnell, J.E., Martin, M.E., Madigan, J.E., Stuen, S. and Dumler J.S. (2000) Comparative pathology, and immunohistology associated with clinical illness after *Ehrlichia phagocytophila*-group infections. *Am. J. Trop. Med. Hyg.* **62**, 29-37.

Madigan, J.E. and Gribble, D.H. (1987) Equine ehrlichiosis in northern California: 49 cases (1968-1981). *J. Am. vet. med. Ass.* **90**, 445-448.

Madigan, J.E., Hietala, S., Chalmers, S. and DeRock, E. (1990) Seroepidemiologic survey of antibodies to *Ehrlichia equi* in horses of northern California. *J. Am. vet. med. Ass.* **196**, 1962-1964.

Madigan, J.E., Richter, P.J., Kimsey, R.B., Barlough, J.E., Bakken, J.S. and Dumler, J.S. (1995) Transmission and passage in horses of the agent of human granulocytic ehrlichiosis. *J. Infect. Dis.* **172**, 1141-1144.

Madigan, J.E., Barlough, J.E., Dumler, J.S., Schankman, N.S. and DeRock, E. (1996) Equine granulocytic ehrlichiosis in Connecticut caused by an agent resembling the human granulocytic ehrlichiosis. *J. clin. Microbiol.* **34**, 434-435.

Munderloh, U.G., Madigan, J.E., Dumler, J.S., Goodman, J.L., Hayes, S.F., Barlough, J.E., Nelson, C.M. and Kurtti, T.J. (1996) Isolation of the equine granulocytic ehrlichiosis agent, *Ehrlichia equi*, in tick cell culture. *J. clin. Microbiol.* **34**, 664-670.

Nyindo, M.B., Ristic, M., Lewis, G.E. Jr, Huxsoll, D.L. and Stephenson, E.H. (1978) Immune response of ponies to experimental infection with *Ehrlichia equi*. *Am. J. vet. Res.* **39**, 15-18.

Ogden, N.H., Woldehiwet, Z. and Hart, C.A. (1998) Granulocytic ehrlichiosis: an emerging or rediscovered tick-borne disease. *J. Med. Microbiol.* **47**, 475-482.

Pusterla, N., Huder, J.B., Leutenegger, C.M., Braun, U., Madigan, J.E. and Lutz, H. (1999) Quantitative real-time PCR for detection of members of the *Ehrlichia phagocytophila* genogroup in host animals and *Ixodes ricinus* ticks. *J. clin. Microbiol.* **37**, 1329-1331.

Pusterla, N., Chae, J.S., Kimsey, R.B., Berger Pusterla, J., DeRock, E., Dumler, J.S. and Madigan, J.E. (2002) Transmission of *Anaplasma phagocytophila* (human granulocytic ehrlichiosis agent) in horses using experimentally infected ticks (*Ixodes scapularis*). *J. Vet. Med. B* **49**, 484-488.

Reubel, G.H., Kimsey, R.B., Barlough, J.E. and Madigan, J.E. (1998) Experimental transmission of *Ehrlichia equi* to horses through naturally infected ticks (*Ixodes pacificus*) from northern California. *J. clin. Microbiol.* **36**, 2131-2134.

Van Andel, A.E., Magnarelli, L.A., Heimer, R. and Wilson, M.L. (1998) Development and duration of antibody response against *Ehrlichia equi* in horses. *J. Am. vet. med. Ass.* **212**, 1910-1914.

Vredevoe, L.K., Richter, P.J., Madigan, J.E. and Kimsey, R.B. (1999) Association of *Ixodes pacificus* (Acari: Ixodidae) with the spatial and temporal distribution of *equine granulocytic ehrlichiosis* in California. *J. Med. Entomol.* **36**, 551-561.

Walls, J.J., Greig, B., Neitzel, D.F. and Dumler, J.S. (1997) Natural infection of small mammal species in Minnesota with the agent of human granulocytic ehrlichiosis. *J. clin. Microbiol.* **35**, 853-855.

CRYPTOSPORIDIOSIS

T. S. Mair*, N. D. Cohen† and G. R. Pearson‡

Bell Equine Veterinary Clinic, Mereworth, Maidstone, Kent ME18 5GS, UK; †Department of Large Animal Clinical Sciences, College of Veterinary Medicine and Biomedical Sciences, Texas A&M University, College Station, Texas 77843-4475, USA; and ‡Department of Clinical Veterinary Science, School of Veterinary Science, Bristol University, Langford House, Langford, Bristol BS40 5DU, UK.

Keywords: horse; coccidia; *Cryptosporidium parvum*; cryptosporidiosis; zoonosis; diarrhoea

Summary

Cryptosporidium parvum is a coccidian parasite that infects the microvilli of intestinal epithelial cells. Strains that infect horses and cattle can also infect man, and therefore cryptosporidiosis is a zoonotic disease. In horses, cryptosporidiosis is most commonly seen in foals (most frequently 1–4 weeks of age) and is associated with diarrhoea and weight loss. Immunocompromised foals (including foals with severe combined immunodeficiency syndrome) are particularly at risk.

Introduction

Cryptosporidium is increasingly gaining attention as a human and an animal pathogen mainly due to its dominant involvement in worldwide waterborne outbreaks (Grinberg *et al.* 2003; Karanis *et al.* 2007; Smith *et al.* 2007). Diarrhoea in horses, primarily foals, caused by *Cryptosporidium parvum* is also being increasingly recognised (Xiao and Herd 1994; Cohen 2002; Sellon 2007). *C. parvum* infects the microvilli of intestinal epithelial cells in many domestic and wild animal species. Strains that infect calves, horses and man are cross-transmissible (Moon and Woodmansee 1986; Hajdusek *et al.* 2004; Chalmers *et al.* 2005; Grinberg *et al.* 2008). Cryptosporidiosis is therefore a zoonotic disease (Levine *et al.* 1988).

Aetiology

The genus *Cryptosporidium* belongs to the phylum *Apicomplexa* and currently comprises 16 valid species: *C. andersoni*, *C. baileyi*, *C. bovis*, *C. canis*, *C. felis*, *C. galli*, *C. hominis*, *C. meleagridis*, *C. molnari*, *C. muris*, *C. parvum*, *C. saurophilum*, *C. scophthalmi*, *C. serpentis*, *C. suis* and *C. wrairi* (Xiao *et al.* 2004; Sunnotel *et al.* 2006). *C. hominis* (formerly known as the *C. parvum* human genotype or genotype I) almost exclusively infects man, while *C. parvum* (formerly known as the *C. parvum* bovine genotype or genotype II) infects man, ruminants and other animal species (Morgan-Ryan *et al.* 2002). It is classically known to be responsible for the majority of the zoonotic cryptosporidial infections. More recently, other species including *C. meleagridis*, *C. suis*, *C. felis* and *C. canis* have been detected in man, which emphasises the risk posed due to the zoonotic transmission of the parasite (Xiao *et al.* 2001, 2004; Cama *et al.* 2007; Llorente *et al.* 2007).

Although classically described as 'unusual' or 'unique' coccidia, *Cryptosporidium* species are probably better considered as a distantly related lineage of apicomplexan parasites that are not in fact coccidia but that do occupy many of the same ecological niches (Barta and Thompson 2006).

Epidemiology

The prevalence of cryptosporidiosis in horses in different geographical locations is poorly documented. Prevalence varies with the method of detection used and the population studied. The prevalence of faecal shedding of oocysts by horses is low (Reinemeyer *et al.* 1984; Coleman *et al.* 1989; Olson *et al.* 1997; Cole *et al.* 1998; Atwill *et al.* 2000; Majewska *et al.* 2004; Chalmers *et al.* 2005; Bakheit *et al.* 2008). In contrast, a serological survey in the UK indicated that 20 of 22 horses (91%) were seropositive, suggesting that sub-

*Author to whom correspondence should be addressed.

clinical infection may be common (Tzipori and Campbell 1981). In another study, the prevalence of faecal shedding of *C. parvum* oocysts in 152 horses in Texas was found to be 8.5% (Cole *et al.* 1998). Specific risk factors for faecal shedding in this study included residence on specific breeding farms, age <6 months and a history of diarrhoea within the preceding 30 days. Prevalence may be 100% among diarrhoeic foals at farms during an outbreak.

Horses become infected by ingesting infective *C. parvum* oocysts. Transmission occurs either via the faecal-oral route or by ingestion of contaminated food or water. In people, contaminated water supplies are an important source of infection (Smith *et al.* 2006), and a similar route may be important in horses. Three features of *Cryptosporidia* ensure a high level of environmental contamination and enhance the likelihood of waterborne transmission. Firstly, they are responsible for disease in a broad range of hosts including man, and have a low infectious dose enhancing the possibility of zoonotic transmission. Secondly, their transmissive stages are small in size and environmentally robust. Thirdly, they are insensitive to the disinfectants commonly used in the water industry (Smith and Nichols 2006). The oocyst stage can remain infective under cool, moist conditions for many months, especially where water temperatures in rivers, lakes, and ponds remain low but above freezing (Frayer 2004). Exposure of foals to cattle and adult horses was not found to be a risk factor for cryptosporidiosis (Cole *et al.* 1998). Likewise, there is little evidence to suggest that mares are an important source of infection of their foals, although infection of calves from their dams at birth has been reported (Pearson and Logan 1978). Inapparently-infected foals may represent a source of infection for other foals.

Pathogenesis

Unlike typical coccidia, *Cryptosporidium* oocysts are sporulated and infectious from the time they are excreted into the faeces (Huang and White 2006). The oocysts exsheath and sporozoites are released during passage through the gastrointestinal tract, allowing infection of enterocytes. Cryptosporidia develop at the apical surfaces of gastrointestinal epithelial cells, beneath the cell membrane, but separate from the host cell cytoplasm (intracellular but extracytoplasmic) (Marcial and Madara 1986) (**Fig 1**). They are closely associated with the

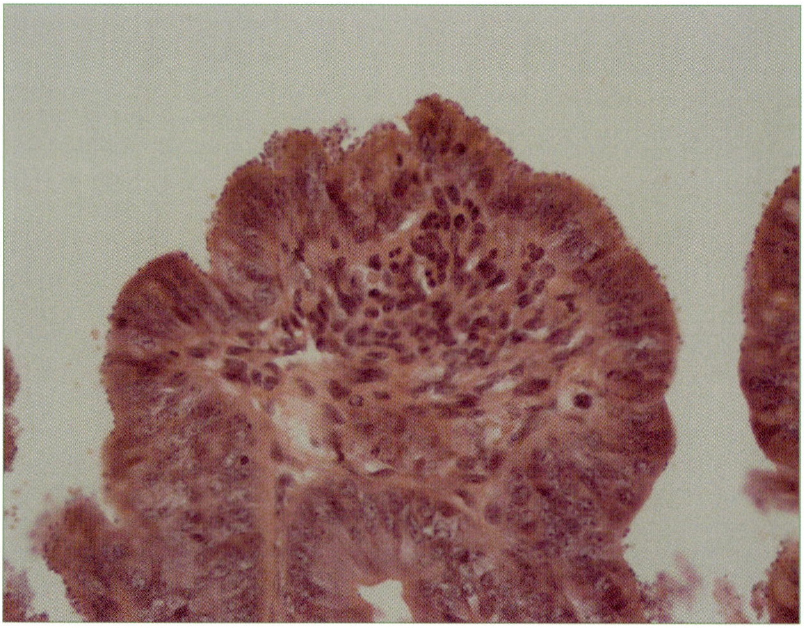

FIGURE 1: Photomicrograph of the small intestine of a foal with cryptosporidiosis. Tip of a villus with attached cryptosoridia on the surface of epithelial cells. Haematoxylin and eosin.

microvillous border of the epithelial cells (Levine 1973; Pearson and Logan 1978, 1983). They damage the intestinal microvilli, resulting in malabsorption, maldigestion and diarrhoea. Amplification occurs through asexual and sexual multiplication. Oocysts are formed that are capable of autoinfection prior to excretion (thin-walled oocysts) or that are immediately infectious when shed in faeces (thick-walled oocysts) (Moon and Woodmansee 1986). In foals with severe combined immunodeficiency, sites other than the small intestine may be infected, including the stomach, common bile duct, colon and pancreatic ducts (Field 2002).

The severity of clinical signs may be related to agent factors (inoculum size, virulence), host factors (age, immunocompetence), and environmental factors (water source, housing practices).

Clinical signs

In horses, clinical disease due to cryptosporidiosis is most commonly reported in foals, particularly from 1–4 weeks of age, although cryptosporidial diarrhoea has occasionally been diagnosed in younger foals (at age 2 days) and in weanlings and yearlings (Netherwood *et al.* 1996). The relatively naïve or immature immune system of newborn foals is likely a predisposing factor for cryptosporidiosis. Cryptosporidial diarrhoea is rare in mature horses; however, subclinical infection is probably common in both healthy foals and adult horses (Cohen and Snowden 1996). The incubation period of cryptosporidiosis is 3–7 days. The clinical features include persistent diarrhoea, with associated dehydration, weakness and death in some cases if untreated (Grinberg *et al.* 2003). Clinical signs usually persist for 5 to 14 days (Mayhew and Greiner 1986), but in older foals (i.e. 3–6 months) the diarrhoea may be more chronic and persist until the foals are aged 9–12 months. Reports of *Cryptosporidium* oocyst shedding in adult horses with diarrhoea are rare (McKenzie and Diffay 2000).

Cryptosporidiosis has been recognised in foals that are hospitalised for other problems, suggesting that the stress of hospitalisation and other disease can predispose them to develop clinical disease. Cryptosporidiosis is also common in foals with severe combined immunodeficiency syndrome (Snyder *et al.* 1978; Gibson *et al.* 1983; Mair *et al.* 1990). Although the disease will generally be more severe in immunocompromised foals, severe or fatal diarrhoea can also occur in immunocompetent foals. Concurrent infection with other enteropathogens (including *Salmonella spp*, *rotavirus*, *coronavirus*, *adenovirus*) can occur, particularly in immunocompromised animals (Mair *et al.* 1990).

Some farms experience epidemics of cryptosporidial diarrhoea, although recurrence during subsequent years is rare. A high density of foals, a municipal water source, foaling in stalls (vs. pasture), and poor hygiene may be risk factors for infection and disease (Cohen 2002).

Diagnosis

Diagnosis is based on the detection of oocytes in the faeces. However, *C. parvum* oocysts are small (4–5 μm in diameter) and are difficult to identify by light microscopy using routine faecal parasitological examinations. Faecal samples should be submitted as fresh material or in recommended preservative (10% formalin or sodium acetate-acetic acid-formalin). Oocysts can be detected using either concentration or staining techniques. Concentration of oocysts may be accomplished by flotation or sedimentation. Regardless of technique, distinguishing oocysts from yeast is an important diagnostic issue.

A number of different diagnostic techniques are available, and include:

- Flotation of oocysts
- Acid-fast staining of oocysts (Cole *et al.* 1999)
- Detection of oocysts using an immunofluorescence assay (IFA) (Cole *et al.* 1999)
- Flow cytometery (Cole *et al.* 1999)
- ELISA (Werner *et al.* 2004)
- PCR and loop-mediated isothermal amplification of DNA (LAMP) (Bakheit *et al.* 2008).

Sedimentation techniques are rarely used. Of the flotation techniques used, flotation in Sheather's sugar solution is most common. Prompt processing is important because oocysts collapse and lose their spherical shape when left in Sheather's sugar solution.

Acid-fast staining of faecal specimens is widely used for detection of *C. parvum*. The organisms appear as red spheres (4–6 mm in diameter) against a dark, counter-stained background, while yeasts generally do not appear red. The technique has relatively poor specificity making it a poor choice as a screening test. However, it is useful clinically as a diagnostic test because of its good sensitivity, availability and low cost.

The IFA test has relatively low sensitivity but excellent specificity. A commercial immunofluorescence assay is available[1] that simultaneously detects cryptosporidial and giardial organisms. The high cost relative to staining techniques and specialised microscopic equipment needed are limitations of the IFA. To date, reliable enzyme-linked immunosorbent assays have not been developed and validated for detecting *C. parvum* in samples from horses. Flow cytometric methods are more sensitive than IFA or acid-fast staining, but are not widely available.

The pattern of oocyst shedding by foals is variable in duration (from days to many weeks) and can be intermittent. Shedding may be antecedent, concurrent or subsequent to the onset of diarrhoea. In view of the variable duration and the intermittent pattern of shedding, multiple samples (at least 3) should be submitted for detecting *C. parvum* in faeces from foals. It may be easier to detect oocysts in unformed than formed faeces.

Treatment

Although numerous different treatments have been tested in a variety of animals, to date no specific chemotherapy or immunotherapy has been proven to be convincingly effective for treating *C. parvum* in people and other mammals, and none has been evaluated in a controlled clinical trial among foals (Cohen 2002). In man, the most commonly used drugs for the treatment of cryptosporidiosis include paromycin, nitazoxanide and azithromycin (Farthing 2006; Gargala 2008). A recent study of the prophylactic and therapeutic use of nitazoxanide in calves did not show the expected positive effect on the course of the *Cryptosporidium* infection, neither on reducing the clinical severity, nor on oocyst excretion (Schnyder *et al.* 2008). Those treatments that may have greatest potential for use in foals include paromomycin and bovine colostrum.

Paromomycin is an aminoglycoside antibiotic that is poorly absorbed from the gastrointestinal tract. Paromomycin reduced the duration and severity of diarrhoea and eliminated oocyst shedding in neonatal calves experimentally infected with *C. parvum*. Doses used in calves have ranged from 50–100 mg/kg bwt administered orally once or twice daily. No data exist for the use of this drug in foals. Adverse effects of paromomycin in man include diarrhoea, nausea and abdominal cramps. As for all other agents used to treat cryptosporidial infection, experimental and clinical evidence also exists indicating a lack of effectiveness of paromomycin. No antibiotic approved for use in horses has been demonstrated to be effective in the treatment of cryptosporidial diarrhoea.

Hyperimmune bovine colostrum has been used with varying success as a means of prophylaxis and therapy of cryptosporidiosis in animals and patients with AIDS. A factor limiting the use of hyperimmune bovine colostrum is its availability. Pooled bovine colostrum, however, is more readily available. Pooled bovine colostrum from nonimmunised animals also may be protective in controlling cryptosporidiosis; non-immunoglobulin factors in the colostrum may provide protection. Use of hyperimmune or pooled bovine colostrum has not been uniformly successful (Cohen 2002). The benefits of administration of colostrum or hyperimmune colostrum to foals, regardless of their age, with cryptosporidiosis are unknown.

Treatment of foals with severe combined immunodeficiency is likely to be unsuccessful. In immunocompetent foals, infection is often subclinical or mild and self-limiting; in these foals no treatment or supportive care is needed. In more severely affected foals further treatment may be necessary.

Control and prevention

The prevention and control of cryptosporidiosis can be difficult. Currently, immunisation effective at preventing cryptosporidiosis in horses and foals is lacking. Although some chemotherapeutic agents have shown preventive potential, the cost-effectiveness of such prophylaxis is often a limiting factor. Oocysts shed in feces are infective, extremely resistant to environmental factors, and can survive for months if not exposed to extremes of temperature or desiccation. Oocysts are highly resistant to most chemical disinfectants (Tzipori 1983). Moist heat (pasteurisation to >55°C or live steam), freezing, or thorough drying may be the most effective means of killing oocysts (Anderson 1985). Exposure to 5% ammonia solution or 10% formalin for 18 h will also kill oocysts (Tzipori 1983). Good sanitation may help by decreasing the oocyst burden in the foals' environment. Specific sanitation strategies would include providing uncontaminated water, rigorous cleaning (preferably with steam) and disinfecting foaling stalls, removing all the bedding, and isolating diarrhoeic foals.

Zoonotic considerations

Ingestion of oocysts can cause gastrointestinal disease in immunocompetent and immunosuppressed human patients. Those working with animals, including farmers and veterinarians, are considered to be at increased risk (Moon and Woodmasnee 1986; Konkle *et al.* 1997; Mahdi and Ali 2002). Cryptosporidiosis has occurred in veterinary students exposed to infected calves and foals (Anderson *et al.* 1982; Pohjola *et al.* 1986; Levine *et al.* 1988; Gait *et al.* 2008). *Cryptosporidium hominis* is spread only among humans, but the major reservoir for *C. parvum* is domestic livestock, predominantly cattle, and direct contact with infected cattle is a major transmission pathway along with indirect transmission through drinking water (Hunter and Thompson 2005). Efforts to minimise transmission in people handling infected foals should include instruction regarding, and rigorous attention to, hygiene, protective clothing (possibly to include face mask, gloves, gown or coveralls, and boots) and efforts to disinfect contaminated areas. Those with primary or acquired immunodeficiency should not be exposed to foals with diarrhoea in which a diagnosis of cryptosporidiosis is possible. In view of the low prevalence of infection, mature horses do not appear to be an important source of environmental contamination (Johnson *et al.* 1997; Atwill *et al.* 2000).

Over the past decade molecular methods have enabled the characterisation and identification of species and genotypes within the *Cryptosporidium* genus. The taxonomy is under continual review, but so far 20 valid species and numerous genotypes have been described. Recently, a long-term genotyping study in the United Kingdom identified 3 unusual *Cryptosporidium* genotypes (skunk, horse and rabbit) in human patients with diarrhoea (Robinson *et al.* 2008). The horse genotype was found in a 30-year-old immunocompetent woman from a rural area of southwest England, who reported swimming and foreign travel (destination unknown) but no contact with animals during the incubation period. A genetic study of 9 *C. parvum* isolates from diarrheic foals in New Zealand were genetically diverse, markedly similar to human and bovine isolates, and carried GP60 IIaA18G3R1 alleles, indicating a zoonotic potential (Grinberg *et al.* 2008).

Manufacturer's address

[1]Meridian Diagnostics Inc., Cincinnati, Ohio, USA.

References

Anderson, B.C., Donndelinger, T., Wilkins, R.M. and Smith, J. (1982) Cryptosporidiosis in a veterinary student. *J. Am. vet. med. Ass.* **180**, 408-409.

Anderson, B.C. (1985) Moist heat inactivation of *Cryptosporidium sp. Am. J. Public Health* **75**, 1433-1434.

Atwill, E.R., McDougald, N.K. and Perea, L. (2000) Cross-sectional study of faecal shedding of *Giardia duodenalis* and *Cryptosporidium parvum* among packstock in the Sierra Nevada Range. *Equine vet. J.* **32**, 247-252.

Bakheit, M.A., Torra, D., Palomino, L.A., Thekisoe, O.M., Mbati, P.A., Ongerth, J. and Karanis, P. (2008) Sensitive and specific detection of *Cryptosporidium* species in PCR-negative samples by loop-mediated isothermal DNA amplification and confirmation of generated LAMP products by sequencing. *Vet. Parasitol.* **158**, 11-22.

Barta, J.R. and Thompson, R.C. (2006) What is *Cryptosporidium*? Reappraising its biology and phylogenetic affinities. *Trends Parasitol.* **22**, 463-468.

Cama, V.A., Ross, J.M., Crawford, S., Kawai, V., Chavez-Valdez, R., Vargas, D., Vivar, A., Ticona, E., Navincopa, M.,Williamson, J., Ortega, Y., Gilman, R.H., Bern, C. and Xiao, L. (2007) Differences in clinical manifestations among *Cryptosporidium* species and subtypes in HIV-infected persons. *J. Infect. Dis.* **196**, 684-691.

Chalmers, R.M., Thomas, A.L., Butler, B.A. and Morel, M.C. (2005) Identification of *Cryptosporidium parvum* genotype 2 in domestic horses. *Vet. Rec.* **156**, 49-50.

Cohen, N.D. (2002) Equine cryptosporidial diarrhea. In: *Manual of Equine Gastroenterology,* Eds: T. Mair, T. Divers and N. Ducharme, W.B. Saunders, Edinburgh. pp 504-507.

Cohen, N.D. and Snowden, K. (1996) Cryptosporidial diarrhea in foals. *Comp. cont. Educ. pract. Vet.* **18**, 298-306.

Cole, D.J., Cohen, N.D., Snowden, K. and Smith, R. (1998) Prevalence and risk factors for fecal shedding of *Cryptosporidium parvum* oocysts in horses. *J. Am. vet. med. Ass.* **213**, 1296-1302.

Cole, D.J., Snowden, K., Cohen, N.D. and Smith, R. (1999) Detection of *Cryptosporidium parvum* in horses: thresholds of acid-fast stain, immunofluorescence assay, and flow cytometry. *J. clin. Microbiol.* **37**, 1999.

Coleman, S.U., Klei, T.R., French, D.D. Chapman, M.R and Corstvet, R.E. (1989) Prevalence of *Cryptosporidium* sp in equids in Louisiana. *Am. J. vet. Res.* **50**, 575-577.

Farthing, M.J. (2006) Treatment options for the eradication of intestinal protozoa. *Nat. Clin. Pract. Gastroenterol. Hepatol.* **3**, 436-445.

Field, A.S. (2002) Light microscopic and electron microscopic diagnosis of gastrointestinal opportunistic infections in HIV-positive patients. *Pathol.* **34**, 21-35.

Frayer, R. (2004) *Cryptosporidium*: a water-borne zoonotic parasite. *Vet. Parasitol.* **126**, 37-56.

Gait, R., Soutar, R.H., Hanson, M., Fraser, C. and Chalmers, R. (2008) Outbreak of cryptosporidiosis among veterinary students. *Vet. Rec.* **162**, 843-845.

Gargala, G. (2008) Drug treatment and novel drug target against *Cryptosporidium*. *Parasite* **15**, 275-281.

Gibson, J.A., Hill, M.W.M. and Huber, M.J. (1983) Cryptosporidiosis in Arabian foals with severe combined immunodeficiency. *Aust. vet. J.* **60**, 378-379.

Grinberg, A., Oliver, L., Learmonth, J.J., Leyland, M., Roe, W. and Pomroy, W.E. (2003) Identification of *Cryptosporidium parvum* 'cattle' genotype from a severe outbreak of neonatal foal diarrhoea. *Vet. Rec.* **153**, 628-631.

Grinberg, A., Learmonth, J., Kwan, E., Pomroy, W., Lopez Villalobos, N., Gibson, I. and Widmer, G. (2008) Genetic diversity and zoonotic potential of *Cryptosporidium parvum* causing foal diarrhea. *J. clin. Microbiol.* **46**, 2396-2398.

Hajdusek, O., Ditrich, O. and Slapeta, J. (2004) Molecular identification of *Cryptosporidium* spp. in animal and human hosts from the Czech Republic. *Vet. Parasitol.* **122**, 183-192.

Huang, D.B. and White, A.C. (2006) An updated review on *Cryptosporidium* and *Giardia*. *Gastroenterol. Clin. North Am.* **35**, 291-314.

Hunter, P.R. and Thompson, R.C. (2005) The zoonotic transmission of *Giardia* and *Cryptosporidium*. *Int. J. Parasitol* **35**, 1181-1190.

Johnson, E., Atwill, E.R., Filkins, M.E. and Kalush, J. (1997) The prevalence of shedding of *Cryptosporidium* and *Giardia* spp. based on a single fecal sample collection from each of 91 horses used for backcountry recreation. *J. vet. Diagn. Invest.* **9**, 56-60.

Karanis, P., Kourenti, C. and Smith, H. (2007) Waterborne transmission of protozoan parasites: a worldwide review of outbreaks and lessons learnt. *J. Water Health* **5**, 1-38.

Konkle, D.M., Nelson, K.M. and Lunn, D.P. (1997) Nosocomial transmission of *Cryptosporidium* in a veterinary hospital. *J. vet. Intern. Med.* **11**, 340-343.

Levine, N.D. (1973) *Protozoan Parasites of Domestic Animals and of Man*, 2nd edn., Burgess Publishing, Minneapolis. p 229.

Levine, J.F., Levy, M.G., Walker, R.L. and Crittenden, S. (1988) Cryptosporidiosis in veterinary students *J. Am. vet. med. Ass.* **193**, 1413-1414.

Llorente, M.T., Clavel, A., Goni, M.P., Varea, M., Seral, C., Becerril, R., Suarez, L. and Gomez-Lus, R. (2007) Genetic characterization of *Cryptosporidium* species from humans in Spain. *Parasitol. Int.* **56**, 201-205.

Mahdi, N.K. and Ali, N.H. (2002) Cryptosporidiosis among animal handlers and their livestock in Basrah, Iraq. *East Afr. Med. J.* **79**, 550-553.

Mair, T.S., Taylor, F.G., Harbour, D.A. and Pearson, G.R. (1990) Concurrent *Cryptosporidium* and coronavirus infections in an Arabian foal with combined immunodeficiency syndrome. *Vet. Rec.* **126**, 127-130.

Majewska, A.C., Solarczyk, P., Tamang and Graczyk, T.K. (2004) Equine *Cryptosporidium parvum* infections in western Poland. *Parasitol. Res.* **93**, 274-278.

Marcial, M.A. and Madara, J.L. (1986) *Cryptosporidium*: cellular localization, structural analysis of absorptive cell-parasite membrane-membrane interactions in guinea pigs, and suggestion of protozoan transport by M cells. *Gastroenterology* **90**, 583-594.

Mayhew, I.G. and Greiner, E.C. (1986) Protozoal diseases. *Vet. Clin. N. Am.: Equine Pract.* **2**, 439-459.

McKenzie, D.M. and Diffay, B.C, (2000) Diarrhoea associated with cryptosporidial oocyst shedding in a quarterhorse stallion. *Aust. vet. J.* **78**, 27-28.

Moon, H.W. and Woodmansee, D.B. (1986) Cryptosporidiosis. *J. Am. vet. med. Ass.* **189**, 643-646.

Morgan-Ryan, U.M., Fall, A., Ward, L.A., Hijjawi, N., Sulaiman, I., Fayer, R., Thompson, R.C., Olson, M., Lal, A. and Xiao, L. (2002) *Cryptosporidium hominis n.* sp. (*Apicomplexa: Cryptosporidiidae*) from *Homo sapiens*. *J. Eukaryot. Microbiol.* **49**, 433-440.

Netherwood, T., Wood, J.L., Townsend, H.G., Mumford, J.A. and Chanter, N. (1996) Foal diarrhoea between 1991 and 1994 in the United Kingdom associated with *Clostridium perfringens*, rotavirus, *Strongyloides westeri* and *Cryptosporidium* spp. *Epidemiol. Infect.* **117**, 375-383.

Olson, M.E., Thorlakson, C.L., Deselliers, L., Morck, D.W. and McAllister, T.A. (1997) *Giardia* and *Cryptosporidium* in Canadian farm animals. *Vet. Parasitol.* **68**, 375-381.

Pearson, G.R. and Logan, E.F. (1978) Demonstration of cryptosporidia in the small intestine of a calf by light, transmission electron and scanning electron microscopy. *Vet. Rec.* **103**, 212-213.

Pearson, G.R. and Logan, E.F. (1983) Scanning and transmission electron microscopic observations on the host-parasite relationship in intestinal cryptosporidiosis of neonatal calves. *Res. vet. Sci.* **34**, 149-154.

Pohjola, S., Oksanen, H., Jokipii, L. and Jokipii, A.M. (1986) Outbreak of cryptosporidiosis among veterinary students. *Scand. J. Infect. Dis.* **18**, 173-178.

Reinemeyer, C.R., Kline, R.C. and Stauffer, G.D. (1984) Absence of *cryptosporidium* oocysts in faeces of neonatal foals. *Equine vet. J.* **16**, 217-218.

Robinson, G., Elwin, K. and Chalmers, R.M. (2008) Unusual *cryptosporidium* genotypes in human cases of diarrhea. *Emerg. Infect. Dis.* **14**, 1800-1802.

Schnyder, M., Kohler, L., Hemphill, A. and Deplazes, P. (2008) Prophylactic and therapeutic efficacy of nitazoxanide against *Cryptosporidium parvum* in experimentally challenged neonatal calves. *Vet. Parasitol.* **160**, 149-154.

Sellon, D.C. (2007) Miscellaneous parasitic diseases. In: *Equine Infectious Diseases*, Ed: D.C. Sellon and M.T. Long, W.B. Saunders, St Louis. pp 473-480.

Snyder, S.P., England, J.J. and McChesney, A.E. (1978) Cryptosporidiosis in immunodeficient Arabian foals. *Vet. Pathol.* **15**, 12-17.

Smith, A., Reacher, M., Smerdon, W., Adak, G.K., Nicuols, G. and Chalmers, R.M. (2006) Outbreaks of waterborne infectious disease in England and Wales 1992-2003. *Epidemiol. Infect.* **134**, 1141-1149.

Smith, H.V., Caccio, S.M., Cook, N., Nichols, R.A. and Tait, A. (2007) *Cryptosporidium* and *Giardia* as foodborne zoonoses. *Vet. Parasitol.* **149**, 29-40.

Smith, H. and Nichols, R.A. (2006) Zoonotic protozoa – food for thought. *Parassitologia.* **48**, 101-104.

Sunnotel, O., Lowery, C.J., Moore, J.E., Dooley, J.S., Xiao, L., Millar, B.C., Rooney, P.J. and Snelling, W.J. (2006) *Cryptosporidium*. *Lett. Appl. Microbiol.* **43**, 7-16.

Tzipori, S. (1983) Cryptosporidiosis in animals and humans. *Microbiol. Rev.* **47**, 84-96.

Tzipori, S. and Campbell, I. (1981) Prevalence of *Cryptosporidium* antibodies in 10 animal species. *J. clin. Microbiol.* **14**, 455-456.

Werner, A., Sulima, P. and Majewska, A.C. (2004) Evaluation and usefulness of different methods for detection of *Cryptosporidium* in human and animal stool samples. *Wiad. Parazytol.* **50**, 209-220.

Xiao, L. and Herd, R.P. (1994) Review of equine *Cryptosporidium* infection. *Equine vet. J.* **26**, 9-13.

Xiao, L., Fayer, R., Ryan, U. and Upton, S.J. (2004) *Cryptosporidium* taxonomy: recent advances and implications for public health. *Crit. Rev. Microbiol.* **17**, 72-97.

Xiao, L., Bern, C., Limor, J., Sulaiman, I., Roberts, J., Checkley, W., Cabrera, L., Gilman, R.H. and Lal, A.A. (2001) Identification of 5 types of *Cryptosporidium* parasites in children in Lima, Peru. *J. Infect. Dis.* **183**, 492-497.

EQUINE TRYPANOSOMIASIS

P. Van den Bossche*[‡], S. Geerts and F. Claes[†§]

Departments of Animal Health and [†]Parasitology, Institute of Tropical Medicine, Antwerp, Belgium; [‡]Department of Veterinary Tropical Diseases, University of Pretoria, Onderstepoort, South Africa; and [§]Department of Biosystems, KULeuven, Belgium.

Keywords: horse; mule; donkey; trypanosomiasis; nagana; dourine; surra

Summary

Equine trypanosomiases are acute or chronic infectious diseases caused by protozoan blood parasites. Depending on the parasite species involved 3 diseases can be distinguished: nagana, surra and dourine.

Introduction

Nagana

Trypanosomes causing nagana (or tsetse-transmitted trypanosomiasis) belong to the subgenera *Nannomonas* (*Trypanosoma congolense*, *T. simiae*, *T. godfreyi*), *Trypanozoon* (*Trypanosoma brucei brucei*, *T. b. rhodesiense* and *T. b. gambiense*) and *Dutonella* (*Trypanosoma vivax*). With the exception of *T. vivax* that can also be found outside the African continent, they occur in sub-Saharan Africa (**Fig 1**). In wild animals these parasites cause mild infections. In domestic animals, however, the infection can be fatal depending on the host and parasite species involved. Nagana is a major direct and indirect constraint to livestock and rural development in sub-Saharan Africa. Nagana in horses, is caused by an infection with *T. congolense*, *T. vivax* and/or *T. b. brucei*.

Surra

Trypanosoma evansi is the causal agent of surra. There are numerous natural hosts of *T. evansi*. They include domestic animals such as horses, donkeys, mules, camels, goats, sheep, pigs, cattle and water buffalo but also a broad range of game animals (e.g. Indian elephant, capybara, lions, tiger and antelope) and pets (cats and dogs). Surra occurs mainly in north and northeast Africa, Latin America (except Chile), the Middle East and Asia and causes considerable economic losses as a result of a reduction in reproduction, working performance, milk yield and/or meat production of cattle, horses, pigs and buffalo (**Fig 1**).

Dourine

Dourine is the result of an infection with *Trypanosoma equiperdum*. Solipeds are the natural hosts of *T. equiperdum*. Because of the difficulties in detecting and isolating *T. equiperdum*, there has been doubt about it being the causative organism of the disease. The parasite is cosmopolitan, but nowadays, western Europe, Australia and the USA are considered to be free from dourine (**Fig 1**).

Aetiology

Trypanosomes, the causal agents of equine trypanosomiases, are elongated extracellular Protozoa with a forwards pointing flagellum for locomotion. They usually possess a kinetoplast, a specific structure that is situated near the base of the flagellum. Trypanosomes have been found in many species of mammals, reptiles, fish, birds as well as in vectors such as insects, ticks, leeches and vampire bats. Some trypanosomes can infect various animal species, while others are species-specific.

Transmission of trypanosomes can be the result of inoculation of infected blood (e.g. during vaccination campaigns) but they are usually transmitted cyclically, mechanically or sexually. Cyclical transmission occurs when the trypanosome undergoes a developmental cycle in the insect vector, the tsetse fly. In mechanical transmission, a

*Author to whom correspondence should be addressed.

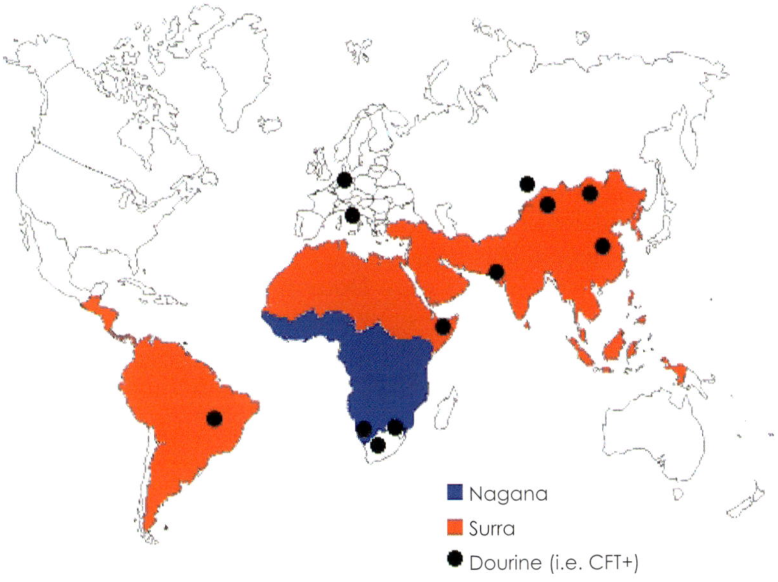

FIGURE 1: Distribution of nagana, surra and dourine.

haematophagous insect becomes contaminated with an infectious agent during normal feeding and the agent may persist on the mouthparts until the next feed without undergoing any biological development. On the African continent, cyclical transmission is the main mode of transmission for *T. congolense*, *T. brucei s.l.* and, to a lesser extent, *T. vivax*. Mechanical transmission is the only mode of transmission for *T. evansi*, but it can also occur with trypanosome species that are normally transmitted cyclically (i.e. *T. congolense* and *T. b. brucei*) and it is a common mode of transmission for *T. vivax*. *T. equiperdum* is transmitted sexually, during copulation, from the stallion to the mare or *vice versa* (Laveran and Mesnil 1912).

Nagana

Nagana caused by *T. congolense*, *T. brucei s.l.* and/or *T. vivax* is the result of a bite of an infected tsetse fly (*Glossina* spp.) that injects the parasite along with its saliva before taking its blood meal. For a few days, the trypanosomes will multiply locally at the site of the bite thereafter they invade the lymphatic system and blood vessels and, especially in the case of *T. brucei s.l.*, invade other tissues and organs, including the central nervous system.

Surra

Trypanosoma evansi does not undergo cyclical transmission, thus, no specific insect stages occur. Two different bloodstream forms can be observed. The long slender form is seen most of the time; the short and stumpy form is scarce but present. The morphology of this trypanosome species is indistinguishable from that of *T. b. brucei*.

Dourine

The morphology of this parasite is identical to the bloodstream forms of *T. b. brucei*. Transmission of the parasite occurs during copulation. After entering the host through the genital tract, *T. equiperdum* first migrates to the bloodstream of the host but converts rapidly into a tissue parasite.

Epidemiology

Nagana

The epidemiology of nagana is complex and, because of the focal nature of the disease, varies spatially and is determined by a number of tsetse-related variables. Generally speaking, the probability of a host contracting trypanosomiasis depends on the rate at which it is fed upon by infected male or female tsetse flies (Rogers 1988). The trypanosomal infection rate of a tsetse population is generally low with a large proportion of the flies being refractory to infection with trypanosomes. The attraction of tsetse flies to a host, such as a horse, and subsequently the proportion of tsetse that feed and challenge a host is the result of a number of visual and olfactory stimuli.

Although the horse population in tsetse-infested Africa is relatively small, the prevalence of nagana in horses can take considerable proportions. For example, at a gate-clinic in The Gambia, 61% of all horses presented were infected with trypanosomes (Dhollander *et al.* 2006). Using more sensitive molecular tools, Faye *et al.* (2001) and Pinchbeck *et al.* (2008) detected a much higher overall prevalence for any trypanosome species reaching up to 93% with a high proportion of mixed infections. In many tsetse-infested African game parks, horseback safaris cannot be sustained because of the high prevalence of trypanosomal infections.

Surra

Trypanosoma evansi is transmitted mechanically by haematophagous insect vectors such as *Tabanidae*, *Stomoxys*, *Haematopota*, *Chrysops* and *Lyperosia*. Vampire bats, *Desmodus rotundus*, are also reported to spread the disease in Latin America (Stephen 1986). Little is known about the epidemiology of *T. evansi* in Africa since more attention is given to tsetse-transmitted trypanosome species. Epidemiological data of surra in equids are scarce apart for Ethiopia where a recent survey showed that equine trypanosomiasis is highly endemic in the highlands (F. Claes, unpublished data). From Eastern Africa, the disease probably spread further into the Middle East and later to Asia. Nowadays, surra can be found in feral camelids in Oman and occasionally in commercially bred camels and horses. Surra is endemic throughout central Asia (India, Mongolia, Kazakstan), southeast Asia and the Indonesian archipelago with the possible exception of Western New Guinea (Singh *et al.* 1995; Reid 2002; Clausen *et al.* 2003). Unfortunately most prevalence data are from camels, cattle and buffalo rather than equids. It is possible that the parasite is more prevalent in the former species that may act as a reservoir and subsequently causes outbreaks in the horse population. In South America also, little is known of the prevalence and spread of *T. evansi*. During a survey in Venezuela, 12% of horses were found seropositive. In Colombia, French Guyana, Argentina and the north of Brazil, no prevalences are recorded but the parasite seems enzootic and high mortality was observed in *T. evansi* outbreaks in horses in these regions (Desquesnes 2004). Only Chile seems to be free from *T. evansi*, possibly due to the natural barrier of the Andes.

Dourine

Since the 19th century, dourine has occurred only sporadically in Europe. Around 1918, the disease was reported in Russia, Turkey, Hungary and Spain. During World War II, however, *T. equiperdum* was re-introduced into western Europe (Saurat 1946). After the war, the disease was eradicated in western Europe through stringent control measures. Nevertheless, sporadic cases of seropositive animals are still reported (e.g. in Italy and recently in Germany). The latest official reports of dourine were from China, Kazakhstan, Kyrgyzstan, Pakistan, Ethiopia, Botswana, Namibia, South Africa, Brazil, Italy and Germany.

Clinical signs

Nagana

Although horses are susceptible to infections with all 3 salivarian trypanosome species, the most common infections are those with *T. congolense* followed by infections with *T. vivax*. Infections with *T. b. brucei* are rare. On the other hand, mixed infections with different species are common.

The clinical signs of nagana in horses differ little from those seen in cattle. They can vary from lethargy and anorexia to no abnormalities detected on clinical examination. Parasitic peaks with large numbers of parasites in the peripheral blood are observed usually in the early phase of infection accompanied by pyrexia (rectal temperature may reach 40.5°C), tachycardia and tachypnoea. Animals with acute nagana are very depressed. Severe anaemia may develop with the packed cell volume (PCV) declining to low levels with increasing weakness and signs of ataxia. Small skin nodules (urticaria) and oedematous plaques may form on the flanks. Progressive oedema of the ventral parts such as sternum, belly, prepuce and especially the legs can be very pronounced but is not a common feature

(Pinchbeck *et al.* 2008). The mucous membranes of the eye, the gums or vagina may become icteric as a result of the rapid destruction of red blood cells.

Equine trypanosomiasis due to *T. b. brucei* (in a single or mixed infection) is often acute and can lead to death in 2 weeks to 3 months with little or no evidence of involvement of the central nervous system (Taylor and Authié 2004).

Infections with *T. congolense* or *T. vivax* have a more chronic nature. In the chronic phase of the infection the parasitaemia is usually low and parasites are difficult to detect using parasitological diagnostic tools. The anaemia progresses with mucous membranes becoming pale. Animals further lose condition and weight and become extremely weak and show signs of ataxia. In the chronic phase of infection, the subcutaneous oedema may extend to the head. Animals may become severely emaciated. In chronic *T. b. brucei* infections, the disease is often associated with nervous symptoms and the presence of the parasite in the cerebrospinal fluid and macroscopically visible lesions of the meninges and the brain leading to ataxia and paralysis (Neitz and McCully 1971; McCully and Neitz 1971). Up to 20% of the horses infected with *T. brucei* may develop keratitis and corneal opacity (Neitz and McCully 1971).

Surra

There are 2 forms of this disease. An acute form, which occurs mostly in horses and camels and a chronic form, which is mostly seen in cattle and water buffalo.

The pathognomonic signs of surra are similar in the different host species but not always readily observed. In acute infections, animals suffer from high pyrexia, progressive anaemia, loss of general body condition and exhaustion, finally resulting in death. In chronic infections, subsequent waves of fever, associated with the parasitaemia peaks, are observed. Oedema, mainly of the lower legs, urticarial plaques and petechial haemorrhages on the mucous membranes can develop (Stephen 1986). The principal clinical signs of the acute form of the disease in horses are pyrexia associated with peaks in the parasitaemia, oedema of the belly, anaemia and muscular weakness. However, *T. evansi* is notorious for its variable pathogenicity so not all signs may be observed and differences may occur from one horse to another.

The mortality rate in horses can be very high (80–100%) (Stephen 1986). In cattle, water buffalo, sheep and goats the mortality rate is much lower (10–40%).

Dourine

Trypanosoma equiperdum causes a chronic infection in horses that can persist for 1–2 years. The incubation period is highly variable. Clinical signs usually appear within a few weeks of infection but, in some cases, may not be evident until after several years. The appearance of clinical signs may be accelerated by stress in infected animals (Barrowman 1976).

An infection with *T. equiperdum* can generally be divided into 3 phases, although the clinical course can vary considerably under different conditions. The first phase is characterised by oedema, tumefaction and damage to the genitalia. In mares, the first sign of infection is usually a small amount of vaginal discharge, which may remain on the tail and hindquarters. Swelling and oedema of the vulva develop later and extend along the perineum to the udder and ventral abdomen. Vulvitis and vaginitis with polyuria may occur. Significant abortion losses can be observed in infected herds. In stallions, the initial signs are variable oedema of the prepuce and glans penis, spreading to the scrotum and perineum and to the ventral abdomen and thorax (**Figs 2** and **3**). Swellings may resolve and reappear periodically. Vesicles or ulcers on the genitalia may heal and leave permanent white scars (leucodermic patches). Conjunctivitis and keratitis are often observed in outbreaks of dourine and may be the first

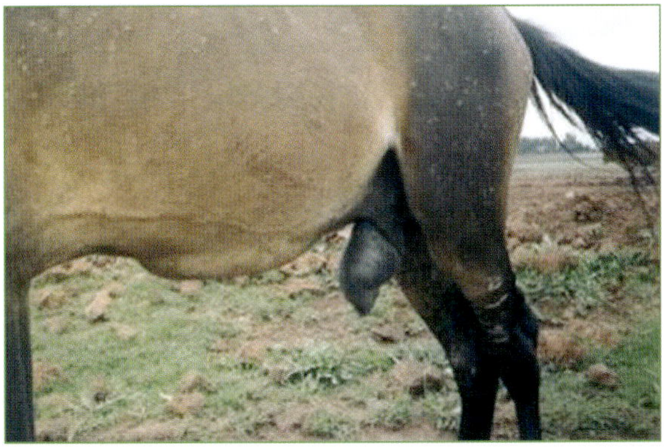

FIGURE 2: Genital and ventral abdominal oedema in an Ethiopian horse affected by dourine.

signs noted in some infected herds. The second phase of the infection is considered to be pathognomonic for dourine. In this period typical cutaneous 'plaques' or areas of thickened skin can occur with variable sizes ranging from very small to the size of a hand and a thickness of one centimeter (Laveran and Mesnil 1912). These plaques usually appear over the ribs, although they may occur anywhere on the body, and usually persist for 3–7 days. Such plaques have also been observed sporadically in animals infected with *T. evansi* (Brun *et al.* 1998). The final phase of dourine is characterised by progressive anaemia and by disorders of the nervous system. Initially these signs consist of restlessness and a tendency to shift weight from one leg to another followed by progressive weakness and incoordination (**Fig 4**). Ultimately, paralysis (mainly of the hind legs), paraplegia and death occur (Stephen 1986).

At *post mortem* examination, gelatinous exudates can be found under the skin. In the stallion, the scrotum, sheath and testicular tunica may be thickened and infiltrated. In some cases the testes are embedded in a tough mass of sclerotic tissue. In the mare, the vulva, vaginal mucosa, uterus, bladder and mammary glands can be thickened with gelatinous infiltration. The lymph nodes, particularly in the abdominal cavity, are hypertrophied, softened and, in some cases, haemorrhagic. The spinal cord of animals with paraplegia is often soft, pulpy and discoloured, particularly in the lumbar and sacral regions.

Acute equine trypanosomiasis must be distinguished from African horse sickness and anthrax. Repeated examination of blood allows for the differential diagnosis with other causes of severe pyrexia in horses such as equine babesiosis (*Babesia caballi*) and theileriosis (*Theileria equi*).

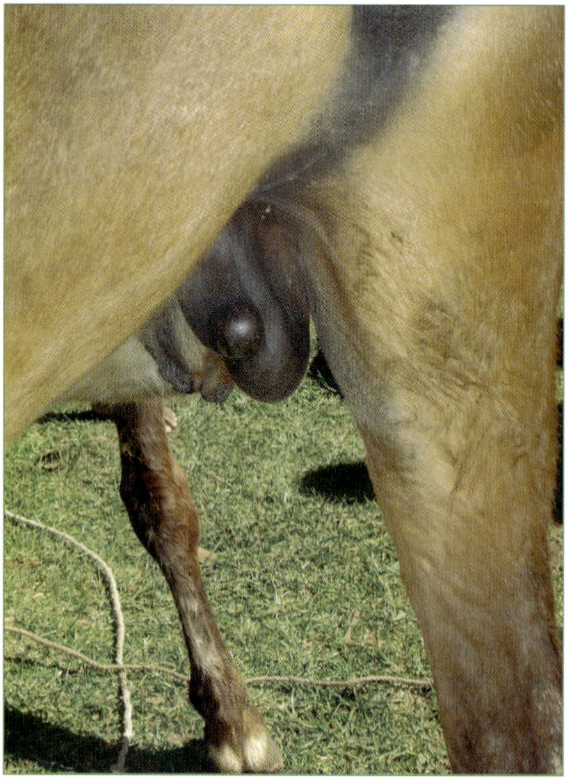

FIGURE 3: Genital oedema in an Ethiopian horse affected by dourine.

Diagnosis

Nagana

Diagnosing nagana is difficult because there are no specific clinical signs and parasitaemias are usually low making parasitological detection of the parasites difficult. As a result, parasitological detection methods have high specificity but low sensitivity (Paris *et al.* 1982). The body fluid most commonly examined is blood. Lymph, aspirated from a punctured superficial lymph node (usually not easily palpable), provides useful supplementary diagnostic material. The simplest parasitological diagnostic techniques are the examination of wet or Giemsa-

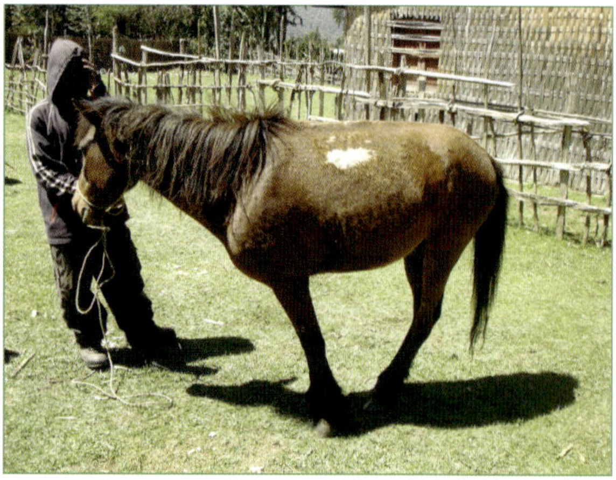

FIGURE 4: Apathy, depression and incoordination in a horse affected by dourine.

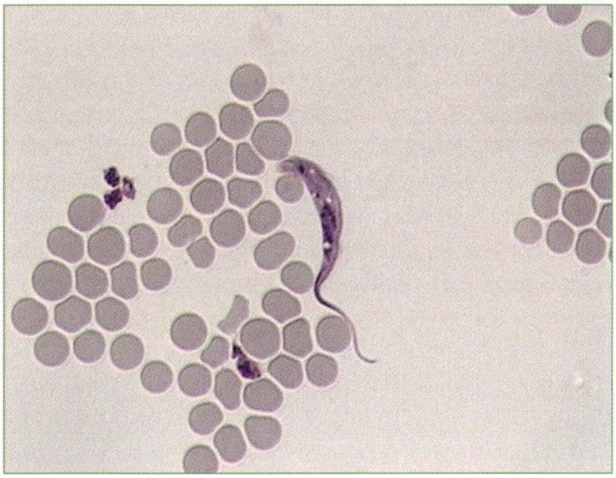

FIGURE 5: Giemsa-stained thin smear of blood infected with Trypanosoma vivax.

stained thick or thin films of fresh blood. Wet blood films are simple, inexpensive and give immediate results. Depending on the trypanosome size and the parasite's movements, a presumptive diagnosis can be made of the trypanosome species involved:

Trypanosoma vivax: Large, extremely active, traverses the whole field very quickly, pausing occasionally.

Trypanosoma brucei: Various sizes, rapid movement in confined areas.

Trypanosoma congolense: Small, sluggish, adheres to red blood cells by the anterior end.

The Giemsa-stained thin smear permits accurate determination of the species of the parasites involved. Trypanosome species can be identified by the following morphological characteristics:

Trypanosoma vivax: 20–27 µm long, undulating membrane is not obvious, free flagellum present at the anterior end, posterior end rounded, kinetoplast large and terminal (**Fig 5**).

Trypanosoma brucei: is a polymorphic trypanosome species. Two distinctly different forms can be distinguished, i.e. a long slender form and a short stumpy form. Often, intermediate forms, possessing characteristics of both the slender and stumpy forms, are observed. The cytoplasm often contains basophilic granules in stained specimens (**Fig 6**).

The long slender form is 17–30 µm long and about 2.8 µm wide, undulating membrane is conspicuous, free flagellum present at the anterior end, posterior end pointed, kinetoplast small and subterminal. The short stumpy form is 17–22 µm long and about 3.5 µm wide, undulating membrane is conspicuous, free flagellum absent, posterior end pointed, kinetoplast small and subterminal.

Trypanosoma congolense: 8–25 µm (small species), undulating membrane not obvious, free flagellum

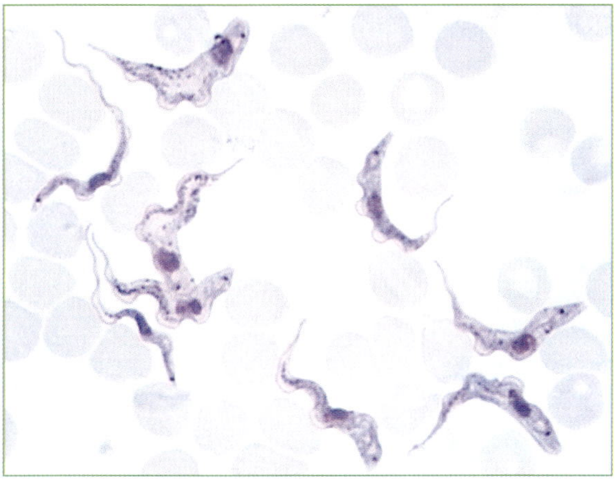

FIGURE 6: Giemsa-stained thin smear of blood infected with long slender and stumpy forms of Trypanosoma brucei brucei.

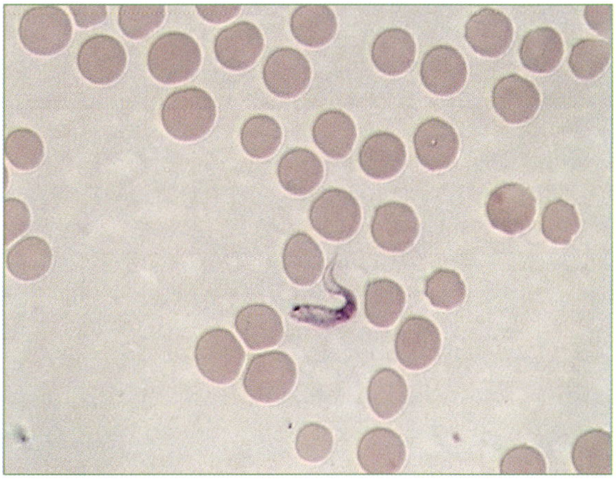

FIGURE 7: Giemsa-stained thin smear of blood infected with Trypanosoma congolense.

absent, posterior end rounded, kinetoplast is medium sized and terminal, often laterally positioned (**Fig 7**). Although *T. congolense* is considered to be monomorphous, a degree of morphological variation is sometimes observed. Within *T. congolense*, different types or subgroups exist (savannah, forest, kilifi, tsavo) that have a different pathogenicity. However, these types can only be distinguished using polymerase chain reaction (PCR).

The diagnostic sensitivity can be improved by increasing the volume of blood to be examined and concentrating the trypanosomes. The microhaematocrit centrifugation technique or Woo-method (Woo 1970) is more sensitive but identification of trypanosome species is difficult. Alternatively, the buffy coat and the uppermost layer of red blood cells can be extruded onto a clean microscope slide and covered with a cover slip (buffy coat technique or Murray method: Murray *et al.* 1977). The methods are particularly useful in that the PCV can be assessed after centrifugation.

Xenodiagnosis or the subinoculation of blood into rodents such as mice or rats, can be used to detect *T. brucei* and *T. congolense* infections (Uilenberg 1998). However, since rodents are refractory to *T. vivax* and not all *T. congolense* and *T. brucei* infections become established in the new host, this method has serious limitations. Mixed trypanosomal infections may also remain undetected. The mini-anion exchange centrifugation technique (mAECT), the most sensitive parasitological test, is seldom applied in animals due to its high cost (Lumsden *et al.* 1979).

As an alternative to parasitological tests, DNA-detection based on PCR is used frequently. These molecular tests usually have high diagnostic sensitivity and specificity. Several *Trypanozoon* specific primers have been designed; including TBR primers, pMUTEC primers, ORPHON primers and ESAG6/7 (Moser *et al.* 1989; Wuyts *et al.* 1994; Pereira de Almeida *et al.* 1998; Holland *et al.* 2001). Specific PCR tests have also been developed for detecting *T. congolense* and *T. vivax*, (Majiwa and Otieno 1990; Morlais *et al.* 2001) Moreover, several molecular tests, such as PCR-RFLP analysis (Geysen *et al.* 2003) and ITS-1 PCR (Davila and Silva 2000; Claes *et al.* 2004) are available that differentiate between trypanosomes of the *Trypanozoon* subgroup, *T. congolense* and *T. vivax.*

The development of anti-trypanosomal antibody detection techniques has been a major improvement in the serodiagnosis of nagana. The indirect fluorescent antibody test (IFAT) (Luckins and Mehlitz 1978) and different ELISA systems (Luckins 1977; Greiner *et al.* 1997; Hopkins *et al.* 1998) have been evaluated and are being used in the field. Most tests, however, have been developed for bovine trypanosomiasis and need to be adapted for use in horses.

Surra

The same parasitological techniques used for the diagnosis of nagana can be applied for the diagnosis of *T. evansi*. For serodiagnosis, the RoTat 1.2 VSG might serve as a marker for *T. evansi*. Several antibody detection tests have been developed and applied in the field based on this antigen; mostly used is the CATT/*T. evansi* test, a card agglutination test (Bajyana Songa and Hamers 1988). Other tests, based on the same antigen, are the ELISA, the LATEX/*T. evansi* and the immune trypanolysis (Verloo *et al.* 2001).

For molecular diagnosis, kinetoplast DNA (kDNA) probes based on mini-circle sequences have been developed (Gibson *et al.* 1983; Borst *et al.* 1987). Unfortunately, this method is not suitable for dyskinetoplastic *T. evansi* strains. To overcome this problem, a species-specific PCR based on the RoTat 1.2 VSG gene is available (Claes *et al.* 2004).

Dourine

Clinical signs of dourine can provide strong indication of the disease, as can its chronic evolution. However, since differential diagnosis with nagana and surra is very difficult, confirmatory diagnosis is needed. It is very difficult to detect *T. equiperdum* in the body fluids of infected horses. Therefore, diagnosis of *T. equiperdum* infection is based on serological evidence. Although antibody and antigen ELISAs have been developed for *T. equiperdum* (Alemu *et al.* 1997), the only internationally recommended serological test remains the complement fixation test (CFT) (Watson 1915), which does not distinguish between *T. equiperdum*, *T. evansi* and *T. brucei* (Robinson 1926; Hoare 1956; Richardson and Kendall 1957). Indeed, possible cross-reactions with *T. evansi* and *T. brucei* may occur and consequently the latter parasites cannot be distinguished from *T. equiperdum* unless the samples originate from *T. evansi* and *T. brucei* free regions. Unfortunately, countries where dourine is currently reported often lie within the distribution area of *T. evansi*.

Currently, the main difficulty with diagnosing dourine is to distinguish *T. equiperdum* from *T. evansi*. Some authors mention the absence of maxicircles in the kDNA of *T. evansi* to be a major difference between *T. evansi* and *T. equiperdum* (Riou and Saucier 1979; Frasch *et al.* 1980). However, since dyskinetoplastic strains exist in both *T. evansi* and *T. equiperdum*, the validity of this characteristic can be questioned. So far, neither isoenzyme analysis (Lun *et al.* 1992), nor southern blot analysis (Hide *et al.* 1990; Zhang and Baltz 1994) or microsatellite markers (Biteau *et al.* 2000) can distinguish *T. equiperdum* from *T. evansi*. Recent characterisation studies indicated a heterogeneity in *T. equiperdum* isolates. In general, most *T. equiperdum* are very similar to *T. evansi* while two strains (OVI and BoTat 1.1) resemble *T. b. brucei* (Claes *et al.* 2003).

Treatment and prevention

Nagana

A number of trypanocidal drugs can be used to treat horses infected with a *T. congolense*, *T. vivax* and/or *T. b. brucei* infection (Connor and Van den Bossche 2004; Holmes *et al.* 2004) (**Table 1**). All these drugs are toxic and have a narrow safety margin.

Isometamidium chloride is the drug that is tolerated best (Connor and Van den Bossche 2004; Dhollander *et al.* 2006; Auty *et al.* 2008) on condition that it is administered correctly, i.e. deeply i.m. and avoiding any leakage of the drug to subcutaneous tissues which may cause sloughing of the skin. This is because the drug causes coagulative necrosis at the injection site, which is encapsulated after some weeks by fibrous tissue (Kinabo and Bogan 1988). For curative and prophylactic purposes the recommended dose is 0.5 mg/kg bwt i.m. It is advised not to exceed this dosage (Uilenberg 1998). The prophylactic cover is highly variable and depends on many factors. Dehoux *et al.* (1996) mention a protection period of 2.5 months in a moderately tsetse-infested environment. Isometamidium chloride can also be injected i.v., which is well tolerated by the horses if administered correctly without any leakage (Dehoux *et al.* 1996). Diminazene aceturate mainly has a curative effect, although the drug provides a short protection period of about 18 days (Faye *et al.* 2001). It is effective against *T. vivax* and *T. congolense* at 3.5 mg/kg bwt i.m. and against *T. brucei* at 7 mg/kg bwt. Although Uilenberg (1998) does not recommend to use the drug in horses because of occasional severe reactions at the injection site, Dhollander *et al.* (2006), who treated more than 1000 *T. vivax* and *T. congolense* infected horses in The Gambia, did not observe any side effects at 3.5 mg/kg bwt. Horses in good condition received the drug in one dose, whereas in animals with a high parasitaemia or severe anaemia the drug was divided over 2 or 3 portions with a 4 h interval. Awan and Johnston (1979), however, reported adverse effects (prostration, staggering gait, appetite loss and marked reactions at the injection site) after treatment at 3.5 mg/kg bwt in 7 horses infected with *T. brucei*.

Quinapyramine is used mainly for the treatment of *T. b. brucei* (and *T. evansi*) in horses and camels.

TABLE 1: Currently available trypanocidal drugs for use in horses

Compound	Dosage (mg/kg bwt)	Route	Use	Active against	Side effects
Isometamidium	0.5	i.m./i.v.	C, P	Tc, Tv, Tb, Te	(+)
Diminazene	3.5	i.m.	C	Tc, Tv, Te	+
Quinapyramine sulphate	3-5	s.c.	C	Tc, Tv, Tb, Te	++
Quinapyramine sulphate and chloride (prosalt)	3-5	s.c.	P	Tc, Tv, Tb, Te	++
Homidium bromide or chloride	1	i.m./i.v.	C, (P)	Tc, Tv, Te	+
Suramin	7–10 g/a*	i.v.	C, (P)	Te	(+)

Tb = *Trypanosoma brucei*; Tc = *T. congolense*; Tv = *T. vivax*; Tv = *T. evansi*; C = curative; P = prophylactic; * = g/animal, to be repeated after a week.

Quinapyramine dimethylsulphate has therapeutic activity whereas a mixture of dimethylsulphate and chloride (3:2 w/w) has a prophylactic effect against *T. congolense*, *T. brucei* and to a lesser extent *T. vivax* (Uilenberg 1998). The dosage is 3–5 mg/kg bwt subcutaneously (based on the sulphate in case of the mixture). Unfortunately, quinapyramine is poorly tolerated by horses and severe albeit transient (in 1–3 h) side effects usually occur (Awan and Johnston 1979; Connor and Van den Bossche 2004; Auty *et al.* 2008). The most commonly observed side effects are restlessness, salivation, sweating, fasciculations, diarrhoea and abdominal discomfort. Sometimes the animals become recumbent and roll. Therefore, it is recommended that: 1) the animals should be well rested before treatment: 2) the dose be split into 2 or 3 portions, which are injected with an interval of 4–6 h (particularly in weakened animals); and 3) the injection site is massaged to minimise local reactions and nodule formation (Connor and Van den Bossche 2004). Quinapyramine has been withdrawn from the market for use in cattle because of problems with the fast development of resistance and cross-resistance to all other trypanocides (Geerts and Holmes 1998). Although the drug is currently available only for use in horses and camels, the remark about (cross)-resistance development remains valid.

Finally, homidium bromide (ethidium bromide) or homidium chloride can also be used in horses. However, these drugs are highly mutagenic and are therefore not recommended. If no other drugs are available they can be used at 1 mg/kg bwt deeply i.m. or i.v. for the treatment of animals infected with *T. congolense* or *T. vivax*. Since horses are very susceptible to the irritant effect at the injection site, Uilenberg (1998) recommends to inject the drug i.v. avoiding any leakage into the tissues surrounding the jugular vein. After i.m. injection Stephen and Mackenzie (1958) observed some development of oedema in the ventral and inguinal regions, which disappeared after 2 weeks. Both drugs are known to have a short prophylactic effect (about one month) in cattle, although this has not been documented in horses.

Up to now drug-resistant strains of *T. congolense*, *T. b. brucei* or *T. vivax* from horse origin have not yet been reported most probably because scientists did not look for them. However, there was some suspicion of resistance of *T. vivax* to diminazene in The Gambia (Dhollander *et al.* 2006). To delay the development of drug resistance the same principles should be applied as for other livestock species (see Geerts and Holmes 1998). As mentioned above, the regular use of quinapyramine should be avoided. If isometamidium is used several times a year in a strategic prophylactic scheme it should be alternated with diminazene (as a sanative pair).

A programme of integrated disease control combining tsetse control techniques and trypanocidal or trypanoprophylactic drugs usually yields greater benefits than a single method alone (Holmes 1997). Particularly in areas with heavy tsetse challenges it is important to cut the thick vegetation around the horse stables and to use insecticide treated targets or insecticide sprays or pour-ons (Van den Bossche and De Deken 2004). Although synthetic pyrethroids are highly effective against tsetse flies even at low concentrations, they may not prevent horses from some contact with the flies and thus possible infection. Sprays or pour-ons also reduce nuisance by other biting insects, which can be quite important in the tropics.

Surra

Most commonly used drugs to treat *T. evansi* infections are diminazene aceturate, isometamidium chloride, quinapyramine sulphate and suramin (**Table 1**). Suramin is recommended since it has a low toxicity in equids (Luckins 1994). As an alternative drug melarsomine (cymelarsan) can be used. This drug was developed initially for the treatment of surra in camelids but evidence shows that at a dose of 0.25 mg/kg bwt it is not toxic for horses and effective in clearing *T. evansi* infections. Trypanocidal drug resistance also occurs in *T. evansi*. Chinese *T. evansi* strains resistant to isometamidium have been reported (Brun and Lun 1994).

Due to the large spectrum of transmitting insect vectors and wild animal reservoir species, control at that level is almost impossible. Therefore, the control of surra is mainly based on diagnosis and treatment of infected animals.

Dourine

There is no officially approved drug to treat horses suffering from dourine, although some older publications mention experimental treatment of horses with suramin and neoarsphenamine

(Novarsenobenzol; Ciuca 1933) or quinapyramine sulphate (Vaysse and Zottner 1950). Nowadays, international regulations of the World Organization for Animal Health (OIE) impose the slaughtering of CFT positive horses. Nevertheless, Zhang *et al.* (1992) and Brun and Lun (1994) reported on the *in vitro* sensitivity of different *T. equiperdum* strains to treatments with suramin, diminazene aceturate, quinapyramine sulphate or melarsomine. However, *in vivo* treatment failure may occur as a result of cryptic infections. The effectiveness of new drugs such as cymelarsan for treatment of dourine has not yet been evaluated. Drug resistance of *T. equiperdum* strains in the laboratory has been observed (Zhang *et al.* 1993), but resistant field cases are rare (or not studied).

References

Alemu, T., Luckins, A.G., Phipps, L.P., Reid, S.W.J. and Holmes, P. (1997) The use of enzyme linked immunosorbent assays to investigate the prevalence of *Trypanosoma equiperdum* in Ethiopian horses. *Vet. Parasitol.* **71**, 239-250.

Auty, H., Mundy, A., Fyumagma, R.D., Picozzi, K., Welburn, S. and Hoare, R. (2008) Health management of horses under high challenge from trypanosomes: A case study from Serengeti, Tanzania. *Vet. Parasitol.* **154**, 233-241.

Awan, M.A.Q. and Johnston, R.S. (1979) Some observations on an outbreak of trypanosomiasis in horses in the Republic of Zambia. *Bull. Anim. Health Afr.* **27**, 177-179.

Bajyana Songa, E. and Hamers, R. (1988) A card agglutination test (CATT) for veterinary use based on an early VAT RoTat 1/2 of *Trypanosoma evansi. Ann. Soc. Belge Méd. Trop.* **68**, 233-240.

Barrowman, P.R. (1976) Experimental intraspinal *Trypanosoma equiperdum* infection in a horse. *Onderstepoort J. vet. Res.* **43**, 201-202.

Biteau, N., Bringaud, F., Gibson, W., Truc, P. and Baltz, T. (2000) Characterization of Trypanozoon isolates using a repeated coding sequence and microsatellite markers. *Mol. Biochem. Parasitol.* **105**, 185-201.

Borst, P., Fase-Fowler, F. and Gibson, W.C. (1987) Kinetoplast DNA of *Trypanosoma evansi. Mol. Biochem. Parasitol.* **23**, 31-38.

Brun, R. and Lun, Z.-R. (1994) Drug sensitivity of Chinese *Trypanosoma evansi* and *Trypanosoma equiperdum* isolates. *Vet. Parasitol.* **52**, 37-46.

Brun, R., Hecker, H. and Lun, Z-R. (1998) *Trypanosoma evansi* and *T. equiperdum*: distribution, biology, treatment and phylogenetic relationship (a review). *Vet. Parasitol.* **79**, 95-107.

Ciuca, A. (1933) La dourine. *Bull. Off. Int. Epiz.* **7**, 168-172.

Claes, F., Agbo, E.E.C., Radwanska, M., Baltz., T., De Waal, D.T., Goddeeris, B.M. and Büscher, P. (2003) How does *Trypanosoma equiperdum* fit into the Trypanozoon group? A cluster analysis by random amplified polymorphic DNA (RAPD) and the multiplex-endonuclease genotyping approach. *Parasitol.* **126**, 425-431.

Claes, F., Radwanska, M., Urakawa, T., Verloo, D., Magnus, E., Majiwa, P.A.O., Goddeeris, B.M. and Büscher., P. (2004) Development of a PCR based on the *Trypanosoma evansi* RoTat 1.2 VSG DNA sequence. *Kinetoplastid Biol. Dis.* **3**, 3-15.

Clausen, P.H., Chuluun, S., Sodnomdarjaa, R., Greiner, M., Noeckler, K., Staak, C., Zessin, K.H. and Schein, E. (2003) A field study to estimate the prevalence of *Trypanosoma equiperdum* in Mongolian horses. *Vet. Parasitol.* **115**, 9-18.

Connor, R.J. and Van den Bossche, P. (2004) African animal trypanosomoses. In: *Infectious Diseases of Livestock*, Vol 1, 2nd edn., Eds. J.A.W. Coetzer, and R.C. Tustin, Oxford University Press, Cape Town. pp 251-296.

Davila, A.M. and Silva, R.A., (2000) Animal trypanosomiasis in South America. Current status, partnership, and information technology. *Ann. N.Y. Acad. Sci.* **916**, 199-212.

Dehoux, J.P., Diaw, M. and, Buldgen, A. (1996) Observation d'une flambée de trypanosomose équine due à *Trypanosoma vivax* en zone urbaine au Sénégal. *Tropicultura* **14**, 35-36.

Desquesnes, M. (2004) *Livestock Trypanosomoses and their Vectors in Latin America.* World Organisation for Animal Health, Paris.

Dhollander, S., Jallow, A., Mbodge, K., Kora, S., Sanneh, M., Gaye, M., Bos, J., Leak, S., Berkvens, D. and Geerts S. (2006) Equine trypanosomosis in the Central River Division of the Gambia: A study of veterinary gate-clinic consultation records. *Prev. vet. Med.* **75**, 152-162.

Faye, D., Pereira de Almeida, P.J.L., Goossens, B., Osaer, B., Ndao, M., Berkvens, D., Speybroeck, N., Nieberding, F. and Geerts, S. (2001) Prevalence and incidence of trypanosomosis in horses and donkeys in the Gambia. *Vet. Parasitol.* **101**, 101-104.

Frasch, A.C.C., Hajduk, S.L., Hoeijmakers, J.H.J., Borst, P., Brunel, F. and Davidson, J. (1980) The kinetoplast DNA of *Trypanosoma equiperdum. Biochim. Biophys. Acta.* **607**, 397-410.

Geerts, S. and Holmes, P.H. (1998) *Drug Management and Parasite Resistance in Animal Trypanosomiasis in Africa,* Food and Agriculture Organization, Rome.

Geysen, D., Delespaux, V. and Geerts, S. (2003) PCR-RFLP using Ssu-rDNA amplification as an easy method for species-specific diagnosis of *Trypanosoma* species in cattle. *Vet. Parasitol.* **110**, 171-180.

Gibson, W.C., Wilson, A.J. and Moloo, S.K., (1983) Characterization of *Trypanosoma* (Trypanozoon) *evansi* from camels in Kenya using isoenzyme electrophoresis. *Res. vet. Sci.* **34**, 114-118.

Greiner, M., Kumar, S. and Kyeswa, C. (1997) Evaluation and comparison of antibody ELISAs for serodiagnosis of bovine trypanosomosis. *Vet. Parasitol.* **73**, 197-205.

Hide, G., Cattand, P., LeRay, D., Barry, D.J. and Tait, A. (1990) The identification of *Trypanosoma brucei* subspecies using repetitive DNA sequences. *Mol. Biochem. Parasitol.* **39**, 213-226.

Hoare, C.A. (1956) Morphological and taxonomic studies on mammalian trypanosomes. VIII. Revision of *T. evansi. Parasitol.* **46**, 130-172.

Holland, W.G., Claes, F., My, L.N., Thanh, N.G., Tam, P.T., Verloo, D., Büscher, P., Goddeeris, B. and Vercruysse, J. (2001) A comparative evaluation of parasitological tests and a PCR for *Trypanosoma evansi* diagnosis in experimentally infected water buffaloes. *Vet. Parasitol.* **97**, 23-33.

Holmes, P.H. (1997) New approaches to the integrated control of trypanosomosis. *Vet. Parasitol.* **71**, 121-135.

Holmes, P.H., Eisler, M.C. and Geerts, S. (2004) Current chemotherapy of animal trypanosomiasis. In: *The Trypanosomiasis*, 1st edn., Eds: I. Maudlin, P.H. Holmes and M.A. Miles, CABI Publishing, Wallingford. pp. 431-444.

Hopkins, J.S., Chitambo, H., Machila, N., Luckins, A.G., Rae, P.F., van den Bossche, P. and Eisler, M.C. (1998) Adaptation and validation of the antibody trapping ELISA using dried blood spots on filter paper, for epidemiological surveys of tsetse transmitted trypanosomosis in cattle. *Prev. vet. Med.* **37**, 91-99.

Kinabo, L.D.B. and Bogan, J.A. (1988) Pharmacokinetic and histopathological investigation of isometamidium in cattle. *Res. vet. Sci.* **44**, 267-269.

Laveran, A. and Mesnil, F. (1912) *Trypanosomes et Trypanosomiasis*, Masson et Co., Paris.

Luckins, A.G. (1994) Equine trypanosomiasis. *Equine. vet. Educ.* **6**, 259-262.

Luckins, A.G. and Mehlitz, D. (1978) Evaluation of an indirect fluorescent antibody test, enzyme-linked immunosorbent assay and quantification of immunoglobulins in the diagnosis of bovine trypanosomiasis. *Trop. An. Health Prod.* **10**, 149-159.

Luckins, A.G. (1977) Detection of antibodies in trypanosoma-infected cattle by means of a microplate enzyme-linked immunosorbant assay. *Trop. An. Health Prod.* **9**, 53-62.

Lumsden, W.H.R., Kimber, C.D., Evans, D.A. and Doig, S.J. (1979) *Trypanosoma brucei*: miniature anion-exchange centrifugation technique for detection of low parasitaemias: adaptation for field use. *Trans. R. Soc. Trop. Med. Hyg.* **73**, 312-317.

Lun, Z.R., Allingham, R., Brun, R. and Lanham, S.M. (1992) The isoenzyme characteristics of *Trypanosoma evansi* and *Trypanosoma equiperdum* isolated from domestic stocks in China. *Ann. Trop. Med. Parasitol.* **86**, 333-340.

Majiwa, P.A. and Otieno, L.H. (1990) Recombinant DNA probes reveal simultaneous infection of tsetse flies with different trypanosome species. *Mol. Biochem. Parasitol.* **40**, 245-253.

McCully, R.M. and Neitz, W.O. (1971) Clinicopathological study on experimental *Trypanosoma brucei* infections in horses. Part 2. Histopathological findings in the nervous system and other organs of treated and untreated horses reacting to nagana. *Onderstepoort J. vet. Res.* **38**, 141-176.

Morlais, I., Ravel, S., Grébaut, P., Dumas, V. and Cuny, G. (2001) New molecular marker for *Trypanosoma* (*Duttonella*) *vivax* identification. *Acta. Trop.* **80**, 207-213.

Moser, D.R., Cook, G.A., Ochs, D.E., Bailey, C.P., McKane, M.R. and Donelson, J.E. (1989) Detection of *Trypanosoma congolense* and *Trypanosoma brucei* subspecies by DNA amplification using the polymerase chain reaction. *Parasitol.* **99**, 57-66.

Murray, M., Murray, P.K. and McIntyre, W.I.M. (1977) An improved parasitological technique for the diagnosis of African trypanosomiasis. *Trans. R. Soc. Trop. Med. Hyg.* **71**, 325-326.

Neitz, W.O. and McCully, R.M. (1971) Clinicopathological study on experimental *Trypanosoma brucei* infections in horses. Part 1. Development of clinically recognizable nervous symptoms in nagana-infected horses treated with subcurative doses of antrypol and berenil. *Onderstepoort J. vet. Res.* **38**, 127-140.

Paris, J., Murray, M. and McOdimba, F. (1982) A comparative evaluation of the parasitological techniques currently available for the diagnosis of African trypanosomiasis in cattle. *Acta. Trop.* **39**, 307-316.

Pereira de Almeida, P.J.L., Ndao, M., van Meirvenne and N., Geerts, S. (1998) Diagnostic evaluation of PCR on dried blood samples from goats experimentally infected with *Trypanosoma brucei brucei*. *Acta. Trop.* **70**, 269-276.

Pinchbeck, G.L., Morrison, L.J., Tait, A., Langford, J., Meehan, L., Jallow, S., Jallow, J., Jallow, A. and Christley, R.M. (2008) Trypanosomosis in The Gambia: prevalence in working horses and donkeys detected by whole genome amplification and PCR, and evidence for interactions between trypanosome species. *BMC vet. Res.* **4**, 1-7.

Reid, S.A. (2002) *Trypanosoma evansi* control and containment in Australasia. *Trends Parasitol.* **18**, 219-224.

Richardson, U.F. and Kendall, S.B. (1957) *Veterinary Protozoology*, Oliver & Boyd, Edinburgh.

Riou, G.F. and Saucier, J.M. (1979) Characterization of the molecular components in kinetoplast-mitochondrial DNA of *Trypanosoma equiperdum*. *J. Cell. Biol.* **82**, 248-263.

Robinson, E.M. (1926) Serological investigation into some diseases of domesticated animals in South Africa caused by trypanosomes. *Repts Direct vet. Educ. Res., Dept. Agric., S. Afr.* **9**, 11-12.

Rogers, D.J. (1988) A general model for the African trypanosomiasis. *Parasitol.* **97**, 193-212.

Saurat, P. (1946) La dourine: son existence actuelle en France. *Rec. Méd. Vét.* **122**, 7, 289-309.

Singh, V., Chaudhari, S.S., Kumar, S. and Chhabra, M.B. (1995) Polyclonal antibody-based antigen-detection immunoassay for diagnosis of *Trypanosoma evansi* in buffaloes and horses. *Vet. Parasitol.* **56**, 261-267.

Stephen, L.E. (1986) *Trypanosomiasis. A Veterinary Perspective*, Pergamon Press, Oxford.

Stephen, L.E. and Mackenzie C.P. (1958) *Trypanosoma vivax* infection in a mare: treatment with ethidium bromide. *Vet. Rec.* **70**, 293-294.

Taylor, K. and Authié, E.M.L. (2004) Pathogenesis of animal trypanosomiasis. In: *The Trypanosomiasis*, 1st edn., Eds. I. Maudlin, P.H. Holmes and M.A. Miles, CABI Publishing, Wallingford. pp 331-353.

Uilenberg, G.A. (1998) *Field Guide for the Diagnosis, Treatment and Prevention of African Animal Trypanosomosis.* Food and Agriculture Organization, Rome.

Van den Bossche, P. and De Deken, R. (2004) The application of bait technology to control tsetse. In: *The Trypanosomiasis*, 1st edn., Eds: I. Maudlin, P.H. Holmes and M.A. Miles, CABI Publishing, Wallingford. pp 525-532.

Vaysse, J. and Zottner, G. (1950) Contribution à l'étude de la chimiothérapie et de la chimioprévention de la dourine par l'antracyde. *Bull. Off. Int. Epiz.* **34**, 172-179.

Verloo, D., Magnus, E. and Büscher, P. (2001) General expression of RoTat 1.2 variable antigen type in *Trypanosoma evansi* isolates from different origin. *Vet. Parasitol.* **97**, 183-189.

Watson, E.A. (1915) Dourine and the complement fixation test. *Parasitol.* **8**, 156-183.

Woo, P.T.K. (1970) The haematocrit centrifuge technique for the diagnosis of African trypanosomiasis. *Acta. Trop.* **27**, 384-386.

Wuyts, N., Chokesajjawatee, N. and Panyim, S. (1994) A simplified and highly sensitivity detection of *Trypanosoma evansi* by DNA amplification. *Southeast Asian J. Trop. Med. Public Health* **25**, 266-271.

Zhang, Z.Q. and Baltz, T. (1994) Identification of *Trypanosoma evansi, Trypanosoma equiperdum* and *Trypanosoma brucei brucei* using repetitive DNA probes. *Vet. Parasitol.* **53**, 197-208.

Zhang, Z.Q., Giroud, C. and Baltz, T. (1993) *Trypanosoma evansi: in vivo* and *in vitro* determination of trypanocide resistance profiles. *Exp. Parasitol.* **77**, 387-94.

Zhang, Z.Q., Giroud, C. and Baltz, T. (1992) *In vivo* and *in vitro* sensitivity of *Trypanosoma evansi* and *Trypanosoma equiperdum* to diminazene, suramin, MelCy, quinapyramine and isometamidium. *Acta Trop.* **50**, 101-110.

EQUINE MANGE

S. Paterson* and S. Shaw

Rutland House Referral Hospital, Abbotsfield Road, St Helens, Merseyside WA9 4HU, UK.

Keywords: horse; mange; *Chorioptes bovis*; chorioptic mange; *Demodex equi*; *Demodex caballi*; demodicosis; *Psoroptes equi*; *Psoroptes natalensis*; *Psoroptes ovis*; *Psoroptes cuniculi*; psoroptic mange; sarcoptic mange

Summary

Equine mange describes chronic skin diseases caused by parasitic mites. Chorioptic mange caused by *Chorioptes bovis* is a common variably pruritic skin condition of the horse. The mites are surface browsing parasites. Clinical signs are most commonly seen in heavy horses with feathered fetlocks. Lesions usually extend from the fetlock to the pastern and consist of thick scale and crust with associated self-inflicted trauma. Demodicosis is a very rare condition. Two forms of demodex mite are recognised: *Demodex equi*, a short-bodied mite found on the body, and *Demodex caballi,* a long-bodied mite that lives in the eyelid and muzzle. Both mites are normal residents of the equine skin. Psoroptic mange is also rare. Four species of psoroptes mite have been reported to parasitise the horse: *Psoroptes equi*, *P. natalensis*, *P. ovis* and *P. cuniculi*. Sarcoptic mange is also very rare. Equine scabies is a very rare disease caused by the *Sarcoptes scabiei* var. *equi*.

Introduction

Equine mange is a broad term used to describe any of several chronic skin diseases of the horse caused by parasitic mites. Mites are found within the order Acarina which is part of the Arachnida class. Within the Acarina family, the principal equine mites are found in the 3 suborders (**Fig 1**); Astigmata, which contains the Sarcoptidae, Psoroptidae and Acaridae families; Prostigmata, which contains the Trombiculidae and Demodicidae families; and Mesostigmata containing the family Dermanyssidae.

The most common mite found in equids in the UK is *Chorioptes bovis*, which is recognised as the cause of leg mange especially in heavy horses. Uncommon environmentally derived mite infestations include *Neotrombicula autumnalis*, the harvest mite; *Dermanyssus gallinae*, the poultry mite and forage mites such as *Acarus*, *Pyemotes* and *Tyrophagus*. Demodicosis is a rare finding in horses with immunosuppression. Psoroptic and sarcoptic mange are very rare if not eliminated in the UK.

Chorioptic mange

Chorioptic mange caused by *Chorioptes bovis* is a common variably pruritic skin condition of the horse. The mites are surface browsing parasites that are approximately 0.3–0.5 mm in length (**Fig 2**). The life cycle takes 3 weeks and is completed on the horse. Mites can survive in the environment under favourable conditions for periods of up to 10 weeks providing they are accompanied by a food supply of epidermal debris (Sweatman 1957). Populations of mites tend to be larger during cold weather leading to an increased incidence of disease in the winter months. As temperature and humidity rise in the spring mite numbers drop and many animals' disease will spontaneously regress, leading in some cases to an asymptomatic carrier state in the summer (Liebisch *et al.* 1985). Clinical signs are most commonly seen in heavy horses with feathered fetlocks. Lesions usually extend from the fetlock to the pastern and consist of thick scale and crust with associated self-inflicted trauma (**Figs 3** and **4**). Horses are often seen to stamp their feet and kick out due to the intense irritation caused by the mites. Where a carrier state exists pruritus can be minimal or nonexistent. Occasionally horses will present with generalised disease where clinical signs extend to the trunk, head, neck and perianal areas (Scott and Miller 2003) (**Figs 5** and **6**). The differential

*Author to whom correspondence should be addressed.

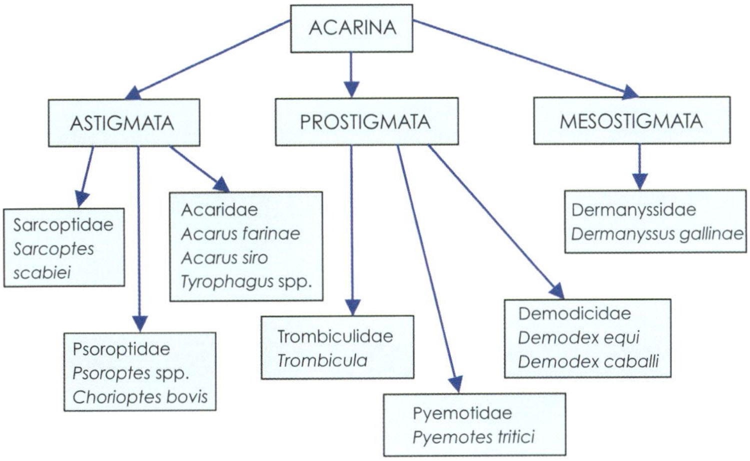

CHART 1: Classification of equine mange mites.

diagnosis of pastern dermatitis includes a variety of infectious and immune-mediated diseases (**Table 1**). Differential diagnosis of generalised disease includes insect hypersensitivity, atopy, food intolerance and ectoparasites especially lice.

A variety of different techniques can be employed to successfully collect the mites. As chorioptic mange mites are active, rapidly moving parasites it has been suggested that a small amount of parasiticide is added to the mounting medium to kill mites and prevent them escaping from the slide (Scott and Miller 2003; Bergvall 2005). Mites can be collected by superficial skin scrapings into liquid paraffin or potassium hydroxide, scrapings using a wooden tongue depressor, acetate tape strips or coat brushings (Littlewood 1999a). **Table 2** details the different techniques and **Table 3** denotes each mite and techniques suitable for each.

Management of chorioptic mange should include, in addition to the affected horse, all in-contact horses. A range of both systemic and topical medications have been suggested for therapy (Littlewood *et al.* 1995; Curtis 1999; Littlewood 1999b, 2000; Rendle *et al.* 2007; Paterson and Coumbe 2008). Topical treatments are labour intensive, but are generally accepted as being more effective than systemic medication (Scott and Miller 2003). A 2% selenium sulphide shampoo (Curtis 1999); lime sulphur (Ackerman 1989; Paterson

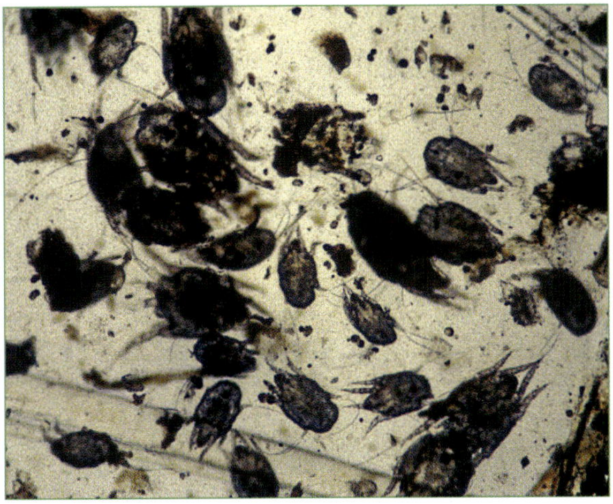

FIGURE 2: Chorioptic mange mites.

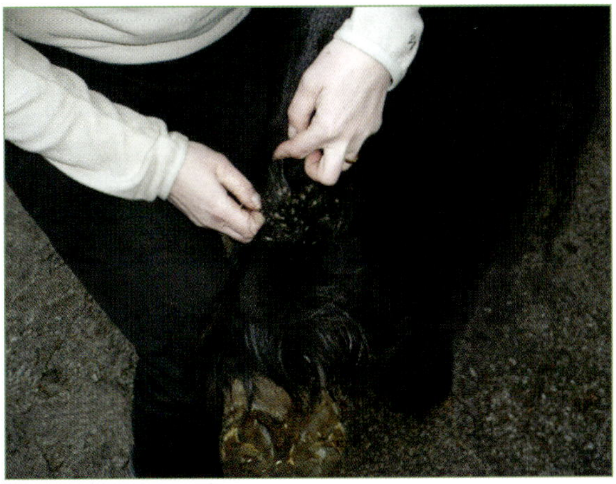

FIGURE 3: Crusting and scaling on the leg of a Friesian with chorioptic mange.

and Coumbe 2008); fipronil (Littlewood 2000); and ivermectin solution (Fadok 1987; Littlewood 1999b) have been used topically for therapy. See **Table 4** for details of dose rates and frequency of application. Topical therapy with products such as selenium sulphide or lime sulphur have the advantage of their keratolytic properties, which help remove crust and scale to physically remove mites as well as making the horse more comfortable. Where systemic medication is used this keratolytic activity is lost and horses will benefit from the use of adjunctive shampoo therapy with products containing such actives as benzoyl

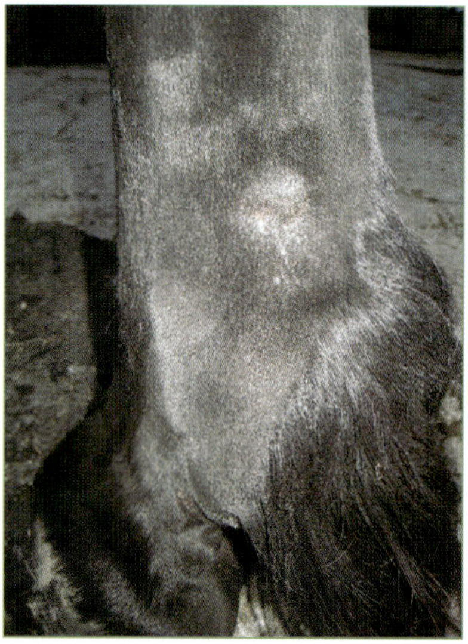

FIGURE 4: Scale on the leg of a Friesian with chorioptic mange.

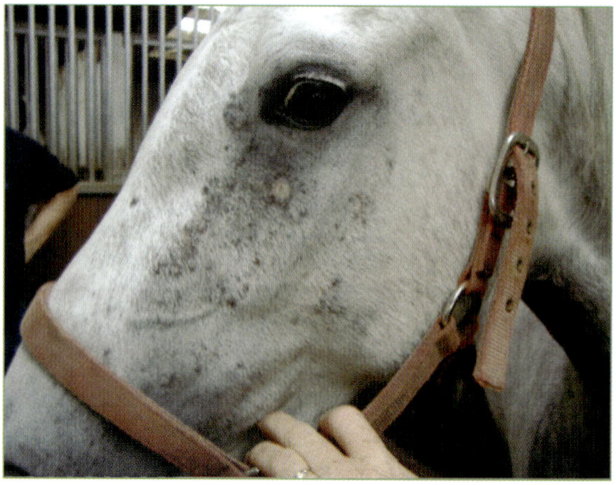

FIGURE 5: Scale and self inflicted trauma on the face of a horse with generalised chorioptic mange.

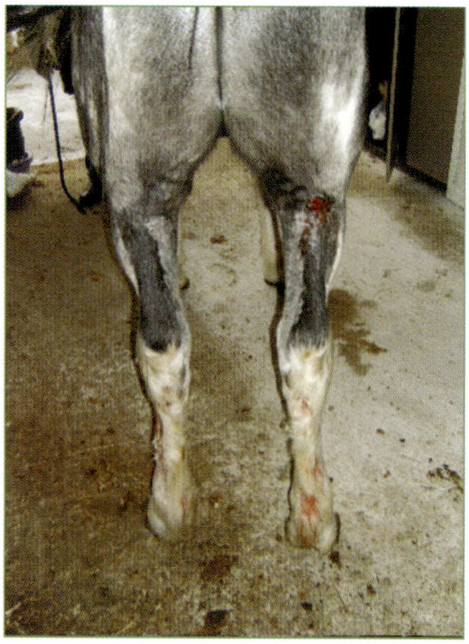

FIGURE 6: Severe self inflicted trauma down the hind legs of a horse with chorioptic mange.

TABLE 1: Differential diagnosis of equine pastern dermatitis

Differential diagnosis of equine pastern dermatitis
Bacterial infection – *Staphylococcus*, *Dermatophilus*
Dermatophytosis
Trombiculidiasis
Contact irritant dermatitis
Photo-induced dermatitis
Leucocytoclastic vasculitis
Lymphoedema

TABLE 2: Diagnostic techniques for collection of mites

Techniques
Superficial skin scrapes of crust using a blunted scalpel blade coated in mineral oil into mineral oil or a wooden tongue depressor scraped across the crust and mounted similarly.
Deep skin scrape of crust and superficial layers of epidermis to produce capillary ooze mounted in potassium hydroxide or liquid paraffin. Where scrapings are taken to identify demodex mites, the skin should be squeezed to express mites from follicles.
Acetate tape strips pressed repeatedly onto the coat and then mounted directly onto a slide.
Coat brushing with toothbrush directly into a Petri dish. Parasites can be visualised directly under a microscope under low power.
Hair plucks of coat mounted in liquid paraffin or potassium hydroxide from areas where there is evidence of comedones.
Examination of cerumin (ear wax) mounted unstained directly onto a microscope slide.

peroxide, sulphur and salicyclic acid. Systemic regimens have been described using injectable doramectin (Rendle *et al.* 2007) and oral ivermectin (Littlewood 1995). **Table 4** details dose rates and frequency for these. Environmental therapy is useful where possible but does require a high degree of owner compliance. Stables should be thoroughly cleaned and disinfected as should all grooming tools, tack and other fomites (Scott and Miller 2003).

Demodectic mange

Demodicosis is a very rare skin condition of the horse. Two forms of demodex mite are recognised: *Demodex equi*, a short-bodied mite found on the body, and *Demodex caballi*, a long-bodied mite that lives in the eyelid and muzzle. Both mites are normal residents of the equine skin, are host specific and live their whole life on the animal (Bennison 1943). The life cycle is thought to be 20–35 days (Scott and Miller 2005). Equine demodicosis is most commonly seen in association with long-term glucocorticoid treatment (Scott and White 1983) but can also be seen in horses with pituitary *pars intermedia* dysfunction (PPID, Cushing's syndrome) (Bergvall 2005) or in old or debilitated horses with malignancies or other severe diseases. The severity of the clinical signs tends to mirror the degree of immunosuppression. Horses

TABLE 3: Equine mites and diagnostic methods of identification

Parasite	Methods that are most useful for identification
Chorioptes bovis	Superficial skin scrape, acetate tape strip, coat brushing.
Demodex caballi	Deep skin scrapes, hair plucks, skin biopsy.
Demodex equi	Superficial skin scrapes, acetate tape strip, skin biopsy.
Neotrombicula autumnalis	Superficial skin scrape, tape strip.
Psoroptes equi	Superficial skin scrape especially from edge of lesions, acetate tape strip.
Psoroptes cuniculi	Superficial skin scrape especially from edge of lesions, acetate tape strip, cerumin examination.
Sarcoptes scabiei	Deep skin scrape.
Acaris siro, Pyemotes spp.	Superficial skin scrape, acetate tape strip, coat brushing.
Dermanyssus gallinae	Superficial skin scrape, acetate tape strip, coat brushing.

TABLE 4: Drugs for therapy of equine mange

Product	Trade name	Treatment regime	Conditions
1.87% w/v Ivermectin paste	Eqvalan paste for horses (Merial Animal Health)[1]	300 µg/kg bwt orally 3 x at 14 day intervals.	Chorioptes Sarcoptes
1% w/v Doramectin	Dectomax (Pfizer Animal Health)[2]	0.3 mg/kg by subcutaneous injection 2 x at 14 day intervals.	Chorioptes Sarcoptes
0.25% w/v Fipronil spray	Frontline (Merial Animal Health)[1]	Solution sprayed onto affected area. Chorioptes 125 ml each leg from elbow to stifle down. Repeat 3–4 weeks.	Chorioptes Trombicula
2% Selenium sulphide shampoo	Seleen shampoo (Sanofi Animal Health)[3]	Shampoo diluted 50:50 with water and used as whole body wash 3 x at 5 day intervals with 10 min contact time.	Chorioptes
5% Lime sulphur solution	Lime Plus Dip (Dermapet)[4]	Stock solution (97%) diluted 25 ml in 1 litre and sprayed and left on affected area 4 x at 7 day intervals (Sarcoptes 6 x 7 days).	Chorioptes, Sarcoptes Trombicula
1% w/v Ivermectin solution	Ivomec injection (Merial Animal Health)[1]	Apply solution directly to the affected area at a dose of 200 µg/kg (1 ml/50 kg body wt).	Chorioptes
5% w/v Cypermethrin	Barricade (Sorex)[5] Deosan Deosect (DiverseyLever)[6]	Single application sufficient providing environmental infestation is removed.	Poultry mite Trombicula

NB. There are, to the authors' knowledge, no veterinary medicines that have been licensed for the treatment of equine mange. As such veterinary surgeons may prescribe an unlicensed product but should follow cascade guidelines. Where a veterinary product is used outside of its data sheet recommendations or a human product is used, then owners should be informed and where possible informed consent should be sought.

present with varying degrees of nonpruritic alopecia often with mild scaling (**Fig 6**). Signs are most commonly seen on the face and neck and occasionally over the shoulder and forelimbs. Principal differential diagnoses include other follicular diseases such as bacterial folliculitis, especially with *Staphylococcus* and *Dermatophilus*, dermatophytosis and alopecia areata. *Demodex caballi* can be isolated from deep skin scrapings (**Table 2**) and also on biopsy, and *Demodex equi* can be found on superficially taken samples. There are only anecdotal reports in the literature of therapy for demodectic mange in the horse. Treatment or removal of any immunosuppressive factors is essential to allow clinical cure and some authors suggest spontaneous remission will occur when the underlying cause is corrected (Scott and White 1983). Drug therapy that has been described includes oral ivermectin or doramectin (Ute Brauer 1997), see **Table 4**. Note that amitraz has no place in the treatment of any disease in the horse.

Trombiculidiasis

Trombiculidiasis, also referred to as chiggers, harvest mites, leg itch mites or heel bugs, is commonly encountered in the horse. Trombiculid adults are free-living parasites that usually feed on invertebrate hosts or plants (Scott and Miller 2003). The larval forms usually feed on the tissue fluids of small rodents but are not host-specific and will attack both horses and people. Mites are relatively large (0.2–0.4 mm) and can be seen with the naked eye (**Fig 7**), characteristically they have six legs. They vary in colour from red to orange to yellow. In Europe, the principal mite is *Neotrombicula autumnalis* which inhabits chalky soils, grasslands and cornfields. The larvae tend to be most active during autumn and feed most vigorously in late afternoon and early evening. Skin lesions such as papules and wheals with secondary self-inflicted trauma are seen at the site of the larval mite attachment. The distal limbs are most commonly affected, but the muzzle, nares, face, ears and neck may also be involved. The horse's reaction to the larvae is quite variable and in pruritic animals hypersensitivity reaction to larval feeding is likely. This is reinforced by the fact that pruritus in some animals may persist for some time after the larvae have detached and fallen off sometimes making a definitive diagnosis difficult. Where larvae attach to the nares or ears, the horse may present with sneezing or head shaking (Mair 1994).

Diagnosis is simple if the larvae can be seen attached to the skin, but in cases where the mites have fallen off differential diagnoses should include chorioptic, sarcoptic and psoroptic mange; forage mites; insect hypersensitivity; atopy and bacterial skin infection. Mites can be difficult to identify on skin scrapings and are best trapped by acetate tape impression smears so they can be mounted directly on a microscope slide. Therapy is often not necessary

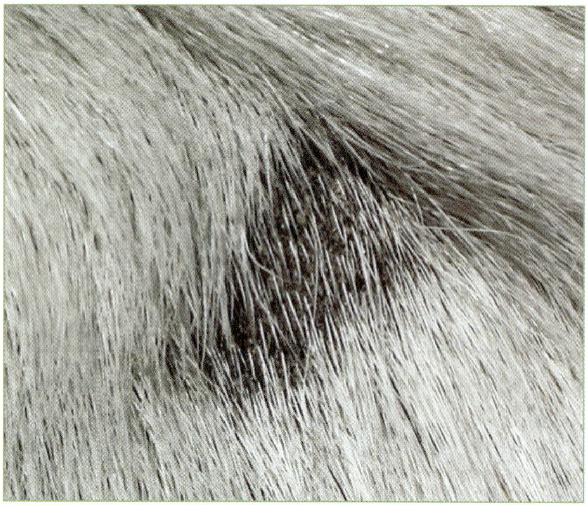

FIGURE 6: Nonpruritic alopecia due to demodicosis in a horse with pituitary pars intermedia dysfunction (picture courtesy of K. Bergvall).

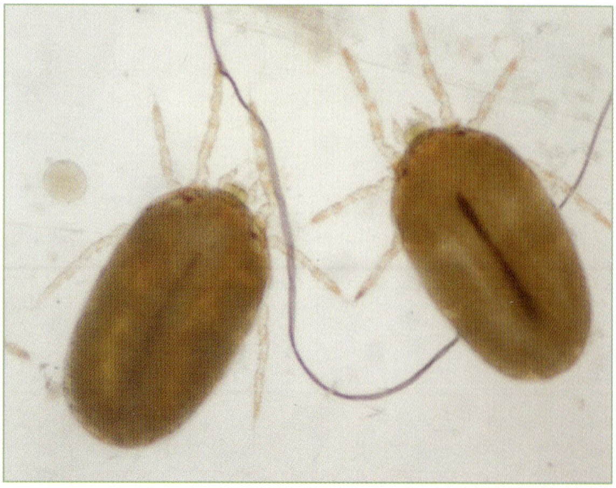

FIGURE 7: **Neotrombicula autumnalis** *mite.*

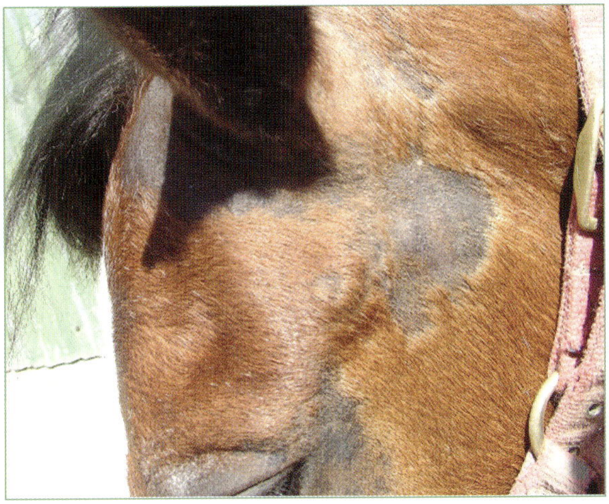

FIGURE 8: Irritation on face of horse after contact with forage mites from feed.

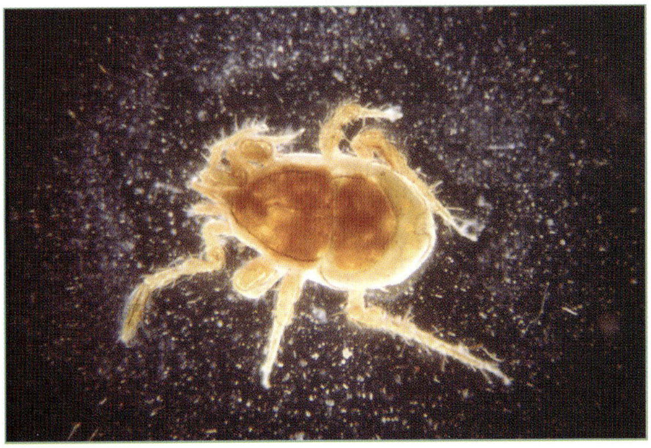

FIGURE 9: Dermanyssus gallinae - poultry mite.

as the disease is self-limiting if horses are prevented from further contact with the mites. Where avoidance is impossible, horses may be treated with any one of a range of products including fipronil, which has been shown to have good activity against trombicula (Nuttall *et al.* 1998). Littlewood (1999b) suggests the spray could be applied every 4 weeks during high risk periods at the same volumes as recommended for chorioptic mange. Other topical medications with activity against trombiculids include cypermethrin and lime sulphur (**Table 4**). Where pruritus is severe, horses benefit from short-term therapy over a few days with glucocorticoids.

Forage mites

Forage mites are free-living mites that normally feed on organic matter (*Acarus siro*, *Acarus farinae* – forage mites) or the larvae of insects in hay or grain (*Pyemotes tritici* – straw itch mite). The life cycle of these mites takes place in the environment and is dependent on temperature and humidity. Mite numbers tend to be lowest in the winter months in the UK (Kunkle and Greiner 1982; Norvall and McPherson 1983). Clinical signs are typically seen as papulocrustous lesions in areas such as the head and muzzle (**Fig 8**) that come into contact with contaminated foodstuffs. Pruritus is variable. Differential diagnoses include sarcoptic, psoroptic or chorioptic mange, contact dermatitis, trombiculidiasis and insect hypersensitivity. Mites can be identified by collection of samples from the lesional areas either by coat brushing, tape stripping or surface skin scrapes. Removal of the contaminated food sources can lead to spontaneous remission of the clinical signs. In severe cases, animals may benefit from 3–5 days of systemic glucocorticoid therapy.

Poultry mites

Horses who have contact with poultry or are housed in areas previously used for poultry can be affected by *Dermanyssus gallinae*, the red poultry mite (Scott and Miller 2003). Adult mites lay their eggs in the cracks and crevices in the walls of poultry houses and in birds' nests. The mites emerge from their microenvironments at night to feed. Sampling of horses during the day time is often fruitless as mites may not be present on scrapings. Adult mites are red in colour and 0.6–1.0 mm in length (**Fig 9**). Where mites can not be identified on the horses but there is a history of possible poultry contacts, the environment and any poultry may be sampled for parasites. Lesions consist of nonspecific papules and crusting in contact areas. Important differential diagnoses include trombiculidiasis, mange in all its different forms, contact dermatitis and insect hypersensitivity. Environmental therapy is important with an appropriate ectoparasiticide. Horses may be treated with such drugs as cypermethrin (**Table 4**).

Sarcoptic mange

Equine scabies is a very rare notifiable disease caused by *Sarcoptes scabiei* var. *equi* (Scott and Miller 2003).

The equine form of scabies is largely a disease of the past and has not to the authors' knowledge been reported in the UK since the late 1990s. Sarcoptes mites burrow through the skin causing severe pruritus in affected horses. The disease is contagious to man, but, as the mite can not complete its life cycle in human skin, man is considered to be a dead-end host. The mite is 0.25–0.6 mm with a spherical body. Its life cycle is completed on the host in 2–3 weeks. The mites are susceptible to dessication and can only survive for several hours under normal environmental conditions, but can for live for a few weeks if colder conditions are present. Mites preferentially feed on areas around the head, neck and ears, but their distribution can become more generalised. Lesions consist of papules, crusts, excoriation and alopecia. In chronic disease, crusts are often accompanied by lichenification. *Sarcoptes scabiei* var. *canis* has been reported to affect parts of Europe. This canine form of sarcoptic mange has been described in horses that have had contact with foxes, either out at pasture or in stables. Lesions in this disease tend to affect the legs and ventral abdominal skin. The disease is self-limiting as the horse is not the natural host for the mite. For therapy of scabies see **Table 4**.

Psoroptic mange

Psoroptic mange is another very rare disease in the horse in the UK. Four species of psoroptes mites have been reported to parasitise the horse. These are *Psoroptes equi*, *P. natalensis*, *P. ovis* and *P. cuniculi* (Scott and Miller 2003). The mites are slightly larger than chorioptes mites (0.4–0.8 mm) and have a slightly more pointed head (**Table 5**). It is likely that, as the different species appear to be genetically homogenous, no one specific clinical presentation can be ascribed to any one species of mite. Psoroptes mites can infest the ears of horses where they can cause intense irritation. Horses may become head shy, show signs of otitis externa or present with head shaking. Psoroptes mites prefer thickly haired areas and are commonly isolated from areas such as the mane, shoulders and intermandibular region. When their activity leads to traumatically-induced alopecia, the mites will abandon a site to move to other haired areas. For this reason, skin scrapings should be taken from the periphery of lesions where possible. Where mites are thought to be a cause of ear disease heavy sedation is necessary to take samples from the ear canals. Important differential diagnoses for psoroptic mange include chorioptic mange, insect bite hypersensitivity and atopic dermatitis. Therapy of ear mite infestation is best accomplished by the use of systemic drugs (Osman *et al.* 2006) such as ivermectin or doramectin as most horses will not tolerate drops in their ears. Treatment of generalised disease is as for chorioptic mange as detailed in **Table 4**.

TABLE 5: Differences between chorioptes and psoroptes mites

	Chorioptes	Psoroptes
Size of mite	0.3–0.5 mm	0.4–0.8 mm
Shape of head	Rounded head	Elongated head
Pedicles	Short unsegmented pedicles	Long segmented pedicles
Suckers	Present	Present

Manufacturers' addresses

[1]Merial Animal Health, Harlow, Essex, UK.
[2]Pfizer Animal Health, Sandwich, Kent, UK.
[3]Sanofi Animal Health, Watford, Hertfordshire, UK.
[4]Dermapet, Potomac, Maryland, USA.
[5]Sorex, Widnes, Cheshire, UK.
[6]DiverseyLever, Northampton, UK.

References

Ackerman, L.J. (1989) Parasitic skin disorders. In: *Practical Equine Dermatology,* American Veterinary Publications Ltd, Goleta. pp 37-41.

Bennison, J.C. (1943) Demodicosis with special reference to equine members of the genus *Demodex*. *J. Royal Army Vet. Corps.* **14**, 34.

Bergvall, K. (2005) Advances in acquisition, identification and treatment of equine ectoparasites. *Clin. tech. Equine Pract.* **4**, 296-301.

Curtis, C.F. (1999) Pilot study to investigate the efficacy of 1% selenium sulphide shampoo in the treatment of equine chorioptic mange. *Vet. Rec.* **144**, 677-675.

Fadok, V.A. (1987) Ectoparasites. In: *Current Veterinary Therapy in Equine Practice,* Ed: N.E. Robinson, W.B. Saunders, Philadelphia. pp 622-624

Kunkle, G.A. and Greiner, E.C. (1982) Dermatitis in horses and man caused by the straw itch mite. *J. Am. vet. med. Ass.* **181**, 467.

Liebisch, A., Olbrich, S. and Deppe, M. (1985) Survival of *Psoroptes ovis*, *Psoroptes cuniculi* and *Chorioptes bovis* away from the host. *Deutsche Tierarztliche Wochenschrift* **92**, 181-185.

Littlewood, J.D. (1999a) *Equine Chorioptic Mange: an Epidemiological Study and Controlled Clinical Trial.* Diploma in Veterinary Dermatology Thesis, Royal College of Veterinary Surgeons.

Littlewood, J.D. (1999b) Control of ectoparasites in the horse. *In Practice* **21**, 418-424

Littlewood, J.D. (2000) Chorioptic mange: successful treatment of a case with fipronil. *Equine vet. Educ.* **12**, 144-146.

Littlewood, J.D., Rose, J.F. and Paterson, S. (1995) Oral ivermectin paste for the treatment of chorioptic mange in horses. *Vet. Rec.* **137**, 661-663.

Mair, T.S. (1994) Headshaking associated with *Trombicula autumnalis* larval infestation in two horses. *Equine vet. J.* **26**, 244-245.

Norvall, J. and McPherson, E.A. (1983) Dermatitis in the horse caused by *Acarus farinae*. *Vet. Rec.* **112**, 385.

Nuttall, T., French, A.T., Cheatham, H.C. and Proctor, F.J. (1998) Treatment of *Trombicula autumnalis* infestation in dogs and cats with a 0.25% fipronil pump spray. *J. Small anim. Pract.* **39**, 237-239.

Osman, S.A., Hanafy, A. and Amer, S.E. (2006) Clinical and therapeutic studies on mange in horses. *Vet. Parasitol.* **10**, 191-195.

Paterson, S. and Coumbe, K. (2008) An open study to evaluate topical lime sulphur solution as treatment for equine chorioptic mange. In: *Proceedings of the 6th World Congress on Veterinary Dermatology*. In press.

Rendle, D.I., Cottle, H.J., Love, S. and Hughes, K.J. (2007) Comparative study of doramectin and fipronil in the treatment of equine chorioptic mange. *Vet. Rec.* **161**, 335-338.

Scott, D.W. and White, K.K. (1983) Demodicosis associated with systemic glucocorticoid therapy in two horses. *Equine Pract.* **5**, 31-32.

Scott, D.W. and Miller, W.H. (2003) Parasitic disease. In: *Equine Dermatology*, W.B. Saunders, Philadelphia. pp 321-375.

Sweatman, G.K. (1957) Life history, non-specificity and revision of the genus *Chorioptes*, a parasitic mite of herbivores. *Can. J. Zool.* **35**, 641-689.

Ute Brauer, V.E.U. (1997) Klinischer Fall einer generalisierten Demodikose bei einem Pferd und deren Behandlung mit Doramectin. *Tierarztl. Umschau.* **52**, 131.

CYSTIC ECHINOCOCCOSIS IN HORSES (HYDATID DISEASE)

A. E. Durham

Liphook Equine Hospital, Forest Mere, Liphook, Hampshire GU30 7JG, UK.

Keywords: horse; *Echinococcus granulosus*; metacestaode; liver; ultrasonography

Summary

Cystic echinococcosis in horses is caused by the metacestode stage of *Echinococcus granulosus* G4. It is rare in the USA and Scandinavia and relatively common in the rest of Europe (especially the UK) and is seen most frequently in the liver as an incidental finding at *post mortem* or during ultrasonographic examination. It is strongly host-adapted and is highly unlikely to have any zoonotic implications. Occasional cases are encountered where clinical relevance is suspected although firm establishment of such may often be difficult. In those cases where treatment is indicated surgical removal, PAIR (puncture-aspiration-injection-reaspiration) and systemic albendazole and/or praziquantel appear to represent the best therapeutic options in horses, although experience with all of these choices is limited.

Introduction

Cystic echinococcosis (CE) refers to visceral infection with hydatid cysts, the intermediate metacestode stage of tapeworms of the *Echinococcus* genus (Thompson and McManus 2001). Hydatid cysts are usually found in various anatomic locations in numerous species of omnivorous and herbivorous mammals that are predated or scavenged by the definitive hosts but may also be found in aberrant hosts, such as man, that do not play a role in the lifecycle of the parasite. Thus in addition to its impact on animal health, CE represents an important zoonosis in several parts of the world (Anon 2001; Pawlowski *et al.* 2001; Budke 2006).

Lifecycle

Small (2–7 mm), adult tapeworms live in the small intestine of dogs. Following a prepatent period of approximately 6–7 weeks, gravid segments are shed which release eggs that are immediately infective and may remain so for as long as one year in a moist environment. After accidental ingestion by a grazing horse or donkey, oncospheres are released from eggs and they penetrate the intestinal veins and/or lymphatics and travel to target organs. Most oncospheres are retained and develop in the liver. Some may reach the heart and lungs and even fewer may pass through the lungs to reach the systemic circulation and reach further sites. Once fixed, the oncosphere develops into a metacestode at its final destination reaching maturity over about 12 months.

Mature, fertile hydatid cysts shed 'brood capsules' by asexual reproduction from the inner germinal epithelium, each containing several protoscolices that may float freely within the cystic fluid contents and are often referred to as 'hydatid sand'. Hydatid cysts may also shed 'daughter cysts' internally giving rise to secondary chambers that may be separate or communicate with the main chamber. Brood capsules and protoscolices might also develop into further hydatid cysts if the parent cyst is ruptured or punctured within the intermediate host (Pawlowski *et al.* 2001). Each protoscolex is capable of developing into an adult tapeworm following ingestion during carcass consumption by the definitive canid host completing the lifecycle as new tapeworms develop in the small intestine.

One report quoted hunt personnel describing that 'cysts were relished by the hounds' perhaps implying evolutionary development to promote ingestion by the definitive host (Thompson and Smyth 1975). Some hydatid cysts do not produce brood capsules or protoscolices and are referred to as sterile. More than half of hydatid cysts in horses and donkeys may be sterile (Thompson 1977; Abo-Shehada 1988; Mukbel *et al.* 2000; Bardonnet *et al.* 2003) although in some studies it has been found that all cysts were viable and fertile (Dixon *et al.* 1973; Daniel Mwambete *et al.* 2004). Horse breeds were more likely to be infected with viable cysts than ponies and cobs in two studies (Cranley 1982; Edwards 1982). Cysts may remain viable for at least 24 years in infected horses (Binhazim *et al.* 1992).

Host-restriction of *Echinococcus* species

There has been considerable debate regarding the taxonomy of *Echinococcus* species, subspecies, genotypes, strains and variants (Williams and Sweatman 1963; Lymbery and Thompson 1996; Thompson and McManus 2001, 2002; Thompson 2008). There were originally 16 species and 13 subspecies that were later condensed into 4 morphologically distinct species: *E. granulosus*, *E. multilocularis*, *E. oligarthus* and *E. vogeli*. Apparent host-restriction of the equine strain then lead to its designation as a subspecies *E. granulosus equinus* (Williams and Sweatman 1963) or a separate species *E. equinus* (Thompson 2008). Various distinct strains/genotypes of *E. granulosus* have been further defined and have also been referred to as G1–G10, with the 'horse strain' being designated as G4 (**Table 1**). Thus the majority of equine CE infections occur from an equine-adapted *Echinococcus* species that may be referred to as *E. granulosus equinus*, *E. equinus* or *E. granulosus* G4 ('horse strain').

Domesticated hunting dogs that are fed on raw horse offal (e.g. fox hounds) are the main definitive host for *E. granulosus* G4 tapeworms (Thompson and Smyth 1975). The red fox (or other wild canids) might also act as a definitive host although access to infected horse offal is likely to be limited (Williams and Sweatman 1963; Thompson and Smyth 1975). Oncospheres shed from dogs infected with *E. granulosus* G4 appear to be highly host-adapted to horses and donkeys although they may also be infective in rats and mice. They do not appear to be infective in deer, hedgehogs, rabbits, monkeys or man and show a very poor infection or survival capability in sheep (Williams and Sweatman 1963; Hatch and Smyth 1975; Thompson and Smyth 1975; McManus and Smyth 1986; Thompson and McManus 2001). Some reports have suggested that the metacestode stage of *E. multilocularis* (= '*alveolar echinococcosis*') might also rarely cause CE in horses and *E. felidis* may infect zebra with the definitive stage existing in lions (Lymbery and Thompson 1996; Chiou *et al.* 2001; Eckert *et al.* 2001a,b; Thompson and McManus 2001; Azlaf and Dakkak 2006; Thompson 2008). Williams and Sweatman (1963) found that neither of 2 experimental horses were susceptible to CE infection by the ovine-adapted *E. granulosus* strain G1 although Azlaf and Dakkak (2006) and Varcasia *et al.* (2008) have reported naturally occurring infections of horses and donkeys with G1 cysts although these appeared to be sterile.

The majority of human CE cases have been shown to derive from the ovine-adapted strain *E. granulosus* G1 with infection arising from contact with dogs although cases involving other strains of *E. granulosus* as well as other *Echinococcus* species are also recognised (**Table 1**, Ekhert *et al.* 2001b; Pawlowski *et al.* 2001; Thompson and McManus 2001; Daniel Mwambete *et al.* 2004; Carmena *et al.* 2008). Notably the equine strain *E. granulosus* G4 has not been reported in man.

TABLE 1: Probable host adaptation of genotypes/strains of *Echinococcus granulosus* (Thompson and McManus 2001; Thompson 2008)

E. granulosus genotype/strain	Definitive hosts	Intermediate/aberrant hosts
G1 (Sheep strain)	Dog, wild canids	Sheep, cow, pig, camel, goat, macropod, human
G2 (Tasmanian sheep strain)	Dog, wild canids	Sheep, human
G3 (Buffalo strain)	Dog, wild canids	Buffalo, human
G4 (Horse strain)	Dog	Horse, donkey
G5 (Cattle strain)	Dog	Cow, human
G6 (Camel strain)	Dog	Camel, goat, cow, human
G7 (Pig strain)	Dog	Pig, human
G8 (Cervid strain)	Dog, wild canids	Cervids
G9	Dog	Pig, human
G10 (Cervid strain)	Dog, wild canids	Cervids

Morphology of hydatid cysts

Cystic echinococcosis in horses is usually caused by large and unilocular cysts (typically 30–70 mm diameter) although small (2–20 mm) unilocular or multilocular cysts are rarely encountered (Williams and Sweatman 1963; Dixon *et al.* 1973; Edwards 1981, 1982; Ronéus *et al.* 1982; Gelberg *et al.* 1984; Binhazim *et al.* 1992; Hoberg *et al.* 1994; Ponce Gordo and Cuesta Banderas 1998). It is not possible to predict the age of cysts accurately from their size.

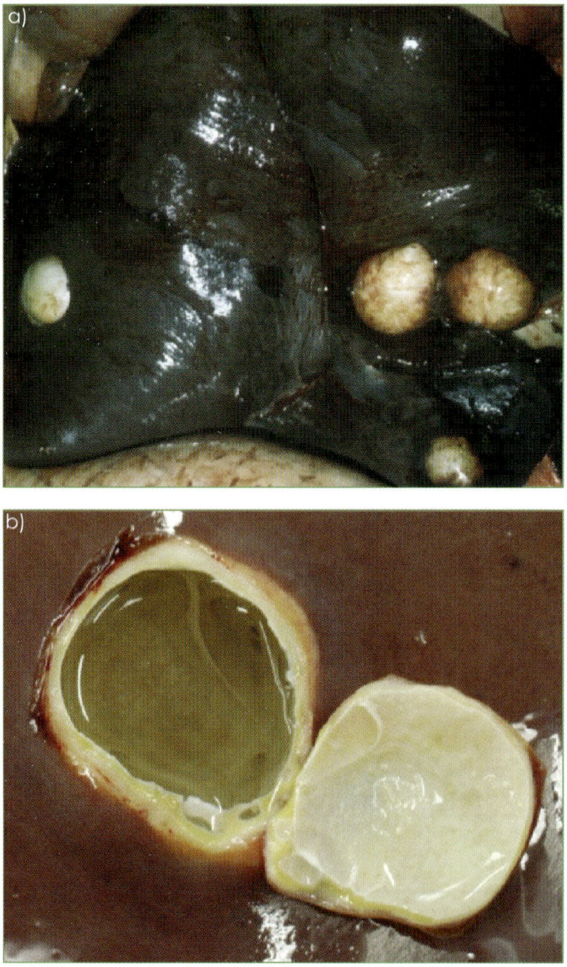

FIGURE 1: a) An equine liver showing 4 superficial hydatid cysts. b) A superficial hydatid cyst in a horse's liver with the upper capsule removed to reveal the thick wall, intracystic fluid and deposit of brood capsules on floor of cyst (Fig 1b. courtesy of Richard Irvine, Division of Pathological Sciences, University of Glasgow).

Williams and Sweatman (1963) described a cyst found 15 months after experimental infection in a horse liver to measure 36 x 15 x 20 mm whereas Ronéus *et al.* (1982) described a similar-sized viable cyst measuring 30 mm diameter that had been present in a horse's liver for at least 15 years. Similarly human cysts may show no active growth at all or may grow at rates anywhere between 1 mm and 160 mm per annum (Pawlowski *et al.* 2001). Pulmonary cysts tended to be smaller than hepatic cysts in one report of equine CE (Williams and Sweatman 1963). *E. equinus* cyst walls are often thick (e.g. 2–4 mm) and laminated combining both parasite- and host-derived parts (Edwards 1982; Rezabeck *et al.* 1993; Chiou *et al.* 2001; Azlaf and Dakkak 2006; Varcasia *et al.* 2008) (**Fig 1**). The outer layer is referred to as the ectocyst or pericyst and is composed of dense, host-derived connective tissue that may become calcified; the middle layer is composed of an acellular lamellated elastic layer; and the inner layer is the germinative layer that produces brood capsules and the fluid within the cyst. The combination of the middle and inner layers are called the endocyst (Thompson and McManus 2001; Turgut *et al.* 2007). The fluid filling the cyst is usually watery although gelatinous content is seen

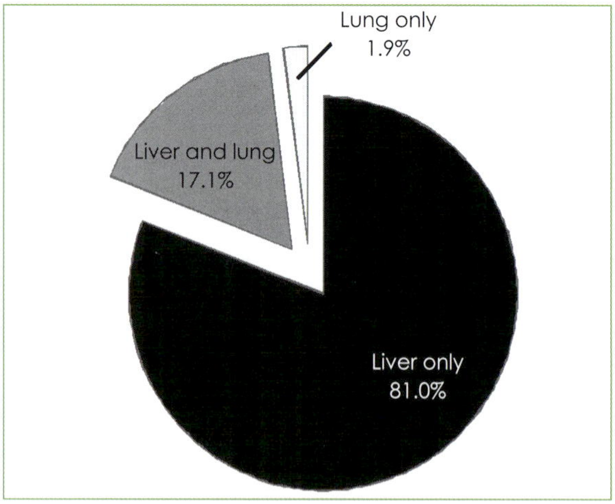

FIGURE 2: Chart representing the commonest anatomic locations of cystic echinococcosis in horses and donkeys (data derived from 2832 cases reported by Williams and Sweatman 1963; Dixon et al. 1973; Cranley 1982; Edwards 1982; Abo-Shehada 1988; Ponce Gordo and Cuesta Bandera 1998; Daniel Mwambete et al. 2004; Azlaf and Dakkak 2006; Varcasia et al. 2008).

in some more longstanding (degenerate?) cases (Chiou *et al.* 2001). Some cysts are reported with little or no wall and it has been suggested that these are not of the *E. equinus* species (Ponce Gordo and Cuesta Bandera 1998; Varcasia *et al.* 2008).

Anatomic distribution of CE

In more than 98% of CE cases in horses and donkeys, hydatid cysts will be found in the liver. The lungs will be affected in approximately 17% cases, usually concurrently with hepatic cysts and only in rare instances are the lungs the sole site of CE infection (**Fig 2**). CE has very rarely been found at other anatomic sites in horses such as the heart, pericardium, brain, pleura, spleen, kidneys and uterus (Williams and Sweatman 1963; Edwards 1982; Eckert *et al.* 2001a). Barnett *et al.* (1988) and Summerhays and Mantell (1995) reported retrobulbar hydatid cysts in 2 horses with a further case cited by Barnett *et al.* (1988) creating suspicion of this as a minor predilection site in the horse.

Geographic distribution and prevalence of *E. granulosus* G4

Equine CE has been recognised most frequently in Europe, Russian Federation states, Africa, South America, Australia, China and the Middle East (Williams and Sweatman 1963; Thompson and McManus 2001; Eckert *et al.* 2001b). CE in the horse appears to be especially rare in several areas including USA, Central America and Scandinavia and probably absent from other countries such as New Zealand, Iceland and Greenland despite the presence of CE in some other species in those countries. In contrast, in Ireland *E. granulosus* G4 appears to be the only species of *Echinococcus* present with nonequid species unaffected by CE (Eckert *et al.* 2001b). In those countries where equine CE is rare, reported clinical cases tend to have been imported from other European states (Williams and Sweatman 1963; Ronéus *et al.* 1982; Gelberg *et al.* 1984; Binhazim *et al.* 1992; Rezabeck *et al.* 1993). Hoberg *et al.* (1994), however, reported hepatic CE found incidentally *post mortem* in a horse born in Virginia and raised with foxhounds in Maryland. McFarlane *et al.* (1994) reported a case of granulomatous pleuritis in a gelding native to southern USA associated with numerous small (<8 mm) aberrant metacestodes although these were not identifiable as being from the *Echinococcus* genus. A query submitted to diplomates of the American College of Veterinary Internal Medicine revealed 4 further unpublished cases of equine CE in the USA all of which were in horses imported from Europe. Eight of 12 US respondents had never seen a case of CE in a horse. This author has seen a single case of hepatic CE in a pony recently imported from Texas to the UK (**Fig 3a**) although further enquires confirmed that the pony originated in the UK.

Surveys of CE in horses in the UK have revealed markedly differing prevalences varying between 0.03% and 61.7% of horses examined and possibly influenced by national geographic and temporal factors as well as perhaps ages and types of horse (Sweatman and Williams 1963; Dixon *et al.* 1973; Thompson and Smyth 1974, 1975; Cranley 1982). In contrast, with few exceptions CE has been reported in only a small percentage of horses from other European countries (Williams and Sweatman 1963; Ponce Gordo and Cuesta Bandera 1998; Carmena *et al.* 2008; Varcasia *et al.* 2008). Prevalence of CE in north Africa and the Middle East may be greater with recent studies reporting approximately 20% of donkeys to be infected (Abo-Shedada 1988; Mukbel *et al.* 2000; Azlaf and Dakkak 2006) and prevalences as high as 60% reported by older studies (Dailey and Sweatman 1965). The prevalence of CE appears to increase with increasing age in endemic areas suggesting poor development of immune resistance (Thompson and Smyth 1975; Cranley 1982; Edwards 1982; Abo-Shehada 1988; Mukbel *et al.* 2000; Bardonnet *et al.* 2003; Azlaf and Dakkak 2006). In a study of 1388 horses, Edwards (1982) found 0/377 horses aged <2 years to be infected with hydatid cysts and a steadily increasing prevalence up to 56/257 (22%) horses aged >8 years. There is no consistent gender predilection reported for CE (Mukbel *et al.* 2000).

Diagnosis of CE

Hepatic CE in horses is invariably initially suspected on the basis of ultrasonographic appearance or *post mortem* examination. Pulmonary cysts are less likely to be diagnosed *ante mortem* although may be seen radiographically as well-defined round or oval radiodensities. The ultrasonographic appearance of human CE was described by Gharbi *et al.* (1981) and has been modified more recently by the World Health Organisation (Anon 2001) (**Table 2**).

In this author's experience CE1s and CE1m cysts are the commonest to be found in equine cases although all types have been reported. The 'snowflake sign' of moving hydatid sand is not frequently seen in horses in this author's experience even when subsequent aspiration confirms the presence of the same. Most often only one or 2 cysts are imaged in horses but occasionally as many as 6 or more might be seen. Most cysts are imaged deep within the hepatic parenchyma but occasionally superficial cysts are also imaged bulging from the hepatic surface (**Fig 3**). More than 500 small cysts have been reported in a single horse in exceptional cases (Edwards 1982; Ronéus *et al.* 1982; Rezabek *et al.* 1993; Mukbel *et al.* 2000; Bardonnet *et al.* 2003). Given the limited ultrasonographic access to the cranial hepatic parenchyma, it is probable that ultrasonography is not a completely sensitive technique for detection hepatic CE in horses. In a study conducted in sheep and goats, only 23/36 (64%) cases of hepatic CE were correctly identified using ultrasonography (compared with *post mortem* examination) with a far lower sensitivity demonstrated for pulmonary CE (Sage *et al.* 1998). All but one of the false negative hepatic CE examinations was associated with cysts in the cranial liver masked by aerated lung.

Definitive diagnosis requires cyst aspiration and examination of the cystic fluid for evidence of protoscolices, hooks or brood capsules (Summerhays and Mantell 1995). However, given the possibility of false negative findings from a 'sterile' cyst and the potential risk associated with leakage, anaphylaxis

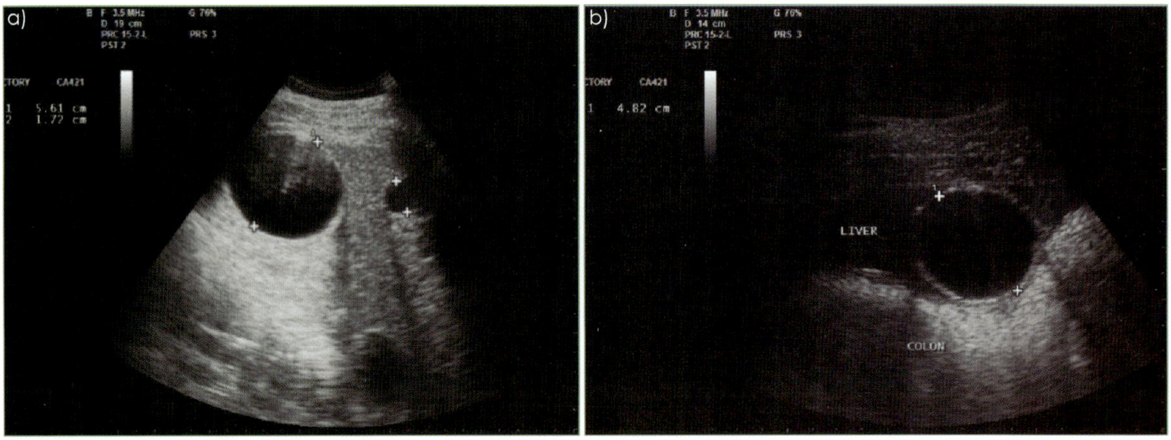

FIGURE 3: Ultrasonographic images of hepatic cystic echinococcosis showing thick-walled, anechoic, spherical cysts with acoustic enhancement distal to the cyst images. a) Image of 3 cysts of varying size within the hepatic parenchyma of a 9-year-old pony recently imported from Texas. b) Image of cyst bulging from the hepatic surface.

TABLE 2: Ultrasonographic classification of human cystic echinococcosis. Each type is further classified according to size: 's' (<5 cm); 'm' (5–10 cm); and 'l' (>10 cm) (e.g. CLs, CE3m etc.) (Anon 2001)

Type	Ultrasonographic appearance
CL (cystic lesion)	Unilocular with uniform anechoic content *without* a visible wall. Usually circular but may be ovoid.
CE1	Unilocular with uniform anechoic content *with* a visible wall. Fine moving echoes may be seen due to moving hydatid sand ('snowflake sign').
CE2	Multivesicular, multiseptate cysts forming wheel-like, rosette-like or honeycomb structures due to daughter cysts.
CE3	Well defined contour containing anechoic fluid although less rounded and 'sagging' in places with a detached wall visible at the cyst periphery or floating within the cystic fluid ('water lily sign').
CE4	An approximately round mass with irregular contour and heterogenous hypo- and hyperechogenicity.
CE5	A hyperechoic contour with acoustic shadow related to calcification.

and further seeding of 'daughter cysts', this does not appear to be a necessary strategy in most cases where characteristic cysts are imaged in typical locations. Specific antibodies against *Echinococcus* cyst antigens may be detected in the cyst fluid and/or sera of human CE patients (Pawlowski *et al.* 2001; Carmena *et al.* 2006) although this approach has not been used or validated in horses (Eckert *et al.* 2001a).

Clinical significance of CE

In the majority of cases of CE the host and the metacestode coexist well and the infection remains subclinical during the whole life of the intermediate host (Eckert *et al.* 2001a). Published reports of CE in horses have generally comprised abattoir studies and clinical cases in which hydatid cysts were discovered incidentally at *post mortem* examination. Hydatid cysts have rarely been reported in association with signs of clinical disease except when arising at a site intolerant of a space occupying mass such as the retrobulbar area (Barnett *et al.* 1988; Summerhays and Mantell 1995). However, Hermann *et al.* (1988) reported a case of CE as a cause of hepatic failure in a heavily infected horse although it would appear that such cases are rarely encountered.

Clinical dilemmas arise when hydatid cysts are found in the liver of horses with clinical and/or laboratory evidence of hepatic disease or in the lungs of horses with pulmonary disease. For example if hydatid cysts are imaged in the liver of a horse showing signs of weight loss and increased serum concentrations of liver derived enzymes the following possible interpretations exist:

a) The hydatid cysts may be entirely incidental and nonpathogenic and liver disease is being caused by another unrelated condition (e.g. hepatotoxicity).
b) The hydatid cysts may be nonpathogenic but acting as a distractor. They may well be the cause of the increase in liver-derived enzymes but are not clinically relevant and weight loss is being caused by a further extra-hepatic disease process (e.g. enteropathy).
c) The hydatid cysts are pathogenic (as a cause of hepatopathy and/or chronic inflammatory disease) and are the primary cause of both the weight loss and the increase in liver-derived enzymes.

In practice it is difficult, and often impossible, to solve this dilemma with certainty although liver biopsy is undoubtedly helpful in many cases. In such a scenario it is this author's practice to collect liver biopsies under real-time ultrasound guidance from hepatic parenchyma both adjacent to and distant from the imaged cysts. If both biopsies show similar degrees of pathological change then this might support a). If both biopsies are unremarkable then it is reasonable to assume that b) is the case. If the pericystic biopsy shows significantly greater inflammatory and/or degenerative change than the biopsy collected distant from the cyst(s) then this might be supportive of c). Other diagnostic findings supportive of the clinical relevance of the hydatid cysts might include increased systemic inflammatory indicators such as globulins, fibrinogen or serum amyloid A in addition to indicators of hepatic functional compromise (e.g. serum bile acids). Hypergammaglobulinaemia occurs in about 30% of human CE cases. In man eosinophilia tends to be absent to moderate ($<1 \times 10^9$/l) except following cyst rupture whereupon marked eosinophilia usually occurs (Pawlowski *et al.* 2001).

Treatment of CE

Most published evidence relating to treatment of hydatid cysts derives from human cases and specific treatment of CE has rarely been reported in horses. Summerhays and Mantell (1995) successfully treated a retrobulbar hydatid cyst with repeated aspiration and systemic albendazole therapy although most cases seen at other anatomic sites are incidental and do not merit specific treatment.

Surgical excision is often favoured in cases of human infection as a means of complete removal of metacestode material and is applicable in about 90% of human CE cases. However, in subjects with multiple cysts or in areas with poor access to surgical facilities then this approach is less favoured. In any case, surgery is almost invariably performed in combination with systemic chemotherapy (see below) (Pawlowski *et al.* 2001; el-On 2003; Ezer *et al.* 2006).

PAIR (puncture-aspiration-injection-reaspiration) therapy is proposed as a simpler alternative to surgical excision in humans usually using 95% alcohol or 15% saline as a protoscolicidal agent following partial aspiration of cyst contents (Akhan and Ozmen

1999; Anon 2001). The technique is not suitable for pulmonary cysts, superficial cysts in other organs (where spillage of contents is likely), multiloculated cysts or calcified cysts. The possible existence of cystobiliary communications (Pawlowski *et al.* 2001; Silva *et al.* 2004) may make this approach potentially hazardous although rapid testing of aspirated contents for presence of bilirubin (e.g. urine dipstick) may serve to detect unsuitable cases prior to injection of agents that might otherwise result in a chemical (sclerosing) cholangitis. As with surgical treatment, peri-interventional systemic chemotherapy is recommended from 4 days before until a month after PAIR (Pawlowski *et al.* 2001). This author has used the PAIR technique without incident on a few occasions in horses with hepatic CE although on one occasion the treated horse collapsed showing signs of acute pain immediately following ultrasound-guided intracystic injection of hypertonic saline. Full recovery followed within a few minutes. Testing of cyst contents for bilirubin was not performed and it is possible that this reaction may have been caused by cystobiliary communication. Studies conducted in sheep have proposed intracystic injection of anthelmintics such as ivermectin and albendazole without reaspiration to be an effective and simpler approach (Deger *et al.* 2000; Hokelek *et al.* 2002).

Systemic chemotherapy of hydatid cysts generally comprises a prolonged course of albendazole and/or praziquantel. Both drugs have good *in vitro* activity against *Echinococcus* metacestodes although *in vivo* efficacy may be limited by diffusion across the cyst wall (Richards *et al.* 1988; el-On 2003). Typical doses of albendazole administered to human CE patients are 10–15 mg/kg bwt daily in a divided dose. Cyclic treatments were once advised but currently continuous therapy for at least 3–6 months is considered to be safe and more efficacious (Horton 1997; Pawlowski *et al.* 2001; el-On 2003). Potential adverse effects of albendazole therapy in man include neutropenia, proteinuria, gastrointestinal disturbances, mild hepatotoxicity, embryotoxicity and teratogenicity, and therefore haematology and liver enzymes should be monitored every 2 weeks during the first 3 months of therapy (Horton 1997; Pawlowski *et al.* 2001). In a review of 665 cysts in human subjects, Horton (1997) described a favourable response to albendazole in approximately 75% of cases. This author has treated several equine subjects with albendazole at 10 mg/kg bwt daily for 3 months with a good clinical response in almost all cases (albeit clinical relevance of the cysts may sometimes have been equivocal). Praziquantel has also been used in human CE patients, most commonly at a dose of 25–50 mg/kg bwt once or twice weekly (Pawlowski *et al.* 2001; el-On 2003; Jamshidi *et al.* 2008). Combination therapy including both albendazole and praziquantel is favoured by several studies (Mohamed *et al.* 1998; Urrea-París *et al.* 2000; Pawlowski *et al.* 2001; Jamshidi *et al.* 2008). Concurrent praziquantel therapy increases plasma levels of albendazole metabolites by 4.5 times, which may increase the risk of adverse effects in addition to improving efficacy (Pawlowski *et al.* 2001). Assessment of response to treatment is difficult as it has been found in man that even when systemic chemotherapy is effective, ultrasonographic changes in the cyst appearance may not develop for at least a year (Nahmias *et al.* 1994).

Acknowledgements

The author would like to thank the following diplomates of the ACVIM for contributing their experience (or lack of experience) of CE in USA: Drs Nick Frank (Tenessee), Christopher Brown (Michigan), Peter Constable (Indiana), Wendy Duckett (Prince Edward Island), Michelle Barton (Georgia), Doug Byars (Kentucky), Pam Wilkins (Illinois), Mary-Rose Paradis (Massachusetts), Dianne McFarlane (Oklahoma), Jill McClure (Louisiana), Rose Nolen-Walston (Pennsylvania) and Virginia Reef (Pennsylvania).

References

Abo-Shehada, M.N. (1988) Prevalence of hydatidosis in donkeys from central Jordan. *Vet. Parasitol.* **30**, 125-130.

Akhan, O. and Ozmen, M.N. (1999) Percutaneous treatment of liver hydatid cysts. *Eur. J. Radiol.* **32**, 76-85.

Anon (2001) *PAIR: Puncture, Aspiration, Injection, Re-aspiration. An option for treatment of cystic echinococcosis.* http://whqlibdoc.who.int/hq/2001/WHO_CDS_CSR_APH_2001.6.pdf

Azlaf, R. and Dakkak, A. (2006) Epidemiological study of the cystic echinococcosis in Morocco. *Vet. Parasitol.* **137**, 83-93.

Bardonnet, K., Benchikh-Elfegoun, M.C., Bart, J.M., Harraga, S., Hannache, N., Haddad, S., Dumon, H., Vuitton, D.A. and Piarroux, R. (2003) Cystic echinococcosis in Algeria: cattle act as reservoirs of a sheep strain and may contribute to human contamination. *Vet. Parasitol.* **116**, 35-44.

Barnett, K.C., Cottrell, B.D. and Rest, J.R. (1988) Retrobulbar hydatid cyst in the horse. *Equine vet. J.* **20**, 136-138.

Binhazim, A.A., Harmon, B.G., Roberson, E.L. and Boerner, M. (1992) Hydatid disease in a horse. *J. Am. vet. med. Ass.* **200**, 958-960.

Budke, C.M. (2006) Global socioeconomic impact of cystic echinococcosis. *Emerg. Infect. Dis.* **12**, 296-303.

Carmena, D., Benito, A. and Eraso E. (2006) Antigens for the immunodiagnosis of *Echinococcus granulosus* infection: An update. *Acta. Trop.* **98**, 74-86.

Carmena, D., Sánchez-Serrano, L.P. and Barbero-Martínez, I. (2008) *Echinococcus granulosus* infection in Spain. *Zoonoses Public Health* **55**, 156-165.

Chiou, M.T., Wang, F.I., Chang, P.H., Liu, C.H., Jeng, C.R., Cheng, C.H., Jou, J. and Pang, V.F. (2001) Hydatidosis in a Chapman's zebra (*Equus burchelli antiquorum*). *J. vet. Diagn. Invest.* **13**, 534-537.

Cranley, J.J. (1982) Survey of equine hydatidosis in Great Britain. *Equine vet. J.* **14**, 153-157.

Dailey, M.D. and Sweatman, G.K. (1965) The taxonomy of *Echinococcus granulosus* in the donkey and dromedary in Lebanon and Syria. *Ann. Trop. Med. Parasitol.* **59**, 463-477.

Daniel Mwambete, K., Ponce-Gordo, F. And Cuesta-Bandera, C. (2004) Genetic identification and host range of the Spanish strains of *Echinococcus granulosus*. *Acta. Trop.* **91**, 87-93.

Deger, E., Hokelek, M., Deger, B.A., Tutar, E., Asil, M. and Pakdemirli, E. (2000) A new therapeutic approach for the treatment of cystic echinococcosis: Percutaneous albendazole sulphoxide injection without reaspiration. *Am. J. Gastroenterol.* **95**, 248-254.

Dixon, J.B., Baker-Smith, J.K. and Greatorex, J.C. (1973) The incidence of hydatid cysts in horses in Great Britain. *Vet. Rec.* **93**, 255.

Eckert, J., Deplazes, P., Craig, P.S., Gemmell, M.A., Gottstein, B., Heath, D., Jenkins, D.J., Kamiya, M. and Lightowlers, M. (2001a) *Echinococcosis* in animals: clinical aspects, diagnosis and treatment. In: *WHO/OIE manual on echinococcosis in humans and animals: A public health problem of global concern.* pp 73-100. http://whqlibdoc.who.int/publications/2001/9290445 22X.pdf

Eckert, J., Schantz, P.M., Gasser, R.B., Torderson, P.R., Bessonov, A.S., Movsessian, S.O., Thakur, A., Grimm, F. and Nikogossian, M.A. (2001b) Geographic distribution and prevalence. In: *WHO/OIE manual on echinococcosis in humans and animals: A public health problem of global concern.* pp 101-143. http://whqlibdoc.who.int/publications/2001/929044522X.pdf

Edwards, G.T. (1981) Small fertile hydatid cysts in British horses. *Vet. Rec.* **108**, 460-461.

Edwards, G.T. (1982) Observations on the epidemiology of equine hydatidosis in Britain. *Vet. Rec.* **110**, 511-514.

el-On, J. (2003) Benzimidazole treatment of cystic *echinococcosis*. *Acta. Trop.* **85**, 243-252.

Ezer, A., Nursal, T.Z., Moray, G., Yildirim, S., Karakayali, F., Noyan, T. and Haberal, M. (2006) Surgical treatment of liver hydatid cysts. *HPB (Oxford)* **8**, 38-42.

Gelberg, H.B., Todd, K.S., Duckett, W.M. and Sanecki, R.K. (1984) Hydatid disease in a horse. *J. Am. vet. med. Ass.* **184**, 342-343.

Gharbi, H.A., Hassine, W., Brauner, M.W. and Dupuch, K. (1981) Ultrasound examination of the hydatic liver. *Radiol.* **139**, 459-463.

Hatch, C. and Smyth, J.D. (1975) Attempted infection of sheep with *Echinococcus granulosus* equinus. *Res. vet. Sci.* **19**, 340.

Hermann, M., Eckert, J., Howald, B., Strickler, B. and Gottstein, B. (1988) Klinisch manifeste echinokokkose bei einem pferde. *Pferdeheilkunde* **4**, 263-267.

Hoberg, E.P., Miller, S. and Brown, M.A. (1994) *Echinococcus granulosus* (Taeniidae) and autochthonous echinococcosis in a North American horse. *J. Parasitol.* **80**, 141-144.

Hokelek, M., Deger, B.A., Deger, E., Tutar, E. and Sunbul, M. (2002) Ivermectin used in percutaneous drug injection method for the treatment of liver hydatid disease in sheep. *Gastroenterology* **122**, 957-962.

Horton, R.J. (1997) Albendazole in treatment of *human cystic echinococcosis*: 12 years of experience. *Acta. Trop.* **64**, 79-93.

Jamshidi, M., Mohraz, M., Zangeneh, M. and Jamshidi, A. (2008) The effect of combination therapy with albendazole and praziquantel on hydatid cyst treatment. *Parasitol. Res.* **103**, 195-199.

Lymbery, A.J. and Thompson, R.C. (1996) Species of *Echinococcus*: pattern and process. *Parasitol. Today* **12**, 486-491.

McFarlane, D., Mann, K.A., Harmon, B.G. and Williamson, L.H. (1994) Pleural effusion secondary to aberrant metacestode infection. *Comp. Cont. Educ. Pract. Vet.* **16**, 1032-1035.

McManus, D.P. and Smyth, J.D. (1986) Hydatidosis: changing concepts in epidemiology and speciation. *Parasitol. Today* **2**, 163-168.

Mohamed, A.E., Yasawy, M.I. and Al Karawi, M.A. (1998) Combined albendazole and praziquantel versus albendazole alone in the treatment of hydatid disease. *Hepatogastroenterology* **45**, 1690-1694.

Mukbel, R.M., Torgerson, P.R. and Abo-Shehada, M.N. (2000) Prevalence of hydatidosis among donkeys in northern Jordan. *Vet. Parasitol.* **88**, 35-42.

Nahmias, J., Goldsmith, R., Soibelman, M. and el-On, J. (1994) Three- to 7-year follow-up after albendazole treatment of 68 patients with cystic *echinococcosis* (hydatid disease). *Ann. Trop. Med. Parasitol.* **88**, 295-304.

Pawlowski, Z.S., Eckert, J., Vuitton, D.A., Ammann, R.W., Kern, P., Craig, P.S., Dar, K.F., De Rosa, F., Filice, C., Gottstein, B., Grimm, F., Macpherson, C.N.L., Sato, N., Todorov, T., Uchino, J., von Sinner, W. And Wen, H. (2001) *Echinococcosis* in humans: clinical aspects, diagnosis and treatment. In: *WHO/OIE manual on echinococcosis in humans and animals: A public health problem of global concern.* pp 20-72. http://whqlibdoc.who.int/publications/2001/929044522X.pdf

Ponce Gordo, F. and Cuesta Bandera, C. (1998) Observations on the *Echinococcus granulosus* horse strain in Spain. *Vet. Parasitol.* **76**, 65-70.

Rezabek, G.B., Giles, R.C. and Lyons, E.T. (1993) *Echinococcus granulosus* hydatid cysts in the livers of two horses. *J. vet. diagn. Invest.* **5**, 122-125.

Richards, K.S., Morris, D.L., Daniels, D. and Riley, E.M. (1988) *Echinococcus granulosus*: the effects of praziquantel, *in vivo* and *in vitro*, on the ultrastructure of equine strain murine cysts. *Parasitology* **96**, 323-336.

Ronéus, O., Christensson, D. and Nilsson, N.G. (1982) The longevity of hydatid cysts in horses. *Vet. Parasitol.* **11**, 149-154.

Sage, A.M., Wachira, T.M., Zeyhle, E.E., Weber, E.P., Njoroge, E. and Smith, G. 1998 Evaluation of diagnostic ultrasound as a mass screening technique for the detection of hydatid cysts in the liver and lung of sheep and goats. *Int. J. Parasitol.* **28**, 349-353.

Silva, M.A., Mirza, D.F., Bramhall, S.R., Mayer, A.D., McMaster, P. And Buckels, J.A.C. (2004) Treatment of hydatid disease of the liver. *Dig. Surg.* **21**, 227-234.

Summerhays, G.E.S. and Mantell, J.A.R. (1995) Ultrasonography as an aid to diagnosis and treatment of a retrobulbar hydatid cyst in a horse. *Equine vet. Educ.* **7**, 39-42.

Thompson, R.C. (1977) Growth, segmentation and maturation of the British horse and sheep strains of *Echinococcus granulosus* in dogs. *Int. J. Parasitol.* **7**, 281-285.

Thompson, R.C. (2008) The taxonomy, phylogeny and transmission of *Echinococcus. Expt. Parasitol.* **119**, 439-446.

Thompson, R.C.A. and McManus, D.P. (2001) Aetiology, parasites and lifecycles. In: *WHO/OIE manual on echinococcosis in humans and animals: A public health problem of global concern.* pp 1-19. http://whqlibdoc.who.int/publications/2001/929044522X.pdf

Thompson, R.C. and McManus, D.P. (2002) Towards a taxonomic revision of the genus *Echinococcus. Trends Parasitol.* **18**, 452-457.

Thompson, R.C.A. and Smyth, J.D. (1974) Potential danger of hydatid disease of horse/dog origin. *Br. med. J.* **3**, 807.

Thompson, R.C.A. and Smyth, J.D. (1975) Equine hydatidosis: a review of the current status in Great Britain and the results of an epidemiological survey. *Vet. Parasitol.* **1**, 107-127.

Turgut, A.T., Altin, L., Topçu, S., Kiliçoglu, B., Aliinok, T., Kaptanoglu, E., Karademir, A. and Kosar, U. (2007) Unusual imaging characteristics of complicated hydatid disease. *Eur. J. Radiol.* **63**, 84-93.

Urrea-París, M.A., Moreno, M.J., Casado, N., Rodriguez-Caabeiro, F. (2000) *In vitro* effect of praziquantel and albendazole combination therapy on the larval stage of *Echinococcus granulosus. Parasitol. Res.* **86**, 957-964.

Varcasia, A., Garippa, G., Pipia, A.P., Scala, A., Brianti, E., Giannetto, S., Battelli, G., Poglayen, G. and Micagni, G. (2008) Cystic *echinococcosis* in equids in Italy. *Parasitol. Res.* **102**, 815-818.

Williams, R.J. and Sweatman, G.K. (1963) On the transmission, biology and morphology of *Echinococcus granulosus equinus*, a new subspecies of hydatid tapeworm in horses in Great Britain. *Parasitol.* **53**, 391-407.

FUNGAL INFECTIONS: SUPERFICIAL, SUBCUTANEOUS, SYSTEMIC

A. J. Stewart

Equine Section, JTVLATH, Department of Clinical Sciences, College of Veterinary Medicine, Auburn University, Auburn, Alabama 36849-5522, USA.

Keywords: horse; granuloma; antifungal; fluconazole; immunodeficiency

Summary

There are more than 70,000 species of fungi, but only 50 have been identified as causing disease in mammalian species. Important fungal infections in horses include dermatophytosis ('ringworm'), a highly contagious fungal infection caused most commonly by *Trichophyton equinum*. Transmission occurs by direct contact or through co-sharing of tack etc. Lesions appear as spreading circular patches of alopecia surrounded by scaling and erythema. Papules and pustules may also be evident. Sporotrichosis (*Sporothrix schenckii* infection) can result in single to multiple, firm, nonpainful cutaneous nodules on the distal limbs, head, neck or trunk. Pythiosis caused by *Pythium insidiosum* infection can affect horses in tropical and subtropical climates; it classically causes large, proliferative, ulcerated, pyogranulomatous, cutaneous and subcutaneous lesions of the extremities, ventral abdomen and face. Fungal organisms such as *Conidiobolus coronatus*, *Cryptococcus neoformans* and *Coccidioides immitis* can form granulomatous mass like lesions in the mucosal tissues of the upper respiratory tract while *Aspergillus* spp. tend to form superficial mycotic plaques. Fungi can also occasionally cause discrete or diffuse pulmonary granulomas, or fungal pleuropneumonia.

Introduction

The fungal kingdom comprises moulds, yeasts, rusts and mushrooms. Fungi are eukaryotic organisms with a cell wall made up of chitins, mannans and glucans. The plasma membrane contains ergosterol, a sterol that is targeted by several antifungal agents. There are more than 70,000 species of fungi, but only 50 species have been identified as causing disease in mammalian species. Dermatophytosis is the most commonly encountered fungal infection in horses, frequently causing large outbreaks within a stable. Subcutaneous and systemic fungal infections in horses tend to be sporadic and are relatively uncommon, although geographic prevalence is highly variable.

Until recently the prognosis for subcutaneous and systemic fungal infections has been guarded to poor. However, the pharmacokinetic profiles of several antifungal agents have been reported for horses, and as affordable formulations become increasingly available, successful outcomes are likely to become more common.

Diagnosis

Fungal hyphae may be identified in impression smears obtained from biopsied masses or in body fluid. The presence of fungal organisms may be insignificant when cellular cytology is normal. Nonpathogenic barn fungus (*Alternaria* spp.) is often present in tracheal aspirates from healthy horses. Some fungi, such as *Cryptococcus* spp. (**Fig 1**), have characteristic morphological features that can provide a rapid cytological diagnosis. Cytological descriptions of various fungal organisms affecting horses are described in **Table 1**. Histopathology slides should be stained with periodic acid Schiff (PAS), Gridley's fungus stain (**Fig 2**) and Grocott-Gomori methenamine-silver nitrate (GMS) to help identify fungal hyphae. Immunohistochemistry, fluorescent *in situ* hybridisation and DNA probes can be used to positively diagnose fungal organisms in histopathology sections.

Some fungi have fastidious growth requirements and may be outcompeted by contaminant bacteria. Samples should be placed in commercially available microbiological transport media[1] and transported at room temperature. Specific culture media such as Sabouraud's dextrose agar, inhibitory mould agar containing cycloheximide and chloramphenicol are useful, but some fungi may take up to several weeks to grow. A Pan-fungal real-time PCR assay[2] can be used to detect a variety of fungal organisms in body fluids and fungal isolates, followed by species specific real-time PCR to positively identify the organism (Pusterla *et al.* 2005).

Serological tests that utilise radioimmunoassays, immunodiffusion, complement fixation and ELISA are available to detect circulating antibodies against several fungal organisms. These titres often decrease with resolution of disease, so repeated measurements can be used to help monitor response to treatment.

Immune function testing

Several fungal infections have been associated with host immune suppression caused by severe malnutrition, congenital immunodeficiency or acquired immunodeficiency. Serum immunoglobulin quantification, lymphocyte subpopulation phenotyping and lymphocyte proliferation assays can be performed (MacNeill *et al.* 2003; Clark-Price *et al.* 2004).

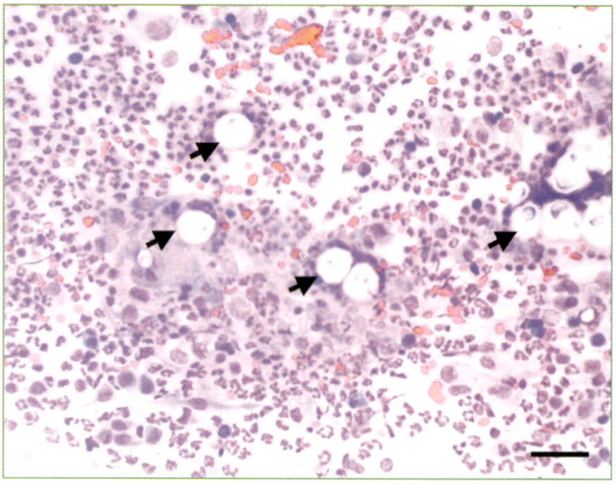

FIGURE 1: Transtracheal wash specimen collected from a horse with pneumonia. Cryptococcus neoformans organisms are identified by their characteristic wide, nonstaining capsules (arrows). (Modified Wright's stain; bar = 60 µm; courtesy of Elizabeth G. Welles, Auburn University).

Treatment

Treatment of subcutaneous fungal granulomas of the skin and upper respiratory tract may involve surgical (debulking, laser or cryotherapy) and/or medical (systemic, topical or intralesional) therapy. *Aspergillus* spp. pneumonia is usually fatal, but successful therapy has been reported for other causes of fungal pneumonia (Stewart *et al.* 2008). Several pharmacokinetic studies of antifungal agents have been recently performed (Prades *et al.* 1989; Latimer *et al.* 2001; Davis *et al.* 2004, 2006). The success rate of therapy is likely to increase as these medications

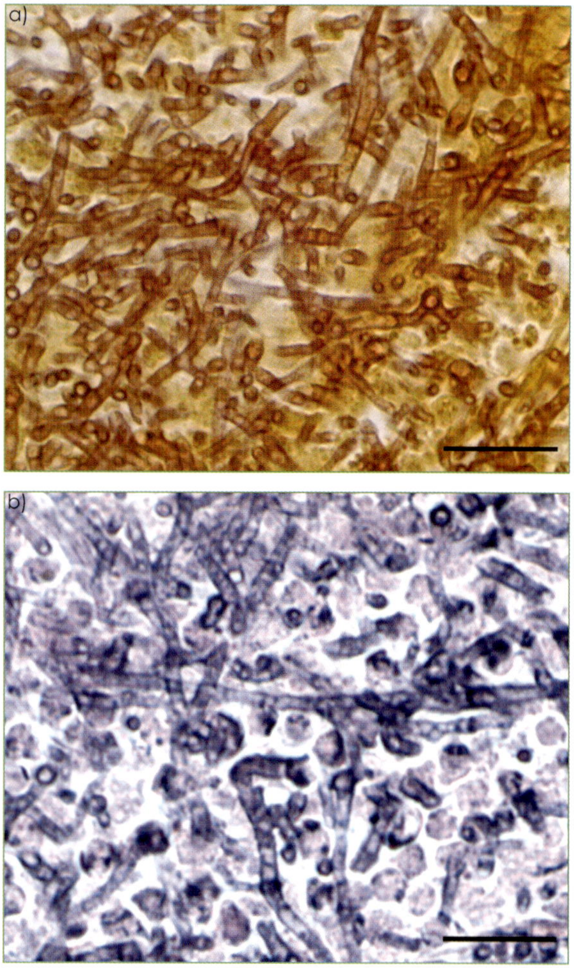

FIGURE 2: Lung sample from a foal with Aspergillus Spp. pneumonia. a) Stained metachromatic with Gridley stain; bar = 30 µm. b) Haematoxylin stain; bar = 20 µm; courtesy of Calvin Johnson, Auburn University.

TABLE 1: Characteristic morphological features and availability of serological tests for fungal organisms reported to cause fungal granulomas in the horses

Agent	Cytological appearance	Diagnostic tests	Recommended treatment
Dermatophytes: *Trichophyton, Microsporum*	Arthrospores can be detected within the hair in approximately 50% of affected horses. Potassium hydroxide (KOH) can be used to clear cellular material. Add a few drops of 10–20% KOH and incubate with gentle heating for 5–10 min. Arthrospores appear as linear chains of small, round to rectangular, highly refractile structures within and on the surface of the hair shaft.	Recommend culture on Sabouraud dextrose agar (more accurate) and dermatophyte test medium (DMT). Wipe skin with alcohol before plucking hairs for culture.	Usually self limiting without therapy. Topical treatment of affected and in-contact horses with 2% enilconazole rinses, natamycin-based suspension, povidone-iodine, thiabendazole ointment, captan or 2% lime sulphur are all anecdotally effective.
Sporothrix schenckii	Yeast-like organisms that are usually round to cigar-shaped, 3–5 µm in diameter, and 5–9 µm in length.	Cytology and histopathology can be difficult as organisms can be sparse. Culture is recommended. Serology by latex and tube agglutination with titres >8 are supportive of a diagnosis.	Iodide has traditionally been used. Amphotericin B and itraconazole are used in man, although some strains are resistant. Fluconazole and voriconazole have high MICs.
Pythium insidiosum	Sparsely-septated hyphae within eosinophilic granulomatous lesions.	Serology	Pythium vaccine
Cryptococcus neoformans and *C. gatti*	Round, thin-walled, yeast-like fungus (5–10 µm) with a large heteropolysaccharide capsule (1–30 µm in diameter) that does not take up common cytological stains (**Fig 1**). Capsule is best stained using Mayer's mucicarmine stain or India ink. Organisms show narrow based budding and lack endospores. Cytology is sufficient for diagnosis.	Cytology and histopathology are very reliable. Culture Serology: capsular antigen ELISA or latex agglutination (Begg *et al.* 2004).	Amphotericin B* (Begg *et al.* 2004), fluconazole, itraconazole or voriconazole
Conidiobolus coronatus	Broad, thin walled highly septate, irregularly branched hyphae (5–13 µm in diameter). Often surrounded by acidophilic staining glycoprotein antigen-antibody complex known as Splendore-Hoeppli material.	Cytology, histopathology and culture are all recommended. Serological tests not commercially available but immunodiffusion is highly sensitive and specific. Decreasing titre correlates to disease resolution in horses (Kaufman *et al.* 1990; Steiger and Williams 2000).	Fluconanzole *per os* (Taintor *et al.* 2004) or amphotericin B intralesionally (**Fig 8**) or topically in combination with DMSO (French *et al.* 1985); (Zamos *et al.* 1996). Iodide
Pseudallescheria boydii	Hyaline, nonpigmented, septate, randomly branched hyphae (2–5 µm in diameter) with regular hyphal contours. Asexual form has nonbranching conidiophores with terminal conidia. Sexual form in culture has cleistothecium (large round body) and ascospores (Davis *et al.* 2000).	Cytology, histopathology and culture are recommended.	Miconazole 2% vaginal cream (Davis *et al.* 2000). Possibly topical natamycin. Voriconazole, ketaconazole or itraconazole. Resistance to amphotericin B and itraconazole is reported.

Coccidioides immitis	Spherules have a double-contoured wall, are variable in size, but can be large (typically 20–80 µm, but up to 200 µm). The mature spherules (sporangia) contain endospores (sporangiospores) 2–5 µm in diameter. In the environment, mycelium are thick-walled with barrel shaped arthroconidia.	Cytology, histopathology, culture and serology are all recommended. Serology to detect IgM and IgG antibodies by AGID is the best method (Ziemer *et al.* 1992; Higgins *et al.* 2005); however, enzyme immunoassay and latex agglutination are available. CF (antibody) (Smith *et al.* 1956; Foley and Legendre 1992; Ziemer *et al.* 1992). May have some false positive results (Higgins *et al.* 2005).	Fluconazole (Higgins *et al.* 2006), itraconazole (Foley and Legendre 1992) (ketoconazole), voriconazole or amphotericin B.
Aspergillus spp.	Broad (2–4 µm diameter) septate hyphae with parallel sides and acute right angled branching (**Figs 2** and **3**).	Cytology, histopathology and culture. Coexisting inflammation makes contamination less likely. Serology not very useful in horses due to environmental exposure. *Aspergillus* Galactomannan EIA (sandwich immunoassay) has cross reactivity to *Penicillium*, *Alternaria* and *Paecilomyces*. AGID (antibody) to *A. fumigatus* only.	Amphotericin B*, voriconazole or itraconazole (Foley and Legendre 1992). Minimal activity to fluconazole. Superficial plaques can be treated with topical miconazole, natamycin, enilconazole or nystatin.
Blastomyces dermatitidis	Yeasts are spherical (15–17 µm in diameter) with basophilic protoplasm and unstained, uniformly shaped refractile walls. Unilateral, broad-based budding is characteristic. Yeasts are often located within multinucleated giant cells.	Cytology, histopathology, culture and serology are all recommended. AGID (antibody) (Toribio *et al.* 1999).	Amphotericin B*, itraconazole or voriconazole.
Histoplasma capsulatum	Yeasts (2–4 µm in diameter) have a thin clear halo surrounding a round or crescent-shaped basophilic cytoplasm.	Cytology, histopathology, culture and serology are all recommended. AGID (antibody) (Rezabek *et al.* 1993).	Amphotericin B* (Cornick 1990), itraconazole or voriconazole. *In vitro* susceptibility to fluconazole is poor.
Acremonium strictum	Mononuclear cells contain single, spherical, intracytoplasmic encapsulated spores 3–5 µm in diameter (Pusterla *et al.* 2005).		Fluconazole was successful in one horse (Pusterla *et al.* 2005), but has poor activity against *A. strictum in vitro* (Guarro *et al.* 1997), and it is uncertain if the fluconazole assisted in disease resolution (Pusterla *et al.* 2005).
Candida spp.	Ovoid budding yeast cells (2–4 µm in diameter) with thin walls, or they can occur in chains that produce septate pseudohyphae when blastospores remain attached after budding division. Filamentous, regular, true hyphae also may be visible.	Cytology, histopathology and culture.	Fluconazole (Reilly and Palmer 1994) although *C. krusei* is resistant. Amphotericin B (Reilly and Palmer 1994) and voriconazole are effective. *Candida glossitis* – mouth wash of potassium permanganate

			(0.025% q. 24 h) or nystatin (0.3 g in 10 mls of water, q. 8 h)
Pneumocystis carinii	Trophozoite (yeast form) is 2–5 µm diameter ameboid with filopodia that attach to the surface of type I pneumocytes. Sporangia (cystic form)are encapsulated spores (4–6 µm in diameter) containing 8 uninuclete spores (intracytic bodies).	Cytology from bronchoalveolar lavage is preferred to transtracheal wash. Organism can not be cultured. PCR can be performed on BAL or TTW samples or lung tissue. Immune function testing is warranted.	Trimethoprim-sulphamethoxazole (25–30 mg/kg bwt *per os* q. 12 h) is the treatment of choice (Flaminio *et al.* 1998). Dapsone[5] (3 mg/kg bwt *per os* daily for 2 months) successfully treated a foal that developed *Salmonella* enterocolitis after TMS treatment (Clark-Price *et al.* 2004).

MIC = minimal inhibitory concentration; ELISA = Enzyme linked immunosorbant assay; AGID = Agar gel immunodiffusion; CF = Complement fixation. *In man i.v. amphotericin B is often administered for 2 weeks prior to prolonged oral azole therapy.

become more affordable. Specific antifungal agents used in horses have been recently reviewed (Stewart 2005; Davis 2008) and dosages are summarised in **Table 2**. Treatment options are dependent on the site and extent of the infection, potential accessibility to surgical intervention, aetiological agent, known antifungal susceptibilities, evidence-based studies from human medicine and financial resources of the owner. Often a multimodal approach is successful, but the relative benefits of each of the individual treatment components are unknown. Recommended treatments used for various fungal infections in horses are summarised in **Table 1**.

Superficial fungal infections: Dermatophytes

Dermatophytosis ('ringworm') is a highly contagious fungal infection caused most commonly by *Trichophyton equinum*, but also by *T. verrucosum*, *T. mentagrophytes*, *Microsporum equinum*, *M. canis* and *M. gypseum*. Transmission occurs by direct contact or through co-sharing of saddle blankets, girths and halters, which remain contaminated for up to 12 months. Insects may also spread infections, while infected soil can be the source of *M. gypseum*. Some species of dermatophytes are zoophilic occasionally spreading between infected horses, cats, cattle and people. Risk factors such as age (<3 years), stress (training), commingling, and concurrent disease can all predispose to infection.

Lesions appear as spreading circular patches of alopecia (**Fig 3**), surrounded by scaling and erythema. Papules and pustules may also be evident. It is important to confirm the diagnosis by culture, because the majority of horses that clinically appear to have ringworm are subsequently diagnosed with bacterial infections such as *Dermatophilus* and *Staphylococcus*. Cytology can provide a diagnosis in 50% of cases.

Ringworm is usually self limiting without therapy. Treatment of affected and in-contact horses with 2% enilconazole rinses, natamycin-based suspension, povidone-iodine, thiabendazole ointment, captan or 2% lime sulphur are all anecdotally effective. In an outbreak situation, all in-contact horses should be treated topically irrespective of presence of clinical signs. Horses can be subclinical carriers and affected animals may still be contagious

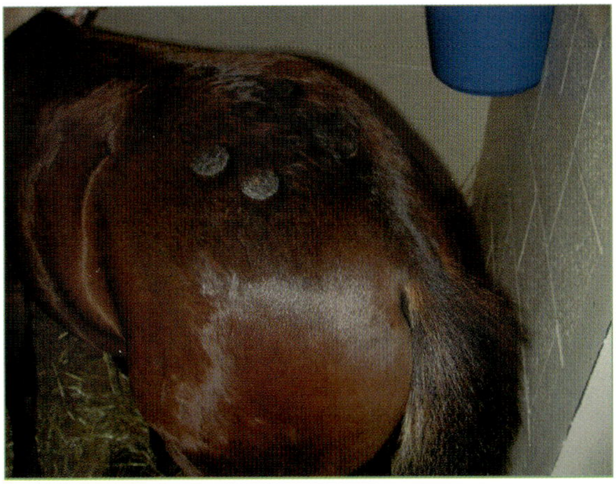

FIGURE 3: Characteristic circular patches of alopecia on the rump of a foal that was being treated for concurrent Rhodococcus equi pneumonia.

TABLE 2: Antifungal drugs used in horses

Drug and relative cost	Class and mechanism of action	Dosage	Susceptible organisms and equine reports	Side effects and comments
Griseofulvin $	Fungistatic. Disrupts the cell's mitotic spindle, arresting the cell in metaphase of cell division.	Adults: 10 mg/kg bwt/day 1–3 weeks. Foals: 1 mg/kg bwt/day *per os* 2–4 weeks.	Only moderately efficacious against *Trichophyton*, *Epidermophyton* and *Sporotichum* and less active against *Microsporum*. Not effective against other pathogenic fungi.	Rarely recommended. Toxic effects include anorexia, diarrhoea, hepatopathy and cutaneous reactions (Rochette *et al.* 2003).
Ketoconazole $$	Azole antifungals are fungistatic, by inhibiting ergosterol biosynthesis. They inhibit cytochrome P450-dependent	30 mg/kg bwt q. 12 h mixed with 0.2 N HCl via nasogastric intubation (Prades *et al.* 1989).	*Scopulariopsis* (Nappert *et al.* 1996), *Coccidioides, Cryptococcus, Candida, Histoplasma, Sporthrix, Malassezia, Microsporum, Trichophyton*.	Absorbed poorly in the nonacidified form.
Itraconazole $$$	14α–sterol demethylase, which is essential for the formation of ergosterol.	5 mg/kg bwt/day solution *per os*: bioavailability 60%, compared to 12% for capsules (Davis *et al.* 2004).	*Aspergillus* (Davis and Legendre 1994; Korenek *et al.* 1994), *Coccidioides* (Foley and Legendre 1992), *Cryptococcus, Histoplasma, Bastomyces, Candida, Scopulariopsis, Parracoccidia, Paecilomyces, Sporothrix, Alternaria, Sporotrichum, Prototheca*. Not active against *Fusarium, Mucor, Rhizopus*.	Very unstable (requires low pH) and lipophilic, therefore compounded formulations are not recommended. Sporanox solution is absorbed well orally.
Fluconazole $$		14 mg/kg bwt *per os* loading followed by 5 mg/kg bwt/day *per os* (Latimer *et al.* 2001).	*Coccidioides* (Higgins *et al.* 2006), *Cryptococcus, Candida* (Reilly and Palmer 1994), *Conidiobolomycosis* (Taintor *et al.* 2003), *Histoplasma, Bastomyces, Scopulariopsis, Mucor, Rhizopus Parracoccidia, Paecilomyces, Sporothrix, Alternaria, Sporotrichum, Prototheca*. Minimal activity against *Aspergillus* and *Fusarium*.	Concentrations achieved in plasma, CSF, synovial fluid, aqueous humor and urine above the MIC reported for several equine fungal pathogens (Latimer et al. 2001). Compounded formulations very stable.
Voriconazole $$$$		3 mg/kg bwt *per os* q. 12 h (Colitz *et al.* 2007). 4.0 mg/kg bwt/day *per os* (Davis *et al.* 2006).	Drug of choice for invasive *Aspergillus, Candida, Cryptococcus, Scedosporium apiospermum* and *Fusarium* species in human patients who are unable to tolerate or are	Concentrations achieved in plasma, CSF, synovial fluid and tear film above the MIC reported for several equine fungal pathogens (Colitz *et al.* 2007).

			refractory to other therapeutic agents.	
Miconazole 2% vaginal cream $		Topical for GPM: 400 mg daily for 7 days, then eod for 14 days, then twice/week for 21 days (Giraudet 2005).	*Aspergillus*, *Candida*, *Malassezia*, *Microsporum*, *Trichophyton* are susceptible. (Ford 2004) Used to treat *Psuedoallescheria boydii* (Davis *et al.* 2000).	For topical use only.
Miconazole 1% solution for injection $$		Topical for GPM: 70 mg diluted in 10 ml 0.9% saline daily for 7 days, then eod for 14 days (Giraudet 2005).		
Enilconazole $		60 ml sprayed directly on guttural pouch lesion daily (Davis and Legendre 1994; Carmalt and Baptiste 2004). Aerosolisation: 1.2 mg/kg in 125 ml normal saline q. 12 h. (Nappert *et al.* 1996).	*Aspergillus*, *Scopulariopsis* (Nappert *et al.* 1996). *Microsporum*, *Trichophyton*,	Available in Europe and in the USA for poultry only. Very effective against superficial *Aspergillus* plaques in the nasopharynx.
Amphotericin B $$$	Polyene macrolide. Fungicidal by irreversibly binding to ergosterol, increasing membrane permeability, leading to cell death.	0.3 mg/kg bwt in 5% dextrose, increasing every 3 days by 0.1 mg/kg bwt until a dose of 0.9 mg/kg bwt i.v. infusion is given for 30 days (Chaffin *et al.* 1995). Local injection or topical therapy: 50 mg in 10 ml sterile water with 10 ml DMSO (Chaffin *et al.* 1995).	*Aspergillus* (Guillot *et al.* 1999) *Candida*, (Reilly and Palmer 1994), *Coccidioides*, *Sporthrix*, *Mucor*, *Rhizopus*, *Cryptococcus* (Begg *et al.* 2004), *Blastomyces*, *Histoplasma*, *Conidiobolus*, *Pythium* are susceptible. *Trichosporon* and *Pseudoallescheria* are often resistant (Ford 2004).	Broadest spectrum of all antifungal agents. Poor oral bioavailability and limited penetration into the CSF, eye and joint fluid. Nephrotoxicity and phlebitis can occur. Nephrotoxicity reduced by pretreatment with sodium chloride and administration of diluted drug over 1–5 h. Monitor renal function using serum creatinine, urine specific gravity and presence of occult blood or tubular casts in urine. No adverse effect on pregnancy (Chaffin *et al.* 1995).
Nystatin suspension, cream $ powder $$		Use topically or by insufflation.	*Cryptococcus*, *Prototheca*, *Aspergillus*, *Trichophyton* are susceptible (Ford 2004).	
20% sodium iodide $	Exact mode of action of iodides is unknown. Very little, if any direct *in vitro* antibiotic	20–40 mg/kg bwt i.v. for 7–10 days or 65 mg/kg bwt i.v. twice weekly (Chaffin *et al.* 1995).	Although several successful cases are reported in which iodides were used as primary or adjunctive therapy,	Iodide toxicity is characterised by excessive lacrimation, nonproductive cough, increased respiratory

	effect. Beneficial effect on the granulomatous inflammatory process (Plumb 2002).		overall efficacy is considered limited at best.	secretions and dermatitis (Steiger and Williams 2000).
Ethylenediamine dihydroiodide (EDDI) 80% iodine $		1–2 mg/kg bwt *per os* of the active ingredient (or approximately 20–40 mg/kg bwt day of the 4.57% dextrose powdered form) q. 12–24 h for 1 week followed by 0.5–1 mg/kg bwt q. 12–24 h, 1.3 mg/kg bwt *per os* q. 12 h for 4 months, then q. 24 h for 1 year, then once/week).		Administration of iodine in the diet of pregnant mares may cause congenital hypothyroidism in foals.
Potassium iodide (76% iodine) $		As for EDDI.		

$ = inexpensive; $$ = moderately expensive; $$$ = very expensive; $$$$ = prohibitively expensive. GPM = guttural pouch mycosis; CSF = cerebral spinal fluid; MIC = minimal inhibitory concentration.

even when hair regrowth is underway. Three negative consecutive cultures collected 2-weeks apart are necessary to confirm resolution. Systemic therapy is no longer recommended. Pharmacokinetics and efficacy of griseofulvin have never been reported and side effects of treatment can occur.

After self-clearance of dermatophyte infection immunity occurs and horses rarely experience reinfection. Some horses appear to be unable to elicit an effective cell-mediated immunity and are prone to recurrent infections unless the organisms are completely eliminated from their environment. Barns and tack can be disinfected with bleach diluted at 1:40 or enilconazole.

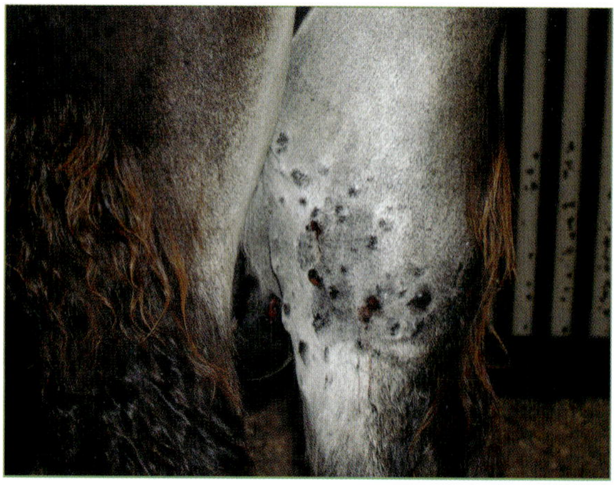

FIGURE 4: Sporotrichosis lesions on the caudal gaskin and scrotum of a donkey stallion. Courtesy of Rebecca Funk, Auburn University.

Subcutaneous fungal infections

Sporotrichosis

Sporothrix schenckii is a saphrophytic dimorphic organism that has worldwide distribution, but occurs more commonly in tropical and subtropical climates. Sporotrichosis causes a chronic lymphocutaneous infection in mammals. Inoculation of traumatised skin leads to infection of the skin, subcutis, lymphatics and lymph nodes. Single to multiple, firm, nonpainful cutaneous nodules can be observed on the distal limbs, head, neck or trunk (**Fig 4**).

Nodules may ulcerate, heal and reoccur over months to years. Differentials include epizootic lymphangitis (*Histoplasma farciminosum*), glanders (*Pseudomonas mallei*), ulcerative lymphangitis (*Corynebacterium pseudotuberculosis*), leishmaniasis and bacterial lymphangitis of other causes. Zoonotic infections have occurred between infected cats and people; therefore the use of gloves when handling lesions is recommended.

Pythiosis

Pythium insidiosum is an aquatic oomycete, and is more closely related to algae than true fungi. Pythiosis affects mammalian species living in tropical and subtropical climates. In horses, pythiosis causes large, proliferative, ulcerated, pyogranulomatous, cutaneous and subcutaneous lesions of the extremities, ventral abdomen and face (**Fig 5**). Occasionally infection can disseminate to arteries, bones, intestines, liver, spleen and lungs, all of which have a poor prognosis. Pythiosis can be diagnosed using serology (ELISA, immunodiffusion or western blot), histopathology with immunohistochemical staining, culture or PCR (Mendoza *et al.* 1997, 2003; Poole and Brashier 2003). *P. insidiosum* hyphae (**Fig 6**) resemble those of fungi in the class Zygomycetes (*Conidiobolus* and *Basidiobolus* sp.), but *P. insidiosum* does not have ergosterol in its cell membrane and is therefore not a true fungus. This explains why most antifungal drugs are generally ineffective at treating pythiosis (Mendoza *et al.* 2003).

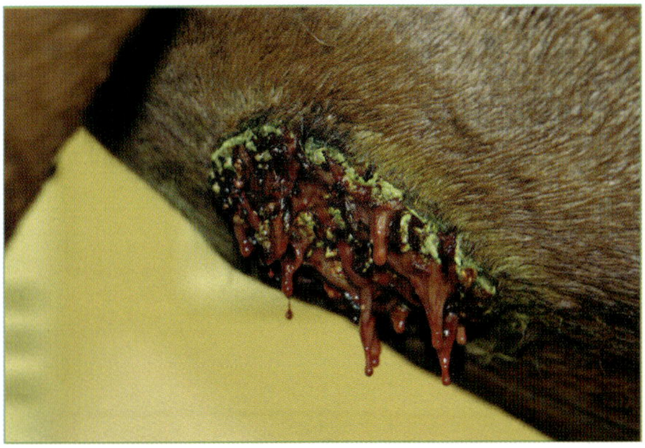

FIGURE 5: Large ulcerative mass on the ventrum of a horse caused by Pythium insidiosum*. The viscous discharge and yellow 'kunkers' are typical. Courtesy of Nicole Passler, Auburn University.*

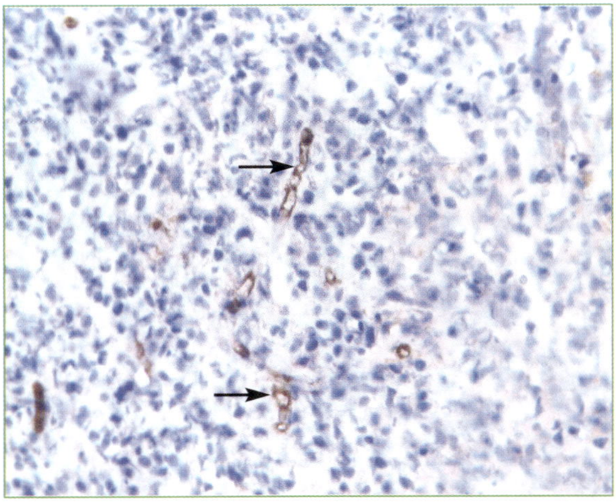

FIGURE 6: Pythium insidiosum *hyphae (arrows) stained brown. Note the nonparallel walls and rare septation. (Streptavidin-HRP conjugated to horseradish peroxidase with rabbit anti-*P. insidiosum *as the primary antibody, and horse anti-rabbit as the secondary antibody).*

An improved pythiosis vaccine[3] containing exoantigens plus cytoplasmic immunogens showed a 72% success rate in the treatment of cutaneous pythiosis (Mendoza *et al.* 2003). The vaccine is injected intramuscularly, and a strong (>10 cm) reaction at the injection site is associated with a greater likelihood of successful outcome.

Upper respiratory tract granulomas

Fungal organisms such as *Conidiobolus coronatus*, *Cryptococcus neoformans* and *Coccidioides immitis* can form granulomatous mass like lesions in the mucosal tissues of the upper respiratory tract while *Aspergillus* spp. tend to form superficial mycotic plaques. The most common clinical signs of upper respiratory fungal infection include unilateral or bilateral mucopurulent or serosanguinous nasal discharge and inspiratory or expiratory noise. Other clinical signs include facial deformation, coughing and dyspnoea caused by partial obstruction of nasal passages by granulomatous masses. Differentials for mycotic granulomas of the respiratory tract include squamous cell carcinoma, ethmoidal haematoma, amyloidosis or exuberant granulation tissue.

Horses with guttural pouch mycosis usually present with episodic serosanguinous nasal discharge that may progress to potentially fatal epistaxis as the fungal plaques are frequently located over an artery. Horses may also present with cranial nerve abnormalities. The duration of clinical signs can vary from days to many months.

Endoscopic examination can be used to observe lesions in the nasal passages, nasopharynx, guttural pouch, trachea and bronchioles directly, while masses in th eparanasal sinuses and lungs may be observed radiographically. Computed tomography or magnetic resonance imaging can be used to determine the extent of lesions and bony invasion in the skull. A sterile rigid arthroscope or flexible endoscope can be passed into the conchal or maxillary sinus via a hole drilled using an 8–20 mm trephine to directly view lesions and obtain biopsy samples.

Large biopsy samples for cytology, histopathology and culture can be obtained from the nasal passages or nasopharynx using a uterine biopsy instrument passed nasally with visual guidance from a flexible endoscope. Excisional biopsy or surgical debulking may be performed through a sinus flap or via laryngotomy.

Differentials for upper respiratory tract fungal granulomas

Conidiobolomycosis

Conidiobolus coronatus is a saprophytic fungus that causes single to multiple granulomatous lesions in the nasal passages, soft palate or trachea (**Fig 7**). Conidiobolomycosis lesions can be treated with surgical excision, laser or cryotherapy or long-term administration of intralesional (**Fig 8**) or systemic antifungals. It is important to remember that long-term therapy and re-evaluation is essential, as recurrence can occur (Zamos *et al.* 1996).

Pseudallescheriosis

Pseudallescheria boydii is a saprophytic ascomycete. Resolution of *P. boydii* lesions in the nasal cavity and sinus of a horse with chronic, malodorous nasal discharge was achieved after surgical debridement, followed by twice daily topical application of miconazole cream that was infused for 4 weeks through lavage tubing placed through the frontal bone and into the sinuses. Adjunctive iodide therapy was also administered (Davis *et al.* 2000).

Cryptococcus, *coccidioides* and *pithiosis* can also form upper respiratory tract granulomas while *Aspergillus* can form plaques in the upper respiratory tract. These organisms are discussed below.

Pulmonary and systemic fungal infections

Horses with discrete or diffuse pulmonary fungal granulomas, or fungal pleuropneumonia can present with signs similar to bacterial pneumonia. Fever, cough, nasal discharge, tachypnoea, respiratory distress, haemoptysis and, if chronic, weight loss may be observed. Radiographic appearance of fungal pneumonia can be variable, although miliary patterns or patchy bronchopneumonia is most common (**Fig 9**). Differentials include bacterial pneumonia, neoplasia, recurrent airway obstructive disease, granulomatous disease complex or silicosis. Fungal infections can affect multiple organ systems and body cavities. Weight loss, colic or diarrhoea can often occur with infection within the abdominal cavity.

Fungal pneumonia may be diagnosed from samples obtained by tracheal wash or bronchoalveolar lavage fluid, or via a lung biopsy. Lung biopsy is associated with significant risk of

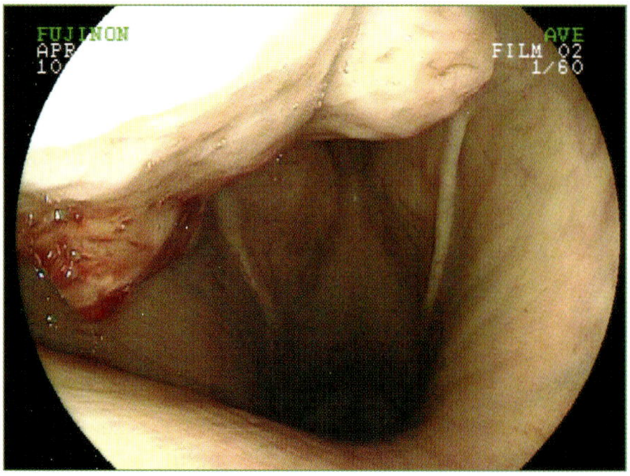

FIGURE 7: Endoscopic image of mycotic granulomas caused by C. coronatus on the dorsal nasopharynx of a pony.

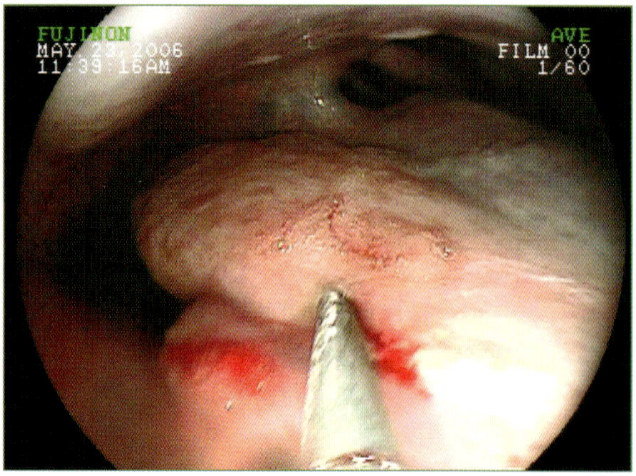

FIGURE 8: Endoscopically guided injection of amphotericin B solution into a C. coronatus granuloma located rostral to the ethmoids.

haemorrhage. The biopsy should ideally be performed after radiographic evaluation or with concurrent ultrasound guidance and should be obtained from the periphery of the lung. The lung is rich in plasminogen, so bleeding complications may be severe. Spring-loaded biopsy needles[4] are safer for lung biopsy compared to Tru-Cut biopsy instruments (Venner *et al.* 2006). Ultrasound evaluation can be used to monitor for bleeding after the procedure.

Differentials for fungal pneumonia or systemic fungal infections

Aspergillosis

Aspergillus spp. are ubiquitous in the environment, especially in mouldy feed and bedding. As opportunistic pathogens they often cause disease in horses that are immunosuppressed from debilitating disease, or that have been treated with immunosuppressive drugs (Slocombe and Slauson 1988; Blomme *et al.* 1998; Johnson *et al.* 1999; Sweeney and Habecker 1999; Tunev *et al.* 1999). Infection is by inhalation of spores or by translocation of organisms across an inflamed gastrointestinal tract (Slocombe and Slauson 1988; Sweeney and Habecker 1999).

Aspergillus spp. pneumonia is almost uniformly fatal, often with no or mild respiratory signs. In human medicine, 50–90% of patients with invasive aspergillosis die despite treatment. The traditional treatment in man has been amphotericin B, but nephrotoxicity occurs in about 50% of cases. Voriconazole is now considered the drug of choice against human aspergillosis.

Treatment of *Aspergillus* sinusitis and rhinitis in horses has been more successful using oral itraconazole (Korenek *et al.* 1994), topical natamycin or enilconazole (lavaged via an endoscope or indwelling catheter placed into the paranasal sinus) and nystatin powder (insufflated up the nostril) (Greet 1981).

Candidiasis

Systemic candidiasis was diagnosed and successfully treated in 4 neonatal septic foals that had been aggressively treated with numerous antibiotics and parenteral nutrition. Two of the foals were treated with i.v. amphotericin B, while oral fluconazole was used on the other 2 foals (Reilly and Palmer 1994). Glossitis, panophthalmitis and cystitis can be associated with systemic candidiasis and should be carefully investigated.

Coccidiomycosis

Coccidioides immitis is a soil saprophyte that grows in sandy, alkaline soils in semiarid areas. Inhaled arthroconidia enlarge to form nonbudding spherules,

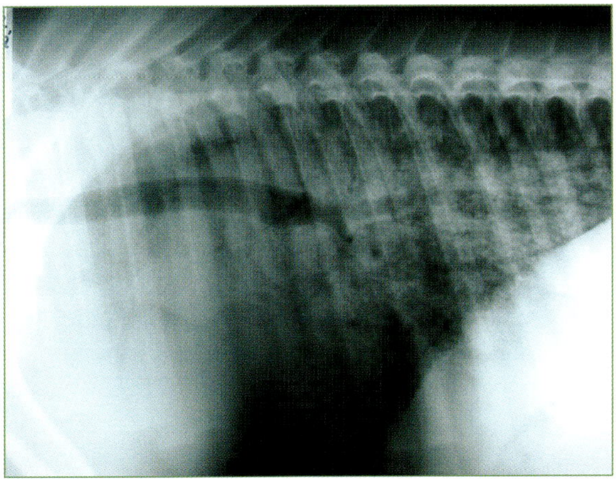

FIGURE 9: Predominately alveolar infiltrate in the caudodorsal lung field of a foal with Histoplasma capsulatum pneumonia (courtesy of Carol Clark, Peterson and Smith Equine Hospital, Florida).

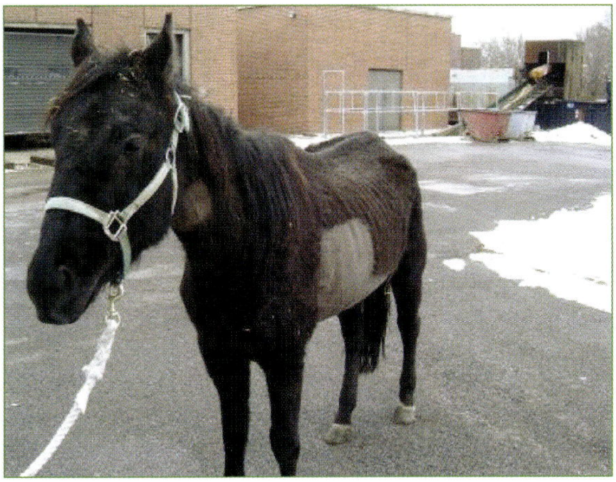

FIGURE 10: Coccidiomycosis in a Quarter Horse mare that presented for severe weight loss after a 3 month period in Arizona and Colorado (courtesy of Jamie Murphy, Califon, New Jersey).

which incite an inflammatory reaction in the lungs and lymph nodes. Horses have weight loss, fever, colic and signs of respiratory disease (**Fig 9**). Diffuse infections, with granulomas in the lungs, liver, kidney or spleen have a grave prognosis (Ziemer *et al.* 1992). Localised, recurring nasal granulomas also have been reported (Hodgin *et al.* 1984). Przewalski's horses may be more susceptible (Terio *et al.* 2003).

Coccidioides immitis is difficult to culture, and spherules may not be observed histologically from *ante mortem* lung biopsies. However, serology is very useful to diagnose infection, and decreasing titres are associated with clinical improvement (Ziemer *et al.* 1992; Higgins *et al.* 2006). Serum antibodies are detected rarely in healthy horses (Higgins *et al.* 2005). Antifungal agents successful in treatment of infected horses include fluconazole and itraconazole (Foley and Legendre 1992; Higgins *et al.* 2006).

Pneumocystosis

Pneumocystis carinii has been reclassified from a protozoan to a saprophytic fungus, but some researchers even consider it to be a plant because it lacks ergosterol. *P. carinii* cannot be cultured, and diagnosis is based on the cytological identification in bronchoalveolar lavage fluid.

Pneumocystosis is common in human AIDS patients, and those undergoing immunosuppressive therapy after organ transplantation. *P. carinii* causes diffuse interstitial pneumonia, especially in immunocompromised patients, such as Arabian foals with severe combined immunodeficiency. It also has been diagnosed in immunocompromised adult horses (Franklin *et al.* 2002; MacNeill *et al.* 2003), as well as an immunocompetent foal (Perron LePage *et al.* 1999). Trimethoprim-sulphamethozazole is the treatment of choice.

Histoplasmosis

Histoplasmosis is caused by the saprophytic fungus *Histoplasma capsulatum*, and is most prevalent in moist soil containing bird or bat waste. *H. capsulatum* may occur in an enteric, pulmonary or disseminated form (**Fig 10**). Successful treatment with amphotericin B was reported in a filly with pulmonary histoplasmosis diagnosed by cytological identification of the organism on a tracheal wash smear and from a lung aspirate (Cornick 1990).

Blastomycosis

Blastomycosis is caused by inhalation of *Blastomyces dermatitidis conidiae.* Systemic blastomycosis has been reported in 2 horses, both of which were subjected to euthanasia (Toribio *et al.* 1999; Dolente *et al.* 2003). Serology is useful for diagnosis.

Cryptococcosis

Cryptococcosis is caused by *C. neoformans* var *grubii* (serotype A), *C. neoformans* var *neoformans* (serotype D) and *C. gattii* (serotypes B and C), which are ubiquitous, saprophytic, round, yeast-like fungi with large capsules that do not take up common cytological stains (**Fig 1**). Cytological or histopathological identification is very reliable for diagnosis because of the characteristic morphology (Jubb *et al.* 1985). There is an epidemiological relationship between *C. gattii* and the Australian river redgum tree (*Eucalyptus camaldulensis*), while *C. neoformans* var *neoformans* has historically been associated with bird (particularly pigeon) excreta. Serological testing with latex agglutination to identify cryptococcal capsular antigen is useful, with resolution of lesions correlated with declining serum titres (Begg *et al.* 2004).

Cryptococcosis in horses is associated primarily with pneumonia, rhinitis, meningitis and abortion. Successful medical treatment, however, has been reported rarely. Surgical removal of a localised jejunal lesion was successful in one horse (Boulton and Williamson 1984). *Cryptococcus gattii* pneumonia diagnosed by transtracheal wash and lung mass aspirates, was treated successfully with daily infusions of amphotericin B over one month (Begg *et al.* 2004). The recent availability of affordable fluconazole tablets is likely to increase the success rate of treatment of equine cryptococcosis.

Rare causes of fungal pneumonia

Scopulariopsis pleuropneumonia was diagnosed in a horse by culture of bronchoalveolar lavage fluid. The infection was successfully treated with a combination of ketaconazole and aerosolisation of enilconazole (Nappert *et al.* 1996).

Acremonium strictum pneumonia was diagnosed by cytological evaluation, culture and PCR testing of bronchoalveolar lavage fluid in a horse. The horse recovered after supportive treatment, which included one month of fluconazole. However, fluconazole has been shown to generally have poor activity against *A. strictum in vitro*, and it uncertain if the fluconazole assisted in disease resolution (Pusterla *et al.* 2005).

Adiaspiromycotic miliary fungal pneumonia caused by the soil mould *Emmonsia crescens* was diagnosed in a horse by percutaneous lung biopsy. Euthanasia was performed without treatment (Pusterla *et al.* 2002).

Manufacturers' addresses

[1]Becton, Dickinson and Company, Sparks, Maryland, USA.
[2]University of California Davis, California, USA.
[3]Pan American Veterinary Labs, Hutto, Texas, USA.
[4]Temno Products Group International, Lyons, Colorado, USA.
[4]CR Bard Inc, Covington, Georgia, USA.
[5]Jacobus Pharmaceutical Co. Inc., Princeton, New Jersey, USA.

References

Begg, L.M., Hughes, K.J., Kessell, A., Krockenberger, M.B., Wigney, D.I. and Malik, R. (2004) Successful treatment of cryptococcal pneumonia in a pony mare. *Aust. vet. J.* **82**, 686-692.

Blomme, E., Del Piero, F., La Perle, K.M.D. and Wilkins, P.A. (1998) Aspergillosis in horses: a review. *Equine vet. Educ.* **10**, 86-93.

Boulton, C.H. and Williamson, L. (1984) Cryptococcal granuloma associated with jejunal intussusception in a horse. *Equine vet. J.* **16**, 548-551.

Carmalt, J.L. and Baptiste, K.E. (2004) Atypical guttural pouch mycosis in three horses. *Pferdeheilkunde* **20**, 542-548.

Chaffin, M.K., Schumacher, J. and McMullan, W.C. (1995) Cutaneous pithiosis in the horse. *Vet. Clin. N. Am.: Equine Pract.* **11**, 91-103.

Clark-Price, S.C., Cox, J.H., Bartoe, J.T. and Davis, E.G. (2004) Use of dapsone in the treatment of *Pneumocystis carinii* pneumonia in a foal. *J. Am. vet. med. Ass.* **224**, 407-410.

Colitz, C.M.H., Latimer, F.G., Cheng, H., Chan, K.K., Reed, S.M. and Pennick, G.J. (2007) Pharmacokinetics of voriconazole following intravenous and oral administration and body fluid concentrations of voriconazole following repeated oral administration in horses. *Am. J. vet. Res.* **68**, 1115-1121.

Cornick, J.L. (1990) Diagnosis and treatment of pulmonary histoplasmosis in a horse. *Cornell Vet.* **80**, 97.

Davis, E.W. and Legendre, A.M. (1994) Successful treatment of guttural pouch mycosis with itraconazole and topical enilconazole in a horse. *J. vet. intern. Med.* **8**, 304-305.

Davis, J.L. (2008) Therapeutics in practice: The use of antifungals. *Compend. Equine* **3**, 128-132.

Davis, J.L., Salmon, J.H. and Papich, M.G. (2006) Pharmacokinetics of voriconazole after oral and intravenous administration to horses. *Am. J. vet. Res.* **67**, 170-175.

Davis, J.L., Gilger, B.C. and Papich, M.G. (2004) The pharmacokinetics of itraconazole in the horse. *J. vet. intern. Med* **18**, 458.

Davis, P.R., Meyer, G.A., Hanson, R.R. and Stringfellow, J.S. (2000) *Pseudallescheria boydii* infection of the nasal cavity of a horse. *J. Am. vet. med. Ass.* **217**, 707-709.

Dolente, B.A., Habecker, P., Chope, K., MacGillivray, K. and Schaer, T. (2003) Disseminated blastomycosis in a miniature horse. *Equine vet. Educ.* **15**, 139-142.

Flaminio, M., Rush, B.R., Cox, J.H. and Moore, W.E. (1998) CD4+ and CD8+ T-lymphocytopenia in a filly with *Pneumocystis carinii* pneumonia. *Aust. vet. J.* **76**, 399-402.

Foley, J.P. and Legendre, A.M. (1992) Treatment of *coccidioidomycosis osteomyelitis* with itraconazole in a horse: a brief report. *J. vet. Intern. Med.* **6**, 333.

Ford, M.M. (2004) Antifungals and their use in veterinary ophthalmology. *Vet. Clin. N. Am.: Small Anim. Pract.* **34**, 669-691.

Franklin, R.P., Long, M.T., MacNeill, A., Alleman, R., Giguere, S., Uhl, E., Lopez-Martinez, A. and Wilkerson, M. (2002) Proliferative interstitial pneumonia, *Pneumocystis carinii* infection, and immunodeficiency in an adult Paso Fino horse. *J. vet. Intern. Med.* **16**, 607-611.

French, D.D., Haynes, P.F. and Miller, R.I. (1985) Surgical and medical management of rhinophycomycosis (conidiobolomycosis) in a horse. *J. Am. vet. med. Ass.* **186**, 1105-1107.

Giraudet, A.J. (2005) Medical treatment with miconazole in four cases of guttural pouch mycosis. *J. vet. Intern. Med.* **19**, 485-485.

Greet, T.R.C. (1981) Nasal aspergillosis in 3 horses. *Vet. Rec.* **109**, 487-489.

Guarro, J., Gams, W., Pujol, I. and Gene, J. (1997) Acromonium species: new emerging fungal opportunists: *in vitro* antifungal susceptiilities and review. *Clin. Infect. Dis.* **25**, 1222-1229.

Guillot, J., Sarfati, J., de Barros, M., Cadore, J.L., Jensen, H.E. and Chermette, R. (1999) Comparative study of serological tests for the diagnosis of equine aspergillosis. *Vet. Rec.* **145**, 348-349.

Higgins, J.C., Leith, G.S., Pappagianis, D. and Pusterla, N. (2006) Treatment of *Coccidioides immitis* pneumonia in two horses with fluconazole. *Vet. Rec.* **159**, 349-351.

Higgins, J.C., Leith, G.S., Voss, E.D. and Pappagianis, D. (2005) Seroprevalence of antibodies against *Coccidioides immitis* in healthy horses. *J. Am. vet. med. Ass.* **226**, 1888-1892.

Hodgin, E.C., Conaway, H. and Ortenburger, A.I. (1984) Recurrence of obstructive nasal coccidioidal granuloma in a horse. *J. Am. vet. med. Ass.* **184**, 339-340.

Johnson, P.J., Moore, L.A., Mrad, D.R., Turk, J.R. and Wilson, D.A. (1999) Sudden death of two horses associated with pulmonary aspergillosis. *Vet. Rec.* **145**, 16-20.

Jubb, K.V.F., Kennedy, P.C. and Palmer, N. (1985) *Pathology of Domestic Animals*, 3rd edn., Academic Press, Orlando. pp 516-518.

Kaufman, L., Mendoza, L. and Standard, P.G. (1990) Immunodiffusion test for serodiagnosing subcutaneous zygomycosis. *J. clin. Microbiol.* **28**, 1887-1890.

Korenek, N.L., Legendre, A.M. and Andrews, F.M. (1994) Treatment of mycotic rhinitis with itraconazole in three horses. *J. vet. Intern. Med.* **8**, 224-227.

Latimer, F.G., Colitz, C.M.H., Campbell, N.B. and Papich, M.G. (2001) Pharmacokinetics of fluconazole following intravenous and oral administration and body fluid concentrations of fluconazole following repeated oral dosing in horses. *Am. J. vet. Res.* **62**, 1606-1611.

MacNeill, A.L., Alleman, A.R., Franklin, R.P., Long, M., Giguere, S., Uhl, E., Lopez-Martinez, A. and Wilkerson, M. (2003) Pneumonia in a Paso-Fino mare. *Vet. clin. Pathol.* **32**, 73-76.

Mendoza, L., Mandy, W. and Glass, R. (2003) An improved *Pythium insidiosum*-vaccine formulation with enhanced immunotherapeutic properties in horses and dogs with pythiosis. *Vaccine* **21**, 2797-2804.

Mendoza, L., Kaufman, L., Mandy, W. and Glass, R. (1997) Serodiagnosis of human and animal pythiosis using an enzyme-linked immunosorbent assay. *Clin. Diagn. Lab. Immunol.* **4**, 715-718.

Nappert, G., VanDyck, T., Papich, M. and ChirinoTrejo, M. (1996) Successful treatment of a fever associated with consistent pulmonary isolation of *Scopulariopsis* sp. in a mare. *Equine vet. J.* **28**, 421-424.

Perron LePage, M.F., Gerber, V. and Suter, M.M. (1999) A case of interstitial pneumonia associated with *Pneumocystis carinii* in a foal. *Vet. Pathol.* **36**, 621-624.

Plumb, D. (2002) *Veterinary Drug Handbook*, 4th edn., Iowa State University Press, Ames.

Poole, H.M. and Brashier, M.K. (2003) Equine cutaneous pythiosis. *Comp. cont. Educ. pract. Vet.* **25**, 229-235.

Prades, M., Brown, M.P., Gronwell, R. and Houston, A.E. (1989) Body fluid and endometrial concentrations of ketaconazole in mares after intravenous injection or repeated gavage. *Equine vet. J.* **21**, 211-214.

Pusterla, N., Holmberg, T.A., Lorenzo-Figueras, M., Wong, A. and Wilson, D.A. (2005) *Acremonium strictum* pulmonary infection in a horse. *Vet. clin. Pathol.* **43**, 413-416.

Pusterla, N., Pesavento, P.A., Leutenegger, J.H., Lowenstine, L.J., Durando, M.M. and Magdesian, K.G. (2002) Disseminated pulmonary adiaspiromycosis caused by *Emmonsia crescens* in a horse. *Equine vet. J.* **34**, 749-752.

Reilly, L.K. and Palmer, J.E. (1994) *Systemic candidiasis* in four foals. *J. Am. vet. med. Ass.* **205**, 464-466.

Rezabek, G.B., Donahue, J.M., Giles, R.C., Petrites-Murphy, M.B., Poonacha, K.B., Rooney, J.R., Smith, B.J., Swerczek, T.W. and Tramontin, R.R. (1993) Histoplasmosis in horses. *J. comp. Pathol.* **109**, 47-55.

Rochette, F., Engelen, M. and vanden Bossche, H. (2003) Antifungal agents of use in animal health - practical applications. *J. vet. Pharmacol. Therap.* **26**, 31-53.

Slocombe, R.F. and Slauson, D.O. (1988) Invasive pulmonary aspergillosis of horses - an association with acute enteritis. *Vet. Pathol.* **25**, 277-281.

Smith, C.E., Saito, M.T. and Simons, S.A. (1956) Pattern of 39,500 serologic tests in *coccidioidomycosis*. *J. Am. vet. med. Ass.* **160**, 546-552.

Steiger, R.R. and Williams, M.A. (2000) *Granulomatous tracheitis* caused by *Conidiobolus coronatus* in a horse. *J. vet. intern. Med.* **14**, 311-314.

Stewart, A.J. (2005) Antifungal therapy for horses. *Comp. cont. Educ. vet. Pract.* **27**, 871-876.

Stewart, A.J., Welles, E.G. and Salazar, T. (2008) Pulmonary and systemic fungal infections. *Compend. Equine* **3**, 260-272.

Sweeney, C.R. and Habecker, P.L. (1999) Pulmonary aspergillosis in horses: 29 cases (1974-1997). *J. Am. vet. med. Ass.* **214**, 808-811.

Taintor, J., Schumacher, J. and Newton, J. (2003) Conidiobolomycosis in horses. *Comp. cont. Educ. pract. Vet.* **25**, 872-876.

Taintor, J., Crowe, C., Hancock, S., Schumacher, J. and Livesey, L. (2004) Treatment of conidiobolomycosis with fluconazole in two pregnant mares. *J. vet. Intern. Med.* **18**, 363-364.

Terio, K.A., Stalis, I.H., Allen, J.L., Stott, J.L. and Worley, M.B. (2003) *Coccidioidomycosis* in Przewalski's horses (*Equus przewalskii*). *J. Zoo Wildlife Med.* **34**, 339-345.

Toribio, R.E., Kohn, C.W., Lawrence, A.E., Hardy, J. and Hutt, J.A. (1999) Thoracic and abdominal blastomycosis in a horse. *J. Am. vet. med. Ass.* **214**, 1357-1360.

Tunev, S.S., Ehrhart, E.J., Jensen, H.E., Foreman, J.H., Richter, R.A. and Messick, J.B. (1999) Necrotizing mycotic vasculitis with cerebral infarction caused by *Aspergillus niger* in a horse with acute *typhlocolitis*. *Vet. Pathol.* **36**, 347-351.

Venner, M., Schmidbauer, S., Drommer, W. and Deegen, E. (2006) Percutaneous lung biopsy in the horse: Comparison of two instruments and repeated biopsy in horses with induced acute interstitial pneumopathy. *J. vet. Intern. Med.* **20**, 968-973.

Zamos, D.T., Schumacher, J. and Loy, J.K. (1996) Nasopharyngeal conidiobolomycosis in a horse. *J. Am. vet. med. Ass.* **208**, 100-101.

Ziemer, E.L., Pappagianis, D., Madigan, J.E., Mansmann, R.A. and Hoffman, K.D. (1992) Coccidioidomycosis in horses - 15 cases (1975-1984). *J. Am. vet. med. Ass.* **201**, 910-916.

EPIZOOTIC LYMPHANGITIS

C. Scantlebury* and K. Reed†

Horse Trust Scholar in Equine Epidemiology, Department of Veterinary Clinical Science, University of Liverpool, Leahurst, Cheshire CH64 7TE; and †Society for the Protection of Animals Abroad (SPANA) 14 John Street, London WC1N 2EB, UK.

Keywords: horse; epizootic lymphangitis; *Histoplasma capsulatum* var. *farciminosum*; fungal disease of equines; EL

Summary

Epizootic lymphangitis (EL) is caused by the fungal agent *Histoplasma capsulatum* var. *farciminosum* and affects horses, mules and donkeys. The disease commonly develops into a chronic debilitating condition, primarily affecting the skin, and treatment is difficult even in early cases. EL has been eradicated from large areas of the world but is still a major cause of morbidity and mortality in various countries particularly in Africa and Asia. The condition has a serious effect on the health and welfare of severely affected animals.

This article outlines the clinical presentation of the disease, current knowledge on the pathogenesis, epidemiology and options for control and aims to give an overview of the available literature.

Introduction

Epizootic lymphangitis (EL) is a debilitating equine disease that in its classical form is characterised by chronic discharging cutaneous nodules. It is often associated with mass gatherings of equids, hence there are a number of accounts of the condition amongst army horses from the British campaigns in the late 19th and 20th centuries (Pallin 1904; Plunkett 1949). The disease was introduced into the British Isles by military horses returning to the country and a mass surveillance and slaughter policy was enforced resulting in eradication of EL from the UK by 1906. Further details of this outbreak can be found in an account by Captain W.A. Pallin (1904).

Epizootic lymphangitis has also been eradicated from other areas of Europe. Currently the disease remains endemic in parts of North, East and West Africa, the Middle East and Far East. However, up-to-date surveillance information is scarce. The World Organisation for Animal Health (OIE) reported figures for 2005 only show notification of cases in Ethiopia, South Africa and Senegal (Anon 2005).

The disease is contagious and can be transmitted between body sites within an infected animal and to other uninfected equids via contact with infected discharge, fomites and fly vectors.

The authors' experience of EL derives from contact with cases in Ethiopia presented to the Society for the Protection of Animals Abroad (SPANA) veterinary mobile clinics. Therefore, parts of this article will focus on this region. Additionally, much of the recent published research on EL has originated from studies conducted in Ethiopia and a section highlighting this is also included.

Clinical details

Al-Ani's literature review (1999) reported 4 different forms of EL: cutaneous, ocular, respiratory and asymptomatic carriers. These are not necessarily considered distinct clinical entities and combinations may occur with one form of the disease leading to development of another. Therefore, whilst for simplicity we discuss each of these presentations in turn, readers should be aware of the overlapping spectrum of signs that might occur.

Cutaneous EL

The cutaneous form is the most widely reported in the literature. The disease is insidious in onset, with a variable incubation lasting weeks to months. Clinically, the disease is characterised by a chronic,

*Author to whom correspondence should be addressed.

a)

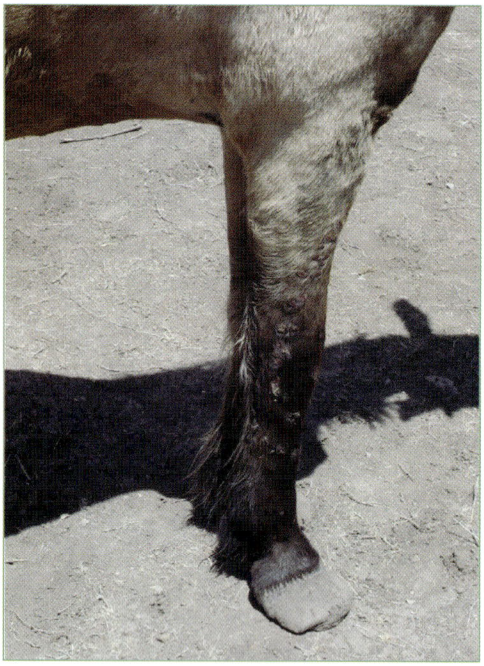

b)

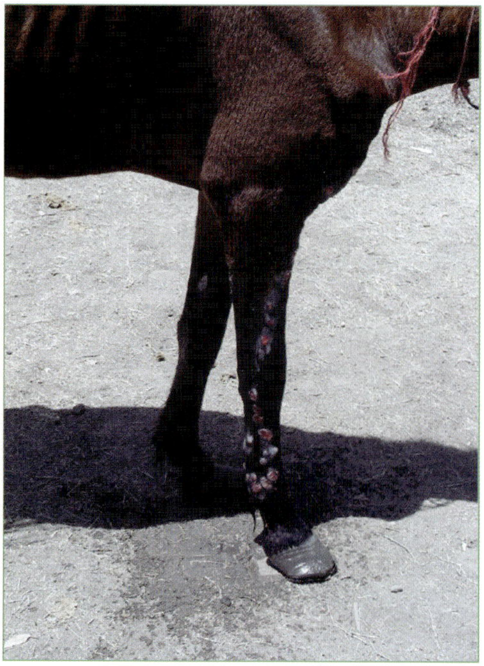

FIGURE 1: The lesions spread along the lymphatics creating a characteristic cording pattern on the affected limbs. The nodules can appear anywhere on the body. The lesions in (b) have been lanced and infused with tincture of iodine solution leaving an ulcerated appearance.

suppurative, ulcerating pyogranulomatous dermatitis and lymphangitis. Nodules may appear on any part of the body but most commonly originate around the lower limbs (**Figs 1** and **2**), chest, neck (**Fig 3**) and face (**Fig 4**). Initially there may be a single intradermal swelling that develops to a nodule around 1.5–2 cm diameter. This usually ruptures and discharges thick, purulent material leaving an ulcerated skin lesion. Spread of lesions occurs radially from the primary site along the lymphatics (**Fig 5**) and many nodules may eventually develop with some coalescing (**Figs 2** and **6**). The fungus also migrates to the local lymph nodes, which become grossly swollen (**Fig 7**) and contain viscid pus, from here the organism may further disseminate to other regions of the body. There is a repeated cycle of nodule development, discharge and ulceration. Healing of the ulcers eventually results in scar formation. The clinical appearance of the cutaneous form must be distinguished from discharging and nondischarging nodules caused by *Burholderia mallei* (glanders), *Sporothrix schenkii* (sporotrichosis), fungal granuloma (e.g. black grain mycetoma due to *Curvularia geniculata*), skin lesions of *Histoplasma capsulatum* var. *capsulatum* (HCC), ulcerative lymphangitis (due to *Corynebacterium* spp.) and strangles (*Streptococcus equi* var. *equi*).

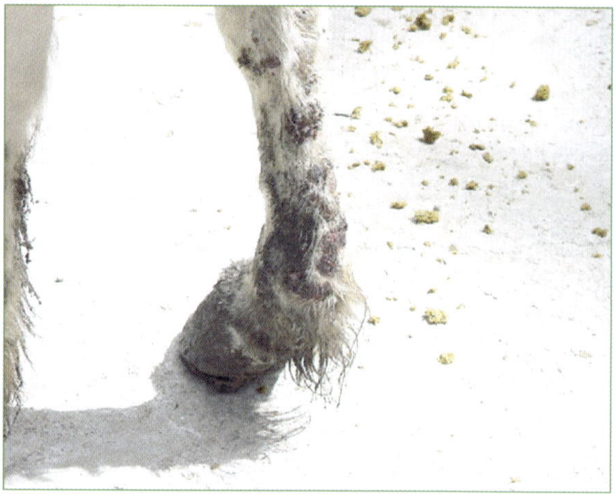

FIGURE 2: The ruptured nodules may become secondarily infected with opportunistic bacteria/fungi; the smell from these lesions is pungent.

In early cases animals remain well and have a near normal appetite. However in severe advanced cases where there is secondary infection present, or if there is joint involvement, the animal gradually becomes debilitated and lameness, anorexia and loss of condition are common.

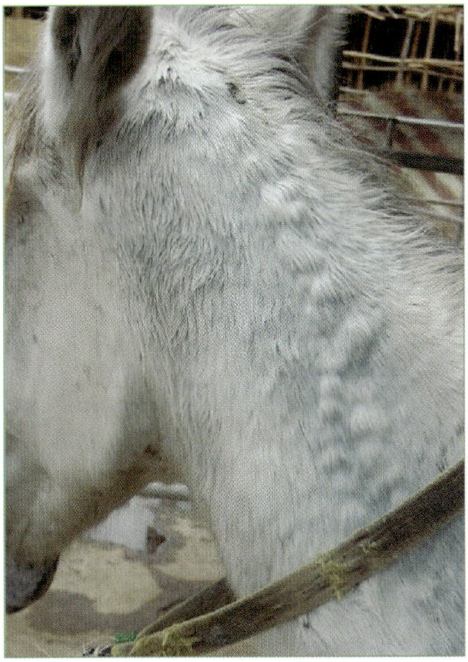

FIGURE 3: Appearance of pre-ruptured nodules following the lymphatics on the lateral neck of a cart-horse.

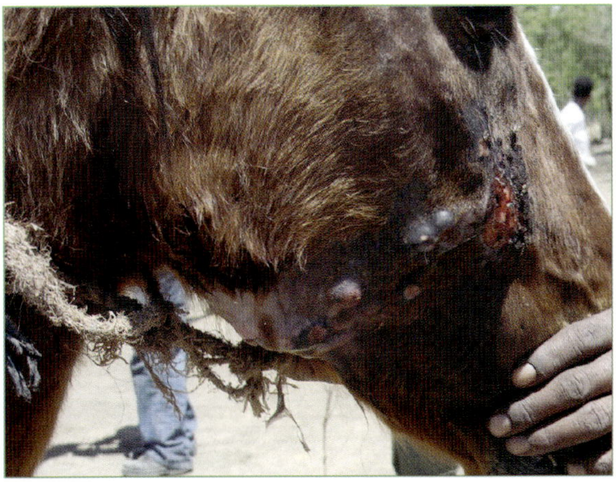

FIGURE 4: EL lesions on the face. The initial lesion is on the rostral end of the maxillary crest and satellite nodules have developed in the lymphatics draining from the area.

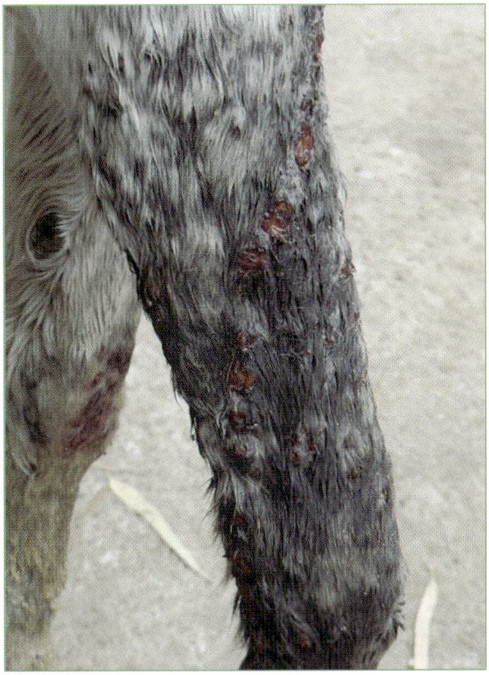

FIGURE 5: Close up of nodules following lymphatics on forelimb.

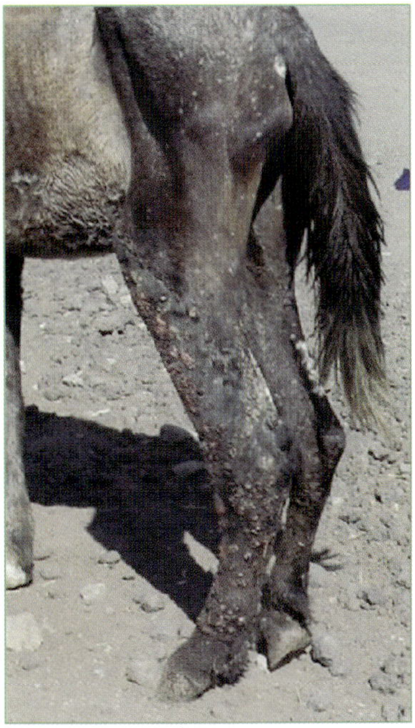

FIGURE 6: Chronic, severe case showing extensive involvement of the hindlimb. This animal was lame on the affected limb.

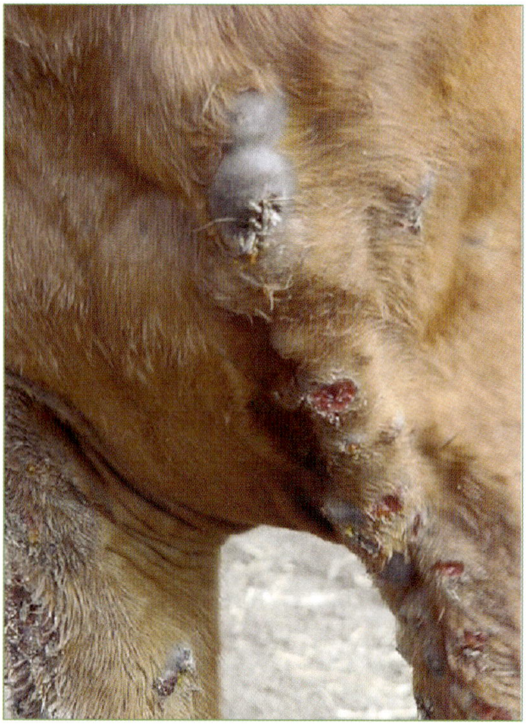

FIGURE 7: The infected lymphatics become fibrosed leading to a 'cording' appearance. In this case the infection had spread to involve the pre-scapular lymph nodes which were swollen and painful.

Ocular EL

The ocular form is characterised by a kerato-conjunctivitis with a serous to mucopurulent discharge. There may also be intradermal swellings within the palpebrae. There may be characteristic button ulcers on the outer margins of the conjunctivae. Extension of infection may occur to the periorbital tissues where a granulomatous reaction may develop (**Fig 8**), and to the lachrymal ducts where infection can progress to communicate with the external skin of the face. The ocular form has been reported as common in donkeys in Egypt in particular (Saleh 1986) but also commonly occurs in horses and mules. The secondary effects of the condition include corneal ulceration, lachrymal duct occlusion, panophthalmitis, myiasis and bacterial infection.

Respiratory EL

Respiratory cases are thought to occur through inhalation of the organism either as spores from the environment or through extension of infection from the external mucous membranes of the nares or from the naso-lachrymal duct. Nodules can be present around the mucocutaneous junction of the nose (**Fig 9**) and at *post mortem* are commonly seen to extend from the nasal passages, through the trachea and into the lung parenchyma. There is often an accompanying viscid mucopurulent nasal discharge and in advanced stages, affected animals will show increased respiratory effort and have a stertuous noise during respiration. This form causes severe debility, cough and progressive weakness and is difficult to differentiate clinically from glanders.

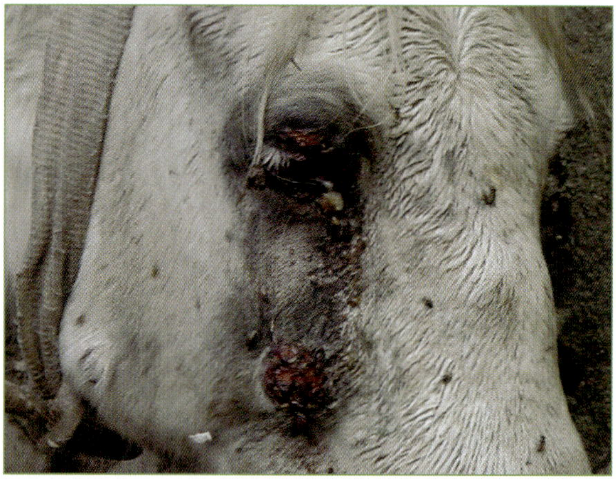

FIGURE 8: Ocular form. Granulomatous lesion on the upper eyelid with mucopurulent conjunctivitis. Further nodules are visible around the medial canthus.

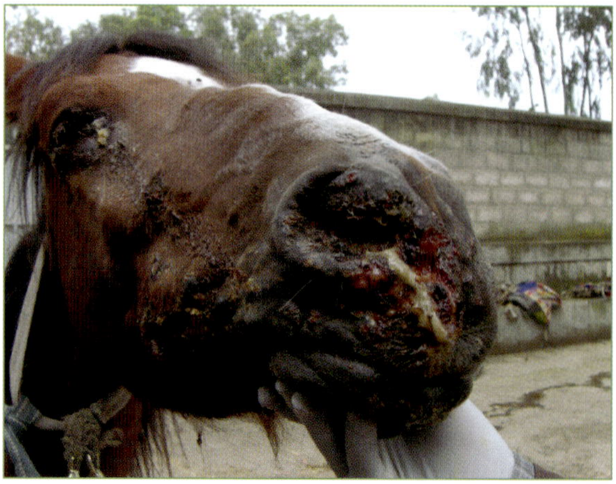

FIGURE 9: Respiratory form. The pictured case shows extensive involvement of the external nares and ocular discharge.

Asymptomatic carriers

Although this is a form reported by Al-Ani (1999), there is a lack of immunological studies investigating the presence and role of these animals. Whilst the organism induces both a humoural and cell-mediated immune response (Gabal and Khalifa 1983), information on the duration of immunity in cases that either heal spontaneously or are successfully treated is not currently available. The duration of the incubation period can vary greatly but it is uncertain whether an animal incubating EL can transmit the disease during this period. It may be possible through the use of the 'histofarcin' test (Soliman *et al.* 1985) or serological antibody tests (see later) to examine this more closely, but this would require long-term cohort studies to derive any firm conclusions. This is certainly an area that warrants further investigation as this is a potentially important aspect of the pathogenesis of disease in endemic areas.

Fungal characteristics

The aetiological agent of EL is the dimorphic fungus *Histoplasma capsulatum* var. *farciminosum* (HCF) previously known as *Cryptococcus farciminosus*. It is considered a variety of *H. capsulatum* var. *capsulatum* (HCC) and *H. capsulatum* var. *duboisii* as they are morphologically alike having similar microconidia, macroconidia and yeast forms and are antigenically similar (Weeks *et al.* 1985). Immunological studies found that HCF reacts similarly to HCC as it possesses common H and M antigens (Standard and Kaufman 1976). More recently, phylogenetic studies have investigated the relatedness of different strains of these organisms and found a close link with HCC. Kasuga *et al.* (1999) suggested that HCF is a variant of HCC acquired by equines originating from South America. HCF is thought to only infect equids and can have varying presentations whereas HCC can infect both horses and man.

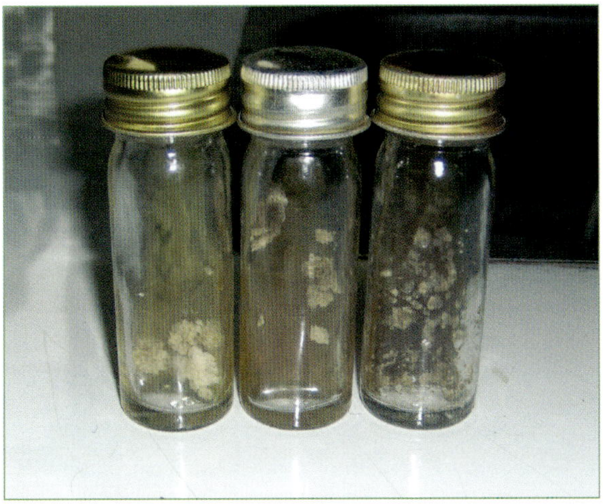

FIGURE 10: Mycelial colonies of Histoplasma capsulatum var farciminosum on Sabouraud dextrose agar slopes supplemented with chloramphenicol and glycerol (photographed in the laboratory of Dr Gobena Ameni, Addis Ababa University).

The fungus has 2 distinct phases, the mycelial form is present in the environment and the yeast is the pathogenic phase found in lesions.

The mycelial phase favours humid, moist environments and is thought to persist in the environment where the disease is endemic. Dissemination of the organism from discharging lesions of affected animals is likely to contribute to the environmental contamination. The soil phase is considered to be an important part of the organism's pathogenesis. However, unlike the case with HCC, formal studies investigating the presence or survival of HCF in the environment have not yet been conducted (HCC is known to grow in soil contaminated with bird/bat droppings where inhalation of spores leads to pulmonary histoplasmosis in man). Survival of HCF in soil has been investigated *in vitro*. Gabal and Hennager (1983a) showed that both temperature and moisture influenced the survival of the mycelial phase in soil and water with a minimum survival of 6–8 weeks in nonsterile soil at 26 and 37°C, respectively. In 1927, Bardelli and Ademollo found the organism remained viable after natural desiccation in the laboratory for 25 months.

Diagnostics

The organism may be identified in pus (or mucopurulent ocular discharge) through staining with Gram, Giemsa or periodic acid Schiff reagents. This is a useful initial tool in differentiating between other pathogens such as *Corynebacterium pseudotuberculosis* and *Burkholderia mallei*. The yeast form is characterised as a Gram-positive pleomorphic ovoid to globose structure (2–5 µm in diameter) with a 'halo' appearance due to a nonstaining capsule. The yeast may be seen intracellularly within macrophages or extracellularly. It is preferable to aspirate a sample from an unruptured nodule after clipping and disinfecting the skin to reduce contamination. It is also possible to visualise the organism in stained histological sections of matured or developing lesions.

Culture of the organism is necessary to confirm the presence of *Histoplasma* species but this is not without difficulty as the organism is slow growing and care must be taken to reduce overgrowth by contaminants. Various protocols to culture the mycelial phase have been documented in the literature (Bullen 1949; Gabal 1983; Weeks 1985). The research group based at Addis Ababa University have been using Sabouraud dextrose agar supplemented with chloramphenicol and glycerol (Ameni and Terefe 2004) (**Fig 10**). It is reported that it is possible to convert the mycelia to the yeast phase within the laboratory by altering culture conditions to 15–30% CO_2 and 37°C (Bullen 1949).

A skin test known as the 'Histofarcin' Test, was developed by Soliman *et al.* (1985). This test has been investigated recently for use in the field (Ameni *et al.* 2006) and could prove a valuable tool in diagnosing the condition. It is similar in principle to the 'tuberculin' or 'mallein' skin test, where a delayed, intradermal, *type IV* hypersensitivity reaction depicts previous exposure to the organism. Ameni *et al.* (2006) found a sensitivity of the histofarcin test in the field to be 90.3%; however, specificity in endemic areas was 69%. They concluded that this large number of false positives may have been due to preclinical stages of the infection causing reaction to the antigen. It is difficult to differentiate between positive reactors as either early preclinical cases or those that have been exposed and acquired immunity with this test alone. The authors acknowledged that there was a need for further study to improve the sensitivity and specificity of the test. They concluded that, after proper validation, the test could play a significant role in detecting early infection and differentiating EL from glanders, ulcerative lymphangitis and sporotrichosis. However, a comparison standard test to demonstrate specificity for the organism is advisable. This is because cross-reactivity with other pathogens may be possible, leading to false interpretation of test results, especially in the case of HCC, which is antigenically similar (Standard and Kaufman 1976).

Serological techniques for diagnosis that have been published include an ELISA (Gabal and Mohammed 1985) and indirect or direct fluorescent antibody techniques (Fawi 1969; Gabal *et al.* 1982 respectively). These tests may have greater sensitivity and specificity than those described previously but they are currently not commercially available. Within the research field, PCR has been used to identify *Histoplasma* spp. (Matos Guedes *et al.* 2003). This could prove a useful tool to investigate the molecular epidemiology of the organism for the purpose of understanding host species strains and endeminicity. However its applicability for field use is currently limited.

Epidemiology of disease in Ethiopia

Epizootic lymphangitis is commonly encountered in equidae in some areas of Ethiopia, and a number of studies have been published over the past decade.

Various cross-sectional studies of EL in Ethiopia identified the prevalence of disease as 26.2% in cart horses (Ameni and Siyoum 2002) and 21% in cart-mules (Ameni and Terefe 2004). In 2003–2004 Ameni (2006) conducted a wider cross-sectional study on 19,082 carthorses in 28 Ethiopian towns and found an overall EL prevalence of 18.8%, varying from 0–39% between individual towns. In this study a higher prevalence was observed in towns in mid-altitude regions (between 1500 and 2300 m above sea level). This effect is recognised locally in Ethiopia and people transport horses to the highlands (>2300 m) reporting that clinical cure is possible at higher altitudes (SPANA Clinic Ethiopia, personal communication). This phenomenon was also mentioned by Pallin (1904) who stated "a cure can be affected by removing animals to a high level i.e. to 7,500 feet" (2286 m). Ameni (2006) showed a significant association between prevalence and average annual temperature, but not with mean annual rainfall. They also found that an increasing horse population in the town was associated with a higher prevalence of EL.

Although EL is known as a disease of equids, traditionally it has been thought that donkeys are less susceptible to infection than horses and mules (Seifert 1996). In Ethiopia, donkeys had previously been considered to be immune to the disease. A cross-sectional study by Bojia and Roger (2003) did not find any cases of EL in donkeys among the study animals. Data from donkeys presented for treatment at The Donkey Sanctuary clinic in Debre Zeit between 2000 and 2002 showed annual EL case numbers in donkeys presented to be less than 5 (Donkey Sanctuary, Debre Zeit, unpublished data 2005). However, in 2003 and 2004 respectively, 40 and 32 cases of cutaneous EL were seen in donkeys attending the clinics (Powell *et al.* 2006), perhaps suggesting that EL is an emerging problem in donkeys in this area.

The cutaneous form of the disease is the most common form presented at veterinary clinics in Ethiopia. Ameni and Siyoum (2002), found a higher percentage of lesions on the forelimbs (33.18%) compared to the hindlimbs (26.2%). Ameni and Terefe (2004), described the distribution of lesions in the scrotal, axillary, facial and cervical regions.

Risk factors

There have been a number of risk factors reported in the literature as associated with particular forms of the disease (see below); however, no large-scale epidemiological cohort studies have been carried out to provide further evidence for these.

Cutaneous EL

Experimental transmission studies and reports from cases in military horses in India (Singh 1965, 1966) observed that the organism required a point of trauma to gain entry through the skin. Infection is acquired through contact with discharges from an infected animal, fomite transmission or through soil contaminated with the organism. Consequently the distributions of the initial lesions are commonly in any areas prone to trauma such as limb extremities/fetlock, chest/girth region, neck and head. However, it is clear that lesions may initiate on any part of the body. Histopathological studies have shown that once the organism is inoculated into the skin, an immunological chain of events leads to the eventual clinical appearance of a nodule (Singh *et al.* 1967).

Flies have been implicated in the spread of EL. Singh (1965) demonstrated that *Musca* spp. and *Stomxys* spp. flies were able to carry HCF within their digestive tract for at least 20 days and were able to transmit disease. The flies act as mechanical vectors and there does not appear to be any development of the organism or its virulence within the fly. Ameni and Terefe (2004) found a positive association between tick infestation (*Amblyoma* and *Boophilus genera*) and the disease suggesting that these could also be involved in spread of the organism. However, no dissection studies were reported. Fly transmission could perpetuate the disease within the same individual by initiating spread of infection from one infected body site to another. Alternatively, the horse may distribute lesions itself through grooming if there is irritation by flies around the lesion.

Discharge from an infected case may lead to contamination of fomites. Stable walls and floors, feed bowls, harness equipment, headcollars and grooming equipment can all be potential sources of spread of the organism. The role of various fomites has been alluded to in the literature. Although the presence or duration of survival of organism on these different materials has not been demonstrated, it would seem logical that these could act as sources of infection.

Ocular

The ocular form of the disease can be transmitted by flies feeding on discharge from infected eyes. Animals with pre-existing trauma/eye infections are at increased risk through attraction of flies to that area. The use of cloths to clean discharge from eyes has been known to distribute the disease from one animal to another (report from India 1899 quoted in Pallin 1904).

Respiratory

The evidence for the route of infection for the respiratory form is not definitive; it has been postulated that inhalation of spores from the environment could lead to seeding of infection in the lung, which would seem plausible (Awad 1960). Trauma to the external nares can also lead to the organism gaining entry to the respiratory tract.

Economic effect of disease in Ethiopia

The use of horse-drawn taxis and carts to generate an income are a means of survival for a significant number of Ethiopian families. They offer a source of sustainable daily income for family expenses (Jones 2006) and often provide the only affordable transportation service in many towns (Ameni 2006). Abebaw (2007) reported on the economics of cart horse work in Ethiopia and noted that the market price of a carthorse was 1402 Ethiopian Birr (EB: approximately £83) and the daily income for a cart horse driver was 21.59 EB (£1.27). The losses to the owner due to morbidity of a horse with EL (reduced working hours, clients reluctant to use horse with lesions) resulted in more than 50% reduction in daily earnings. Therefore the effect of this disease on resources of poor families, as well as animal welfare, can be devastating. Treatment costs to the owner in Abebaw's study were not included since they were borne by the equine welfare charity SPANA. The current cost of treating each infected animal is approximately £24 (400 EB) (SPANA, unpublished data).

Treatment

Intravenous sodium iodide, oral potassium iodide, surgical excision/firing of lesions, topical treatments and administration of modern antifungals have all been attempted, either alone or in combination, in various countries.

Al Ani's review (1999) reported that some cases heal spontaneously without treatment and that these are reputedly then immune for life. This has not been confirmed but there is a belief, in some endemic areas, that horses bearing characteristic scars are immune and are consequently being bought for premium prices (personal communication, SPANA Debre Zeit). However, reports from SPANA clinics in Ethiopia have identified recurrence of the disease up to a year later in some cases suggesting that immunity is not complete.

In vitro testing of amphotericin B (at a concentration of 50-100 μg/ml) and nystatin (at 50 u/ml) strongly inhibited the growth of HCF (Gabal 1984). Amphotericin B is also the listed drug of choice for the treatment of clinical cases of EL by the OIE (Anon 2004) and has been used successfully in some areas. However, the use of antifungal preparations in Ethiopia is currently limited by financial constraints, as well as the practical problems of sourcing the drugs.

Getachew (2004) carried out a clinical trial on the use of iodides combined with local excision and treatment in infected cart horses presented for treatment at SPANA clinics in Ethiopia. This study compared the use of oral potassium iodide with i.v. sodium iodide and found no significant difference in efficacy. This study has lead to the development of the following standard treatment protocol used by SPANA in the field in Ethiopia.

On the initial day of presentation the animal is sedated, all nodules are incised and treated with topical 4% tincture of iodine. Potassium iodide (KI, 30 g) in solution is administered by stomach tube (for a horse of 200–250 kg).

Ideally cases are seen daily, nodules treated topically and any new lesions incised. Oral KI is given at the same dose daily for 5 days and then every other day for a further 3–4 weeks, or as long as there is compliance from the owner. This treatment protocol is very labour intensive and prolonged and only efficacious in the early stages of the disease. Owners are encouraged to permit euthanasia of severely affected animals that do not respond to treatment. This is important not only in reducing environmental contamination with discharge from infected animals, but also to improve welfare of chronic cases that are often left abandoned by the roadside when they are no longer able to work (**Fig 11**).

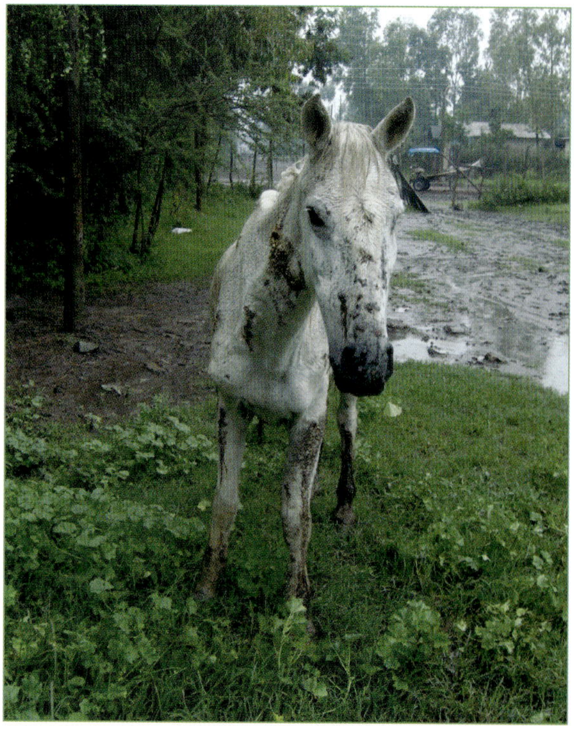

FIGURE 11: Chronic case left abandoned at clinic site.

Signs of iodinism have been rarely encountered. Most animals under treatment continue to work, despite the clinical team's efforts at persuading owners to rest them or allow hospitalisation. Compliance with the treatment regime is often difficult, and owners are now commonly given KI in weighed sachets to administer themselves, mixed with feed. It appears to be very palatable, particularly in horses rarely provided with hard feed (Jones 2006).

In 2001 and 2002, Ameni and Tilahun studied the *in vitro* effect of a local medicinal plant known as endod on the growth of HCF and attempted to evaluate its potential *in vivo*. An initial study found a positive effect of treatment with endod and concluded that further study to extract the active ingredient and evaluate it further would be justified (Ameni and Tilahun 2003).

Options for prevention

According to the World Organisation for Animal Health (OIE) recommendations for the control of EL are as follows:

"Control of the disease is usually through elimination of the infection. This is achieved by culling infected horses and application of strict hygiene practices to prevent spread of the organism."

Certainly, in nonendemic areas within developed countries this has been followed successfully. However, culling infected animals in an endemic area, particularly in developing countries is often impracticable and control at present depends on basic hygiene, wound management, infection control and treatment when available.

In Ethiopia, control depends largely on education of horse owners. SPANA mobile veterinary clinics advise owners in the following aspects:

- Presenting cases early for treatment.
- Advice on basic hygiene of harnessing and equipment - avoid sharing tack between animals, or if unavoidable, then good cleaning of tack.
- Fly control - use of repellents such as kerosene.
- Promoting euthanasia in advanced cases with careful disposal of infected carcasses.
- Prevention of wounds - prompt repair and maintenance of harness, general health care of animals with respect to workloads, dehydration, routine worming etc.
- Proper management of wounds - fly control, appropriate dressings.

The possible efficacy of environmental decontamination has not been studied with HCF and is probably impractical on a large scale in endemic regions. Studies investigating survival and favoured microenvironments of the organism in endemic areas have not been conducted. In Ethiopia, horses are often housed on mud floors and this could be an area where the organism persists. Pallin (1904) remarked that stable decontamination should consist of burning deep litter over the floor and then removing at least 7.5–15 cm off the surface before replacing with new material. The removed soil should be mixed with quick lime and buried to 6 feet under the ground.

A live attenuated vaccine tested in China was reported to protect 75.5% of animals inoculated, with immunity persisting for >2 years (Zhang *et al.* 1986). This vaccine is not commercially available and there were some issues of adverse reactions that would need addressing. Other evidence of vaccine use is scarce.

Epizootic lymphangitis, although eradicated in many countries, is continuing to have a significant impact on equine health and welfare in resource poor countries. Economic and social losses in developing countries due to working equine morbidity are important not only on an individual level, but also to local communities. Further research is required to increase understanding, particularly within the areas of the immunology and epidemiology of EL, in order to define effective and practical control strategies in endemic countries.

Acknowledgements

C. Scantlebury's Scholarship is funded by The Horse Trust. Many thanks to the staff of the mobile veterinary clinics of SPANA and The Donkey Sanctuary, Debre Zeit, Ethiopia for time spent with the authors on clinics and sharing their knowledge of EL.

Thank you to Dr Gina Pinchbeck, Professor Derek Knottenbelt and Dr Rob Christley for comments during proof reading.

References

Abebaw, Z. (2007) *Assessment of Socioeconomic Impact of Epizootic Lymphangitis (EL) on Horse Drawn Cart Taxi Business in Selected Towns of Central Ethiopia: (Debre Zeit and Debre Berhan).* Submitted as Thesis for BA to Addis Ababa University, Faculty of Business and Economics (Unpublished).

Al-Ani, F.K. (1999) Epizootic Lymphangitis in horses: A review of the literature. *Rev. Sci. Tech. Off. int. Epiz.* **18**, 691-699.

Ameni, G. (2006) Epidemiology of Equine histoplasmosis (epizootic lymphangitis) in carthorses in Ethiopia. *Vet. J.* **172**, 160-165.

Ameni, G. and Siyoum, F. (2002) Study on histoplasmosis (epizootic lymphangitis) in cart-horses in Ethiopia. *J. vet. Sci.* **3**, 135-140.

Ameni, G. and Terefe, W. (2004) A cross-sectional study of Epizootic lymphangitis in cart-mules in Western Ethiopia. *Prev. vet. Med.* **66**, 93-99.

Ameni, G. and Tilahun, G. (2003) Preliminary laboratory and field trials on the effect of endod on Epizootic lymphangitis. *Bull. anim Health. Prod. Afr.* **51**,153-160.

Ameni, G., Terefe, W. and Hailu, A. (2006) Histofarcin test for the diagnosis of Epizootic lymphangitis in Ethiopia: development, optimisation and validation in the field. *Vet. J.* **171**, 358-362.

Anon (2004) Epizootic lymphangitis, In: *OIE Manual of Diagnostic Tests and Vaccines for Terrestrial Animals,* Chapter 2.5.13, updated 23.07.2004. http://www.oie.int/eng/normes/mmanual/A_00091.htm

Anon (2005) *WAHID Interface.* http://www.oie.int/wahid-prod/public.php?page=disease_status_map

Awad, F.I. (1960) Studies on epizootic lymphangitis in the Sudan. *J. comp. Pathol.* **70**, 457-463.

Bardelli, P. and Ademollo, A. (1927) Sulla resistenza delle conture di *Cryptococcus farcimnosus* Rivolta agli agenti fisci e chimici. *Annual Igiene* **37**, 81-85.

Bojia, E. and Roger, F. (2003) Comparative studies on the occurrence and distribution of Epizootic lymphangitis and ulcerative lymphangitis in Ethiopia. *Int. J. App. R. Vet. Med.* **1**, (3).

Bullen, J.J. (1949) The yeast-like form of *Cryptococcus farciminosus* (Rivolta) (*Histoplasma farciminosum*). *J. Pathol. Bacteriol.* **61**, 117-120.

Fawi, M.T. (1969) Fluorescent antibody test for the serodiagnosis of *Histoplasma farciminosum* infections in *equidae*. *Br. vet. J.* **125**, 231-234.

Gabal, M.A. (1984) The effect of amphotericin-B, 5-fluorocytosine and nystatin on *Histoplasma farciminosum in vitro. Zbl. vet. Med. B.* **31**, 46-50.

Gabal, M.A. and Hennager, S. (1983a) Study on the survival of Histoplasma farciminosum in the environment. *Mykosen* **26**, 481-487.

Gabal, M.A. and Khalifa, K. (1983c) Study on the immune response and serological diagnosis of equine histoplasmosis (Epizootic lymphangitis). *Zbl. vet. Med. B.* **30**, 317-321.

Gabal, M.A. and Mohammed, K.A. (1985) Use of enzyme-linked immunosorbent assay for the diagnosis of equine *Histoplasmosis farciminosi* (epizootic lymphangitis) *Mycopathologia* **91**, 31-37.

Gabal, M.A., Al-Bana, A. and El-Gendi, M. (1982) The use of fluorescent antibody technique for the diagnosis of equine histoplasmosis 'epizootic lymphangitis'. *Mykosen,* **25**, 683-686.

Gabal, M.A., Hassan, F.K., Al-Siad, A.A. and Al-Karim, K.A. (1983b) Study on equine histoplasmosis 'epizootic lymphangitis'. *Mykosen* **26**, 145-151.

Getachew, A. (2004) *Clinical Trial of Iodides Combined with Ancillary Treatment on Epizootic Lymphangitis in Cart Horses at Debre Zeit and Akaki towns.* Submitted as DVM Thesis, Faculty of Veterinary Medicine, Addis Ababa University (Unpublished).

Jones, K. (2006) Epizootic lymphangitis: the impact on subsistence economies and animal welfare. *Vet. J.* **172**, 402-404.

Kasuga, T., Taylor, J.W and White, T.J. (1999) Phylogenetic relationships of varieties and geographical groups of the human pathogenic fungus *Histoplasma capsulatum* Darling. *J. clin. Microbiol.* **37**, 653-663.

Matos Guedes, H.L., Guimaraes, A.J., Medeiros Muniz, M., Pizzini, C.V., Hamilton, A.J., Peralta, J.M., Deepe Jr, G.S. and Zancope-Oliveira, R.M. (2003) PCR assay for Identification of *Histoplasma capsulatum* based on the nucleotide sequence of the M antigen. *J. clin. Microbiol.* **41**, 535-539.

Pallin, W.A. (1904) *A Treatise on Epizootic Lymphangitis,* 2nd edn. Williams and Norgate, Liverpool.

Plunkett, J.J. (1949) Epizootic lymphangitis. *Journal of the Royal Army Veterinary Corps* **20**, 94-99.

Powell, R.K., Bell, N.J., Abreha, T., Asmamaw, K., Bekelle, H., Dawit, T., Itsay, K. and Feseha, G.A. (2006) Cutaneous histoplasmosis in 13 Ethiopian donkeys. *Vet. Rec.* **158**, 836-837.

Saleh, M. (1986) Chapter 10: Lacrimal Histoplasmosis in Donkeys In: *The Professional Handbook of the Donkey,* Ed: E.D. Svendsen, Donkey Sanctuary, Sidmouth. pp 123-129.

Seifert, H.S.H. (1996) Part 3.2.2. In: *Tropical Animal Health,* Kluwer Academic Publishers, Amsterdam.

Singh, T. (1965) Studies on epizootic lymphangitis I. Mode of infection and transmission of equine histoplasmosis (epizootic lymphangitis). *Indian J. vet. Sci.* **35**, 102-110.

Singh, T. (1966) Studies on epizootic lymphangitis (study of clinical cases and experimental transmission). *Indian J. vet. Sci.* **36**, 45-59.

Singh, T., Varmani, B.M.L. and Bhalla, N.P. (1967) Studies on epizootic lymphangitis. II Pathogenesis and histopathology of equine histoplasmsosis. *Indian J. vet. Sci.* **35**, 111-120.

Soliman, R., Saad, M.A. and Refai, M. (1985) Studies on *Histoplasmosis farciminosii* (epizootic lymphangitis) in Egypt. III Application of a skin test ('histofarcin') in the diagnosis of epizootic lymphangitis in horses. *Mykosen* **28**, 457-461.

Standard, P.G. and Kaufman, L. (1976) Specific immunological test for the rapid identification of members of the genus *Histoplasma. J. clin. Microbiol.* **3**, 191-199.

Weeks, R., Padhye, A.A. and Ajello, L. (1985) *Histoplasma capsulatum* variety *farciminosum*: A new combination for *Histoplasma farciminosum. Mycologia* **77**, 964-970.

Zhang, W.T., Wang, Z.R., Liu, Y.P., Zhang, D.L., Liang, P.Q., Fang, Y.Z., Huang, Y.J. and Gao, S.D. (1986) Attenuated vaccine against epizootic lymphangitis of horses. *Chin. J. vet. Sci. Technol.* **7**, 3-5.

MANAGEMENT OF CONTAGIOUS DISEASE OUTBREAKS

J. Traub-Dargatz

Animal Population Health Institute, College of Veterinary Medicine and Biomedical Sciences, Colorado State University, Fort Collins, Colorado 80523-1678, USA.

Keywords: horse; equine contagious disease outbreak investigation and management

Summary

Outbreaks of equine contagious disease can have major impact based on cost of caring for sick horses, movement restrictions implemented to contain the disease and even result in fatalities in affected horses. The veterinarian who is looked to for leadership in best management of such outbreaks needs to be prepared to make a diagnosis and to implement a plan for containment of the disease. There are multiple resources available to the veterinarian related to the topic of outbreak management. These resources are described in this manuscript.

Introduction

The management of outbreaks of equine contagious disease requires that the veterinarian on the scene works in conjunction with the facility manager to develop a plan for containment of the disease to avoid its spread to other horses on the facility or to other facilities. It is optimal if the veterinarian has discussed a general plan with the facility manager prior to the outbreak. In addition, there is value in the veterinarian being aware of sources of information related to diagnostic options and control methods for various types of diseases, such as respiratory infection, neurological disease, abortion, diarrhoeal disease and vesicular disease, in advance of a disease outbreak.

It is critical that the attending veterinarian (the veterinarian who will be initially on the scene when an outbreak occurs) determines what his/her responsibilities and options are in the management of an outbreak of contagious disease. If the veterinarian has no authority to direct the control or prevention of the outbreak or if their opinions were not sought or heard then they certainly do not want to be blamed if and when things go wrong (Lunn 2007). However veterinarians have a natural and appropriate desire to take responsibility for the health and well-being of the animals particularly in the face of clear risk (Lunn 2007). If you are charged with disease prevention at an equine facility or as part of your role as the veterinarian for an equine event such as a show, sale or race, then you will need to clarify with the facility management your role in the planning and implementation of disease control strategies should an outbreak of contagious disease occur. Armed with some key messages the veterinarian can serve as a source of information for equine owners, farm managers and equine event organisers so that they can make informed decisions regarding pre-planning for control of equine contagious diseases and the implementation of that plan when an outbreak occurs (Lunn 2007).

Knowledge of the methods to obtain an aetiological diagnosis, along with supplies necessary to initiate a diagnostic investigation and the initial steps in implementing biosecurity on the first day that a problem is detected, allows for a timely and focused response to the situation. There are diverse situations in which a veterinarian could be asked to assist in the management of a contagious disease outbreak due to the heterogenous nature of equine facilities (Dwyer 2007). There are few scientific studies that have evaluated the efficacy of biosecurity measures on one facility compared to another, and as a result the recommendations for disease control are usually based on the personal experiences of the attending veterinarian, descriptions of disease control methods used in veterinary hospitals, scientific studies in other species or knowledge gained from experimental challenge studies in horses, and colleagues' observations (Dwyer 2007).

Communication is required by the attending veterinarian to the designated animal health regulatory authority in the event that a reportable disease occurs. The list of reportable equine diseases or syndromes varies from state to state in the USA. A list of reportable diseases is generally available on the State Veterinarian's website and should be available upon request from the Animal Health Official in each State. For example, the list of reportable equine diseases in Florida is posted on the website for the State Veterinarian's Office at http://www.doacs.state.fl.us/ai/main/ani_diseases_ main.shtml. A list of State Animal Health Officials in the USA along with their contact information is available from the US Animal Health Association at http://www.usaha.org/StateAnimalHealthOfficials.pdf.

In the USA there may be additional reporting obligations beyond those required by the State or Federal Veterinary official, for example the racing commission may have requirements for reporting to them at venues where they have sanctioned racing. The attending veterinarian is thus responsible for knowing the reporting criteria for infectious diseases for the various situations in which they practice.

In other countries there are also veterinary regulatory requirements for the reporting of various suspect and/or confirmed infectious disease events and these vary by country. For example, in the UK, a list of notifiable equine diseases (a disease named in section 88 of the Animal Health Act 1981 or an Order made under that Act) is available from the Department for Environment, Food and Rural Affairs (Defra) website (http://www.defra.gov.uk/animalh/diseases/notifiable/index.htm). A veterinarian who suspects the presence of any of these notifiable diseases is required to immediately inform the appropriate Defra divisional veterinary manager. Along with the list of diseases, there is information about the each of the notifiable diseases as well as the order giving Defra authority to respond to the notification of the individual diseases. The equine industry in the UK (through the work of the Horserace Betting Levy Board) has an annually updated set of voluntary Codes of Practice (Anon 2008a), which set out minimum recommendations for the prevention of specific equine contagious diseases and for their control, should they occur, during horse or pony breeding activities. The diseases addressed in the Code of Practice include venereally transmitted bacterial diseases caused by contagious equine metritis organism, *Klebsiella pneumonia* and *Pseudomonas aeruginosa*, equine viral arteritis (EVA), equine infectious anaemia (EIA), equine herpesvirus (EHV) and strangles. The recommendations apply to all breeds of horse and pony, and to both natural mating and artificial insemination.

In 2006, the American Association of Equine Practitioners put forward guidelines related to the control of infectious contagious disease outbreaks. The purpose of these guidelines are to promote an effective first response by providing a clear, concise action plan proceeding from generalised signs to specific diagnosis of contagious disease. These guidelines are posted on the website for the AAEP and are available to be viewed by all potential users at the AAEP website (Anon 2006). These guidelines were developed by a task force of AAEP members with expertise related to specific infectious diseases, biosecurity, diagnostic methods for identification of the aetiology of equine infectious disease, use of vaccines in disease control, situations encountered at equine events such as racetracks, and situations encountered in private veterinary practice. The guidelines, once drafted, were then reviewed the executive board of the AAEP, and, once revised based on input from the board, accepted by board. These guidelines are written for use by veterinarians who encounter contagious infectious disease in horses. As new information becomes available related to the diagnosis or control of equine contagious diseases there is the option to readily update the guidelines based on review by the Infectious Diseases Committee of the AAEP.

There are 3 major sections to the AAEP Infectious Disease Guidelines: 1) Pre-outbreak Considerations, 2) When Equine Infectious Disease Is Suspected and 3) Use of These Guidelines. It is difficult to summarise all the information contained in the guidelines but the following is an effort to highlight their content.

Pre-outbreak considerations

The Pre-outbreak Considerations section emphasises preplanning. The implementation of a management programme before an outbreak will maximise the effectiveness of the response plan should an infectious disease occur. An effective programme incorporates risk management, resource management and horse management, and is unique to each equine event.

When an equine infectious disease is suspected

The guidelines suggest that the veterinarian's responsibilities are 1) Do No Harm - do not rush into a stall/barn until you have a plan on how to leave it and 2) respond to the 'worst case scenario' until you have a specific diagnosis. The veterinarian should have an established response plan for control of contagious disease outbreaks - a planned response is the most effective tool for minimising the outbreak impact. Key components of the plan include:

Maintain a log, recording events as they occur, including:

- Case identification - which horse(s) got sick, where, and when.
- Control measures implemented.
- Horse movement - within facility, entering and exiting facility.
- Diagnostic testing results.
- Communications with practitioners, horsemen and regulatory veterinarians.

Establish effective communication, including:

- Regular meetings providing clear information and simple instructions to:
  - o Facility management
  - o Horsemen
  - o Veterinarians
  - o Media
  - o Related industry affiliates.
- Note: Effective communication minimises speculation and establishes expectations.

Manage time effectively:

- Delegate tasks that do not require execution by a licensed veterinarian. (For example, when feasilbe utilise licensed veterinary technicians for sample collection, physical inspections, temperature recording etc.)

Using these guidelines

This section of the guidelines contains a flow chart for initial response to 4 different syndromes, respiratory infection, diarrhoeal disease, neurological disease and vesicular disease. There is also a section for respiratory, diarrhoeal and neurological syndrome that includes a definition of the syndrome, a list of differential diagnoses for each syndrome, establishing biosecurity protocols, communication of the plan and methods that can be used to attempt to make a diagnosis (sample collection, testing, and shipping). There is also a section with guidelines related to several equine infectious diseases that can be used once a specific diagnosis is made; these include: botulism, clostridial diarrhoea, eastern equine encephalitis, equine herpesvirus, EVA, influenza, Potomac horse fever, rabies, salmonellosis, *Streptococcus equi* infection, Venezuelan equine encephalitis, western equine encephalitis and West Nile virus.

The application of the AAEP Infectious Disease Guidelines was featured in an in-depth session at the 53rd annual AAEP convention, and would be of potential use to a veterinarian faced with the management of a contagious equine disease outbreak (Lunn 2007). This proceedings entitled 'Managing Infectious Disease Outbreaks at Events and Farms; Challenges and the Resources for Success' includes sections related to resources available to the equine practitioner (where to find information, where to find materials to implement biosecurity measures, how fast and how easy can a diagnosis be made and how to interpret test results, how useful are screening tests in preventing entry and movement of infection, how useful is vaccination in prevention and intervention, and what is the role of the veterinarian in responding to the infectious disease outbreak), strategies for outbreak management including answering the questions what, when, where, who and ultimately why. The focus of the outbreak investigation should determine the answers to 4 questions: what is the aetiology of the disease? how far has the disease spread? how far could it spread? and what populations are at risk?, in order to most effectively control the outbreak. Multiple case scenarios are included to illustrate outbreak investigation and management. Another proceedings from this same AAEP meeting, entitled 'Aspects of

Equine Infectious Disease Control From the United Kingdom Perspective', featured information related to a mandatory vaccination programme for equine influenza for racehorses attending race meetings, the introduction and evolution of the voluntary code of practice for equine infectious venereal diseases, the increasing acceptance of the carrier state in endemic persistence of strangles and the introduction of the first modified live vaccine in Europe for the control of strangles (Newton 2007). These proceedings are accessible on line to members of the AAEP at www.aaep.org.

Additional sources of information related to equine infectious diseases that can be beneficial to the veterinarian involved in management of outbreaks are available in various textbooks, for example a recently released textbook entitled Equine Infectious Diseases (Sellon and Long 2007) features chapters on specific diseases as well as chapters related to biosecurity and outbreak management. Additional resources related to the management of specific equine infectious diseases are the consensus statements from organisations such as the American College of Veterinary Internal Medicine (ACVIM). Thus far the ACVIM has a consensus statement related to 2 contagious equine disease namely, *Streptococcus equi* infection (Sweeney *et al.* 2005), and equine herpesvirus-1 (Lunn *et al.* 2009). The ACVIM consensus statements include sections related to the diagnosis, treatment, control and prevention and are available at http://www.acvim.org/index. aspx?id=322. There is a recently released report from USDA:APHIS:VS Centers for Epidemiology and Animal Health (CEAH) entitled Equine Herpesvirus Myeloencephalopathy: Mitigation Experiences, Lessons Learned and Future Needs in which there is a summary of interviews with those involved in the investigation and response to recent equine herpesvirus myeloencephalopathy (EHM) outbreaks (Anon 2008b). One of the stated goals of this report is to provide those involved in future outbreaks with information related to how past outbreaks were managed and lessons learned from those involved in the management of these outbreaks.

Acknowledgement

The author would like to extend thanks to the working group led by Dr Mary Scollay-Ward who wrote the AAEP guidelines for management of Infectious Disease Outbreaks and Dr Tim Mair for his review and additions to this article.

References

Anon (2006) *Infectious Disease Guidelines*, American Association of Equine Practitioners (AAEP) accessed 15th October 2008, http://www.aaep. org/control_guidelines_nonmember.htm.

Anon (2008a) *Code of Practice,* Horse Betting Levy Board (HBLB), accessed 16th October 2008, http://www.hblb.org.uk/document.php?id=43

Anon (2008b) *Equine Herpesvirus Myeloencephalopathy: Mitigation Experiences, Lessons Learned and Future Needs.* USDA:APHIS:VS, Centers for Epidemiology and Animal Health, #N522.0708, accessed 15th October 2008 http://www.aphis.usda.gov/vs/nahss/equine/ehv/equine_herpesvirus_nahms_ 2008report.pdf

Dwyer, R.M. (2007) Control of infectious disease outbreaks In: *Equine Infectious Diseases,* Eds: D.C. Sellon and M.T. Long, Saunders Elsevier, St Louis. pp 539-545.

Lunn, D.P. and Traub-Dargatz, J. (2007) Managing Infectious Disease Outbreaks at Events and Farms; Challenges and the Resources for Success. *Proc. Am. Ass. equine Practnrs.* **53**, 1-12.

Lunn, D.P., Davis-Poynter, N., Flaminio, M.B.J.F., Horohov, D.W., Osterrieder, K., Pusterla, N. and Townsend, H.G.G. (2009) Equine herpesvirus-1 consensus statement. *J. vet. int. Med.* **23**, 450-461.

Newton, J.R. (2007) Aspects of equine infection control from the United Kingdom perspective. *Proc. Am. Ass. equine Practnrs.* **53**, 13-21.

Sellon, D.C. and Long, M.T. (2007) *Equine Infectious Diseases*, Saunders Elsevier, St Louis.

Sweeney, C., Timoney, J.F., Newton, J.R. and Hines, M.T. (2005) *Streptococcus equi* Infections in Horses: Guidelines for Treatment, Control, and Prevention of Strangles. *J. vet. Int. Med.* **19**,123-134. accessed 15th October 2008, http://www.acvim.org/uploadedFiles/Consensus_Statements/Strangles.pdf